Monitoring and Intervention for the Critically Ill Small Animal

The Rule of 20

Monitoring and Intervention for the Critically Ill Small Animal

The Rule of 20

Edited by

Rebecca Kirby, DVM, DACVIM, DACVECC

and

Andrew Linklater, DVM, DACVECC

WILEY Blackwell

This edition first published 2017 © 2017 by John Wiley & Sons, Inc.

Editorial Offices: 1606 Golden Aspen Drive, Suites 103 and 104, Ames, Iowa 50010, USA
The Atrium, Southern Gate, Chichester, West Sussex, PO19 8SQ, UK
9600 Garsington Road, Oxford, OX4 2DQ, UK

For details of our global editorial offices, for customer services and for information about how to apply for permission to reuse the copyright material in this book please see our website at www.wiley.com/wiley-blackwell.

Library of Congress Cataloging-in-Publication Data

Names: Kirby, Rebecca, editor. | Linklater, Andrew K. J., editor.
Title: Monitoring and intervention for the critically ill small animal : the rule of 20 / [edited by] Rebecca Kirby, Andrew Linklater.
Description: Ames, Iowa : John Wiley & Sons, Inc, 2016. | Includes bibliographical references and index.
Identifiers: LCCN 2016018620 (print) | LCCN 2016030761 (ebook) | ISBN 9781118900833 (pbk.) | ISBN 9781118900963 (pdf) | ISBN 9781118900840 (epub)
Subjects: LCSH: Dogs–Diseases–Treatment. | Cats–Diseases–Treatment. | Veterinary critical care. | Veterinary emergencies. |
    MESH: Emergencies–veterinary | Critical Care | Dog Diseases | Cat Diseases
Classification: LCC SF991 .M65 2016 (print) | LCC SF991 (ebook) | NLM SF 778 | DDC 636.0896028–dc23
LC record available at https://lccn.loc.gov/2016018620

A catalogue record for this book is available from the British Library.

Wiley also publishes its books in a variety of electronic formats. Some content that appears in print may not be available in electronic books.

Set in 9/11pt Minion by SPi Global, Pondicherry, India

Printed and bound by CPI Group (UK) Ltd, Croydon, CR0 4YY

C9781118900833_060723

Dedication

In loving memory of Douglass K. Macintire and Lesley G. King ... whose beauty, grace, compassion, and wisdom bless our lives and the lives of thousands of animals. We miss you ...

Contents

Contributors

Linda Barton, DVM, DACVECC
BluePearl Specialty and Emergency Medicine for Pets
Renton, Washington

Dawn Merton Boothe, DVM, MS, PhD, DACVIM, DACVCP
Director, Clinical Pharmacology Laboratory
Professor of Physiology and Pharmacology
Department of Anatomy, Physiology, and Pharmacology
College of Veterinary Medicine, Auburn University
Auburn, Alabama

Dennis E. Burkett, VMD, PhD, DACVECC, DACVIM
(CARDIOLOGY)
Hope Veterinary Specialists
Malvern, Pennsylvania

Heather Darbo, CVT, VTS (ECC)
Veterinary Technician
Lakeshore Veterinary Specialists
Glendale, Wisconsin

Jennifer J. Devey, DVM, DACVECC
Consultant
Fox Valley Animal Referral Center
Appleton, Wisconsin

Carol E. Haak, DVM, DACVECC
Milwaukee, Wisconsin

Lee Herold, DVM, DACVECC
Chief Medical Officer
DoveLewis Emergency Animal Hospital
Portland, Oregon

Veronica Higgs, DVM
Metropolitan Veterinary Specialists and Emergency Services
Louisville, Kentucky

Christine Iacovetta, DVM, DACVECC
BluePearl Veterinary Partners
Queens, New York

Lesley G. King, MVB, DACVIM, DACVECC, DECVIM
(COMPANION ANIMALS)†
Professor, Clinical Educator
Director, Intensive Care Unit
Director, Emergency and Critical Care Residency Program
Medical Director, Wards Nursing
School of Veterinary Medicine
University of Pennsylvania
Philadelphia, Pennsylvania

Rebecca Kirby, DVM, DACVIM, DACVECC
(Formerly) Animal Emergency Center
Gainesville, Florida

Jennifer Klaus, DVM, DACVECC
Director
Blue Pearl Veterinary Partners
Phoenix, Arizona

Jan Kovacic, DVM, DACVECC
Horizon Veterinary Services
Four Seasons Veterinary Specialists
Lafayette, California

Susan E. Leonard, DVM, DACVECC
Emergency Veterinarian
Northeast Veterinary Referral Hospital
Plains, Pennsylvania

Andrew Linklater, DVM, DACVECC
Clinical Specialist and Instructor
Lakeshore Veterinary Specialists
Milwaukee, Wisconsin

Natara Loose, DVM, DACVECC
Brooklyn, New York

Adesola Odunayo, DVM, MS, DACVECC
Clinical Assistant Professor of Emergency and Critical Care
University of Tennessee
Knoxville, Tennessee

Cheryl Page, CVT, VTS (ECC)
Veterinary Technician
Lakeshore Veterinary Specialists
Glendale, Wisconsin

Armi Pigott, DVM, DACVECC
Clinical Specialist and Instructor
Lakeshore Veterinary Specialists
Milwaukee, Wisconsin

Christin Reminga, DVM
University of Pennsylvania
Philadelphia, Pennsylvania

Elke Rudloff, DVM, DACVECC
Clinical Specialist and Instructor
Lakeshore Veterinary Specialists
Milwaukee, Wisconsin

†Deceased.

ix

Lauren Sullivan, DVM, MS, DACVECC
Assistant Professor
Small Animal Emergency and Critical Care
Department of Clinical Sciences
Colorado State University
Fort Collins, Colorado

Caroline Tonozzi, DVM, DACVECC
Veterinary Specialist
VCA Aurora Animal Hospital
Aurora, Illinois

Conni Wehausen, DVM, DACVECC
Board-Certified Criticalist
Animal Emergency and Referral Center of Minnesota
St Paul, Minnesota

Ryan Wheeler, DVM
Four Seasons Veterinary Specialists
Lafayette, California

Preface

The Rule of 20: how to keep them alive in the ICU

It is 4:00 in the morning and finally time to go home after a long day. A last look is given to Maggie, the Toy Poodle that had gram-positive rods circulating in her neutrophils, Junior, the Poodle with diabetes, pancreatitis, and seizures, and Shooter, the postoperative gastric dilation-torsion Great Dane. The care of these and other critical patients must be passed on to the on-duty critical care team. How can I be confident that I have addressed the immediate problems of each of these animals? Do I have a plan in place that is sufficient to anticipate, detect, and minimize complications? Will intervention be early enough to make a positive difference in the outcome? These heartfelt concerns led to the creation of the Rule of 20.

The Rule of 20, in its simplest form, is a check-off list. It was created to remind doctors and ICU staff to examine the status of critical organ systems, clinical and laboratory parameters, and treatment goals that are essential for patient survival. While the inciting cause of the critical illness will vary, a common denominator often exists between the most critical patients – systemic inflammation. Most of the pathophysiology is occurring at the capillary level, making every organ at risk for deleterious changes. Damage to one organ can rapidly initiate a cascade of events resulting in multiple organ dysfunction or failure. A multiorgan approach to patient assessment and treatment is required and can be effectively guided by using the Rule of 20.

Monitoring and Intervention for the Critically Ill Small Animal Patient: The Rule of 20 is focused on dogs and cats admitted for intensive care. Each of the 20 parameters of the Rule of 20 has a dedicated chapter, with the final chapter focused on the selection and administration of anesthesia for the critical small animal patient. The authors are veterinary specialists devoted to the critical care of dogs and cats and share their expertise and experiences related to their topic. The book is designed for use as a reference as well as at the cage side, with tables, schematics, algorithms, and drawings provided for quick reference. Common problems and complications encountered in the ICU patient are highlighted within each chapter. A review of the basic physiology and pathophysiology relevant to the topic is presented, with recommendations for the diagnosis, monitoring, and treatment of common disorders. While the book is not meant to be an emergency manual, the basic life-saving concepts and procedures for the emergency patient and the ICU patient are often identical and are highlighted throughout the book.

Veterinary specialists, practicing veterinarians, residents, interns, veterinary nurse technicians, assistants, and veterinary students will find valuable and potentially life-saving ideas, procedures, and tips in this comprehensive patient care book. It is ideal to review the book beginning with the Introduction to SIRS and the Rule of 20 (Chapter 1) to become acquainted with the concepts. You will also gain insight into the consequences of systemic inflammation and the systemic inflammatory response syndrome (SIRS). Chapter 2 (Fluid Balance) should immediately follow since the formulation of an effective fluid resuscitation and maintenance plan is at the core of every ICU treatment sheet. Subsequently, careful review of each chapter in the book is warranted to acquire the knowledge base essential for understanding the complex nature of critical illness.

Acknowledgments

The editors wish to thank the contributing authors for their expertise, as well as Nancy Turner, Erica Judisch, and Susan Engelken at Wiley Publishing for their help and patience through this project. We want to recognize the important contributions of Jan Kovacic, DVM, DACVECC, and Dennis T. Crowe, DVM, DACVS, DACVECCS, for their roles in establishing the Animal Emergency Center as an important training center, setting the stage for the development of the Rule of 20. We also wish to thank each of our mentors for guiding our professional development. Finally, a big thank you to our friends and family for their patience and support.

Becky and Andrew

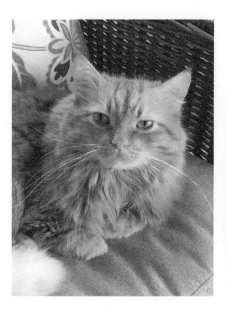 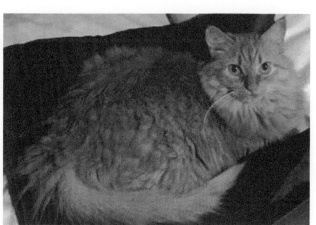

Izzy (left) and Dolly (right) Kirby, hand raised since birth, providing love daily.

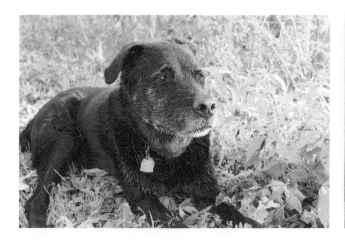 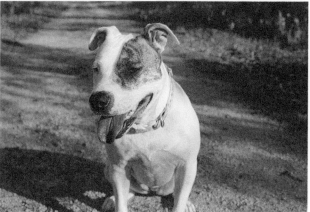

Kiris (left) and Ella (right) Linklater, both rescues from Wisconsin, providing endless support

CHAPTER 1

An introduction to SIRS and the Rule of 20

Rebecca Kirby

(Formerly) Animal Emergency Center, Gainesville, Florida

Introduction to the Rule of 20 and inflammatory response syndromes

Heat stroke, peritonitis, parvovirus diarrhea, systemic lymphosarcoma, leptospirosis, massive trauma, gastric dilation-torsion, aspiration pneumonia, pancreatitis, immune-mediated disease, and postoperative laparotomy are but a sampling of the multitude of potentially life-threatening disorders that can affect the small animal intensive care unit (ICU) patient. These and other disorders share a common pathophysiology: an inciting stimulus initiates the production and release of circulating mediators that cause systemic inflammatory changes.

Inflammation can be defined as a localized protective response elicited by injury or destruction of tissues that serves to destroy, dilute, or wall off both the injurious agent and the injured tissue [1]. Chemical mediators are released in response to an inciting antigen and initiate the innate immune response that causes inflammation. The classic signs of inflammation are heat, redness, swelling, pain, and loss of normal function. These are manifestations of the physiological changes that occur during the inflammatory process: (1) vasodilation (heat and redness), (2) increased capillary permeability (swelling), and (3) leukocytic exudation (pain). The initial inflammatory response to a localized insult is good, serving to localize the problem, destroy an offending pathogen, clean up damaged tissues, and initiate the healing process.

However, many ICU patients develop a negative trajectory when the inflammatory mediators and their response have systemic consequences. When this occurs due to an infection, it is called sepsis, and when it progresses, it often results in multiple organ dysfunction syndrome (MODS) or multiple organ failure (MOF).

It might appear logical that an overwhelming infectious agent could stimulate systemic inflammation. Yet, an almost identical clinical progression has been commonly observed in response to conditions that are not due to infection (such as trauma, surgery, and certain metabolic diseases). The term "sepsis syndrome" was first used to describe this in human patients when they appeared to be septic but had no obvious source of infection [2–4].

By the mid-1990s, sepsis syndrome had evolved into the nomenclature of systemic inflammatory response syndrome (SIRS). It was discovered that the body can respond to noninfectious insults and tissue injury in the same exaggerated manner that it does to microbial pathogens, with an almost identical pathophysiology [5]. In sepsis, pathogen-associated molecular patterns (PAMPs), expressed by the pathogen, stimulate pattern recognition receptors (PRRs) in the host. With noninfectious diseases, damaged tissues also release endogenous mediators, such as alarmins and damage-associated molecular pattern (DAMP) molecules (such as heat shock proteins, HMGB-1, ATP, and DNA). These will stimulate the toll-like receptor, PRRs or other receptor systems that typically respond to microbes and activate immune cell responses [6–8]. A list of proinflammatory cytokines associated with SIRS is provided in Table 1.1. Figure 1.1 provides a schematic of many of the proinflammatory changes that occur in this syndrome.

Soon the one-hit and two-hit models of MODS caused by SIRS were recognized in humans; one hit results from an initial massive insult (traumatic, metabolic, infectious), culminating in early SIRS and MODS. The two hits occur when a severely injured patient is successfully resuscitated, followed by a second inflammatory insult which amplifies SIRS and results in MODS [9,10]. It was discovered that an antiinflammatory response occurred after the initial inflammatory response as well. This compensatory antiinflammatory response syndrome (CARS) is characterized by increased appearance of antiinflammatory cytokines and cytokine agonists found in the circulation [11]. These antiinflammatory mediators were found for days or weeks after the proinflammatory mediators had gone [12]. Macrophage dysfunction is a significant contributor to CARS, with a decreased capacity to present antigens and release proinflammatory cytokines [13]. It was found that the T-cells are defective and depleted due to apoptosis and decreased proliferation [14]. In addition, there is an increase in the suppressor cell populations [15]. Many of the cytokines released during CARS are listed in Table 1.1. Figure 1.2 provides a schematic of many of the antiinflammatory changes that occur during this process.

It was determined that the production of proinflammatory and antiinflammatory cytokines occurs simultaneously, with antiinflammatory gene expression paralleling the increased expression of proinflammatory genes [16]. It was then proposed that the induction of SIRS and CARS occurs simultaneously [17]. The emergence of myeloid-derived suppressor cells (MDSCs) results in suppression of T-cell responses through increased production of nitric oxide and reactive oxygen species. The increase in MDSCs is proportional to the severity of the inflammatory insult [17].

Although the pathophysiology has not been clearly defined for the SIRS-CARS phenomenon, the basic hemodynamic consequences have been identified. Once the mediators have entered the circulation, the progression and complications are similar for each inciting disease: peripheral vascular dilation, increased capillary permeability, and depressed cardiac function. Three forms of shock are known to occur simultaneously in these patients: hypovolemic, distributive, and cardiogenic (see Figure 1.3). Once shock ensues, MODS is likely to occur if aggressive patient support has been delayed.

Monitoring and Intervention for the Critically Ill Small Animal: The Rule of 20, First Edition. Edited by Rebecca Kirby and Andrew Linklater.
© 2017 John Wiley & Sons, Inc. Published 2017 by John Wiley & Sons, Inc.

Table 1.1 Inflammatory and hemostatic mediators of severe sepsis and their effects. Adapted from: Balk RA, Ely EW, Goyette RE. Stages of infection in patients with severe sepsis. In: Sepsis Handbook, 2nd edn. Thomson Advanced Therapeutics Communication, 2004, pp 24–31.

Proinflammatory mediators

Tumor necrosis factor

  IL-6 induction, TF expression, downregulation of TM gene expression and increased catabolism, activation of fibrinolysis, cytotoxicity, upregulation of endothelial cell adhesion molecules, induction of NO synthase, neutrophil activation, antiviral activity, fever, and other effects; circulating soluble receptor is antagonist

Interleukin-1

  Fever, synthesis of acute-phase proteins, induction of IL-6 synthesis, upregulation of TF expression, decreased TM expression, activation of fibrinolysis, and other effects

Interleukin-6

  Induction of acute-phase response, induces B-cell growth and T-cell differentiation, enhances NK-cell activity, promotes maturation of megakaryocytes, can inhibit endotoxin-induced IL-1 and TNF-alpha; circulating soluble receptor is agonist

Interleukin-8

  Release stimulated by TNF, IL-1, IL-2, promotes chemotaxis, enhances neutrophil function, upregulates adhesion molecule expression, level correlates with severity of systemic manifestation of pathology

Interferon-gamma

  Induction of IgG production, potentiation of activity of IL-12, macrophage activation

Antiinflammatory mediators

Interleukin-4

  Stimulation and inhibition of various classes of T-cells, suppression of TNF and IL-1 secretion, upregulation of IgE and IgG secretion

Interleukin-10

  Inhibition of inflammatory cytokine production by mononuclear cells, suppression of monocyte procoagulant activity, downregulation of monocyte killing, share receptor homology with interferon

Transforming growth factor-beta

  Tissue development and repair, other antiinflammatory properties

Soluble receptor and receptor antagonists

  Soluble TNF-1 receptor and IL-1 soluble receptor inhibit function

Hemostatic factors

Tissue factor

  Upregulates expression on monocytes and subset of endothelial cells by TNF and IL-1 leading to stimulation of extrinsic coagulation cascade

Thrombin

Protein C

Protein S

Antithrombin

Plasminogen activator inhibitor-1

Tissue factor pathway inhibitor

Plasmin

Thrombin activatable fibrinolysis inhibitor

Other mediators

Nitric oxide

Bradykinin

Lipopolysaccharide binding protein

Complement

Leukotrienes

Prostaglandins

Superoxide radicals

Platelet activating factor

Myocardial depressant factor

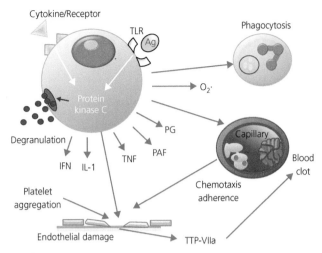

Figure 1.1 A schematic of some of the major consequences of the proinflammatory component of systemic inflammatory response syndrome (SIRS). Many cells produce proinflammatory mediators, including monocytes, macrophages, and endothelial cells. The interaction of an antigen (microbial or tissue based) with its receptor will cause the stimulation of protein kinase C and the production of cytokines. Cytokines in the circulation will interact with their specific receptor on other cells and stimulate the production of more cytokines. In addition to the release of cytokines (IFN, IL-1, TNF), the arachidonic acid cascade is stimulated and produces PG, PAF, and leukotrienes. Reactive oxygen species are produced as well. Some of the consequences include degranulation of white cells, endothelial damage, stimulation of coagulation, white blood cell chemotaxis and adherence in capillaries, and increased phagocytosis of Ags. Ag, antigen; IFN, interferon; IL, interleukin; O_2^-, superoxide radicals; PAF, platelet activating factor; PG, prostaglandins; TNF, tumor necrosis factor; TLR, toll-like receptor; TTP, tissue thromboplastin; VIIa, activated factor VII.

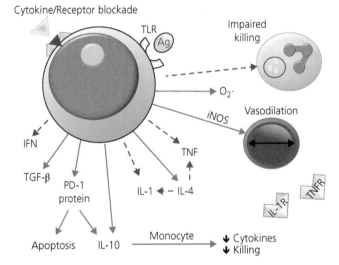

Figure 1.2 A schematic of some of the major consequences of the antiinflammatory component of the compensatory antiinflammatory response syndrome (CARS). Red dotted lines depict inhibitory actions, blue solid lines depict stimulatory action. T-cells, monocytes, and macrophages are the primary cells affected. The same antigens (microbial or tissue based) that stimulate the proinflammatory response can also stimulate the antiinflammatory cascades. The antiinflammatory mediators will block the production of many of the proinflammatory cytokines (*red triangle and red dotted lines*). TNF and IL-1 receptors are found in the circulation and will bind and inactivate TNF and IL-1 proinflammatory mediators. Ag, antigen; IFN, interferon; IL, interleukin; IL-1R, interleukin-1 receptor; iNOS, inducible nitric oxide synthetase; O_2^-, superoxide radicals; PD-1, programmed death-1; TGF-β, tissue growth factor-beta; TLR, toll-like receptor; TNF, tumor necrosis factor; TNFR, tumor necrosis factor receptor.

Many research and clinical trials have been conducted in laboratory animals and humans looking for a single best therapy that would be effective in treating most patients with the SIRS-CARS phenomenon, with minimal success. Since inflammation and immune suppression have been found to be occurring simultaneously, each patient is more likely to be experiencing their own unique combination of immune stimulation and suppression. This makes a standardized protocol for therapy extremely difficult to formulate until further knowledge is acquired. Emphasis is no longer primarily directed at methods to stop exaggerated proinflammatory responses but is instead placed on supporting the patient and searching for new methods that prevent prolonged immunosuppression or restore immune function [18].

Sepsis, the SIRS-CARS phenomenon (referred to simply as SIRS from here on), and MODS remain tremendous obstacles to the successful treatment of critically ill small animals. A "back to basics" approach is critical for any patient with the potential for inflammatory changes. Several basic yet key principles that can be used to guide patient assessment and care are listed in Box 1.1. Problems within the major organ systems should be anticipated in advance, with appropriate diagnostic, therapeutic, and monitoring efforts employed early, rather than waiting for a problem to surface and reacting to it. The Rule of 20 was developed to assist the critical care team in thoughtfully and carefully assessing these patients. Table 1.2 lists common problems to anticipate under each parameter of the Rule of 20 in patients with SIRS. Sample forms that can be used when applying the Rule of 20 are provided in Figures 1.4 and 1.5.

The critical care team must remain open to options for the diagnosis and care of the patient when changes in patient status occur and must reconsider differentials when a patient is not progressing

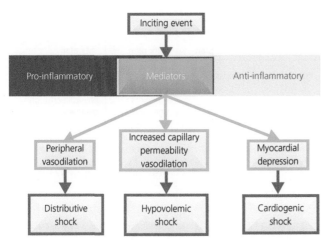

Figure 1.3 A schematic depicting the presence of proinflammatory (*blue*) and antiinflammatory (*yellow*) mediators released concurrently (*green*), causing hemodynamic changes that result in three simultaneous forms of shock.

Box 1.1 Key principles to guide the care of the small animal ICU patient.

- Treat the most life-threatening problem first
- Treat the patient, not the numbers
- Anticipate the worst and be ready for it
- Provide the right treatment, at the right time, in the right amount
- Examine the cause of the problem and the effect on the patient
- Weigh the pros and cons of every drug and procedure
- There is not a drug for every problem – less is best
- If it has not been written down, it has not been done
- Never ignore your gut feeling
- Things are done in the order of importance

Table 1.2 Common problems to anticipate for each parameter of the Rule of 20 in the SIRS patient.

Rule of 20 parameter	Anticipated problems
Fluid balance	Hypovolemia; vasodilation, increased capillary permeability
Albumin, COP	Hypoalbuminemia; loss through capillaries and catabolic state; reduced COP and extravasation of fluid from vasculature
Blood pressure	Hypotension; hypovolemia and impaired cardiac performance, peripheral vasodilation
Glucose	Hypoglycemia; increased consumption, decreased intake; can affect vascular tone and cardiac performance
Electrolytes	Hypokalemia; any disorder is possible with fluid imbalances, catabolic state, and depressed nutritional intake
Acid–base	Metabolic acidosis associated with poor perfusion and elevated lactate is common
Oxygenation/ventilation	Hypoxemia possible if pulmonary edema from inflammatory vascular changes or poor cardiac performance
Coagulation	Thrombocytopenia (declining trend); some form of DIC due to mediator-induced vasculitis, activation of serine proteases, and insufficient antithrombin
Red blood cells	Anemia from disease or erythrocytosis from dehydration; frequent blood sampling can result in anemia
Heart rate, rhythm, contractility	Tachycardia in dogs with poor perfusion, bradycardia in cats with poor perfusion; arrhythmias if poor perfusion; depressed myocardial contractility with circulating mediators
Neurological status	Depressed level of consciousness from perfusion changes, hypoxemia if present, circulating mediators, metabolic changes or underlying disease
Urinary tract status	Azotemia if poor perfusion or dehydration; impaired renal function if prolonged hypotension or nephrotoxic drugs
WBC, immune status	Impaired immune function, lymphopenia possible, susceptible to nosocomial infections
Gastrointestinal status	Gastric paresis, ileus; third body fluid spacing into bowel; bacterial translocation if no enteral feeding
Nutrition	Catabolic state and early malnutrition anticipated; bacterial translocation without enteral feeding
Drugs	Altered volume of distribution, metabolism and excretion
Body temperature	High if active inflammation; low in cats with poor perfusion or dogs with difficult-to-resuscitate shock
Pain control	Pain is anticipated with all critical illness and deserves analgesic support; critical early in shock resuscitation
Wound and bandage care	Possible source of pathogens requiring close monitoring of wound sites and bandage changes
Nursing care and TLC	Must receive the right treatment at the right time in the right amount; anticipate problems, be ready; provide TLC

COP, colloidal osmotic pressure; DIC, disseminated intravascular coagulation; TLC, tender loving care; WBC, white blood cell.

as expected. A problems list for the patient should be established and revised at least daily, with options for diagnostic, therapeutic, and monitoring plans for each problem outlined and considered (Figure 1.6). A differential diagnosis list is prepared for each problem and frequently reevaluated with the goal of finding one diagnosis that could be responsible for all the listed problems.

There are many aspects of critical care that are unique to the cat. Challenges occur when treating the cat due to species differences such as their physiological response to shock, the specific methods required for shock resuscitation and the different drug responses, metabolism, and dosing requirements. Knowledge of the traits specific to the cat is mandatory for optimizing their ability to recover from critical illness. These differences are highlighted in each chapter throughout the Rule of 20.

The successful treatment of SIRS and MODS has lead to the emergence of a new syndrome identified in human medicine, the persistent inflammation/immunosuppression catabolism syndrome (PICS) [17]. Secondary nosocomial infections and severe protein catabolism are hallmarks of PICS. This syndrome presents

the simultaneous challenge of managing chronic inflammation and immunosuppression. These patients are identified in the surgical ICU after ≥10 days and have persistent inflammation defined by findings such as elevated C-reactive protein, lymphopenia (<800/mm³), serum albumin < 3 g/dL, and weight loss >10%.

A study of adult humans suffering severe blunt trauma found that patients with complicated clinical outcomes are exhibiting PICS [19]. These patients were reported as being significantly older and sicker, with persistent leukocytosis but low lymphocyte and albumin levels compared with uncomplicated patients. They expressed significant suppression of myeloid cell differentiation, increased inflammation, decreased chemotaxis, and defective innate immunity compared with uncomplicated patients. Genomic analysis found changes consistent with defects in the adaptive

Problems list	Dx plan	Rx plan	Mx plan
Poor perfusion Tachycardia, Pale MM, CRT 3 sec	Doppler BP CVP when stable	Crystalloids, HES high normal end-points; large volume technique	Doppler BP CVP, UO physical perfusion parameters
Vomiting Yellow liquid	POC database, CBC, UA, biochemistry, radiographs when stable	Fluid therapy NPO anti-emetics ± NG tube	PE for hydration and perfusion frequency of vomiting

Figure 1.6 An example of a worksheet to ensure that each patient problem has a diagnostic, therapeutic, and monitoring plan. The worksheet has some examples of problems to demonstrate the intention of the form. Each of the problems that the patient has that day should be listed in the left-hand column. New and unresponsive problems deserve a diagnostic, therapeutic, and monitoring plan written down. After assessing each problem and possible plan, the task of choosing the most efficient means for patient diagnosis and care can be performed. Dx, diagnostic; Mx, monitoring; Rx, therapeutic.

Rule of 20 Parameters	
☐ Fluid balance	☐ Neurological status
☐ Blood pressure	☐ Urinary tract status
☐ Albumin, COP	☐ WBC, Immune status
☐ Glucose	☐ GI tract status
☐ Electrolytes	☐ Nutritional status
☐ Acid – base	☐ Drug dosing, metabolism
☐ Oxygenation/ventilation	☐ Body temperature
☐ Coagulation	☐ Pain control
☐ Red blood cell status	☐ Wound and bandage care
☐ Heart rate, rhythm, contractility	☐ Nursing care, TLC

Figure 1.4 The Rule of 20. Each parameter should be assessed regularly in any critically ill dog or cat. The order of importance will vary between individual patients. COP, colloidal osmotic pressure; GI, gastrointestinal, TLC, tender loving care; WBC, white blood cell.

Parameter	Patient	Target	Intervention	Parameter	Patient	Target	Intervention
Fluid balance				Heart rate, rhythm, contractility			
Blood pressure				Neurological status			
Oncotic pull /albumin				Urinary tract status			
Glucose				WBC, immune status, antibiotics			
Electrolytes				Gastrointestinal status			
Acid–base				Nutritional status			
Oxygenation & ventilation				Drugs, dosage, metabolism			
Coagulation				Pain			
RBCs				Wounds, bandages			
Temperature				Nursing care			

Figure 1.5 Rule of 20 form for recording current patient status, targeted endpoints, and proposed intervention. RBC, red blood cell; WBC, white blood cell.

immune response and increased inflammation. Clinical data showed persistent inflammation, immunosuppression, and protein depletion.

Unfortunately, at this time, when PICS is recognized, the course correction is difficult. Therapeutic interventions are geared towards supportive care and treating secondary infections. Further research is needed to identify appropriate multimodal therapies that target specific components of the syndrome [16]. The Rule of 20 now becomes even more important for thoroughly assessing and supporting these critical patients.

Diagnostic and monitoring procedures

The practice of medicine is an art that depends on the ability to successfully acquire and integrate the findings from the patient history, physical examination (PE), and cage-side point of care (POC) laboratory database. Patients continuously give important information through their physical changes, progression of illness, and clinical signs. Additional diagnostic testing is done to confirm, deny or better define the clinical impressions gained from evaluation of the patient status and underlying disease(s). It is not uncommon for life-threatening problems to require stabilization before time-consuming or invasive diagnostic and monitoring procedures are employed.

The history and physical examination

The key to taking a great history is organization. A sample format for obtaining a sequential history pertaining to the small animal ICU patient is presented in Table 1.3. The order in which the topics are addressed is specifically arranged to better direct information gathering while allowing the owner to describe their concerns about their pet.

Frequently reported complaints elicited from the history (such as vomiting, inability to walk, diarrhea) require further characterization to localize the disease or indicate the severity of the problem. Discussions about significant historical data pertaining to each of the Rule of 20 topics can be found in the corresponding topic chapter.

Each member of the critical care team will develop his or her own style and routine for performing a PE for individual patients. The key is to be consistent and thorough. A rapid evaluation of the ABCs (Airways, Breathing, Bleeding, Circulation, Consciousness) is the first priority, with intervention provided when potentially life-threatening problems are identified. Developing a head-to-tail system of examination helps to maintain a routine and remain focused. Saving the examination of the body parts most likely related to the presenting complaint to the end of the PE can help prevent distraction and failure to complete the remainder of the PE. It is best to perform the equipment-dependent examinations at the end of the PE to avoid distraction.

As the PE progresses from head to tail, neurological and orthopedic evaluations are done along with the general PE. Any animal that has had head trauma, loss of consciousness, prolonged seizures, or other indication of intracranial edema or hemorrhage must maintain a normal head position throughout the examination. When an area of pain is identified, examination of that area is postponed and the general PE is continued, followed by a closer assessment of the painful region. Significant PE findings relative to each of the Rule of 20 topics are discussed in the corresponding topic chapter.

Table 1.3 Example of a format for obtaining a sequential history relevant to the small animal ICU patient. The recommended sequence of questioning is shown and is directed at controlling the conversation while meeting the needs of the client to tell their story about their pet.

Format for history	Notes
Signalment	Alert for age, breed and intact reproductive tract related disorders
Presenting complaint	Noted by staff at time of presentation and recorded. Best not to start history with this inquiry in order to control the historical sequence of the problem
Last normal	Inquire when patient was last absolutely normal, may be abnormal prior to presenting complaint. Differentiates peracute, acute, chronic, and acute-on-chronic problems
Progression	Outline of sequence of changes occurring in the patient from the time of "Last normal" until the present day
Characterization of problems	Identified problems are characterized (such as volume, rate, consistency, color, sound, intensity, duration). Individual problems in the Rule of 20 are discussed in individual chapters
Systems review	Report on problems or systems not discussed related to the current problems and progression. Examples include: vomiting, diarrhea, coughing, sneezing, nasal or ocular discharge, seizures, fainting, weakness, water intake, urination frequency and effort, urine color, stool consistency
Past medical history	Vaccination, heartworm, and parasite control are listed. Any blood transfusions, problems with anesthesia or sedation are reported. Past medical problems and laboratory results of concern
Medications	List prescribed, over the counter and supplements given to the animal. Medications taken by the owner may be important if patient exposure is possible
Exposure to toxins or infectious disease	Inquire about the patient environment including outdoor habits, ill animals or people, groups of animals, new products or people and other lifestyle habits
Nutrition	Inquire about type, quantity, and brand of food, feeding routine, appetite, access to water, weight gain or loss

Point of care testing

The most important and immediate laboratory assessment of the ICU small animal patient is done at the cage side with POC testing. The minimum database should include the packed cell volume (PCV), plasma total protein (TP), blood glucose, blood urea nitrogen (BUN or creatinine), electrolytes, acid–base status, blood lactate, coagulation profile, blood smear for platelet estimate and red blood cell (RBC) morphology, and urinalysis.

There are several POC data points that, when abnormal, warrant immediate investigation and intervention (indicated by red checkmarks in Table 1.4). The significance of the abnormalities with the possible cause(s), intervention options, and monitoring recommendations are available under the corresponding topic chapters.

The microhematocrit tube provides a great deal of data. Figure 1.7 illustrates information that can be obtained from the spun tube, including the PCV, TP, buffy coat, and serum color. The PCV and

Table 1.4 Point of care (POC) blood values of concern.

Factor	Value
✓PCV	>60% or <20%
✓TP	>9.0 or <5.0 g/dL
✓Glucose	<60 mg/dL (3.3 mmol/L)
	>200 mg/dL (11.1 mmol/L)
✓BUN	>40 mg/dL (14 mmol/L)
	<5 mg/dL (1.8 mmol/L)
✓Lactate	>2.0 mmol/L
✓Electrolytes	Na$^+$ >170 or <135 mEq/L*
	K$^+$ >6.0 or <3.0 mEq/L*
	Cai^{++} >6.0 or <3.0 mmol/L
	Cl$^-$ >125 or <110 mEq/L
✓Acid–base	pH >7.5 or <7.2
	pCO$_2$ >50 or <25 mmHg
✓Urinalysis	Renal tubular cell cast
	White or red cell casts
	Glycosuria with normal blood glucose
	Specific gravity <1.004
	Protein ≥3+

BUN, blood urea nitrogen; PCV, packed cell volume; TP, total protein; i, ionized.

* (mEq/L = mmol/L).

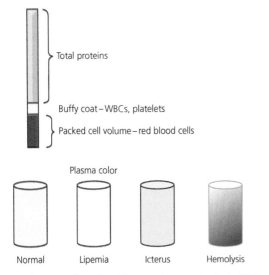

Figure 1.7 Schematic of benefits of the microhematocrit tube in POC testing. After the tube has been centrifuged, the top portion contains the total protein fraction, the small white layer is the buffy coat containing the white blood cells and platelets, and the bottom red portion is the packed cell volume. The lower columns serve as a reminder that the color of the plasma should also be noted: normal (straw colored), lipemia, icterus, or hemolyzed are the most common abnormalities.

TP are evaluated together, with the most common interpretation of changes presented in Table 1.5.

The white layer in the hematocrit tube, between the plasma and the RBCs, consists of the white blood cells (WBCs) and platelets, called the buffy coat. When this is >1–2%, it suggests high WBC counts, and when <1%, low counts. A slide can be made of this layer and the cells examined for morphology, inclusion bodies or parasites. Platelet estimates are best made from a drop of whole heparinized blood rather than the buffy coat. However, if few or no platelets are seen in the buffy coat, further investigation is warranted regarding platelet count. How

to perform a platelet estimate is discussed in Chapter 9, Box 9.3. Even when an acceptable platelet count is found at presentation, a repeated estimate should be made after resuscitation. A declining trend in platelet numbers can be one of the first indications of disseminated intravascular coagulation (DIC). This is to be anticipated in dogs and cats with SIRS.

Urine should be collected prior to fluid resuscitation, when possible, especially for patients with likely infectious or metabolic problems. The ability of the kidneys to concentrate urine is reflected by the specific gravity. Glycosuria without hyperglycemia reflects proximal tubular cell damage, a complication of nephrotoxic drugs or renal hypoxia. Urine sediment is evaluated for casts in animals on nephrotoxic drugs or having experienced severe shock. Urine casts present (from acute to chronic) as cellular casts, followed by coarse granular casts, fine granular casts, and finally hyaline casts. Renal tubular and coarse casts may appear before significant elevations in BUN and creatinine.

Clinicopathological laboratory testing

Blood is collected prior to therapy when possible for a complete blood count and serum biochemical profile to be run at a commercial or in-hospital laboratory. It is often beneficial for the clinical pathologist to look at the blood smear for significant changes in the morphology of the blood cells. These additional data will add to the database and provide more information pertaining to the metabolic status of the patient. Evaluation of renal function, hepatic changes, and white blood cell response to illness is important for every critically ill patient.

Often special tests must be ordered to identify a pathogen, confirm a diagnosis or evaluate the success of treatment in the patient. Common clinicopathological laboratory tests that can be used to better define the cause or impact of a parameter of the Rule of 20 are discussed in each of the corresponding topic chapters.

Diagnostic imaging

Diagnostic imaging will almost always begin with survey radiographs of the affected body area. Orthogonal views are always recommended. Chest and abdominal radiographs are examined for evidence of metastatic disease, organ size, shape and position, and fluid accumulation. Contrast studies can assist in outlining structures or demonstrating dynamic changes.

Ultrasound evaluation provides imaging of the organ structure and differentiation between soft tissue and fluid densities. The focused assessment with sonography in trauma (FAST) techniques for rapid assessment of the chest and abdomen are becoming common triage tools and are outlined in the appropriate topic chapters. Doppler blood flow studies can complement the examination when thrombosis or anomalies of the vasculature are suspected.

Echocardiographic evaluation of the performance and size of the heart chambers provides a noninvasive means of assessing cardiac dynamics. Shunts and heart valve disorders can be more closely evaluated using color flow Doppler techniques. The electrocardiogram (ECG) demonstrates cardiac conduction. Information regarding cardiac assessment is presented in Chapter 11.

Endoscopy, laparoscopy, thoracoscopy, and cystoscopy can each provide images and biopsies and facilitate specific procedures of different organs when indicated. Computed tomography (CT) and magnetic resonance imaging (MRI) with and without contrast can provide more detailed imaging of structures that are poorly defined by ultrasound or radiographs.

Table 1.5 Changes in packed cell volume and total protein and their significance.

Variable value	Cause	Interpretation	Plan
Packed cell volume			
>60%*	General concerns:	Hyperviscosity	Oxygen supplementation
	Hypoxia	Pulmonary disease	Treat cause
	Hemoconcentration	Loss of plasma water	Fluids
	Overproduction	Polycythemia vera	± phlebotomy
<20%	General concerns:	Tissue hypoxia	± transfusion
	Blood loss	Hemorrhage	Hemostasis if warranted,
	Lack of production	Bone marrow problem	treat underlying cause
	RBC destruction	Immune mediated	
Total protein			
>9.0 g/dL	General concerns:	Hyperviscosity	Promote blood flow
	Loss of fluids	Hemoconcentration	Fluids
	Overproduction	Inflammation, cancer	Treat cause
<5.0 g/dL	General concerns:	Loss of COP	Give colloids
	Dilution of plasma	Excessive water	Adjust fluids
	Lack of production	GI or liver disease	Treat cause
	Loss of proteins	Vasculitis, glomerular, hemorrhage	Hemostasis
PCV/TP			
↑↑	Hemoconcentration	Loss of plasma water	Fluids
↑↓ or N	Blood loss	Splenic contraction	Hemostasis
	Hemoconcentration with	SIRS, liver or glomerular disease	Colloids, fluids
	protein loss or poor production		Treat underlying cause
↓↓	Blood loss	Acute hemorrhage	Hemostasis, ± transfusion
	Chronic disease	Liver, glomerular	Treat cause, ± transfusion
N↓	Protein loss	Liver, glomerular, GI	Colloids, treat cause
	Poor production		

COP, colloidal osmotic pressure; GI, gastrointestinal; PCV, packed cell volume; SIRS, systemic inflammatory response syndrome; TP, total protein (plasma).
* PCV between 60% and 70% can be normal for sight hounds, ferrets, and animals at high altitudes.

Recommendations for diagnostic imaging procedures with suggested techniques (such as contrast studies, FAST examination) are presented for each topic of the Rule of 20 in the corresponding topic chapter.

Monitoring procedures

The PE findings will always provide the most important data regarding the status of the patient. Following the trend of change in every monitored parameter affords more accurate information than assessing a single value. Equipment-based monitoring can include indirect and direct blood pressure, ECG, pulse oximetry, end-tidal CO_2, central venous pressure, urine output, body temperature, and body weight and is readily available for the small animal patient. Serial assessment of blood values, such as PCV, TP, acid–base status, coagulation times, electrolytes and lactate, reflects patient progress and can guide therapy. More sophisticated procedures, such as pulmonary artery catheters, $ScvO_2$, and calorimetry, are presented as options in the appropriate chapters, with known advantages and disadvantages highlighted. Each topic in the Rule of 20 will require patient monitoring. The recommended monitoring procedures are discussed in each corresponding topic chapter.

Communications and the Rule of 20

Exceptional communication skills are needed to quickly build a good rapport with the pet owner under very stressful and emotional circumstances. From first contact by telephone to final discharge of the patient and follow-up care, each member of the critical care team must develop a caring and trusting relationship with the pet owner (client). It is important to create an open forum that includes a gentle tone of voice, body language that projects an approachable demeanor, open-ended questions when taking information, attentive listening to owner concerns, and establishing realistic medical and financial expectations. When successful, the decisions made regarding the medical care of the patient can be a shared process between the owner(s) and the critical care team. More information can be found in the Further reading list at the end of the chapter.

The Rule of 20 is a fluid and dynamic monitoring tool that can be utilized to treat any critical patient. As the knowledge pertaining to the pathophysiology of disease expands, new drugs, new treatments, additional diagnostic tools, and state-of-the-art monitoring methods can be easily inserted into the format. The information gained from the Rule of 20 provides a solid foundation for patient care, as well as for communications among staff and with clients. The Rule of 20 assists the critical care team in providing the structured, thorough, and complete evaluation needed for small animal patients with complex medical problems.

Human medicine has coined the term *hospital medicine* to describe the discipline concerned with the medical care of acutely ill hospitalized patients. Physicians whose primary professional focus is hospital medicine are called hospitalists [20]. The term *criticalist* has been used in a similar capacity in veterinary medicine. The hospital medicine concept in some human studies has been associated with decreased mortality and fewer adverse events [21,22]. The Rule of 20 provides an important tool for the critical care team to facilitate reaching similar goals for the veterinary small animal ICU.

References

1. Miller-Keane Encyclopedia and Dictionary of Medicine, Nursing, and Allied Health, 7th edn. St Louis: Saunders, 2003.
2. Waydhas C, Nast-Kolb D, et al. Inflammatory mediators, infection, sepsis, and multiple organ failure after severe trauma. Arch Surg. 1992;127(4);460–7.
3. Nuytinck HK, Offermans XJ, et al. Whole body inflammation in trauma patients: an autopsy study. Prog Clin Biol Res. 1987;236A:55–61.
4. Faist E, Baue AE, et al. Multiple organ failure in polytrauma patients. J Trauma. 1983;23(9);775–87.
5. Matzinger P. The danger model: a renewed sense of self. Science. 2002;296(5566);301–5.
6. Zhang Q, Raoof M, et al. Circulating mitochondrial DAMPs cause inflammatory responses to injury. Nature. 2010;464(7285):104–7.
7. Pugin J. Dear SIRS, the concept of 'alarmins' makes a lot of sense! Intensive Care Med. 2008;34(2);218–21.
8. Tang D, Kang R, et al. PAMPs and DAMPs: signals that spur autophagy and immunity. Immunol Rev. 2012;249(1);158–75.
9. Moore FA, Moore EE. Evolving concepts in the pathogenesis of postinjury multiple organ failure. Surg Clin North Am. 1995;75(2):2577.
10. Moore FA, Sauaia A, et al. Postinjury multiple organ failure: a bimodal phenomenon. J Trauma. 1996;40(4);501–10.
11. Bone RC. Toward a theory regarding the pathogenesis of the systemic inflammatory response syndrome: what we do and do not know about cytokine regulation. Crit Care Med. 1996;24(1):163–72.
12. Rogy MA, Coyle SM, et al. Persistently elevated soluble tumor necrosis factor receptor and interleukin-1 receptor antagonist levels in critically ill patients. J Am Coll Surg. 1994;178(2):132–8.
13. Munoz C, Carlet J, et al. Dysregulation of in vitro cytokine production by monocytes during sepsis. J Clin Invest. 1991;88(5):1747–54.
14. Hotchkiss RS, Osmon SB, et al. Accelerated lymphocyte death in sepsis occurring by both the death receptor and mitochondrial pathways. J Immunol. 2005;174(8):5110–18.
15. Fehervari A, Sakaguchi S.CD4+ Tregs and immune control. J Clin Invest. 2004;114(9):1209–17.
16. Xiao W, Mindrinos MN, et al. A genomic storm in critically injured humans. J Exp Med. 2011;208(13):2581–90.
17. Gentile LF, Cuenca AG, et al. Persistent inflammation and immunosuppression: a common syndrome and new horizon for surgical intensive care. J Trauma Acute Care Surg. 2012;72(6):1491–501.
18. Hotchkiss RS, Coopersmith SM, et al. The sepsis seesaw: tilting toward immunosuppression. Nat Med. 2009;15(5);496–7.
19. Vanzant EL, Lopez CM, et al. Persistent inflammation, immunosuppression, and catabolism syndrome after severe blunt trauma. J Trauma Acute Care Surg. 2014;76(1):21–9.
20. Vazirani S, Lankarani-Fard A, et al. Perioperative processes and outcomes after implementation of a hospitalist-run preoperative clinic. J Hosp Med. 2012 7(9):697–701.
21. Raghavendra M, Hoeg RT, et al. Management of neutrophic fever during a transition from traditional hematology/oncology service to hospitalist care. World Med J. 2014;113(2):53–8.
22. Tadros RO, Raries, PL, et al. The effect of a hospitalist co-management service on vascular surgery inpatients. J Vasc Surg. 2015;61(6):1550–5.

Further reading

Silverman J, Kurtz S, Draper J. Skills for Communicating with Patients, 3rd edn. London: Radcliffe Publishing, 2013.

CHAPTER 2

Fluid balance

Rebecca Kirby[1] and Elke Rudloff[2]
[1] (Formerly) Animal Emergency Center, Gainesville, Florida
[2] Lakeshore Veterinary Specialists, Milwaukee, Wisconsin

Introduction

Water is the most essential nutrient of the body. It is the transport medium that brings oxygen, solutes, and hormones to the interstitium and delivers waste products to the liver, kidneys, and lungs for breakdown and excretion. In the interstitial space, water facilitates movement of these substances between the capillary and the cell. Within the cell, water provides a medium for organelles and for expansion of the cell membrane. Dissipation of heat occurs through the evaporation of water.

Sixty percent of the body mass (0.6 L/kg) is made up of water [1]. The total body water (TBW) is partitioned into segments according to how water is contained. There are two major compartments where water is located: the *intracellular compartment* (66% TBW, 0.4 L/kg) and the *extracellular compartment* (33% TBW, 0.2 L/kg), which are separated by the cell membrane. The extracellular fluid (ECF) compartment is further divided by the vascular membrane into intravascular and interstitial compartments. The interstitial fluid compartment makes up 75% of the ECF compartment (25% of the TBW), and the intravascular fluid compartment makes up 25% of the ECF compartment (8% of the TBW) (see Figure 2.1).

Water moves freely across all membranes (cell and vascular) that separate fluid compartments. Two principles, osmosis and the modified Starling's equation, govern how water remains within or moves between compartments. Osmosis is the process by which fluid diffuses through a semipermeable membrane from a solution with a low solute concentration to a solution with a higher solute concentration until there is an equal solute concentration on both sides of the membrane. Water moves across the cell membrane between the intra- and extracellular compartments by osmosis. Small molecular weight solutes on one side of the semipermeable plasma membrane hold water because they generate osmotic pressure. The primary solutes that generate intracellular osmotic pressure are potassium and magnesium, and the primary solutes that generate extracellular osmotic pressure are sodium, chloride, glucose, and urea [2,3]. When the concentration of solutes changes on one side of the cellular membrane and is no longer equal across the membrane, an osmolar gradient is produced. Water will move from the compartment with the lower solute concentration to the compartment with the higher solute concentration. Any sudden change in osmolality in the intravascular and interstitial compartment can affect the movement of water across the capillary membrane. The capillary membrane is freely permeable to small solutes and water, so any increase in solute concentration (osmolarity) in either extracellular compartment will be short-lived.

The components of the modified Starling's equation produce the forces that dictate water movement within the extracellular space (J_v) across the capillary membrane, defined by the following formula [4,5].

$$J_v = kf\left[\left(P_c - P_{is}\right) - \sigma\left(\pi_c - \pi_{seg}\right)\right] - Q_{lymph}$$

The hydrostatic (hydraulic) pressure within the vessel (P_c) is generated by cardiac output (CO) and systemic vascular resistance. Hydrostatic pressure within the interstitium (P_{is}) is produced by the presence of water within the collagen fibrils and fibroblasts. Colloid osmotic pressure (COP; π) is the osmotic force generated by protein particles (such as albumin, fibrinogen, and globulins) that attract water. The COP within the plasma (π_c) is opposed by the COP within the subglycocalyx space (π_{seg}, virtually zero under normal conditions) (see Figure 4.2 in Chapter 4). The movement of colloid particles across the endothelial membrane will be affected by the osmotic reflection coefficient (σ), and the movement of water and particles will be controlled by the filtration coefficient (kf). In normal tissues, the lymphatic circulation is continuously removing fluid and particles from the interstitium (Q_{lymph}), creating a slight negative interstitial pressure that promotes continuous flow of fluid and particles from the intravascular space through the interstitium into the lymphatic system which deposits them back into the intravascular space (via the thoracic duct). The major contributing forces affecting capillary fluid dynamics are illustrated in Figure 2.1.

Fluid balance refers to the state of TBW homeostasis. *Euvolemia* and *euhydration* refer to a state of normal water content in the intravascular and interstitial fluid compartments, respectively. *Hydration* is the taking in of water, and describes the clinical state of TBW. *Dehydration* is a reduction in water content, when intake through food and water is less than output lost in feces, urine, sweat, and respiratory vapor. Clinically, the term *dehydration* is used to reflect the state of insufficient water content in the interstitial space. *Overhydration* is a condition of excess water content in the interstitial and intracellular spaces.

Transmembrane ion pumps and channels regulate the movement of solutes and water in and out of the cell, maintaining cellular and organelle integrity. The primary active pump for solute transport across the cell membrane is the sodium-potassium pump. Additional membrane pumps and channels regulate the movement of calcium, hydrogen, chloride, magnesium, glucose, and amino acids. These membrane transport systems are present in every cell in every organ, and many require energy to function.

Energy required to drive transmembrane ion exchange is supplied by cleavage of adenosine triphosphate (ATP). In contrast to

Monitoring and Intervention for the Critically Ill Small Animal: The Rule of 20, First Edition. Edited by Rebecca Kirby and Andrew Linklater.
© 2017 John Wiley & Sons, Inc. Published 2017 by John Wiley & Sons, Inc.

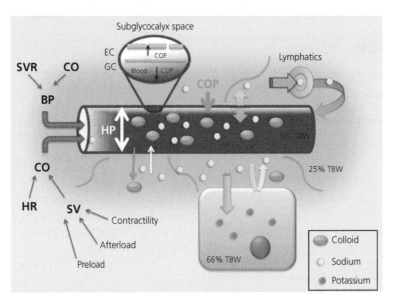

Figure 2.1 Schematic of body water dynamics at the level of the capillary. The Starling's forces across the capillary membrane favor the retention of water in the capillary due to a higher concentration of colloid molecules (*green circles*) in the intravascular space compared to the subglycocalyx space. The Pc is the major force favoring fluid movement from the capillary into the interstitium. It is a result of CO and BP. The stroke volume is dependent on the preload, thereby a driving force behind the Pc. Sodium is the primary component of the osmotic pressure in the capillary and interstitium, and is freely permeable to the capillary membrane. It is not freely permeable to the cell membrane (*yellow arrow*). Potassium provides the major intracellular osmotic force that holds water within the cell. Water is freely permeable to the cellular membrane. The lymphatics pass through the interstitial space and remove water and solutes from the interstitium (creating a negative interstitial pressure) and return them back to the intravascular space via the thoracic duct. The intracellular space contains 66% of the TBW, the interstitium 25% of the TBW and the intravascular space 8% of the TBW. Red cylinder, capillary; blue square, cell; blue arrows, water movement; blue background, interstitial fluid; sodium, yellow circle; potassium, orange circle. CO, cardiac output; COP, colloidal osmotic pressure; EC, endothelial cells; GC, glycocalyx layer; HR, heart rate; Pc, capillary hydrostatic pressure; SV, stroke volume; SVR, systemic vascular resistance; TBW, total body water.

the 38 ATP molecules that are produced during aerobic metabolism, anaerobic metabolism produces lactate and only two ATP molecules per glucose molecule. Oxygen and glucose are transported from the intravascular space to the cell through a fluid medium. Carried by hemoglobin to the capillaries, oxygen normally diffuses with great ease through the capillary membrane and interstitial space, then into the cells, most of which are located less than 50 micrometers from a capillary.

Perfusion is the delivery of oxygen to the tissues. The conduit for fluid that transports oxygen and glucose is the vascular system. The heart serves as the pump of the conduit. Oxygen delivery is the product of arterial flow and arterial oxygen content. Hemoglobin concentration and hemoglobin oxygen saturation are the prime components of arterial oxygen content, with dissolved oxygen content in plasma being a minor component (see Chapters 8 and 10).

Arterial flow is a product of CO and systemic vascular resistance. Cardiac output is a product of myocardial contraction and heart rate. Venous return, as defined by the Frank–Starling law of the heart, increases the stretch of the heart chambers (preload), which increases the force of myocardial contraction. Factors influencing venous return to the heart include mean circulatory filling pressure, right atrial pressure, and resistance of the arteries (see Chapter 11).

Blood flow is also influenced by pressure differences and compliance within the vascular circuit as well as the viscosity of the fluid medium. Extrinsic and intrinsic regulation of the cardiovascular system also affects blood flow to the tissues. Intrinsic metabolic autoregulation affects local organ blood flow, and is influenced by oxygen availability and the accumulation of metabolic byproducts.

Continuously produced and utilized, adequate ATP production becomes heavily dependent on oxygen availability during high energy output states of critical illness. Optimum ATP production, therefore, depends on both oxygen delivery (DO_2) to the cell and oxygen utilization (VO_2) by the cell. Other than oxygen supplementation and maintaining adequate hemoglobin concentration, reestablishing and maintaining intravascular fluid volume supports maximum oxygen delivery.

Compensatory neuroendocrine responses are initiated for restoring blood volume and meeting metabolic demands occurring during decreased CO states and increased ATP demands. Hormonal mechanisms control the volume and distribution of TBW and involve the kidney and the brain [6–9]. These mechanisms are continuously adjusting the amount of water retained and lost in response to fluids lost and taken in, balancing TBW. Loss of extracellular water with little or no solute (hypotonic fluid loss) results in an increase in plasma osmolality. This increase is detected by osmoreceptors which send an afferent signal to the hypothalamic paraventricular nuclei and cause the release of antidiuretic hormone (ADH) [10,11]. ADH increases the concentration of aquaporins in the renal collecting ducts, facilitating water reabsorption and therefore concentrating the urine. An increase in plasma osmolality is also detected by the thirst center (near the supraoptic and preoptic nuclei in the anteroventral region of the third ventricle), stimulating the sensation of thirst and an increase in water intake [12].

In the critically ill or injured patient, the mechanisms that balance fluid compartments are challenged and can become impaired. Water deficits result in altered body temperature regulation, neurological dysfunction, electrolyte imbalances, and hypovolemia causing reduced organ perfusion, acute kidney injury, and eventually, death [13,14]. Excess water can result in altered ventilation and lung function, gastrointestinal dysfunction, electrolyte imbalances, and cerebral edema [15]. Movement of water between compartments and into and out of the body can occur rapidly, and is not tolerated in critically ill patients. The normal compensatory responses might not occur as quickly as needed and can be incomplete, inappropriate or ineffective due to end-organ dysfunction. Frequent assessment of the fluid balance in the critical small animal patient is necessary throughout hospitalization to identify the cause(s) of fluid imbalance, and to make appropriate adjustments in the treatment plan.

Diagnostic and monitoring procedures

Monitoring the fluid balance of a patient should occur on a regular basis since changes can be very drastic over relatively short periods of time. The history and physical examination provide initial insight into problems that can affect or be affected by an altered fluid balance. In hospital point of care (POC) testing, clinicopathological laboratory tests, diagnostic imaging, and monitoring procedures are each assessed in light of the physical status of the patient.

History and physical examination

Historical and presenting problems reported by the owner that can be associated with or affect assessment of water balance include vomiting, diarrhea, respiratory problems, blood loss, trauma, toxin exposure, fever, nasal discharge, heart failure, alterations in water intake and urine output, and exposure to environmental heat extremes. A list of prescribed and over-the-counter medications should be reviewed for drugs that might affect water balance (such as diuretics or vasodilators). Recently administered medication (such as ketamine or atropine) can alter mucous membrane moisture without being a reflection of TBW changes.

The physical examination will identify abnormal parameters associated with fluid imbalance, in particular those associated with perfusion and hydration. Parameters that reflect peripheral perfusion include heart rate, mucous membrane (MM) color, capillary refill time (CRT), pulse quality, level of consciousness, and body temperature. Reduction in intravascular volume leads to clinical signs of hypovolemic shock. A progression of shock manifests in alterations in perfusion parameters, listed in Table 2.1. Rectal temperatures represent peripheral body temperatures and are an indirect indicator of the status of peripheral blood flow. Redistribution of blood flow from the periphery to the core with vasoconstriction can give a differential core-to-peripheral temperature (see Chapter 17).

Clinical signs of compensatory shock in the dog can be easily overlooked. The signs of hyperemic mucous membranes, tachycardia, rapid capillary refill time, and normal to increased arterial blood pressure should not be interpreted as normal. The arterial blood pressure is being maintained at the expense of the increased heart rate and mild vasoconstriction. The cat does not typically manifest a compensatory shock response since this stage lasts only seconds to minutes after the initiation of shock in the cat [16].

The state of hydration is in continuous flux, and there is no single parameter that reflects hydration status accurately. Physical examination findings and laboratory indices are used to estimate current hydration status [17]. Physical parameters used to assess hydration include mucous membrane and corneal moisture, skin turgor, and eye position within the orbit (Table 2.2). Two important qualifications must be considered: (1) acute changes in tissue hydration may not be evident on physical examination, since there has not been time for compensatory fluid shifting (underestimating the percentage of dehydration), and (2) older or emaciated animals have poor skin turgor and sunken eyes in their orbit unrelated to their hydration status (overestimating the percentage of dehydration).

Up to 90% of acute changes in body mass can be attributed to a change in TBW, so that in the critically ill patient, a 1 kg change in

Table 2.1 Physical examination and measured parameters that reflect peripheral perfusion in the normal state and during the stages of shock. The presence of three or more variables attributable to a particular stage of shock supports a diagnosis of that state of perfusion.

Physical and measured parameter	Normal	Compensatory stage of shock	Early decompensatory stage of shock (middle)	Late decompensatory stage of shock (terminal)
Level of consciousness	Alert	Normal	Normal to decreased	Decreased to moribund
Heart rate (bpm)	Dogs: 60–120	Dogs: >140	Dogs: >140	Dogs: <140
	Cats: 170–200	Cats: >170	Cats: ≤180	Cats: <160
Mucous membrane color	Pink	Red	Pale	Gray to white
Capillary refill time (seconds)	1–2	<1	>2	>3 to none
Peripheral pulse intensity	Strong	Bounding	Weak	Weak to absent
Rectal temperature °F (°C)	100–102.5 (37.7–39.2)	100–102.5 (37.7–39.2)	Dogs: low normal Cats: <98 (<36.7)	Dogs: 98–100 (36.7–37.7) Cats: <98 (36.7)
Blood pressure (indirect – mmHg)				
Systolic	90–120	>100	<100	<80 may not be
Mean	80–100	>80	<80	<60 detectable
CVP (cmH$_2$O)	−1 to 5	Variable	<5	Variable; can be high with heart failure
Urine output mL/kg/h	1–2	Variable	≤1	≤0.08

bpm, beats per minute.

Table 2.2 Physical examination findings and the associated estimated percent dehydration (interstitial fluid deficits).

Estimated % dehydration	Physical exam findings
0–4	No physical exam changes
4–6	Tacky mucous membranes
6–8	Loss of skin turgor
	Dry mucous membranes
	Slight hemoconcentration
8–10	Loss of skin turgor
	Dry mucous membranes
	Retracted globes within orbits
	Moderate hemoconcentration
10–12	Persistent skin tent due to complete loss of skin elasticity
	Dry mucous membranes
	Retracted globes
	Dull corneas
	Severe hemoconcentration
>12	Persistent skin tent
	Dry mucous membranes
	Retracted globes
	Dull corneas
	Signs of perfusion deficits (see Table 2.1)
	Extreme hemoconcentration

Box 2.1 Common clinical signs associated with excess interstitial fluid (overhydration) in the dog and cat.

Mild signs

Serous nasal discharge
Chemosis
Polyuria
Hypothermia, shivering

Moderate signs

Increased skin turgor (gelatinous nature)
Tissue edema
Increased respiratory rate and effort
Pleural effusion
Abdominal fluid wave, ascites
Diarrhea
Nausea and vomiting
Acute weight gain

Severe signs

Exophthalmos
Hypertension
Pulmonary moist crackles
Cough
Tachy- or bradycardia
Depressed level of consciousness

body weight may be equivalent to a 1 L change in TBW [18–22]. However, due to third body fluid space accumulation (in the abdominal or pleural spaces, or intestines or uterus) or tissue edema, a change in body weight may not occur even though there is loss of fluids from the intravascular or interstitial space(s). Weighing patients, particularly small patients, every six hours is recommended and is a simple monitoring tool to use when assessing trends of change in fluid balance.

Any systemic inflammatory response syndrome (SIRS) disease (such as sepsis, pancreatitis, trauma, immune-mediated disease, neoplasia) will have increased capillary permeability as part of the syndrome that can result in fluid extravasation. This can lead to complications associated with hypovolemia, interstitial edema, and third body space fluid accumulation. Abdominal distension, reduced bowel sounds, and short or shallow breaths due to increased pressure on the diaphragm can provide physical evidence of a large accumulation of abdominal fluid. Fluid waves might be felt during abdominal palpation. Pleural fluid accumulation can produce an elevated respiratory rate and effort, and muffled lungs sounds. Pulmonary edema may cause respiratory distress with a rapid, shallow breathing pattern and moist lung sounds heard on auscultation. Edema of the intestines may result in poor gastrointestinal function, altered borborygmi, vomiting or diarrhea.

Areas of the body that have thin membranes, low muscle mass, and/or lack of fat will demonstrate fluid accumulation first. Conjunctival edema (chemosis) is an early sign of fluid intolerance, followed quickly by subcutaneous fluid accumulation around the common calcaneal tendon, intermandibular space, head and neck, and the distal limbs. Box 2.1 lists common clinical signs of overhydration. Causes of interstitial edema or cavitary effusion unrelated to increased capillary permeability include oliguric kidney failure, right-sided heart failure, and portal hypertension. Hypovolemia may or may not be associated with these problems.

Point of care testing

The minimum POC laboratory database that should be assessed before and during fluid therapy includes the packed cell volume (PCV), total protein (TP) measured by refractometer, creatinine, blood glucose, plasma lactate, serum electrolytes, acid–base status, coagulation times, platelet estimate, and urine specific gravity (USG). Following the trend of change over time is necessary since the infusion of fluids and other forms of therapy will result in changes that may require intervention.

Loss and gain of extracellular water can result in hemoconcentration (increased PCV and TP) or hemodilution (decreased PCV and TP). Hemorrhage should be considered when the PCV and TP are reduced, although patients with acute hemorrhage can have normal or increased PCV as a result of sympathetic-induced splenic contraction releasing red cells back into the circulation. In that situation, a reduction in the initial TP can be a tell-tale sign of hemorrhage in a patient with a compatible history. An initial low TP without hemorrhage might reflect hypoalbuminemia and fluid shifts due to a loss of intravascular COP. As fluid resuscitation and rehydration are performed, hemodilution will result in a decrease in both PCV and TP.

Decreased DO_2 due to inadequate blood flow caused by hypovolemic shock can result in anaerobic metabolism. Hyperlactatemia, metabolic acidosis, and increased base deficit are usually associated with conditions causing tissue hypoxemia.

Intracellular volume changes cannot be identified on physical examination. The clinician must rely on changes in the effective osmolality of ECF (primarily recognized by changes in sodium concentration) to mark changes in cell volume. Hyponatremia will be associated with movement of water from the ECF into the intracellular fluid (ICF) compartment, and a subsequent increase in intracellular volume. Hypernatremia will be associated with a decrease in intracellular volume (see Chapter 6).

Changes in blood glucose can affect water balance. Hyperglycemia increases plasma osmolarity and can result in increased extracellular water if a patient receives or takes in fluid. Hyperglycemia also induces glycosuria, diuresis, and water loss. A significant loss of TBW can occur when water losses exceed intake, and can result in hypovolemia, dehydration, and hypernatremia (see Chapter 5).

Urine specific gravity is a reflection of the kidney's functional ability to concentrate urine. The USG can be used during assessment of fluid balance. A low USG in the patient receiving intravascular fluid (IVF) support can be difficult to interpret by itself. An inappropriately low USG in the clinically dehydrated patient, or one with azotemia, may indicate altered kidney function. If the USG is normal to increased in the patient receiving fluid therapy, fluid losses may be exceeding fluid intake and additional fluids may be warranted.

Abnormal clotting times and platelet estimate can cause internal hemorrhage and signs of hypovolemia, necessitating careful titration of intravascular fluids to prevent a sudden increase in hydrostatic pressure and exacerbation of bleeding (see Chapter 9). Patients with hypercoagulable conditions may benefit from fluid therapy to prevent capillary stasis.

Clinicopathological laboratory testing

An automated complete blood count with a manual differential count, a serum biochemical profile, and urinalysis should be reviewed for changes that might impact fluid balance and fluid therapy. Evidence of liver failure (low BUN, hypoalbuminemia, hypoglycemia, increased coagulation times, alterations in serum cholesterol) can be a cause of portal hypertension and a loss of intravascular COP with fluid extravasation into the intestinal interstitium and peritoneal cavity. An elevation in creatinine and reduced USG support renal disease, which can result in water and electrolyte imbalances. Hypertension and fluid retention will occur if oliguria or anuria develops. Hypoalbuminemia lowers intravascular COP and can potentiate fluid loss from the intravascular space (see Chapter 4). Significant proteinuria may signify altered glomerular function and, when severe, can result in hypertension, a relative oliguria, and interstitial edema.

When investigating for causes of a solute-free water imbalance, the serum osmolarity should be compared to the urine osmolarity. Normal serum osmolarity ranges from 290 to 310 mOsm in the dog and 290 to 330 mOsm in the cat [23]. Urine osmolarity can range between 161 and 2830 mOsm/L in normally hydrated dogs [24] and between 600 and 3000 mOsm/L in normally hydrated cats [25]. As the serum osmolarity rises, the urine osmolarity should also rise when the kidney works to conserve water. When there is an excess of water in the body, the normal kidney will dilute the urine, eliminating extra body water.

Ethylene glycol and other small molecular weight toxins can increase measured plasma osmolarity without increasing calculated plasma osmolarity. This will cause an increased osmolar gap and alter fluid distribution and balance. Many osmolar toxins can be tested for in commercial laboratories.

Diagnostic imaging

Survey thoracic and abdominal radiographs can be examined for signs of intracavitary fluid accumulation. Loss of abdominal detail and abdominal distension on abdominal radiographs are signs suggestive of peritoneal fluid accumulation. Distended pulmonary vessels can be caused by increased pulmonary vascular pressure. Increased interstitial densities and alveolar lung patterns are consistent with fluid accumulation in the lung parenchyma. Pleural

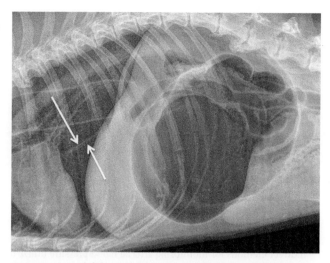

Figure 2.2 Lateral abdominal radiograph of dog with gastric dilation-volvulus. Note the small size of the vena cava (*white arrows*) and the cardiac silhouette supportive of insufficient intravascular volume. Volume replacement is critical prior to induction of anesthesia.

fissure lines and retraction of the lungs from the pleural wall with surrounding soft tissue opacity suggest thoracic fluid accumulation. Small caudal vena cava and heart sizes are compatible with hypovolemia (Figure 2.2).

Ultrasonography is more specific than radiography for demonstrating peritoneal, pleural, and/or pericardial fluid accumulation, organ structure, tissue edema, vessel size and obstructions to blood flow. Thoracentesis or abdominocentesis for fluid retrieval and sampling can be guided using ultrasonography. Echocardiography can provide important information regarding the role that the heart might have in patients with hypotension or fluid imbalance.

Monitoring procedures

Hemodynamic monitoring can be invasive or noninvasive, continuous or intermittent, physical or biochemical. Perfusion parameters and vital signs should be routinely and repeatedly evaluated from the start of fluid resuscitation until the patient leaves the hospital.

Heart rate can be assessed by pulse palpation, continuous ECG monitoring, direct cardiac auscultation, Doppler blood flow monitoring or by pulse oximetry. "Bounding" pulse quality can be associated with compensatory shock, anemia, or pain. Weak pulse quality can be associated with decreased CO from decompensatory shock or heart failure, vasodilation, or severe vasoconstriction. Body temperature is an indirect indicator of peripheral blood flow within the tissues. Pain, anxiety, and abnormal body temperature may influence sympathetic tone and should be taken into consideration when assessing perfusion parameters. Indications of successful resuscitation of perfusion deficits include a normalization of heart rate, improved pulse quality, CRT of 1–2 seconds, pink MM color, normalization of body temperature, and improvement in mentation.

Periodic monitoring of arterial blood pressure, central venous pressure (CVP), oximetry, urine output, blood lactate, and venous blood gas can be performed in those patients requiring more extensive monitoring. Arterial blood pressure is a frequently monitored parameter for documenting hypo- and hypertension and assessing the success of fluid resuscitation. Arterial blood pressure is an indirect estimation of perfusion and can be a reflection of intravascular volume status when cardiovascular function is normal. Arterial blood pressure should always be assessed in conjunction with heart rate and other parameters of perfusion.

Direct arterial blood pressure monitoring is considered to be the "gold standard" for blood pressure monitoring. Persistently unstable patients that require intensive monitoring may benefit from direct arterial blood pressure monitoring (see Chapter 3). This technique is invasive and requires skill and specialized equipment. It can be difficult to place an arterial catheter in the hypovolemic or vasconstricted patient, and the use of a transducer and special monitor is required.

Indirect methods for monitoring arterial blood pressure utilize a Doppler or an oscillometric monitor. The indirect method of measuring arterial blood pressure is the most efficient and least expensive means for monitoring arterial blood pressure, but studies correlating indirect to direct methods have shown inconsistent results, especially in cats [26–31]. Indirect arterial blood pressure does not accurately reflect venous return or regional blood flow [32], so the trend of change in indirect arterial blood pressure in conjunction with improved physical perfusion parameters implies a positive response to therapy. Pain, anxiety, cardiac dysrhythmias, and hypothermia may result in blood pressure readings that do not accurately reflect intravascular volume status.

Urine output volumes can provide a nonspecific estimation of perfusion to the kidneys. Normal urine production depends upon adequate renal blood flow and a mean arterial pressure $\geq$60 mmHg. Mean arterial pressures below this value can result in oliguria. A urine output $\geq$1–2 mL/kg/hour is ideal in the critically ill patient undergoing treatment. If the patient has a decreased urine output, one must evaluate for hypotension, postrenal obstruction, and acute kidney injury.

Central venous pressure is used to assess right ventricular preload. Central venous pressure reflects intravascular volume status when there is normal right heart function and vascular tone with no obstruction to flow. The two main factors that will reduce CVP are hypovolemia and venodilation, and an increase in CVP following a fluid challenge may indicate a fluid-responsive condition. There is controversy regarding the predictability of CVP monitoring for distinguishing fluid responders from nonfluid responders. This necessitates that the CVP be evaluated in light of the entire clinical picture [33–39]. Elevated CVP measurements can correlate with volume overload, right or left cardiac dysfunction, increased intrathoracic pressure or an increase in pulmonary arterial resistance [40]. The goal during fluid resuscitation of the hypovolemic patient is to achieve and maintain a CVP = 5–8 cm H_2O. A brief description of how to set up and manually measure the CVP is provided in Figure 2.3. In-line water manometers or pressure transducers are used to measure CVP.

Successful placement of arterial and jugular venous catheters for direct blood pressure (BP) and CVP monitoring is challenging in the hypovolemic and small patient, and may require cutdown techniques for vascular placement. The supplies needed for placing an arterial catheter are listed in Box 3.2a and the technique outlined in Box 3.2b in Chapter 3. A brief description of how to perform a jugular or cephalic vein cutdown for catheter placement is outlined in Box 2.2. A more detailed and complete description of techniques

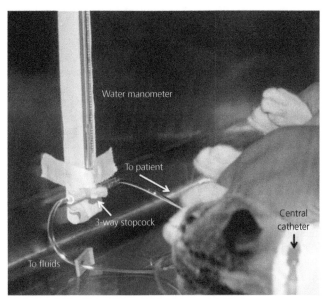

Figure 2.3 General equipment and patient positioning to measure the central venous pressure (CVP) through a central venous catheter using a water manometer. Placement requires the use of sterile technique and equipment. A central catheter is placed with the tip of the catheter located near the base of the heart (with jugular venous placement) or in the intrathoracic caudal vena cava (with femoral vein placement). A water manometer is attached to the central port of a three-way stopcock. The outflow port is attached to a fluid extension set and the inflow port to an intravenous fluid infusion set attached to a bag of isotonic fluids. The water manometer port is closed, the inflow and outflow lines are filled with fluid. The outflow line is attached to the patient. The inflow line is closed to the patient and the water manometer is filled to at least 20 cmH_2O. The apparatus can be held by hand during measurement or can be attached to a solid surface (as in the photograph). Each measurement should be taken with the patient and apparatus in the same position. The "0" point on the manometer should be at the estimated level of the right atrium of the patient. To measure the CVP, the fluid infusion port is closed. Time is allowed for equilibration which is when the fluid column stops falling and the meniscus of the fluid column in the manometer oscillates up and down with ventilation. Once the level is stabilized, the bottom of the meniscus is read at the CVP measurement. Alternatively, CVP can be measured with a transducer and electronic monitor instead of a manometer.

Box 2.2 Cutdown technique for rapid vascular access in the dog and cat with peripheral vascular collapse.

1. Clip the hair and aseptically prepare the insertion site over the cephalic or jugular vein.
2. Administer local anesthetic (lidocaine) if time permits.
3. Make a skin incision at a 45° angle over the targeted vessel. When a small incision is desired there is more success finding the vein with this location of the incision rather than incising parallel to the vein.
4. Dissect through the subcutaneous tissue over the vessel with the tip of Halsted mosquito hemostats to expose the vein.
5. Insert the largest diameter over-the-needle catheter possible into the exposed vein.
6. Flush the catheter with saline and apply an injection cap.
7. Secure the catheter in place using the catheter wings or by using medical tape to make butterfly-type wings that can be sutured to the skin.
8. Suture or staple the open skin if necessary.
9. Place sterile gauze and a protective bandage.
10. Examine the catheter insertion site once to twice daily.

for obtaining vascular access can be found in the Further reading list at the end of this chapter.

Lactate has proven its value as a significant variable associated with mortality, and is part of the Acute Patient Physiological and Laboratory Evaluation (APPLE score) for dogs and cats [41,42]. Data from canine studies of hemorrhagic shock [43,44] and critically ill and injured dogs [45–47] have demonstrated that an increase in initial plasma lactate is correlated with a worse prognosis after blood loss. More importantly, a lack of lactate clearance is associated with an increase in morbidity and mortality [48–57]. Associative data suggest that lactate normalization during resuscitation is a more powerful indicator of resuscitation adequacy than oxygen-derived variables. The goal with fluid resuscitation of the patient with hyperlactatemia is to have a return of lactate to normal. Despite its usefulness in evaluating response to resuscitation efforts and as a prognostic indicator, serum lactate concentration is not a sensitive marker for identifying local tissue hypoperfusion.

The hydration status should be monitored daily by evaluating change in the MM moisture, skin turgor, body weight, and PCV/TP. Clinical signs of dehydration and overhydration are listed in Table 2.2 and Box 2.1. Comparing fluid intake with fluid output at least once daily may identify a patient's response to treatment and the need for adjustment in fluid therapy. In severely compromised small animal patients, advanced monitoring procedures may be indicated for obtaining additional clues to fluid balance status.

Advanced monitoring procedures

Determination of TBW using isotope dilution and neutron activation analysis techniques is considered the "gold standard" but this has not been investigated in the critically ill patient [58]. Multifrequency bioelectrical impedance analysis is a method that has been used to identify acute fluid shifts in critically ill people and racing horses, but controversies exist on its reliability [59–61]. This procedure differentiates extracellular water or intracellular water from TBW by using the electrical properties of body tissues. Extracellular water is quantified using low-frequency current, and TBW is quantified using the data from higher frequencies. Intracellular water can be assessed by subtracting the values measured between the two water compartments [62].

Pulmonary artery (PA) pressure, pulmonary capillary wedge pressure (PCWP), CO, and venous oximetry can be measured for additional information on problems with perfusion status. Venous oximetry can be performed using mixed venous blood (SvO_2) from the PA catheter or distal jugular venous blood ($ScvO_2$) from a central venous jugular catheter. Mixed venous hemoglobin oxygen saturation is considered more specific for global oxygen delivery and utilization compared to $ScvO_2$; however, $ScvO_2$ has been determined to be an accurate and sensitive marker of ongoing hemorrhage and a predictor of success of resuscitation in experimental models of canine hemorrhage [63,64]. In dogs with severe sepsis or septic shock related to pyometra, an admission $ScvO_2 < 52\%$ carries an increased risk of death [65]. Considering dogs in the ICU, an $ScvO_2 < 68\%$ is associated with an increased mortality risk [66]. Jugular venous hemoglobin oxygen saturation must be evaluated in light of other perfusion parameters, body temperature, cardiac function, and arterial oxygen concentration. If normalization of physical perfusion parameters does not correlate with a higher $ScvO_2$, causes of a reduced PCV, PaO_2, and CO need to be investigated, and inotropic therapy considered [67].

Pulmonary artery catheter placement is used to measure not only SvO_2 but also pressures in the right atrium and PA as well as the PCWP. The PCWP reflects left ventricular diastolic pressure, and can be used during assessment of left ventricular function, CO, and fluid responsiveness. The predictability of PCWP in distinguishing fluid responders from fluid nonresponders and the lack of improving mortality with the use of PA catheters have resulted in a significant reduction in their use in human medicine [68–71]. The cost of equipment and supplies, the technical skills required to place and maintain PA catheters, the experience needed to interpret monitored parameters, and the risk to the patient have made the use of PA catheters uncommon in clinical veterinary medicine. This fluid balance monitoring technique is being overshadowed by newer imaging technology.

Ultrasonography can be used to assess intravascular volume by measuring inferior vena cava (IVC) collapsibility and by observing the dynamic changes of the ventricles during systole and diastole. In people, the compliant IVC changes diameter with TBW changes and respiratory cycle [72,73]. A flat IVC diameter during inspiration (<2 cm) has been shown to be an indicator of poor prognosis in trauma patients and acute surgical patients [74]. The collapsibility index is defined as the difference of the IVC diameter measured 2 cm distal to the hepatic vein inlet during inspiration (IVCi) and expiration (IVCe) in relation to expiration value ((IVCi-IVCe)/IVCe) [75–80].

In people, a collapsibility index >50% is supportive of noncardiogenic, nonobstuctive types of shock (such as hypovolemic, distributive) [81], and in spontaneously breathing patients with hypovolemia, a collapsibility index >42% can predict an increase in CO after fluid infusion [82]. This monitoring technique is still under evaluation in people, and has not yet been validated in animals.

Echocardiography can be used to globally assess the heart for pericardial fluid and cardiac tamponade (end-diastolic right ventricular and right atrial collapse). Myocardial contractility should also be evaluated, and characterized as being hyperdynamic, normal, decreased or severely dysfunctional. Hypovolemic and distributive shock can be associated with hyperdynamic myocardial function in the normal heart [83]. The cardiac chambers appear small and contractions are vigorous and hyperkinetic with the endocardial surfaces almost touching during systole ("kissing walls") [84–86].

Newer transcutaneous pulse oximeters (PVI® on MasimoSET®, Masimo, Irvine, CA) may be able to provide additional information regarding cardiovascular dynamic variables that can be measured in patients that are being manually or mechanically ventilated. Variations in pulse amplitude or pulse intensity (PI) of the pulse pressure waveform during respiratory cycles (inspiration or expiration) have been associated with fluid responsiveness. The PI is calculated by indexing the infrared pulsatile signal against the nonpulsatile signal and expressing this number as a percentage. The plethysmography variability index (PVI) is automatically calculated with the following formula:

$$PVI = (PImax - PImin) / PImax \times 100$$

A PVI $\geq 20\%$ is suggestive of hypovolemia, and the hemodynamic instability will likely be responsive to fluid administration [87]. This method is still under investigation in veterinary medicine.

Videomicroscopy with sidestream dark field imaging has also been used to evaluate blood flow in the membranes of the oral cavity. This method estimates total vessel density, proportion of perfused vessels, microcirculatory flow index, and perfused vessel density. It permits visualization of the microcirculation during low flow states, and following therapeutic interventions. This method has been used in anesthetized dogs [88,89] but requires a practiced skill in acquiring views, time for image analysis, and the patient must be very still (anesthetized, sedated or very ill) during image acquisition.

Additional monitors for peripheral perfusion have been evaluated experimentally, but are not available as a bedside test or not commonly used in veterinary medicine. Tissue partial pressure of CO_2 can be measured in highly vascular areas, including sublingual, brain, conjunctiva, skin, and intestinal surfaces. Hypoperfusion leads to an increase in tissue CO_2 levels. The most common areas interrogated are the sublingual and gastric mucosal surfaces. Elevated tonometry values and gradients between mucosal and arterial PCO_2 are associated with impaired perfusion. The use of tonometry has not become routine in human or veterinary medicine [90–93].

Disorders of fluid balance

The most common and persistent problem in the management of the critical small animal patient is establishing and maintaining fluid balance. There is no single test or combination of tests that accurately and consistently identifies fluid balance disorders. Significant changes can happen rapidly and at any time, necessitating frequent patient reassessment and modification of the fluid therapy plan. While guidelines are provided below for establishing resuscitation and maintenance fluid therapy plans, wide variation can occur between patients, necessitating an individualized approach to fluid therapy. Too little and too much fluid can be catastrophic.

Intravascular fluid excess
An acute iatrogenic overexpansion of the intravascular compartment causes stretch of the atria and release of atrial natriuretic peptide (ANP), increasing renal water and sodium excretion [94,95]. However, before excess water can be eliminated, there is an immediate increase in intravascular hydrostatic pressure. A dilutional decrease in the intravascular COP results when the excess volume is from a crystalloid fluid infusion. These changes in Starling's forces will favor the extravasation of fluids from the capillaries into the interstitial compartment, with tissue edema a potentially serious consequence.

The most common cause of fluid overload is the injection of excessive intravenous or subcutaneous fluids. Other causes include an increase in total body sodium content with a subsequent increase in extracellular water, such as occurs with congestive heart failure, kidney failure, liver failure, and oliguria. The intravenous administration of hyperosmolar solutions (such as mannitol, hypertonic saline, diagnostic contrast medium), blood products, and medications dissolved in fluid can also cause an increase in intravascular volume.

The severity of the clinical consequences of intravascular fluid excess is dependent on the organ(s) that are affected and their ability to handle excess fluid. The clinical signs commonly associated with intravascular fluid excess in the dog and cat are listed in Box 2.1. The urgency of treatment is guided by the severity of signs. Treatment of mild signs typically includes restriction of water intake and restriction or discontinuation of fluid administration.

Moderate signs might improve with the administration of diuretics (such as furosemide, 1–2 mg/kg IV) and restriction or discontinuation of the intake of water, fluids, and sodium. Severe signs might require discontinuing fluid administration, the administration of diuretics and the use of vasodilators and positive inotropes to support cardiac output. Dialysis may be indicated if the patient is oliguric or anuric. If pulmonary edema caused by fluid overload is causing hypoxemia, then temporary mechanical ventilation may be necessary.

Intravascular fluid deficits
Circulatory shock is a life-threatening phenomenon of ineffective circulating volume. The most common cause of circulatory shock is loss of intravascular volume (hypovolemic shock) through mechanisms such as hemorrhage, vomiting, diarrhea, decreased water intake, increased metabolic activity, and/or third body fluid spacing. However, there can also be insufficient return of blood to the heart due to peripheral vasodilation (distributive shock) or obstruction of central venous blood flow (obstructive shock). In these two conditions, the blood volume can actually be within "normal limits" but is ineffective at maintaining tissue perfusion. Animals in shock with poor cardiac performance (cardiogenic shock) will also have a reduced CO but the circulating intravascular volume can be variable (high, low or normal). The hemodynamic signs manifesting for each of these forms of shock are essentially the same, but fluid resuscitation is usually only beneficial in patients with hypovolemic and distributive forms of shock.

Intravascular fluid deficits cause a decrease in venous return and CO. A schematic of the basic mechanisms of hypovolemic shock in the dog and cat is presented in Figure 2.4. The renin-angiotensin-aldosterone system will cause an increased fluid retention by the kidneys. A release of ADH stimulates the renal conservation of water and sodium [96]. These mechanisms serve to increase intravascular volume and venous return and improve CO and arterial flow. Energy is required to sustain this compensatory mechanism, and an additional oxygen supply is required for energy production. Substrates required for cellular energy production are provided through the actions of the stress hormones (glucagon, growth hormone, cortisol, and epinephrine).

These natural neuroendocrine responses can be adequate to compensate for mild-to-moderate acute decreases in intravascular volume, and produce the *compensatory stage* of hypovolemic shock commonly recognized in dogs. Cats experience the compensatory stage, but it is short (seconds to minutes) in duration and rarely recognized.

Clinical signs of compensatory shock in the dog (see Table 2.1) include hyperemic mucous membranes, tachycardia, rapid capillary refill time, and normal to increased arterial blood pressure, which should not be interpreted as normal. Maintaining arterial blood pressure occurs at the expense of an increased heart rate and mild vasoconstriction (both energy consuming). Should the natural neuroendocrine mechanisms be inadequate to restore baroreceptor stretch, should cardiac dysfunction exist, or should intravascular volume and systemic vascular resistance be inadequate in restoring oxygen delivery to the tissues, cardiovascular decompensation occurs.

Continued low CO amplifies sympathetic stimulation, clinically manifesting as significant peripheral vasoconstriction and tachycardia. Selective vasoconstriction of the skin, mucous membranes, and splanchnic beds shunts arterial blood flow to preferred organs (heart and brain), maintaining blood flow to those vital organs as

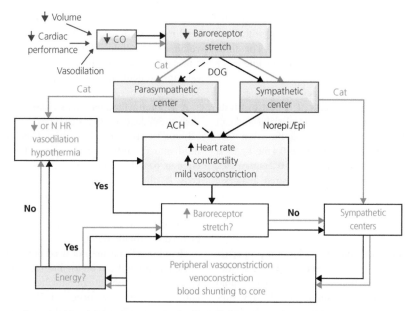

Figure 2.4 Schematic of the mechanism of the shock response in the dog and cat. This simplistic representation shows the response in the dog in blue lines and boxes and the response in the cat in green lines and letters. A decline in cardiac output initiates the process, with decreased stretch of the baroreceptors sending afferent signals to the brainstem. There is an increase in sympathetic output in both the dog and cat, resulting in a release of norepinephrine and epinephrine which increases heart rate and contractility, and causes a mild vasoconstriction. This is the compensatory stage of shock. This is where the clinical signs diverge in the dog and cat. In the dog, there is suppression of the parasympathetic output and heart rate remains elevated, but in the cat, a vasovagal type response is elicited and a normal or slow heart rate develops. If the baroreceptors are still not stretched, more dramatic sympathetic stimulation occurs with shunting of the peripheral blood to the core circulation (dog and cat). This response is the early decompensatory (or middle) stage. Energy is required to maintain these compensatory responses. When energy becomes depleted, the rapid heart rate and vasoconstriction can no longer be maintained. The heart rate slows and vasodilation results. This is the decompensatory (or terminal) stage of shock. Centrally mediated hypothermia plays a role in the middle stage of shock in the cat, resulting in the triad of hypothermia, bradycardia, and hypotension.

long as possible. Cellular oxygen and energy demands increase as vasoconstriction intensifies. Oxygen consumption becomes dependent on oxygen delivery, and anaerobic glycolysis results in lactate production and hydrogen ion release.

This multilevel cellular dysfunction places the animal in the *early decompensatory (middle) stage* of hypovolemic shock. Clinical signs of this stage in the dog include tachycardia, pale mucous membrane color, prolonged capillary refill time, decreased jugular vein distension, hypotension, and oliguria (see Table 2.1).

Cats with hypovolemic shock will present with a subnormal temperature, decreased heart rate, and low arterial blood pressure. In the cat, the neuroendocrine response to hypovolemia appears to promote vasodilation, hypothermia, and bradycardia. Rather than an inhibition of the parasympathetic tone, the cat experiences a response similar to a vasovagal reflex that blunts the typical tachycardic response. Centrally mediated hypothermia is a shock response in the cat that leads to a poor response of adrenergic receptors to the increased catecholamine release, augmenting vasodilation and bradycardia.

Vasoactive substances produced due to local tissue hypoxia at the capillary level cause local vasodilation and increased capillary permeability, resulting in maldistribution of blood flow in the hypoxic tissue beds. When chemical mediators (cytokines) produced locally in hypoxic tissues enter the systemic circulation, they incite a systemic inflammatory response syndrome (SIRS). Significant vasodilation and damage at the endothelial lining resulting in increased capillary permeability further deplete intravascular volume. Redistribution of blood flow away from the heart and the brain occurs, leading to further hypoxic consequences and the stage of *late decompensatory shock*. This effect is compounded when

central pathology blunts the typical compensatory response, intravascular volume loss is massive, earlier compensatory responses are ineffective or inadequately treated, or the insult is severe and overwhelming. The mitochondria are unable to produce enough ATP, and the ensuing circulatory collapse and insufficient arterial flow to the brain and heart cause these and other organs to malfunction, and eventually fail.

Clinical signs of this terminal stage include a relative bradycardia, hypotension, substantially delayed (>3 sec) or no capillary refill time, white or cyanotic MM color, hypothermia, altered mentation, and anuria (see Table 2.1). A positive outcome is optimized with early recognition of the clinical signs, hemostasis when applicable, as well as adequate and timely fluid resuscitation that incorporates specifically selected resuscitation goals for the patient.

Intravascular fluid deficit resuscitation plan

Relative to fluid balance, three presumptions exist: volume overload is bad, inadequate volume is bad, and what we conclude about the fluid balance of the patient may be incorrect. It is important to realize that the presence of fluid responsiveness is not an absolute indication that fluids are necessary. The decision to administer fluid therapy must be supported not just by a proof of volume responsiveness, but also by a need for hemodynamic improvement. Fluid infusion *per se* is not always the correct therapy for hemodynamic instability. Cardiac performance should also be evaluated in animals with a compatible history, physical examination or disease process that suggests abnormal cardiac function (see Chapter 11) prior to infusing large quantities of fluid for resuscitation. Thoughtful consideration must be given to the amount and rate of fluids to be administered in terms of individual patient needs, the underlying problems, and the degree of risk associated with fluid administration when outlining a fluid therapy plan. The fluid therapy plan involves resuscitation, rehydration, and maintenance phases.

Oxygen supplementation (see Chapter 8) and analgesic administration are part of the resuscitation process. It is best to titrate analgesics and sedatives to effect, as responses are variable and can be affected by underlying renal and hepatic dysfunction (see Chapter 19). For all types of pain, methadone (0.2–0.4 mg/kg IV q 2–6 hours), hydromorphone or oxymorphone (0.1–0.2 mg/kg IV), or fentanyl (0.3–0.5 µg/kg) can be titrated to desired analgesic effects with or without a sedative (such as diazepam or midazolam, 0.2 mg/kg IV).

Fluid choices

The choice of fluid(s) to administer will be based on the properties of the specific fluid, the needs of the patient, and any potential side-effects that might negate the selection of that fluid. Crystalloid fluids are typically chosen as the foundation of fluid therapy, supporting both intravascular and interstitial volumes. The addition of synthetic colloids or blood products is often warranted when there are significant intravascular volume deficits, with the goal of extending the duration of intravascular volume expansion. Blood products can provide additional support through the administration of RBCs, albumin, and coagulation factors.

Crystalloids

A crystalloid fluid is a water-based solution with small molecules that are osmotically active in the body fluids and freely permeable to the capillary membrane. The amount that remains in the vessel depends on Starling's forces and the distribution of TBW (see Figure 2.1). The sodium concentration provides the greatest contribution to the osmolarity of the crystalloid solution. Convention has defined an *isotonic* fluid as one that has an osmolarity equal to that of erythrocytes and therefore does not affect the exchange of fluid across the erythrocyte membrane. A *hypertonic* fluid will decrease erythrocyte volume, and a *hypotonic* fluid will increase erythrocyte volume. Crystalloid solutions commonly administered to the dog and cat are listed in Table 2.3 with the sodium, potassium and calcium content, osmolarity, pH, and common indications for selection.

A hypotonic fluid has an osmolarity less than intracellular fluid, such as 5% dextrose in water (D_5W) or half-strength saline (0.45% saline). To prevent red cell lysis from the infusion of hypotonic fluid into the intravascular space, dextrose is added to provide enough osmotic pressure to prevent movement into the blood cells. As the dextrose is metabolized, however, the water travels into the interstitial then the intracellular compartments based on normal TBW distribution. Other solutions with solutes that are metabolized (such as partial parenteral nutrition fluids) can also be used to provide water.

Hypotonic fluids are not used during the resuscitation or rehydration phase but can be used to reestablish solute-free water deficits in treating the patient with hypernatremia, after resuscitation and rehydration have occurred. When serum sodium values are greater than 170 mEq/L in the presence of altered mentation, replacement of free water is indicated (see Chapter 6 for guidelines). The solute-free water deficit is calculated and replaced over 24–48 hours. The rate of sodium decline should be no more than 0.5–1 mEq/h to avoid rapid neuronal osmotic shifts and cell swelling. The volume of fluids is administered in addition to maintenance requirements.

Hypertonic fluids such as 7% and 23% saline have more osmotically active particles per unit volume than intracellular fluid. The dose recommended for rapid intravascular volume resuscitation is 4–6 mL/kg of a 7% saline solution. After administration, water moves through osmosis from the interstitial and intracellular compartments into the intravascular space. There is a rapid increase in intravascular volume until Starling's forces bring the equilibrium back across the capillary membrane. This may be mitigated when hypertonic saline is combined with hydroxyethyl starch (one part

Table 2.3 Common crystalloid solutions used in the critically ill dog and cat.

Crystalloid	Tonicity Osmolarity (mOsm/L)	Na+ (mEq/L)	K+ (mEq/L)	Ca++ (mg/dL) (mmol/L)	pH Buffer	Common indications for selection
Ringer's lactate	Isotonic 273	130	4	2.7 (0.675)	6.7 lactate	Extracellular volume replacement of hyponatremic patient
Plasmalyte-A®	Isotonic 294	140	5	0	7.4 acetate, gluconate	Extracellular volume replacement
Normosol-R®	Isotonic 295	140	5	0	7.4 acetate, gluconate	Extracellular volume replacement
Normal saline (0.9%)	Isotonic 308	154	0	0	5.7 no buffer	Metabolic alkalosis, severe hypochloremia, hypercalcemia
7% hypertonic saline	Hypertonic 2395	1198	0	0	5.0 no buffer	Rapid IV volume resuscitation
0.45% saline with or without 2.5% dextrose	Isotonic then hypotonic (hypotonic without dextrose) 280	77	0	0	4.5 no buffer	Replace solute-free water deficit
Dextrose (5%) in water	Hypotonic 253	0	0	0	5.0 no buffer	Replace solute-free water deficit, drug carrier

Na+, sodium; K+, potassium; Ca++, ionized calcium.

23% hypertonic saline with three parts hydroxyethyl starch, 4–6 mL/kg). Adequate interstitial and intracellular fluid must be available for intravascular volume expansion to occur after the intravenous administration of a hypertonic solution.

Hypertonic saline has been reported to produce a mild inotropic effect [97,98] with mild systemic and pulmonary vasodilation [99], improve immune function [100–102], and rapidly expand intravascular volume [103]. Hypertonic saline can also be administered to reduce intracranial pressure in brain-injured patients [104]. In dogs with a hemoperitoneum, 7% hypertonic saline (HTS) combined with 6% hydroxyethyl starch (up to 8 mL/kg and 10 mL/kg, respectively) significantly reduced time to endpoint resuscitation parameters compared with lactated Ringer's solution (LRS) (up to 90 mL/kg). Centrally mediated hypotension and peripherally mediated bradycardia and vasodilation are possible with infusion rates greater than 1 mL/kg/minute [105]. Extreme caution is used if administering to patients that are severely dehydrated, hyperosmolar, or have little tolerance for rapid intravascular hydrostatic pressure increases (such as those with active hemorrhage or cardiac dysfunction).

Isotonic replacement crystalloids (IRC) contain a sodium concentration similar to that of the normal extracellular fluid compartment, making them the ideal crystalloid for the resuscitation and rehydration phase of the fluid therapy plan. Plasmalyte-A®, Normosol-R®, and lactated Ringer's solution contain buffers and are the preferred choice for restoring intravascular volume in most hypovolemic patients (see Table 2.4). The buffer lactate is converted to bicarbonate by the liver and kidney, and is not likely to cause a clinically sustained change in blood lactate [106]. In patients with severe liver dysfunction or neoplasia, prolonged elevations in lactate may occur after lactated Ringer's administration, but the clinical significance of this is unknown [107–109]. Acetate and gluconate buffers are metabolized to bicarbonate by the liver as well as muscle tissue. Theoretically, the calcium in lactated Ringer's solution may precipitate the citrate anticoagulant when administered through the same line as blood products, but this has not been shown to be relevant when blood products have been prepared according to blood banking standards [110]. Supplemental electrolytes can be added to isotonic fluids according to patient requirements. As a safeguard in preventing acute hyperkalemia, the rate of potassium administration added to resuscitation fluids should not exceed 0.5 mEq/kg/hour unless carefully monitored.

Normal saline (0.9% sodium chloride) solution is an IRC with a high chloride concentration (154 mmol/L) and low pH (5.0) compared to plasma, and it does not contain additional electrolytes or buffer. This acidifying solution is best used for treating hypochloremic metabolic alkalosis or as a carrier fluid.

Under normal conditions, approximately 80% of the crystalloids administered intravenously will filter into the interstitium within an hour, according to normal extracellular TBW distribution. However, IRC can be an effective means of restoring perfusion parameters when the cause of hypovolemia can be rapidly corrected, and the interstitial compartment is capable of handling this additional fluid load. The detrimental effects of rapid, large-volume crystalloid administration increase when moderate-to-severe anemia is present, when increased capillary permeability exists or when the lymphatics cannot manage and the affected organs cannot tolerate additional fluid load (lung, brain, heart). The addition of colloid fluids during resuscitation from hypovolemic shock in these situations becomes important.

Colloids

Colloid fluids are isotonic fluids containing a significant concentration of molecules larger in size than the capillary pore that contribute to COP. Whole blood, plasma, and concentrated albumin have natural colloids in the form of proteins. Hydroxyethyl starches (HES; hetastarch, tetrastarch) are synthetically derived colloids. Table 4.6 and Table 4.7 in Chapter 4 list the natural and synthetic colloids respectively, which are commonly used in the critical small animal ICU patient; dose recommendations are also listed.

Blood products

Blood products are administered when albumin, antithrombin, coagulation factors, platelets, or red blood cells are required. Prior to administering red blood cells, it is ideal to determine the blood type of the patient and to perform a cross-match in order to administer compatible blood and limit transfusion reactions. In the dog, a DEA 1.1-negative transfusion is ideal to administer if blood typing or cross-match is not possible. Since the infusion of incompatible blood products can result in life-threatening reactions (especially in the cat), determining the blood type and performing a cross-match are strongly recommended. Unfortunately, catastrophic situations can arise requiring an immediate infusion of blood to save the life of the patient. The use of DEA 1.1-negative donor blood in the dog, type-specific blood in the cat (see Chapter 10) or an autologous blood transfusion can minimize the incidence of serious transfusion reactions.

Plasma transfusion administration does not require patient blood typing or a cross-match. An in-line 18-micron micropore filter is used during administration of plasma and a 170–210 micron blood administration set for products containing red cells. See Chapters 9 and 10 for additional information on blood products.

Human and canine albumin products can be administered to supplement albumin and to maintain COP in the intravascular space. Plasma transfusions have an albumin concentration equal to normal plasma and may not be an effective colloid when used alone. Large volumes may be needed to affect the albumin concentration, which can be cost prohibitive. A 5 g lyophilized canine albumin product (Animal Blood Resources International, Dixon, CA), has been used at a 5% concentration in the treatment of hypotension and hypoalbuminemia in dogs [111]. It is stored in a dehydrated powder form and reconstituted with isotonic saline to a desired concentration. The high concentration of albumin and COP (200 mmHg) in 25% human albumin has the greatest capability of increasing plasma COP and albumin [112–115] but severe and deadly hypersensitivity reactions have been reported in dogs. Additional information regarding the administration of albumin can be found in Chapter 4.

Synthetic colloids

Synthetic colloid fluids contain large molecular weight particles that effectively increase COP beyond what can be obtained with blood product infusion alone. They maintain intravascular COP because their average molecular size is too large to pass through the normal capillary pores. A list of synthetic colloids and their characteristics is provided in Table 4.7 (Chapter 4).

Synthetic colloids are administered with IRC to restore intravascular volume. Synthetic colloids do not provide albumin, hemoglobin, antithrombin, platelets, or coagulation proteins, but can be administered simultaneously with blood products. They are not used for interstitial volume replacement. Elimination of smaller molecular weight particles is through glomerular filtration. Larger particles are eliminated in bile, stored in tissue, or broken down into smaller particles by the monocyte-macrophage system and tissue or blood enzymes such as amylase.

Hydroxyethyl starch is the parent name of a synthetic polymer of glucose (98% amylopectin), made from a waxy species of either plant starch maize or sorghum. It is a highly branched polysaccharide closely resembling glycogen, formed by the reaction between ethylene oxide and amylopectin in the presence of an alkaline catalyst. The molecular weight and molar substitution can be adjusted by the degree of substitution of hydroxyl groups with hydroxyethyl groups at the C2, C3, and C6 positions on the glucose molecule. The greater the substitution on position C2 in relation to C6 (C2:C6 ratio), the slower the degradation of the molecule by amylase [116].

The number-averaged molecular weight (M_n) is the arithmetic mean of the molecular weights of the polymers in solution. Weight-averaged molecular weight (M_w) is the sum of the number of molecules at each number-averaged molecular weight divided by the total of all molecules. This weight is generally larger when larger polymers are present in solution.

There are two types of HES products clinically available in the US at this time: hetastarch and tetrastarch. Hetastarch can be purchased in 0.9% sodium chloride (Hespan™, B Braun Medical, Inc., Bethlehem, PA; M_w of 600 kD and 0.7 degree of substitution) or in LRS (Hextend™, BioTime, Inc., Alameda, CA; a M_w of 670 kD and 0.75 degree of substitution). The electrolyte and buffer compositions of Hextend may reduce the incidence of hyperchloremic acidosis. Hextend also contains 0.45 mmol/L magnesium and 99 mg/dL (0.99%) dextrose. VetStarch™ (Abbott Laboratories, North Chicago, IL) has a M_w of 130 kD and a 0.4 degree of substitution and Tetraspan™ 6% (Braun Medical, Inc.) has a M_w of 130 kD and a 0.42 degree of substitution. Hydroxyethyl starch (HES) 130/0.4 doses have been recommended up to 50 mL/kg in people.

Hydroxyethyl starch can affect von Willebrand's factor, factor VIII function, and platelet function. However, the coagulation effect of HES is no greater than that of saline, and less than that of HTS solutions at equivolume as well as clinically relevant dilutions [117].

While HES administration can provide important and lasting benefits, potential limitations must be recognized. Hydroxyethyl starches will increase coagulation times, particularly when high doses are administered. Literature has reported evidence for an increased risk for acute kidney injury in critically ill people and people with severe sepsis when treated with HES [116,118–120]. This complication has not been identified in dogs or cats receiving 6% hetastarch or 6% tetrastarch. A retrospective study of dogs receiving 10% HES 250/0.5 (pentastarch) has reported an association between the use of 10% pentastarch and adverse outcome [121]. This may be related to the type and concentration of the HES administered. A study of ovine endotoxemic shock found that saline-based 10% HES 200/0.5 was linked to impaired renal function and more pronounced tubular epithelial injury when compared with 6% HES 130/0.4 and balanced crystalloids [122]. Further research is required to document the incidence and severity of any detrimental responses to 6% hetastarch or tetrastarch in dogs and cats.

Four-step intravascular fluid resuscitation plan

The fluid resuscitation plan should include the following steps: (1) determine whether there is an intravascular volume deficit affecting perfusion, (2) select fluid(s) specific for the patient, (3) determine resuscitation endpoints, and (4) determine the resuscitation technique to be employed (Box 2.3). Careful patient assessment is

---

Box 2.3 The four-step plan for intravascular fluid resuscitation for the dog and cat.

Step 1: Determine whether there is an intravascular fluid deficit affecting perfusion by assessing the physical perfusion parameters (heart rate, pulse intensity, CRT, MM color, body temperature) and arterial blood pressure.

Step 2: Select the appropriate fluid or fluids to replace the intravascular deficit.
Crystalloids are used to replace intravascular and interstitial deficits.
Colloids are used to replace intravascular deficits.
Crystalloid-colloid combination is ideal to simultaneously replace perfusion and hydration deficits.

Step 3: Select the most appropriate resuscitation endpoints.
High normal – SIRS-related diseases, metabolic disease, surgical problems.
Low normal – heart, lung or brain disease, coagulopathy, hemorrhage, oliguric renal failure.

Step 4: Choose fluid infusion technique.
Large volume – dogs with SIRS, metabolic or surgical problems.
Small volume – all cats, dogs requiring low normal targeted endpoints.
The patient should be reassessed after every fluid prescription to determine response to therapy and if further therapy is required.

CRT, capillary refill time; MM, mucous membranes; SIRS, systemic inflammatory response syndrome.

---

essential to detect clues to the underlying cause of the poor perfusion and to identify any important consequences of the inciting disorder. This information will guide the entire resuscitation plan, influencing fluid choice, resuscitation endpoint selection, and, most importantly, the fluid infusion technique.

Step 1

The first step is to identify whether or not there is a problem with perfusion caused by intravascular volume loss. This is quickly assessed by evaluating the physical perfusion parameters, arterial blood pressure, and other monitored indices.

Step 2

The second step of intravascular fluid resuscitation involves fluid selection. Crystalloid fluids with or without colloids are used for rapid intravascular resuscitation. The choice of fluid(s) to infuse will depend on the mode of delivery, which compartment has a deficit, duration of action desired, and the initiating mechanism(s) of circulatory shock. Intravenous or intraosseous fluid administration is recommended when treating hypovolemic shock. Placement of a short, large-diameter catheter in a peripheral vein during the initial stages of resuscitation optimizes laminar flow and infusion rates. Fluids must be administered that will expand and remain in the body fluid compartment where the volume deficit lies.

The changes in blood volume in response to crystalloid infusion compared to HES administration in dogs have been measured [123]. While saline infusion causes the largest immediate increase in blood volume, the change is transient. HES infusion results in an increase in volume that is more sustained. Tetrastarch infusion is also more effective than saline at increasing blood pressure in dogs with septic shock [124]. A combination of both crystalloid and colloid infusion can provide a sustained increase in intravascular volume with the colloid while simultaneously providing fluid support for the intravascular and interstitial spaces through the crystalloid. The selection of the specific crystalloid and colloid to infuse should be based on the immediate needs of the patient and the characteristics of the fluid as described above.

Step 3

The goals of resuscitation should be decided and appropriate resuscitation endpoints (high normal or low normal) assigned (Table 2.4). There are no effective "standard" formulas for crystalloid or colloid infusion that will guarantee complete volume resuscitation without complications in a small animal patient. Variables such as renal function, increased capillary permeability, brain injury, lung injury, heart disease or failure, or closed cavity hemorrhage will require that fluid resuscitation rate and volumes be individualized for the patient. Sufficient fluid quantities should be administered to reach desired endpoints of resuscitation. The endpoints typically reflect the perfusion status of the animal and include heart rate, MM color, CRT, pulse intensity, blood pressure, CVP, and ScvO$_2$.

Shock will rapidly result in cell starvation and a negative energy balance leading to cellular and organ dysfunction. However, restoring the circulation to "normal," with normal oxygenation and normal perfusion parameters, does not guarantee that there will be sufficient ATP production for repair and maintenance of the cells. When a patient is suspected of having a SIRS-related disease process, high normal endpoint resuscitation parameters are chosen. The goal is to maximally deliver oxygen and glucose to the cells to support sufficient energy production for both repair and maintenance of the cells.

There are clinical situations, however, when obtaining high normal endpoint resuscitation parameters can be detrimental to the animal. Increased vascular hydrostatic pressure can dislodge a life-saving clot in a traumatized patient or in an animal with a coagulopathy, resulting in significant hemorrhage. Brain and lung edema or hemorrhage can be worsened by aggressive and sudden increases in vascular hydrostatic pressure. Low normal endpoint resuscitation parameters are at the lower limits of normal. The goal is to administer the smallest volume of fluids possible to successfully resuscitate the intravascular compartment while minimizing extravasation of fluids into the interstitium (especially the brain or lungs). Small-volume resuscitation techniques should be used to reach low normal resuscitation endpoints.

Step 4

An algorithm to guide the selection of specific resuscitation techniques for the dog is shown in Figure 2.5 and for the cat in Figure 2.6. The goal of resuscitation is to reach the targeted endpoints within 15–30 minutes from the initiation of resuscitation. With sepsis and SIRS-related disorders, the use of synthetic colloids during volume resuscitation and fluid maintenance can reduce the overall volume required to meet targeted resuscitation endpoints and maintain intravascular volume until increased capillary permeability has resolved. Larger volumes are usually needed for SIRS patients compared to hypovolemic conditions not associated with SIRS.

Dogs in hypovolemic shock that are targeted for high normal endpoint resuscitation values will benefit from large-volume infusion techniques. Resuscitation from catastrophic hemorrhagic shock may require rapid infusion of large quantities of whole blood, with infusion rates compensating for losses through ongoing hemorrhage. Typically, blood products are administered at 5–15 mL/kg/hour (see Table 10.8, Chapter 10). Care must be taken to stop active hemorrhage. Autologous blood transfusion may be life-saving in these situations (see Chapter 10).

Small-volume resuscitation techniques are chosen for all cats and for dogs with clinical evidence of cardiac dysfunction, brain disease, pulmonary dysfunction, oliguric kidney failure, coagulopathy or hemorrhage. The immediate goal is to administer only the volume of fluids necessary to successfully resuscitate the intravascular compartment. This technique is employed to minimize extravasation of fluids into the interstitium, titrate the amount of preload stretching in a potentially disabled heart, and reduce the probability of disturbing a preexisting clot or clot formation.

Cats with circulatory shock typically present with a triad of problems (hypothermia, bradycardia, hypotension) that increase their sensitivity to rapid fluid infusion. Hypothermia (temperature <98 °F, <36.7 °C) will blunt the normal vasoconstriction that occurs in response to catecholamines. The initial fluid infusions are titrated (as above) until the femoral pulses are readily palpable and an indirect systolic blood pressure reading is ≥50 mmHg. At this time, active external warming with water circulating blankets or forced air heating blankets should begin to raise the body temperature to 98 °F (36.7 °C) or higher (see Figure 2.6). The warming phase of feline resuscitation is important to reduce the incidence of pulmonary edema and pleural effusion from overzealous fluid infusion. However, since the application of surface heat can cause local vasodilation, warming should not occur until the initial fluid infusion has provided some vascular support. Commonly, hypotension present at the beginning of the rewarming period will resolve with little or no additional fluids once the body temperature of the cat is ≥98 °F (36.7 °C). However, should the cat still have hypotension after rewarming, additional colloid or crystalloid can be titrated as needed to reach the targeted endpoints. Warming techniques are continued to maintain the body temperature ≥98 °F (36.7 °C). Small-volume fluid infusion techniques are used in the cat to reach both high normal and low normal endpoint resuscitation targets (see Figure 2.6).

Table 2.4 Resuscitation endpoints targeted with fluid resuscitation in the dog and cat.

Parameter	High normal	Low normal
Level of consciousness	Alert, responsive	Alert, responsive
Heart rate (bpm)		
Dog	80–140	80–140
Cat	>160	>160
Mucous membrane color	Pink	Pale pink
Capillary refill time (seconds)	1–2	≤2
Peripheral pulse intensity	Strong	Palpable central and peripheral pulses
Rectal temperature	99–101 °F	≥98 °F
	37.2–38.3 °C	36.6 °C
Indirect blood pressure (mmHg)		
Systolic	90–120	≥90
Mean	80–100	60–80
Central venous pressure (cmH$_2$O)	8–10	3–6
Urine output (mL/kg/h)	1–2	1.0
Lactate (mmol/L)	≤2.0	Declining trend to ≤2.0
ScvO$_2$ %	>70	>70

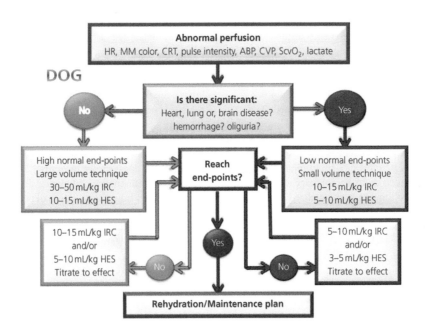

Figure 2.5 An algorithm to guide the fluid resuscitation of dogs in hypovolemic shock. ABP, arterial blood pressure; BP, blood pressure; CRT, capillary refill time; CVP, central venous pressure; HES, hydroxyethyl starch; IRC, isotonic replacement crystalloids; MM, mucous membrane; ScvO$_2$, central venous oxygen saturation.

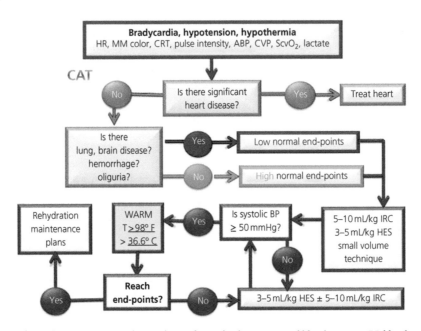

Figure 2.6 An algorithm to guide the fluid resuscitation of cats in hypovolemic shock. ABP, arterial blood pressure; BP, blood pressure; CRT, capillary refill time; CVP, central venous pressure; HES, hydroxyethyl starch; IRC, isotonic replacement crystalloids; MM, mucous membrane; ScvO$_2$, central venous oxygen saturation.

Nonresponsive shock

Once the fluid resuscitation plan has been initiated, continuous monitoring of the patient is critical. This requires a "stand by the cage" approach to patient care at this time. Failure to reach reasonable resuscitation endpoints after multiple titrations of fluids (up to 60–90 mL/kg/hour of IRC and 20–30 mL/kg HES) requires investigation for causes of nonresponsive shock (Figure 2.7).

The most common cause of persistent hypotension and/or tachycardia is inadequate quantity of fluids administered. A fluid challenge can be given when there is a sudden drop in a previously stable blood pressure or the hemodynamic parameters have not been stabilized as a result of the previous fluid infusions. The fluid

challenge typically consists of a 10–15 mL/kg infusion of crystalloids and 5 mL/kg infusion of colloid. If the perfusion parameters improve with this challenge, then insufficient fluid volume may be playing a role in the nonresponsive shock.

When the fluid challenge fails to improve or cannot sustain the hemodynamic parameters, an evaluation is made for POC laboratory database changes. A rapid decline in the PCV (<25%) in the acutely hemorrhaging patient or a PCV <18% in any critically ill dog or cat warrants the administration of packed red blood cells or whole-blood transfusion. Hypoglycemia and electrolyte imbalances are corrected. If further evaluation identifies abnormalities in the respiratory rate or there is evidence of elevated intracranial pressure,

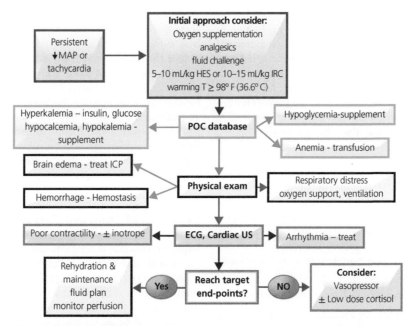

Figure 2.7 Decision-making algorithm to guide the management of persistent hypotension in the small animal ICU patient. When a critically ill patient has persistent signs of hypotension ± tachycardia without having a positive response to fluid infusion, then an assessment is made for causes of nonresponsive shock. A POC database is immediately evaluated and, if present, treatment of hypoglycemia, anemia, and electrolyte disorders is initiated. If examination reveals evidence of increased ICP, treatment is initiated; if respiratory distress exists, oxygen supplementation and/or assisted ventilation is initiated; and if active hemorrhage is occurring, hemostasis is performed and coagulopathy corrected. Following this, if persistent hypotension and/or tachycardia exist, then ECG and cardiac US are evaluated for signs of primary heart disease and antiarrhythmic and/or inotrope treatment administered. If target endpoint parameters are still not reached, then vasopressor and/or low-dose cortisol therapy is initiated. ECG, electrocardiogram; HES, hydroxyethyl starch; ICP, intracranial pressure; IRC, isotonic replacement crystalloids; MAP, mean arterial pressure; POC, point of care; T, rectal temperature; US, ultrasound.

specific interventions are performed to improve oxygenation and ventilation, and reduce intracranial pressure, respectively. The heart is evaluated for arrhythmias and/or hypocontractility. Decreased myocardial contractility can be supported with dobutamine (2.5–10 μg/kg/minute IV as a constant rate infusion (CRI), titrate to effect). If cardiac function is assessed as adequate and hypotension persists, vasopressors such as norepinephrine (1–20 μg/kg/minute IV as CRI) are administered to support the blood pressure. Other inotropic and vasoactive agents are listed with doses in Table 3.4, Chapter 3. If vasopressor therapy does not correct hypotension, then low-dose cortisol therapy is considered (hydrocortisone: 0.5–1 mg/kg IV q 6 hours or 0.08 mg/kg/hour continuous infusion or dexamethasone 0.08 mg/kg IV q 24 hours). The use of vasoactive agents is continued until the blood pressure has been stabilized for at least four hours.

Interstitial volume deficits

Excessive vomiting or diarrhea, polyuria, reduced water intake in relation to output, significant hemorrhage, or loss of water into third body fluid spaces with SIRS-related disorders will result in extracellular isotonic fluid losses. Intravascular and interstitial water content equilibrate easily so that a change in one compartment will affect the other. Acute and rapid intravascular fluid loss can cause hypovolemia without initially causing clinically detectable changes in the interstitial fluid compartment. With time, however, fluid shifting will occur and the interstitial fluid will equilibrate across the intravascular membrane, resulting in signs of dehydration.

As interstitial fluid volume becomes depleted, clinical signs of dehydration develop. The clinician must estimate the degree of dehydration as a percentage of body weight in kilograms based on these patient physical parameters (see Table 2.2). As a general guideline, the minimum degree of interstitial dehydration that can be detected in the average patient is approximately 5% of body weight [125].

As changes to the fluid volume of the interstitial space equilibrate with the intravascular space, all patients with evidence of interstitial dehydration will also have a degree of plasma volume depletion, although interstitial dehydration has to be severe (>10% to 12%) before clinically detectable changes in perfusion are likely to occur [126]. Interstitial dehydration greater than 12% is likely to be fatal. Given that there is substantial clinical variation in the correlation between clinical signs and degree of dehydration, one can only make an estimation of the clinical hydration status.

Excessive intravascular fluid administration or fluid retention due to oliguria will result in increased intravascular hydrostatic pressure, jugular venous distension, and increased CVP. As fluid volumes equilibrate between the interstitial and intravascular compartments, the PCV/TP become decreased and interstitial overhydration ensues. Box 2.1 lists the common clinical signs of overhydration. Pregnancy, increased salt intake, exercise, and malnutrition as well as acute and chronic conditions will affect TBW and the division of water between the fluid compartments [127]. Factors unrelated to hydration status that can alter the physical parameters used to estimate interstitial hydration include atropine administration (which reduces MM moisture), hypersalivation from nausea or pain, advanced age (which reduces skin elasticity), and changes in body fat content. Emaciated animals may appear to have decreased skin turgor even when normally hydrated, and dehydration may be more challenging to appreciate in obese animals. The skin in young animals is very elastic, making changes in skin turgor harder to detect, and therefore it is difficult to accurately assess hydration with this parameter alone.

Changes in body weight may not reliably correspond to clinical parameters of hydration in the small animal ICU population [128].

For example, the critical patient with pleural effusion and pleuritis associated with pyothorax can have a simultaneous collection of fluid in third space fluid compartments and a reduction in interstitial and intravascular water. Although the body weight may not have changed, individual fluid compartment water has changed, with fluid accumulation in the pleural space. Therefore, body weight changes should not be used alone in determining a patient's level of hydration. Frequent reassessment and reevaluation are required to monitor response to treatment and adjust therapy accordingly.

Rehydration

Once perfusion has been restored, interstitial hydration parameters are reassessed (see Table 2.2). Most of the IRC administered during resuscitation will move into the interstitial space and change the hydration status from the initial estimation. Most IRCs are appropriate for rehydration of the interstitial compartment since they have a comparable sodium concentration. The volume of crystalloid to administer to replace hydration deficits is calculated based on the newest estimation of percentage of dehydration.

$$BW\,(kg) \times \%\,dehydration = volume\,interstitial\,fluid\,deficit\,(L)$$

The rehydration rate is added to the hourly maintenance rate (see below) to determine the total fluid volume required.

If the fluid has been acutely lost, the rate of replacement is over 2–4 hours. If the fluid has been chronically lost or there is a significant risk of interstitial fluid overload, the calculated volume is administered over 6–12 hours. Frequent reassessment of clinical hydration status, continuing losses, and metabolic demands is necessary to meet the ongoing needs during this hydration phase.

Maintenance fluids

Normal metabolism uses water in excess of sodium. Sensible water losses are those that can be measured, for example, in urine and feces. Insensible water losses cannot be measured, for example through respiration or sweat. The water used for daily metabolic functions is estimated to be:

$$30 \times body\,weight\,(kg) + 70 = mL\,maintenance\,fluids\,/\,24\,hours$$

For patients weighing <2 or >70 kg, it may be more accurate to use the following equation:

$$70 \times body\,weight\,(kg)^{0.75}$$

Ongoing fluid losses are estimated and added to the daily maintenance fluid requirements. Conditions such as fever, polyuria, vomiting, diarrhea, tissue inflammation, and third body fluid spacing require higher than anticipated fluid volumes to replace loss and maintain metabolism.

The ideal fluid to use for daily maintenance fluid infusion is one that contains lower concentrations of sodium and chloride and higher concentrations of potassium (such as Normosol-M and 5% Dextrose®, Hospira, Lake Forest, IL), containing 40 mEq/L sodium chloride, 13 mEq/L KCl with 5.0% dextrose) compared to IRC. However, since most critically ill patients are receiving IRCs to replace their ongoing losses, it is convenient and less expensive to use the IRC also for the daily maintenance fluid requirements. Daily monitoring of serum sodium will identify significant changes in sodium and any need to alter the concentration of sodium infusion. When a SIRS process is occurring, HES should be continued at 20–30 mL/kg/day to maintain the intravascular COP, with an equivolume reduction made in the daily isotonic crystalloids given. The HES infusion is stopped when blood products are being infused and restarted upon completion of the transfusion to reduce the risk of volume overload.

Maintenance and replacement fluid requirements for the critically ill small animal patient should be estimated, monitored and recalculated at least twice per day. The total volume of fluid infused must include the fluid volume of any drugs administered by CRI, large-volume IV drugs, oral intake and parenteral or enteral nutritional support. Measuring the exact volume of ongoing losses is impossible, but they can be estimated by the quantification of urine output, vomitus, diarrhea, drainage fluids, and nasogatric tube suction. If the patient is tolerant of enteral fluids, administration of fluids orally or by enteral feeding tube can reduce the risk of fluid overload. Placement of a nasogastric or nasoesophageal tube can facilitate enteral fluid administration and permit a continuous rate of infusion, if desired.

Methods of fluid administration

Rapid intravascular volume infusion necessitates peripheral venous access with one or more large-bore shorter catheter(s). Highly experienced veterinarians and technical staff may be able to place a central venous catheter if peripheral venous catheterization is impossible, but this is usually too time-consuming and too stressful for the patient during the initial resuscitation phase. A vascular cutdown technique can be used for rapid venous access if hypotension is severe enough to prevent normal catheterization (see Box 2.2).

Intraosseous needle or catheter placement in the femur, tibia or humerus can be an alternative to intravenous catheterization. It can be rapidly performed with practice, and/or the use of an intraosseous drill. The intraosseous space communicates directly with the venous system. Intraosseous fluid administration is associated with low complication rates and allows for IV fluid expansion and subsequent IV catheter placement [129,130].

Once a critical patient has been stabilized, the benefits of placing a single-lumen or multilumen central venous catheter are considered. These catheters permit blood collection in addition to infusion of multiple fluids simultaneously through the multilumen catheter. The modified Seldinger technique is used to place multilumen catheters (Box 2.4).

There is not an "expiry date" for catheters following placement, and due to the limited number of sites available for venous access, the catheter should not be removed or changed unless there is a known or suspected complication. Guidelines for catheter placement and catheter care can be found in Chapter 20.

Once vascular access has been accomplished, the fluids must be infused at a specific rate and volume. The use of a fluid administration pump or Buretrol® solution set (Baxter Healthcare, Deerfield, IL) can safeguard against erroneous infusion of too much or too little fluid. The techniques used to mark the fluid bags and lines, set up the fluid pumps or Buretrol and add supplements to the fluids are outlined in Chapter 20.

Potential complications of fluid administration

The administration of intravenous fluids is not without the potential for serious consequences. Complications of fluid administration should be anticipated and are discussed through this chapter. Frequently encountered complications along with guidelines for prevention and intervention are summarized in Table 2.5. Frequent comparison of fluid intake volume (intravenous, enteral) with the volume of fluid lost (urine, vomitus, stool, NG tube aspiration, drain production), and frequent monitoring of acute changes in body weight will detect early discrepancies that can be associated with alterations in fluid balance.

Box 2.4 Steps for placing a catheter using the modified Seldinger technique in the jugular vein of the dog and cat.

1. Provide mild-to-moderate sedation and identify the jugular vein.
2. Monitor with ECG, +/- BP, SpO2, ETCO2 (if intubated).
3. Clip and aseptically prepare the insertion site.
4. Secure a sterile field with sterile drapes, use sterile instruments and technique at all times.
5. Occlude the jugular vein and insert an over-the-needle IV catheter in the direction of the heart. Advance catheter after flashback and remove stylet.
6. Advance the guidewire through the catheter toward the heart at least one catheter length past the catheter within the vessel.
7. Pull out the catheter over the guidewire, ensuring that the guidewire remains in place. All portions of the guidewire must remain sterile. Use digital pressure to avoid excessive hemorrhage.
8. Slide the dilator over the guidewire and into the subcutaneous space. A scalpel blade can be used to release the skin to get the dilator into the subcutaneous space.
9. Remove the dilator while keeping the guidewire in place.
10. Remove the injection cap on the most distal port to allow the guidewire to pass out. Thread the multilumen catheter over the guidewire until the guidewire has passed out of the catheter injection port.
11. Grasp the guidewire and feed the catheter over the wire through the skin and into the vessel.
12. Advance the catheter to a predetermined location.
13. Pull out the guidewire.
14. Aspirate the air from the catheter ports and then flush with heparinized saline. Replace injection cap.
15. Secure the catheter by suturing the suture clip of the catheter to the skin. Apply a light sterile bandage.
16. Radiograph to confirm the location of the catheter tip.
17. Inspect catheter insertion site daily for evidence of inflammation or infection.

Table 2.5 Potential complications associated with choice of intravenous fluid(s) and rate and volume of intravenous fluid administration.

Source	Complication	Intervention
Fluid overload	Tachypnea Labored breathing Pleural effusion Nasal discharge Hypotension Hypertension Heart murmur Cardiac arrhythmia Change in mentation Change in level of consciousness Peripheral edema (pitting) Ascites Hypothermia	Careful fluid selection using colloids to support intravascular retention of fluids Reassess total fluid infused vs output Employ careful monitoring procedures Physical perfusion parameters PCV/TP Changes in body weight, urine output Blood pressure, CVP, ECG, SpO_2 Assess cardiac function Reduce fluid input Careful diuretic administration $\pm$ Thoracentesis or abdominocentesis Compression wrap if limb edema Reassess and recalculate fluid needs
Electrolyte alterations	Hyponatremia Hypernatremia Hyperchloremia Acidosis, alkalosis Hypokalemia Change in tonicity of fluids	Choose isotonic, balanced crystalloids Monitor electrolytes, acid–base status Supplement potassium during maintenance fluid therapy Support renal function
Glucose-containing fluids	Hyperglycemia Hyperosmolar fluid shifts causing dehydration Hyponatremia if D5W Cellular swelling if D5W	Use isotonic balanced crystalloids Monitor electrolytes and blood glucose Use D5W only to replace solute-free water or as carrier for CRI drugs
Renal injury	Renal injury reported with dextran use and in humans receiving HES (not seen in dogs and cats) Inadequate fluid resuscitation	Promote GFR Assure adequate blood pressure Use crystalloids with colloids to replace hydration deficits quickly Avoid using dextrans
Anemia	Dilution of RBCs Coagulopathy	Monitor PCV/TP Administer RBCs if necessary
Sudden increase in intravascular hydrostatic pressure	Dislodge clot in damaged vessel or organ Extravasation of intravascular fluids	Choose small-volume resuscitation technique to reach low normal endpoints Careful titration of fluid volume Anticipate potential for vessel injury
Coagulopathy	Dilutional from fluids Interference with coagulation with HES, dextran	Monitor quantity of colloid given Administer plasma if needed

CRI, constant rate of infusion; CVP, central venous pressure; D5W, 5% dextrose in water; ECG, electrocardiogram; GFR, glomerular filtration rate; HES, hydroxyethyl starch; PCV, packed cell volume; RBCs, red blood cells; SpO_2, pulse oximetry; TP, total protein.

References

1. Wamburg S, Sandgaard NCF, Bie P. Simultaneous determination of total body water and plasma volume in conscious dogs by the indicator dilution principle. J Nutr. 2002;132(6 Suppl 2):1711S–13S.

2. Wellman ML, DiBartola S, Kohn CW. Applied physiology of body fluids in dogs and cats. In: Fluid, Electrolyte and Acid-Base Disorders in Small Animal Practice, 3rd edn. DiBartola S, ed. St Louis: Saunders-Elsevier, 2006: pp 3–25.

3. Aronson PS, Boron WF, Boulpaep EL. Physiology of membranes. In: Medical Physiology: A Cellular and Molecular Approach, 2nd edn. Boron WF, ed. Philadelphia: Elsevier-Saunders, 2005: pp 50–86.

4. Starling EH. On the absorption of fluid from the connective tissue spaces. J Physiol (Lond). 1896;19:312–26.

5. Woodcock TE, Woodcock TM. Revised Starling equation and the glycocalyx model of transvascular fluid exchange: an improved paradigm for prescribing intravenous fluid therapy. Br J Anaesth. 2012;108(3):384–94.

6. Schrier RW, Berl T, Anderson RJ: Osmotic and nonosmotic control of vasopressin release. Am J Physiol. 1979;236:F321.

7. Stachenfeld NS, Gleim GW, Zabetakis PM, et al. Fluid balance and renal response following dehydrating exercise in well-trained men and women. Eur J Appl Physiol Occup Physiol. 1996;72(506):468–77.

8. Robertson GL, Athar S. The interaction of blood osmolality and blood volume in regulating plasma vasopressin in man. J Clin Endocrinol Metab. 1976;42:613.

9. Robertson GL, Shelton RL, Athar S. The osmoregulation of vasopressin. Kidney Int. 1976;10:25.

10. Zucker A, Gleason SD, Schneider EG. Renal and endocrine response to water deprivation in dog. Am J Physiol. 1982;242:R296.

11. Metzler GH, Thrasher TN, Keil LC, et al. Endocrine mechanisms regulating sodium excretion during water deprivation in dogs. Am J Physiol. 1986;251:R560.

12. Fitzsimons JT. The physiological basis of thirst. Kidney Int. 1976;10:3.

13. Armstrong LE, Maresh CM, Gabaree CV, et al. Thermal and circulatory responses during exercise: effects of hypohydration, dehydration, and water intake. J Appl Physiol. 1997;82(6):2028–35.

14. Leaf A. Regulation of intracellular fluid volume and disease. Am J Med. 1970;49:291.

15. Lee JY, Rozanski E, Anastasio M, et al. Iatrogenic water intoxication in two cats. J Vet Emerg Crit Care. 2013;23(1):53–7.

16. Rudloff E, Kirby R. Feline circulatory shock. In: The Cat: Clinical Medicine and Management. Little S, ed. St Louis: Elsevier-Saunders, 2012.

17. Rudloff E. Assessment of hydration. In: Small Animal Critical Care Medicine, 2nd edn. Silverstein D, Kopper K, eds. St Louis: Elsevier-Saunders, 2015.

18. Cheuvront, SN, Ely BR, Kenefick RW, Sawka MN. Biological variation and diagnostic accuracy of dehydration assessment markers. Am J Clin Nutr. 2010;92(3):565–73.

19. Shirreffs SM. Markers of hydration status. Eur J Clin Nutr. 2003;57(Suppl 2):S6–9.

20. Kavouras S. Assessing hydration status. Cur Opin Clin Nutr Metab Care. 2002;5(5):519–24.

21. Opplinger RA, Bartok C. Hydration testing of athletes. Sports Med. 2002;32(15):959–71.

22. Armstrong LE. Hydration assessment techniques. Nutr Rev. 2005;63(6 Pt 2):S40–54.

23. DiBartola S. Disorders of sodium and water: hypernatremia and hyponatemia. In: Fluid, Electrolyte and Acid-Base Disorders in Small Animal Practice, 3rd edn. DiBartola S, ed. St Louis: Saunders-Elsevier, 2006: pp 47–79.

24. Van Vonderen IK, Kooistra HS, Rijnberk A. Intra- and interindividual variation in urine osmolality and urine specific gravity in healthy pet dogs of various ages. J Vet Intern Med. 1997;11(1):30–5.

25. Dibartola S, Cottam YH, Caley P, et al. Feline reference values for urine composition. J Nutr. 2002;132:1754S–6S.

26. Grandy JL, Dunlop CI, Hodgson DS, et al. Evaluation of the Doppler ultrasonic method of measuring systolic arterial blood pressure in cats. Am J Vet Res. 1992;53(7):1166–9.

27. Branson KR, Wagner-Mann CC, Mann FA. Evaluation of an oscillometric blood pressure monitor on anesthetized cats and the effect of cuff placement and fur on accuracy. Vet Surg. 1997;26(4):347–53.

28. Pedersen KM, Butler MA, Ersbøll AK, et al. Evaluation of an oscillometric blood pressure monitor for use in anesthetized cats. J Am Vet Med Assoc. 2002;221(5):646–50.

29. Haberman CE, Morgan JD, Kang CW, et al. Evaluation of Doppler ultrasonic and oscillometric methods of indirect blood pressure measurement in cats. Int J Appl Res Vet Med. 2004;2(4):279–89.

30. Gains MJ, Grodecki KM, Jacombs RM, et al. Comparison of direct and indirect blood pressure measurements in anesthetized dogs. Can J Vet Res. 1995;59(3):238–40.

31. Caulkett NA, Cantwell SL, Houston DM. A comparison of indirect blood pressure monitoring techniques in the anesthetized cat. Vet Surg. 1998;27(4):370–7.

32. Greenway CV, Lawson AS. The effect of haemorrhage on venous return and regional blood flow in the anaesthetized cat. J Physiol. 1966;184:856–71.

33. Murphy CV, Schramm GE, Doherty JA, et al. The importance of fluid management in acute lung injury secondary to septic shock. Chest. 2009;136(1):102–9.

34. Osman D, Ridel C, Ray P, et al. Cardiac filling pressures are not appropriate to predict hemodynamic response to volume challenge. Crit Care Med. 2007;35(1):64–8.

35. Marik PE, Baram M, Vahid B. Does central venous pressure predict fluid responsiveness? A systematic review of the literature and the tale of seven mares. Chest. 2008;134(1):172–8.

36. Kumar A, Anel R, Bunnell E, et al. Pulmonary artery occlusion pressure and central venous pressure fail to predict ventricular filling volume, cardiac performance, or the response to volume infusion in normal subjects. Crit Care Med. 2004;32(3):691–9.

37. Boyd JH, Forbes J, Nakada TA, Walley KR, Russell JA. Fluid resuscitation in septic shock: a positive fluid balance and elevated central venous pressure are associated with increased mortality. Crit Care Med. 2011;39(2):259–65.

38. Muller L, Louart G, Bengler C, et al. The intrathoracic blood volume index as an indicator of fluid responsiveness in critically ill patients with acute circulatory failure: a comparison with central venous pressure. Anesth Analg. 2008;107(2):607–13.

39. Hu B, Xiang H, Liang H, et al. Assessment effect of central venous pressure in fluid resuscitation in the patients with shock: a multi-center retrospective research. Chin Med J (Engl). 2013;126(10):1844–9.

40. Gelman S. Venous function and central venous pressure: a physiologic story. Anesthesiology. 2008;4108(4):735–48.

41. Hayes G, Mathews K, Doig G, et al. The acute patient physiologic and laboratory evaluation (APPLE) score: a severity of illness stratification system for hospitalized dogs. J Vet Intern Med. 2010;24(5):1034–47.

42. Hayes G, Mathews K, Doig G, et al. The feline acute patient physiologic and laboratory evaluation (Feline APPLE) score: a severity of illness stratification system for hospitalized cats. J Vet Intern Med. 2011;25(1):26–38.

43. Us MH, Ozkan S, Oral L, et al. Comparison of the effects of hypertonic saline and crystalloid infusions on haemodynamic parameters during haemorrhagic shock in dogs. J Int Med Res. 2001;29(6):508–15.

44. Horton J, Landreneau R, Toggle D. Cardiac response to fluid resuscitation from haemorrhagic shock. Surg Gynecol Obstet. 1985;26(2):168–75.

45. Kitagawa H, Yasuda K, Kitoh K, Sasaki Y. Blood gas analysis in dogs with heartworm caval syndrome. J Vet Med Sci. 1994;56(5):861–7.

46. Jacobson S, Lobetti RG. Glucose, lactate, and pyruvate concentrations in dogs with babesiosis. Am J Vet Res. 2005;66(2):244–50.

47. Nel M, Lobetti RG, Keller N, Thompson PN. Prognostic value of blood lactate, blood glucose, and hematocrit in canine babesiosis. J Vet Intern Med. 2004;18(4):471–6.

48. Green T, Tonozzi C, Kirby R, Rudloff E. Evaluation of initial plasma lactate as a predictor of gastric necrosis and initial and subsequent plasma lactate values as a predictor of survival in dogs with gastric dilatation-volvulus: 84 dogs (2003–2007). J Vet Emerg Crit Care. 2011;21(1):36–44.

49. Zacher LA, Berg J, Shaw AP, et al. Association between outcome and changes in plasma lactate concentration during presurgical treatment in dogs with gastric dilation-volvulus: 64 cases (2002–2008). J Am Vet Med Assoc. 2010;236(8):892–7.

50. Mooney E, Raw C, Hughes D. Plasma lactate concentration as a prognostic biomarker in dogs with gastric dilatation and volvulus. Topics Compan Anim Med. 2014;29(3):71–6.

51. Gower SB, Weisse CW, Brown DC. Major abdominal evisceration injuries in dogs and cats: 12 cases (1998–2008). J Am Vet Med Assoc. 2009;234(12):1566–72.

52. Bright JM, Golden AL, Gompf RE, Walker MA, Toal RL. Evaluation of the calcium channel-blocking agents diltiazem and verapamil for treatment of feline hypertrophic cardiomyopathy. J Vet Intern Med. 1991;5(5):272–82.

53. Parsons KJ, Owen LJ, Lee K, Tivers MS, Gregory SP. A retrospective study of surgically treated cases of septic peritonitis in the cat (2000–2007). J Small Anim Pract. 2009;50(10):518–24.

54. Stevenson CK, Kidney BA, Duke T, Snead EC, Mainer-Jaime RC, Jackson ML. Serial blood lactate concentrations in systemically ill dogs. Vet Clin Pathol. 2007;36(3):234–9.

55. Butler AL, Campbell VL, Wagner AE, Sedacca CD, Hackett TB. Lithium dilution cardiac output and oxygen delivery in conscious dogs with systemic inflammatory response syndrome. J Vet Emerg Crit Care. 2008;18(3):246–57.

56. Holahan ML, Brown AJ, Drobatz KJ. The association of blood lactate concentration without come in dogs with idiopathic immune-mediated hemolytic anemia: 173 cases (2003–2006). J Vet Emerg Crit Care. 2010;20(4):413–20.

57. Buriko Y, vanWinkle TJ, Drobatz KJ, Rankin SC, Syring RS. Severe soft tissue infections in dogs: 47cases (1996–2006). J Vet Emerg Crit Care. 2008;18(6):608–18.

58. Armstrong LE. Assessing hydration status: the elusive gold standard. J Am Coll Nutr. 2007;26(5 Suppl):575S–84S.

59. Baldwin CE, Paratz JD, Bersten AD. Body composition analysis in critically ill survivors: a comparison of bioelectrical impedance spectroscopy devices. J Parenter Enteral Nutr. 2012;36(3):306–15.

60. Savalle M, Gillaizeau F, Maruani G, et al. Assessment of body cell mass at bedside in critically ill patients. Am J Physiol Endocrinol Metab. 2012;303(3):E389–96.

61. Waller A, Lindinger MI. Hydration of exercised Standardbred racehorses assessed noninvasively using multi-frequency bioelectrical impedance analysis. Equine Vet J. 2006;36(Suppl):285–90.

62. Malbrain ML, Huygh J, Dabrowski W, et al. The use of bio-electrical impedance analysis (BIA) to guide fluid management, resuscitation and deresuscitation in critically ill patients: a bench-to-bedside review. Anesth Intensive Ther. 2014;46(5):381–91.

63. Scalea TM, Holman M, Fuortes M, et al. Central venous blood oxygen saturation: an early, accurate measurement of volume during hemorrhage. J Trauma. 1988;28(6):725–32.

64. Reinhart K, Rudolph T, Bredle DL, et al. Comparison of central venous to mixed-venous oxygen saturation during changes in oxygen supply/demand. Chest 1989;95(6):1216–21.

65. Conti-Patara A, de Araújo Caldeira J, de Mattos-Junior E, et al. Changes in tissue perfusion parameters in dogs with severe sepsis/septic shock in response to goal directed hemodynamic optimization at admission to ICU and the relation to outcome. J Vet Emerg Crit Care. 2012;22(4):409–18.

66. Hayes GM, Mathews K, Boston S, et al. Low central venous oxygen saturation is associated with increased mortality in critically ill dogs. J Small Anim Pract. 2011;52(8):433–40.

67. Young BC, Prittie JE, Fox P, Barton LJ. Decreased central venous oxygen saturation despite normalization of heart rate and blood pressure post shock resuscitation in sick dogs. J Vet Emerg Crit Care. 2014;24(2):154–61.

68. Murphy CV, Schramm GE, Doherty JA, et al. The importance of fluid management in acute lung injury secondary to septic shock. Chest. 2009;136(1):102–9.

69. Osman D, Ridel C, Ray P, et al. Cardiac filling pressures are not appropriate to predict hemodynamic response to volume challenge. Crit Care Med. 2007;35(1):64–8.

70. Kumar A, Anel R, Bunnell E, et al. Pulmonary artery occlusion pressure and central venous pressure fail to predict ventricular filling volume, cardiac performance, or the response to volume infusion in normal subjects. Crit Care Med. 2004;32(3):691–9.

71. Wiener RS, Welch HG. Trends in the use of the pulmonary artery catheter in the United States, 1993–2004. J Am Med Assoc. 2007;298(4):423–9.

72. Jardin F, Vieillard-Baron A. Ultrasonographic examination of the venae cavae. Intensive Care Med. 2006;32(2):203–6.

73. Perera P, Mailhot T, Riley D, Mandavia D. The RUSH exam: rapid ultrasound in shock in the evaluation of the critically ill. Emerg Med Clin North Am. 2010;28(1):29–56.

74. Ferrada P, Vanguri P, Anand RJ, et al. Flat inferior vena cava: indicator of poor prognosis in trauma and acute care surgery patients. Am Surg. 2012;78(12):1396–8.

75. Ferrada P, Anand RJ, Whelan J, et al. Qualitative assessment of the inferior vena cava: useful tool for the evaluation of fluid status in critically ill patients. Am Surg. 2012;78(4):468–70.

76. Ando Y, Yanagiba S, Asano Y. The inferior vena cava diameter as a marker of dry weight in chronic hemodialyzed patients. Artif Organs. 1995;19(12):1237–42.

77. Seif D, Perera P, Mailhot T, Riley D, Mandavia D. Bedside ultrasound in resuscitation and the rapid ultrasound in shock protocol. Crit Care Res Pract. 2012;2012:503254.

78. Brennan JM, Blair JE, Goonewardena S, et al. Reappraisal of the use of inferior vena cava for estimating right atrial pressure. J Am Soc Echocardiogr. 2007;20(7):857–61.

79. Sefidbakht S, Assadsangabi R, Abbasi HR, Nabavizadeh A. Sonographic measurement of the inferior vena cava as a predictor of shock in trauma patients. Emerg Radiol. 2007;14(7):181–5.

80. Kent A, Bahner DP, Boulger CT, et al. Sonographic evaluation of intravascular volume status in the surgical intensive care unit: a prospective comparison of subclavian vein and inferior vena cava collapsibility index. J Surg Res. 2013;184(1):561–6.

81. Wu TS. The CORE scan: concentrated overview of resuscitative efforts. Crit Care Clin. 2014;30(1):151–75.

82. Airapetian N, Maizel J, Alyamani O, et al. Does inferior vena cava respiratory variability predict fluid responsiveness in spontaneously breathing patients? Crit Care. 2015;19(1):400–8.

83. Perera P, Lobo V, Williams SR, Gharahbaghian L. Cardiac echocardiography. Crit Care Clin. 2014;30(1):47–92.

84. Roscoe A, Strang T. Echocardiography in intensive care. Contin Educ Anaesth Crit Care Pain. 2008;8(2):46–9.

85. Durkan SD, Rush JE, Rozanski EA, et al. Echocardiographic findings in dogs with hypovolemia. Proceedings of the International Veterinary Emergency and Critical Care Congress, Atlanta, Georgia, 2005. J Vet Emerg Crit Care. 2005;15:S4.

86. DeFrancesco T. Focused or Coast³ – Echo (Heart). In: Focused Ultrasound Techniques for the Small Animal Practitioner. Lisciandro GR, ed. Ames: Wiley Blackwell, 2014: pp 189–205.

87. Muir WW. A new way to monitor and individualize your fluid therapy plan. Vet Med. 2013;Feb:76–82.

88. Silverstein DC, Pruett-Saratan A, Drobatz KJ. Measurements of microvascular perfusion in healthy anesthetized dogs using orthogonal polarization spectral imaging. J Vet Emerg Crit Care. 2009;19(6):579–87.

89. Silverstein DC, Cozzi EM, Hopkins AS, Keefe TJ. Microcirculatory effects of intravenous fluid administration in anesthetized dogs undergoing elective ovariohysterectomy. Am J Vet Res. 2014;75(9):809–17.

90. Weil MH, Nakagawa Y, Tang W, et al. Sublingual capnometry: a new noninvasive measurement for diagnosis and quantitation of severity of circulatory shock. Crit Care Med. 1999;27(7):1225–9.

91. Gutierrez G, Palizas F, Doglio G, et al. Gastric intramucosal pH as a therapeutic index of tissue oxygenation in critically ill patients. Lancet. 1992;339(8787):195–9.

92. Velmahos GC, Alam HB. Advances in surgical critical care. Curr Probl Surg. 2008;45(7)446–51.

93. Miami Trauma Clinical Trials Group. Splanchnic hypoperfusion-directed therapies in trauma: a prospective randomized trial. Am Surg. 2005;71(3):252–60.

94. Ackermann U, Irizawa TG, Milojevic S, et al. Cardiovascular effects of atrial extracts in anesthetized rats. Can J Physiol Pharmacol. 1984;62(7):819–26.

95. Genest J, Cantin M. Atrial natriuretic factor. Circulation. 1987;75(1 Pt 2):118–24.

96. Zucker A, Gleason SD, Schneider EG. Renal and endocrine response to water deprivation in dog. Am J Physiol. 1982;242:R296.

97. Wildenthal K, Mierzwiak DS, Mitchell JH. Acute effects of increased serum osmolality on left ventricular performance. Am J Physiol. 1969;216:898–904.

98. Kien ND, Kramer GC. Cardiac performance following hypertonic saline. Braz J Med Biol Res. 1989;22:245–8.

99. Gazitua MC, Scott JB, Swindall B. Resistance responses to local changes in plasma osmolality in three vascular beds. Am J Physiol. 1971;220:384–91.

100. Coimbra R, Junger WG, Hoyt DB, Liu FC, Loomis WH, Evers MF. Hypertonic saline resuscitation restores hemorrhage-induced immunosuppression by decreasing prostaglandin E(2) and interleukin-4 production. J Surg Res. 1996;64(2):203–9.

101. Rosengren S, Henson PM, Worthen GS. Migration-associated volume changes in neutrophils facilitate the migratory process in vitro. Am J Physiol. 1994;267(6 Pt 1):C1623–32.

102. Coimbra R, Junger WG, Liu FC, Loomis WH, Hoyt DB. Hypertonic/hyperoncotic fluids reverse prostaglandin E2 (PGE2)-induced T-cell suppression. Shock. 1995;4(1):45–9.

103. Wolf MB. Plasma volume dynamics after hypertonic fluid infusing in nephrectomized dog. Am J Physiol. 1971;221:1392–5.

104. Li M, Chen T, Chen Shu-da, et al. Comparison of equimolar doses of mannitol and hypertonic saline for the treatment of elevated intracranial pressure after traumatic brain injury. Medicine (Baltimore) 2015;94(17):e736.

105. Kien ND, Kramer GC, White DA. Acute hypotension caused by rapid hypertonic saline infusion in anesthetized dogs. Anesth Analg. 1991;73(5):597–602.

106. Boysen S, Dorval P. Effects of rapid intravenous 100% L-isomer lactated Ringer's administration on plasma lactate concentrations in healthy dog. J Vet Emerg Crit Care. 2014;24(5):571–7.

107. Kruse J, Zaidi S, Carlson R. Significance of blood lactate levels in critically ill patients with liver disease. Am J Med. 1987;83(1):77–82.

108. Mizock BA, Falk JL. Lactic acidosis in critical illness. Crit Care Med. 1992;20(1):80–93.

109. Vail DM, Ogilvie GK, Fettman MJ, et al. Exacerbation of hyperlactemia by infusion of lactated ringer's solution in dogs with lymphoma. J Vet Intern Med. 1990;4(5):228–32.

110. Lorenzo M, Davis JW, Negin S, et al. Can Ringer's lactate be used safely with blood transfusion? Am J Surg. 1998;175(4):308–10.

111. Craft EM, Powell LL. The effect of canine-specific albumin in dogs with septic peritonitis. J Vet Emerg Crit Care. 2012;22(6):631–9.

112. Mathews KA, Barry M. The use of 25% human serum albumin: outcome and efficacy in raising serum albumin and systemic blood pressure in critically ill dogs and cats. J Vet Emerg Crit Care. 2005;15(2):110–18.

113. Vigano F, Perissinotto L, Bosco VRF. Administration of 5% human serum albumin in critically ill small animal patients with hypoalbuminemia: 418 dogs and 170 cats (1994–2008). J Vet Emerg Crit Care. 2010;20(2):237–43.

114. Trow AV, Rozanski EA, Delaforcade AM, Chan DL. Evaluation of use of human albumin in critically ill dogs: 73 cases (2003–2006). J Am Vet Med Assoc. 2008;233(4):607–12.

115. Horowitz FB, Read RL, Powell, LL. A retrospective analysis of 25% human serum albumin supplementation in hypoalbuminemic dogs with septic peritonitis. Can Vet J. 2015;56(6):591–7.

116. Glover P, Rudloff E, Kirby R. Hydroxyethyl starch: a review of pharmacokinetics, pharmacodynamics, current products, and potential risks, benefits, and use. J Vet Emerg Crit Care 2014;24(6):642–61.

117. Wurlod VA, Howard J, Francey T, et al. Comparison of the in vitro effects of saline, hypertonic hydroxyethyl starch, hypertonic saline, and two forms of Hydroxyethyl starch on whole blood coagulation and platelet function in dogs. J Vet Emerg Crit Care. 2015;25(4):474–87.

118. Myburgh JA, Finfer S, Bellomo R, et al. Hydroxyethyl starch or saline for fluid resuscitation in intensive care. N Engl J Med. 2012;367(20):1901–11.

119. Perner A, Haase N, Guttormsen AB, et al. Hydroxyethyl starch 130/0.42 versus Ringer's acetate in severe sepsis. N Engl J Med. 2012;367(2):124–34.

120. Haase N, Perner A, Hennings LI, et al. Hydroxyethyl starch 130/0.38–0.45 versus crystalloid or albumin in patients with sepsis: systematic review with meta-analysis and trial sequential analysis. BMJ. 2013;346:f839.

121. Hayes G, Benedicenti L, Mathews K. Retrospective cohort study on the incidence of acute kidney injury and death following hydroxyethyl starch (HES 10% 250/0.5/5:1) administration in dogs (2007–2010). J Vet Emerg Crit Care. 2016;26(1):35–40.

122. Ertmer C, Kohler G, Rehberg S, et al. Renal effects of saline-based 10% pentastarch versus 6% tetrastarch infusion in ovine endotoxemic shock. Anesthesiology 2010;112(10):936–47.

123. Silverstein DC, Aldrich J, Haskins KJ, et al. Assessment of changes in blood volume in response to resuscitative fluid administration in dogs. J Vet Emerg Crit Care. 2005;15(3):185–92.

124. Gauthier V, Holowaychuk MK, Kerr CL, et al. Effect of synthetic colloid administration on hemodynamic and laboratory variables in healthy dogs and dogs with systemic inflammation. J Vet Emerg Crit Care. 2014;24(3):251–8.

125. Langston C. Managing fluid and electrolyte disorders in renal failure. In: Fluid, Electrolyte and Acid-Base Disorders in Small Animal Practice, 4th edn. DiBartola S, ed. St Louis: Saunders-Elsevier, 2012: pp 545–56.

126. Francesconi RP, Hubbard RW, Szlyk PC, et al. Urinary and hematological indexes of hypohydration. J Appl Physiol. 1987;62(3):1271–6.

127. Armstrong LE, Kenefick RW, Castellani JW, et al. Bioimpedance spectroscopy technique: intra-, extracellular, and total body water. Med Sci Sports Exerc. 1997;29(12):1657–63.

128. Hansen B, DeFrancesco T. Relationship between hydration estimate and body weight change after fluid therapy in critically ill dogs and cats. J Vet Emerg Crit Care. 2002;12(4):235–43.

129. Giunti M, Otto CM. Intraosseous catheterization. In: Small Animal Critical Care Medicine, 2nd edn. Silverstein DC, Hopper K, eds. St Louis:Elsevier, 2015: pp 1009–13.

130. Lee C, Rattner P, Wu X, Gershengorn H, Acquah S. Intraosseous versus central venous catheter utilization and performance during inpatient medical emergencies. Crit Care Med. 2015;43(6):1223–8.

CHAPTER 3

Blood pressure

Lauren Sullivan
Colorado State University, Fort Collins, Colorado

Introduction

Blood pressure is a measure of the force exerted by blood on the arterial wall. Measurement of arterial blood pressure (ABP) has a wide range of indications and is considered the "fourth vital sign" (temperature, pulse, respiration, blood pressure) in critical care settings. It is a key determinant of tissue perfusion and is responsible for tissue oxygenation, energy substrate delivery, and removal of metabolic byproducts.

The amount of force exerted by blood pressure is measured in millimeters of mercury (mmHg) and is dependent upon cardiac output (CO) and systemic vascular resistance (SVR). The physiological components of CO and SVR are outlined in Box 3.1. A full understanding of these complex factors allows pragmatic identification and timely intervention of blood pressure anomalies in the ICU setting.

Cardiac output is dependent upon heart rate and stroke volume, with stroke volume determined by the preload, afterload, and contractility of the heart. The preload is influenced by the circulating blood volume, sympathetic tone, blood viscosity, and intrathoracic and pericardial pressures. Factors that influence afterload include vascular resistance, blood viscosity, and arterial wall compliance. Various systemic conditions can exert positive or negative inotropic effects on the heart in the critical care setting, including the presence of circulating proinflammatory mediators, catecholamines, acid–base disorders, hypoxemia, hypoglycemia, and electrolyte disorders.

The SVR is the opposition of blood flow through the circulation. The determinants of flow resistance include blood viscosity, length of the vascular bed, and blood vessel diameter (see Poiseuille's law, Box 3.1). Vascular bed length does not change appreciably *in vivo* and therefore does not significantly contribute to SVR. Blood vessel diameter is the most important determinant of vascular resistance in the clinical setting. Small changes in blood vessel diameter lead to large changes in resistance. Vascular tone can vary widely in critical illness, leading to alterations in vessel diameter, vascular resistance, and ultimately blood pressure.

The pulsatile blood flow during ventricular contraction and relaxation results in two arterial blood pressure measurements: systolic (contraction) and diastolic (relaxation) pressures. Systolic arterial pressure (SAP) is the higher ABP measurement and becomes progressively higher towards the distal peripheral arteries. Normal SAP ranges are 154 ± 20 mmHg in dogs and 125 ± 11 mmHg in cats [1,2]. Diastolic arterial pressure (DAP) is the lower ABP measurement, with reported reference ranges of 84 ± 9 mmHg in dogs and 70 ± 9 mmHg in cats [1,2].

The mean arterial pressure (MAP) indicates the time-weighted driving force of the arterial system throughout the cardiac cycle. The duration of systole is typically considered to be one-third and diastole two-thirds of the cardiac cycle. The MAP is approximated using the adjusted equation [MAP = DAP + (SAP-DAP)/3]. This calculation, however, may not be representative in patients with tachycardia. Normal MAP ranges are 107 ± 11 mmHg in dogs and 105 ± 10 mmHg in cats [1,2]. MAP is helpful in hemodynamic assessment and therapeutic decisions because (1) the mean pressures are essentially the same in all parts of the arterial tree, (2) the pulmonary and systemic vascular resistances are derived from mean pressures, (3) the MAP is not significantly affected by machine artifact, and (4) the MAP approximates the pressure within the vital systemic and cerebral capillary beds [3]. Blood pressure is typically recorded as the SAP/DAP, with the MAP in parenthesis.

Large fluctuations in blood pressure that affect tissue oxygenation, energy substrate delivery, and removal of metabolic byproducts will contribute to patient morbidity. Yet vascular beds within many tissues are able to maintain a constant blood flow over a wide range of pressures through a concept known as *autoregulation*. Between mean arterial pressures of approximately 70–175 mmHg, tissues regulate local blood flow by adjusting their vascular resistance, thereby maintaining constant perfusion [4]. Autoregulation helps preserve cellular and organ function in the face of rapid or large ABP changes. This mechanism is particularly important in the brain (autoregulatory range of 60–140 mmHg) and the kidney (autoregulatory range 75–160 mmHg) [4]. When MAP ventures outside these ranges, the autoregulatory response is blunted and tissues may be adversely affected by abnormally low or high MAP. This makes the timely identification and treatment of ABP disorders necessary to optimize tissue perfusion and prevent adverse effects from severe blood pressure alterations.

Diagnostic and monitoring procedures

Important information to define the cause and identify the effects of blood pressure disorders can be obtained through the history, physical examination, point of care (POC) testing, clinicopathological testing, diagnostic imaging, and equipment-based monitoring tools. Direct and indirect methods for monitoring blood pressure can provide SAP/DAP (MAP) values to guide therapeutic intervention. Other markers of tissue perfusion that may indicate poor perfusion and a need for therapeutic intervention include blood lactate concentration, base deficit, central venous oxygen saturation, urine output, and physical examination findings.

Monitoring and Intervention for the Critically Ill Small Animal: The Rule of 20, First Edition. Edited by Rebecca Kirby and Andrew Linklater.
© 2017 John Wiley & Sons, Inc. Published 2017 by John Wiley & Sons, Inc.

Box 3.1 Physiological components of blood pressure.

$BP = CO \times SVR$

$CO = HR \times SV$

- SV depends on:
  - Preload = volume and pressure of blood entering heart
  - Afterload = pressure and volume of blood leaving ventricles
  - Contractility = intrinsic myocardial fiber shortening (inotropy)
- HR depends on:
  - Parasympathetic and sympathetic control
  - Barorecptor and Bainbridge reflexes
- SVR = opposition to blood flow, defined by
  - Poiseuille's equation (law):

$$\Delta P = \frac{8\mu L Q}{\pi r^4}$$

BP, blood pressure; CO, cardiac output (mL/kg/min); d, diameter; HR, heart rate (beats per minute); L, length of vessel; Q, volume flow rate; r, radius; SV, stroke volume (mL); SVR, systemic vascular resistance; ΔP, pressure loss; μ, dynamic viscosity; π, pi.

Table 3.1 Common drugs and toxins that cause vasodilation ad vasoconstriction.

Vasodilation	Vasoconstriction
Aldosterone blocker	**Alpha-adrenergic agonists**
Spironolactone, eplerenone	Epinephrine (high dose)
Alpha-adrenergic antagonists	Norepinephrine
Acepromazine	Dopamine (high dose)
Chlorpromazine	Vasopressin
Phenoxybenzamine	Phenylephrine
Prazosin	Ephedrine
Beta-adrenergic stimulants	Pseudoephedrine
Epinephrine (low dose)	**Central nervous system**
Dopamine (midrange dose)	**stimulants**
Beta-adrenergic antagonists	Cocaine
Propanolol, esmolol, atenolol	Ephedrine
Calcium channel blockers	Amphetamines
Amlodipine, nicarpidine	Nicotine
Dopamine-1 agonist	Caffeine
Fenoldopam	Methylxanthines (chocolate)
Renin-angiotensin-aldosterone	**Other**
system inhibitors	Corticosteroids
Enalapril, benazepril	
Losartan, irbesartan	
Phosphodiesterase inhibitors	
Aminophylline	
Pimobendan	
Nitric oxide release	
Nitroprusside	
Smooth muscle relaxant	
Hydralazine	

History and physical examination

The history will begin with the signalment (age, sex, breed). Breed-associated cardiac disease (such as cardiomyopathy observed with the Doberman Pinscher or Boxer, sick sinus syndrome in Schnauzers) should be considered when managing blood pressure abnormalities in the ICU patient. There is a reported effect of the sex on ABP in dogs, with males having higher and intact females lower values. The difference, however, is less than 10 mmHg [5]. The history continues with the progression of current clinical signs, past medical history (including kidney disease, hyperthyroidism, cardiac disease) and exposure to medications (human and veterinary) and toxins. A list of common drugs and toxins that can affect blood pressure is provided in Table 3.1.

The owners might report clinical signs of weakness, lethargy, and mental depression with either hypo- or hypertension. Clinical signs associated with target organ damage from hypertension can be vague (such as lethargy, hiding). Acute blindness or sudden onset of abnormal mentation might be a consequence of severe hypertension. Any history of significant fluid loss such as vomiting or diarrhea requires further investigation for hypotension from hypovolemia. Polyuria can result from kidney disease and hypertension.

The physical examination begins with the temperature, pulse rate and intensity, oral mucous membrane color, and capillary refill time. These physical findings provide a reasonable assessment of peripheral tissue perfusion and as a group can be called the physical peripheral perfusion parameters.

The various stages of shock can be initially detected through the physical peripheral perfusion parameters. Animals with hypotension (early decompensatory and late decompensatory stages of shock) typically manifest one or more of the following characteristics: tachycardia (dogs) or bradycardia (dogs in late stages and cats), pale mucous membrane color, prolonged capillary refill time, abnormal peripheral pulse palpation (weak, thready or absent), dull mentation, and low body temperature (cats). In the early stages of sepsis or severe hyperthermia, the mucous membranes may appear bright red due to peripheral vasodilation. The presence of hypotension should be confirmed and quantified with ABP measurement in each situation.

Palpation of the femoral pulse has been cited to provide an estimate of ABP; however, the strength of the palpated pulse (pulse pressure) provides a more accurate method of feeling the difference between SAP and DAP. A patient with a normal pulse pressure could have an abnormal SAP or DAP reading, making the actual measurement of ABP the more accurate method of assessment.

Complete physical and neurological examinations are then performed. The finding of jugular vein distension or a jugular pulse can indicate an increase in intrathoracic or pericardial pressure, each a potential cause of inadequate venous return and hypotension. Skin turgor, mucous membrane and corneal moisture and eye position within the orbit are used to estimate the hydration status of the patient; patients with severe dehydration may exhibit concurrent hypovolemia (see Chapter 2). The ophthalmic examination might reveal retinal vascular engorgement or hemorrhage, blindness, hyphema or choroidopathy, each a possible consequence of severe hypertension. Evidence of trauma, third body fluid spacing, vomiting, diarrhea or polyuria could be associated with hypovolemia and hypotension. Auscultation of the heart for a murmur or arrhythmias (pulse deficits, tachy- or bradyarrhythmias) could direct further testing for cardiac disease as a contributor to hyper- or hypotension. Careful palpation for a "thyroid slip" in the cat might demonstrate enlarged thyroid glands with hyperthyroidism and hypertension possible.

Further patient evaluation requires the collection of additional data. Cage-side or POC testing, clinicopathological testing, diagnostic imaging, and equipment-based monitoring can provide valuable information to detect alterations in blood pressure, identify the cause, and reveal any potential consequences.

Point of care testing

A minimum database is provided through POC in-hospital testing and should include the packed cell volume (PCV), total protein (TP), blood glucose, blood urea nitrogen (BUN) electrolyte panel, blood lactate, acid–base status, coagulation profile, and urinalysis.

Blood viscosity is directly related to vascular resistance. As the PCV or hematocrit increases, blood viscosity and vascular resistance also increase. The opposite effects are observed with a low hematocrit. Hypoglycemia can affect SVR, with insufficient energy substrate available resulting in poor contraction of vascular smooth muscle and poor vascular tone. An elevated BUN and isosthenuria on urinalysis might direct further investigation for kidney disease, a frequent cause of hypertension in the dog and cat. Electrolyte disorders affecting sodium (Na^+), potassium (K^+), magnesium (Mg^{++}), ionized calcium (iCa^{++}) or chloride (Cl^-) and severe acidemia or alkalemia could impair cardiac contractility or vascular tone.

A high blood lactate suggests anaerobic metabolism, poor tissue oxygenation, and impaired perfusion. Blood lactate should be assessed during resuscitation and a declining trend documented as evidence of return of blood flow. An elevated blood lactate found with a normal ABP warrants investigation for ischemia localized to an organ or isolated tissue bed as a cause.

Clinicopathological testing

A complete blood count and serum biochemical profile with thyroid panel will provide data pertaining to possible contributions of the internal organs to abnormalities of the blood pressure. An elevation in serum creatinine and BUN directs further investigation for kidney disease and possible renal hypertension. Problems such as liver disease, pancreatitis or hypoadrenocorticism might be found as a cause of hypovolemia from vomiting and diarrhea; this should be interpreted along with a urinalysis. Fecal examination for parasites might find a cause for diarrhea and hypovolemia. Additional testing is often required and could include serology for inciting pathogens (cause of systemic inflammatory response syndrome (SIRS)-related hypotension), fluid analysis with culture and susceptibility, adrenal function testing (for hypoadrenocorticism, hyperadrenocorticism or pheochromocytoma) and diagnostic imaging. Rarely, further clinicopathological testing may be useful in the diagnosis of pheochromocytoma.

Diagnostic imaging

Survey thoracic and abdominal radiographs provide the initial diagnostic imaging data once the patient has been stabilized. Thoracic radiographs can demonstrate the heart size and shape, evidence of heartworm disease or other pulmonary vascular changes, lung parenchymal fluid or masses, pleural fluid or air, and rib or vertebral changes. The size of the caudal vena cava can represent central venous volume and preload to the heart (when no evidence of pleural air or pericardial fluid). Abdominal radiographs could show evidence of peritoneal fluid or air and provide an initial assessment of abdominal organ size, shape, and position.

Abdominal and thoracic ultrasound provides a more in-depth assessment of organ structure and can identify fluid pockets not seen on plain radiographs. Diagnostic and therapeutic centesis can be performed as indicated. Evaluation of the size and structure of the adrenal glands might identify adrenal hypertrophy or a mass, potentially contributing to blood pressure abnormalities. Documentation of primary cardiac disease often requires a combination of thoracic radiography, electrocardiography (ECG), and echocardiography. Echocardiographic findings associated with sepsis-related myocardial dysfunction include biventricular dilation with reduced ejection fraction and reduced fractional shortening [6]. Advanced imaging with computed tomography or nuclear magnetic resonance imaging may be warranted to better define an organ structure or evaluate the tissues of the central nervous system.

Equipment-based monitoring methods

Indications for monitoring ABP are numerous and include any animal with a history of hypo- or hypertension, an underlying physiological derangement that could predispose an animal to a blood pressure disorder or the need for heavy sedation or general anesthesia.

Direct and indirect methods are available to monitor ABP in the dog and cat. Traditional techniques include direct arterial catheterization, Doppler ultrasonography, and oscillometric sphygmomanometry. Alternate techniques include high-definition oscillometry and photoplethysmography.

Direct ABP monitoring

Direct ABP (dABP) monitoring is considered to be the "gold standard" for ABP measurement but requires placement and maintenance of an indwelling arterial catheter. Arterial pressure within the catheterized vessel is detected and converted to an electrical signal by a pressure transducer and amplified and continuously displayed as a waveform (Figure 3.1) and numeric values. Advantages of dABP monitoring include real-time data display, ability for continuous monitoring, reliability, accuracy of measurement, and accessibility for arterial blood gas sampling.

The vast amount of information gleaned from dABP monitoring often balances the time and invasiveness of arterial catheterization. Critically ill animals that might warrant dABP monitoring include severe hypotension related to cardiogenic or vasodilatory shock, severe hypertension requiring pharmacological intervention, and patients requiring general anesthesia that are assessed to have a high physical status classification score (see Table 22.1).

Arterial catheter placement is typically achieved in the dorsal metatarsal, radial, coccygeal or femoral artery of the dog and cat. Catheterization of the femoral artery may carry a greater risk for catheter dislodgment, bleeding or thrombosis compared to the other arterial locations. The materials required for arterial catheterization as well as the steps for the procedure are listed in Box 3.2a. The steps for setting up direct blood pressure monitoring are provided in Box 3.2b with the set-up pictured in Figure 3.2 [7] and steps to perform direct arterial measurement in Box 3.3. Complications associated with dABP monitoring include catheter site hemorrhage,

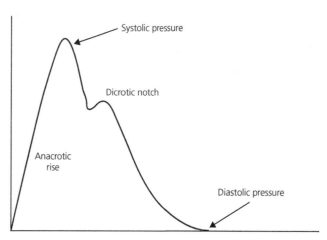

Figure 3.1 Diagram of an arterial pressure waveform. Anacrotic rise = rapid left ventricular ejection related to cardiac inotropy and rate of blood acceleration. Systolic pressure = measured at top of upstroke. Dicrotic notch = elastic recoil from aortic valve closure. Diastolic pressure = measured at baseline.

Box 3.2a Materials for arterial catheter placement.

- Hair clippers
- 4–6 cotton balls soaked in povidone-iodine
- 4–6 cotton balls soaked in 70% isopropyl alcohol
- 1" standard porous adhesive tape
- Over-the-needle intravenous catheter; catheter selection is based on size of patient and artery to be cannulated:
  - 20 gauge, 1.88" or 1.16" length catheter for medium-to-large dogs
  - 22 gauge, 1" length catheter for small dogs and large cats
  - 24 gauge, 0.75" length catheter for small cats
- T-port adaptor or male adaptor
- Syringe with heparinized saline
- Arterial catheter will ultimately be connected to noncompliant tubing flushed with heparinized saline attached to a three-way stopcock.

Box 3.2b Technique for placing arterial catheter.

- Palpate the artery of interest (typically dorsal metatarsal or femoral arteries).
- Clip then aseptic preparation of catheter insertion site (alternating povidone-iodine and isopropyl alcohol scrubs).
- Flush intravenous catheter with heparinized saline.
- Insure catheter and stylet will separate.
- Secure the limb to prevent movement.
- Using a gloved hand, locate and isolate arterial pulse.
- Hold the catheter at a 15–30° angle over artery.
- Insert catheter percutaneously toward palpated pulse.
- Rapid flow of red, pulsating blood indicates entering artery.
- Lower catheter parallel with limb and slowly advance.
- Advance catheter over stylet into the artery.
- Remove stylet, attach T-port flushed with heparinized saline.
- Secure arterial catheter with tape and clearly label.

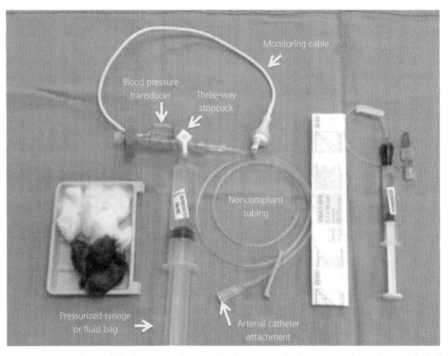

Figure 3.2 Set-up for direct measurement of arterial blood pressure. The arterial catheter is attached to noncompliant tubing preflushed with heparinized saline. The tubing is connected to a three-way stopcock. The stopcock is also connected to a pressurized system of heparinized saline (20 cc syringe in this picture) and the pressure transducer. Note: the pressure transducer is placed at the level of the right atrium. It is connected to the monitor by the monitoring cable.

infection, thrombosis, and accidental intraarterial drug administration. Contraindications to dABP are relative to the need for invasive monitoring but may include coagulopathy, thrombocytopenia or thrombocytopathia, local skin necrosis or infection, or animals receiving anticoagulant or thrombolytic agents.

An arterial pressure waveform is produced by dABP monitoring which visually demonstrates varying arterial pressures obtained throughout the cardiac cycle. The components of this waveform are illustrated in Figure 3.1. The upstroke of the waveform (*anacrotic rise*) is closely related to cardiac inotropy and the rate of blood acceleration during contraction. The SAP is measured at the top of this upstroke. During the downward slope, the aortic valve closes at the onset of diastole, with the elastic recoil causing the *dicrotic notch*. Blood continues to run distally until baseline is reached where the DAP is measured.

Alterations in waveform morphology are most commonly observed with cardiac arrhythmias (sloped anacrotic rise with a lower peak pressure), hypotension (decreased anacrotic rise; rate, slope, and amplitude, lower peak pressure and disappearance of the dicrotic notch), and hypertension (rapid anacrotic rise, higher peak and baseline pressure, enlarged waveform phases) [3].

Waveform changes will prompt immediate assessment of patient perfusion parameters to determine if a true change in the condition of the animal has occurred. Should patient status appear stable, the monitoring system and set-up are checked for problems.

Basic system troubleshooting begins with assessing the patient position relative to the transducer, system lines free of air bubbles or kinks, a patent arterial catheter (flushes easily, no kink or thrombus, positioned within the middle of the arterial lumen) and an adequately pressurized saline bag. Additional conditions inherent to the monitoring system itself (known as *damping*) should then be assessed. Damping is a loss of pulse pressure energy between the catheter tip and the transducer due to frictional resistance and absorption of energy [7]. The effects of overdamping and underdamping are listed in Table 3.2. To determine if the monitoring

system has an adequate dynamic response and is optimally damped, a "square wave" test may be performed. This is done by opening the continuous flush valve (from the pressurized flush system) for a few seconds, creating a square wave and then quickly closing the system [7]. A system with appropriate dynamic response characteristics will return to baseline waveforms within one or two oscillations. If this fails, further troubleshooting of the system is required.

The values for SAP, DAP, and MAP can each be evaluated with the waveforms. Minor variations in ABP will naturally occur in concert with the respiratory cycle. During spontaneous breathing, SAP drops during inspiration as intrapleural pressure becomes more negative, causing cardiac and vessel pressures to fall. The SAP then rises during spontaneous expiration. The phenomenon known as *pulsus paradoxus*, by which abnormally large decreases in SAP (defined as >10 mmHg) are observed during spontaneous inspiration, is often associated with cardiac tamponade or severe respiratory tract disease [8].

When a patient is undergoing mechanical ventilation, the opposite cardiovascular effects are expected during inspiration (increased SAP) and expiration (decreased SAP). Mechanically ventilated animals demonstrate decreased cardiac output and stroke volume as inspiratory-to-expiratory ratio and airway pressure increase [9]. In ventilated animals with consistent tidal volumes, the change in SAP associated with inspiration versus expiration (known as *systolic pressure variation* (SPV)) may be used to predict volume responsiveness. Hypovolemia exacerbates changes in stroke volume, SAP, and subsequently SPV (Figure 3.3). Typical SPV in healthy anesthetized dogs is approximately 5.3±1.8 mmHg. Increases in

Box 3.3 Steps for direct measurement of arterial blood pressure.

1. Place intraarterial catheter, flush and connect T-port (see Box 3.2b for technique).
2. T-port of arterial catheter is connected to noncompliant tubing primed with heparinized saline.
3. Tubing is connected to a three-way stopcock: the pressure transducer is attached to the end of the stopcock directly opposite tubing and placed at level of right atrium.
4. The perpendicular end of the stopcock is connected by an IV administration set attached to a 1 L bag of heparinized saline (0.9% saline with 1–2 U/mL of unfractionated heparin) which can be pressurized.
5. The pressure transducer is connected to the monitoring system by a transducer cable.
6. All air bubbles are evacuated from the system and the bag of saline is pressurized to a pressure greater than the patient SBP.
7. The monitoring system is "zeroed" by opening the transducer stopcock to the external environment and adjusting monitor settings (arterial waveform should flatten).
8. The stopcock is then closed to the environment and the line flushed using the transducer flush valve.
   The arterial waveform should be seen on the monitor screen.

Table 3.2 Effects of "damping" on direct arterial pressure measurement and waveforms. Damping is the loss of pulse pressure energy between the catheter tip and the transducer due to frictional resistance and absorption of energy [7].

Status	Signs	Effect
Overdamping Long or overly compliant tubing, air bubbles, clots or kinks	Less distinct waveform Obscure dicrotic notch	Falsely low SAP, exaggerated DAP
Underdamping Most systems. Due to inadequate frequency response for patient pulsatile signal	Sharp waveform points Display artifacts	Exaggerates SAP, falsely low DAP
Fast flush or square wave test	A square wave form is produced	System with appropriate dynamic response will return to baseline waveform within 1–2 oscillations

DAP, diastolic arterial pressure; SAP, systolic arterial pressure.

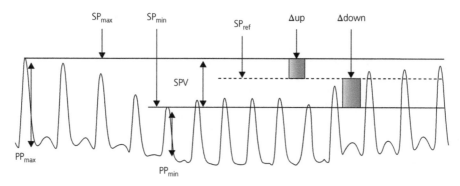

Figure 3.3 Variables used to determine volume responsiveness based on ventilation-associated variation in blood pressure. PP_{max}, maximum pulse pressure; PP_{min}, minimum pulse pressure. SP_{max}, maximum systolic pressure; SP_{min}, minimum systolic pressure; SP_{ref}, reference systolic pressure; SPV, systolic pressure variarion. Source: Cooper E, Cooper S. Direct systemic arterial blood pressure monitoring. In: Advanced Monitoring and Procedures for Small Animal Emergency and Critical Care. Burkitt Creedon JM, Davis H, eds. Ames: John Wiley & Sons, 2012: pp.122–33. Used with permisison of Wiley.

SPV (inspiratory SAP-expiratory SAP) have been associated with ongoing hemorrhage and hypovolemia [10].

A similar calculation known as *pulse pressure variation* (PPV) [12] determines volume responsiveness using a continuous arterial waveform (see Figure 3.3). The PPV is a percentage calculated by dividing the maximum and minimum pulse pressures (PP_{max}–PP_{min}) over a single breath by the mean of the two values [(PP_{max}–PP_{min})/2]. PPV has been found to be more reliable than SPV when determining preload dependency. It controls for changes in extramural pressure during respiration and focuses on changes related to left ventricular stroke volume [13]. Automatic calculation of PPV and other dynamic parameters by modern-day monitors has contributed to their popularity and clinical use. These parameters are not without limitations and it is important to remember that PPV is not useful during spontaneous breathing, cardiac arrhythmias, right-sided heart failure, and large variations in tidal volume [14].

Indirect ABP monitoring

Indirect arterial blood pressure monitoring (also known as noninvasive blood pressure (NIBP) monitoring) is preferred when cardiovascular status is stable and large fluctuations in ABP are unlikely to occur. NIBP measurement allows for rapid determination of ABP without the morbidities associated with intraarterial catheterization. Disadvantages to NIBP measurement are largely due to its indirect nature. These devices estimate ABP through detection of arterial blood flow rather than directly measuring pressure within the artery itself. Accuracy of the device may be affected by dramatic changes in arterial flow or the device's ability to detect that flow.

Noninvasive blood pressure measurements in animals are easily influenced by various patient factors, such as species, anesthetized or conscious state, degree of illness, cuff placement along a limb with varying circumference, size and anatomical accessibility of the artery being occluded, and patient movement during ABP measurement. The American College of Veterinary Internal Medicine (ACVIM) has created veterinary-specific recommendations for the validation of NIBP measurement devices (Box 3.4) [15]. When considering use of a specific NIBP monitor in clinical practice, it is advisable to (1) determine which species and conditions the monitor will be used for, and (2) investigate if the monitor has been validated for the expected circumstances according to peer-reviewed literature or ACVIM recommendations.

A consensus protocol for standardized NIBP measurement in small animals (Box 3.5) has been proposed by the ACVIM [15]. The goal is to obtain reliable values that can be accurately trended over time. Skilled personnel who are comfortable with ABP measurement equipment and animal restraint are essential.

Various forms of NIBP monitoring employ a cuff technique that impedes arterial blood flow when the cuff is inflated. A gradual reduction in the amount of externally applied pressure allows for small increases in flow through the partially deformed artery. Return of blood flow may then be recorded using various devices. Doppler ultrasonography, oscillometric sphygmomanometry and high-definition oscillometry all utilize a cuff technique to measure NIBP in small animal patients.

Doppler ultrasonography and oscillometric sphygmomanometry are the most commonly used NIBP devices in veterinary practice. They each employ slightly different technology for detection of blood flow and measurement of pressure through use of a cuff, and each technique presents unique advantages and disadvantages in the clinical setting.

Doppler ultrasonography requires two pieces of equipment for ABP measurement: a cuff attached to a sphygmomanometer, and ultrasound unit with amplifier and speakers (Figure 3.4). The ultrasound unit consists of a Doppler probe containing piezoelectric crystals, which are placed over the artery of interest. Preferred locations in small animals include the palmar common digital artery, dorsal metatarsal artery, or medial caudal (coccygeal) artery. The pressure cuff is then placed around the limb and proximal to the Doppler probe. Following inflation of the cuff, arterial blood flow is occluded and the piezoelectric crystals cannot detect any flow above the patient's systolic pressure. With gradual cuff deflation

---

Box 3.4 American College of Veterinary Internal Medicine validation criteria for noninvasive blood pressure devices [15].

System efficacy is validated if the following conditions are met.
- The mean difference of paired measurements for systolic and diastolic pressures treated separately is 6 ± 10 mmHg or less, with a standard deviation of 15 mmHg or less.
- The correlation between paired measures for systolic and diastolic pressures treated separately is ≥0.9 across the range of measured values of BP.
- 50% of all measurements for systolic and diastolic pressures treated separately lie within 10 mmHg of the reference method.
- 80% of all measurements for systolic and diastolic pressures treated separately lie within 20 mmHg of the reference method.
- The study results have been accepted for publication in a referred journal.
- The subject database contains no fewer than eight animals for comparison with an intraarterial method or 25 animals for comparison with a previously validated indirect device.

Box 3.5 Standardized protocol for noninvasive blood pressure measurement in small animals provided by the American College of Veterinary Internal Medicine [15].

- Calibrate the BP device semiannually.
- Standardized calibration and BP measurement procedures.
- Environment: isolated, quiet, generally with the owner present. Unsedated patient remains quietly in room for 5–10 minutes prior to measurement.
- Gently restrain with patient in comfortable position. Ventral or lateral recumbency to limit distance from heart base to cuff (if >10 cm, a correction factor of +0.8 mmHg/cm below the heart base can be applied).
- Cuff should be approximately 40% of circumference of the cuff site in dogs and 30–40% in cats. Note cuff size in the medical record.
- Cuff placement can be on a limb or the tail (varies with animal conformation, user preference). Record site for cuff placement in the medical record.
- The same individual (preferably a technician) performs all blood pressure measurements following this standard protocol. Training of this individual is essential.
- The patient should be calm and motionless.
- The first measurement should be discarded. At least three, and preferably 5–7, consecutive, consistent (<20% variability in systolic values) values should be recorded.
- Repeat as necessary, changing cuff placement as needed to obtain consistent values.
- Average all values to obtain the ABP measurement.
- If in doubt, repeat the measurement subsequently.
- Written records should be kept on a standard form and include cuff size and site, values obtained, rationale for excluding any values, the final (mean) result, and interpretation of the results by a veterinarian.

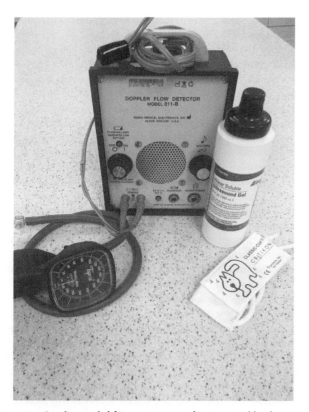

Figure 3.4 Supplies needed for measurement of noninvasive blood pressure using Doppler ultrasonography. From left to right: sphygmomanometer (WelchAllyn, Scaneatelles Falls, NY), ultrasound unit with amplifier and speaker (Doppler Flow Detector®, Parks Medical Electronics, Aloha, OR), Doppler probe containing piezoelectric crystals (placed over artery) and cord, cuff to attach to sphygmomanometer, ultrasound gel (ProAdvantage NDC, La Vergne, TN).

using the sphygmomanometer, the crystals eventually detect an audible flow through the speaker. At the point when flow is heard, a pressure number on the sphygmomanometer is read and is recorded as the SAP. Doppler ultrasonography may be used to assess SAP with good repeatability and reproducibility in healthy awake dogs and cats [16,17].

The DAP and MAP cannot be reliably obtained with Doppler methodology but in situations of low-pressure systems, the audible noise may correlate better with the MAP than the SAP [18]. There exists a large body of literature comparing Doppler ultrasonography to the gold standard (dABP monitoring) in dogs and cats.

Oscillometric sphygmomanometry is an automated device that requires less time than the Doppler methodology. It estimates ABP using pneumatic inflation and detection of arterial wall movement secondary to blood pulsation. The cuff is attached to the machine using two hoses, one which pressurizes the cuff until no arterial wall motion (oscillation) is present and a second that senses oscillations within the inflated cuff. The machine slowly deflates the cuff while searching for return of arterial wall movement against the inflated cuff. As the cuff is deflated, oscillations rapidly increase at the SAP, reach a maximum amplitude at the MAP, and then rapidly decrease to a low amplitude at the DAP [18]. For most device microprocessors, MAP is measured and the nonmeasured values (SAP and DAP) are then calculated using internal algorithms.

Cuff selection and placement are key to obtaining accurate values when using oscillometric technology. The cuff bladder should be placed directly over the artery of measurement (typically the radial or dorsal metatarsal artery). False readings may occur with improper cuff selection; inappropriately large cuffs result in falsely low ABP values and small cuffs in falsely high ABP values. In addition, error(s) in measurement may be suspected when the NIBP values obtained do not correspond with the clinical status of the patient, when the pulse rate on the oscillometric unit does not match the patient's heart rate, or there is identification of confounding factors that interfere with oscillometric technology (severe vasoconstriction, rapid fluctuations in ABP or heart rate, patient shivering or restlessness, or lack of pulsatile blood flow to the region of measurement).

High-definition oscillometry (HDO®) represents a newer type of NIBP measurement that allows for continuous, real-time ABP measurement due to its high-speed data acquisition and graphical analysis. Rapidity of measurement is helpful in circumstances that typically preclude standard oscillometric techniques (tachycardia, cardiac arrhythmias) and advanced technical features allow for ABP measurement over a wide range of pressures [18]. Compared to standard oscillometric units, HDO follows each signal as the artery repetitively opens and analyzes it for SAP, DAP, and MAP and permits evaluation of pulse pressure. Literature regarding the use of HDO in small animals demonstrates mixed results regarding its accuracy and precision, but more recent work in cats supports its superiority when compared to dABP monitoring [19]. Additional studies are needed to assess the appropriateness of HDO in a larger variety of clinical contexts.

Other forms of NIBP monitoring have undergone limited evaluation in veterinary medicine. Photoplethysmography is a simple and low-cost optical technique that can be used to detect blood volume changes in a microvascular bed of tissue [20]. A familiar application of photoplethysmography is the continuous waveform created with pulse oximetry [21,22]. Other photoplethysmographic devices have been created specifically for NIBP measurement, utilizing an inflatable finger cuff that measures the arterial pressure waveform on a beat-by-beat basis. These devices gained some veterinary interest and publication [23–25] but their clinical implementation remains relatively sparse compared to other NIBP measurement techniques.

Additional monitoring tools

Central venous pressure (CVP), ECG, echocardiography, pulse oximetry, end-tidal CO_2, urine output, blood lactate, and repeating the minimum database can all provide value when monitoring the ICU small animal patient with hypotension or hypertension. The CVP reflects the pressure in the vena cava. This is a function of the central venous volume (preload) when there is normal right heart function and normal pleural and pericardial pressures. The trend of change in CVP can guide fluid infusion rate and volume during resuscitation from hypovolemia and hypotension. The blood lactate and urine output provide a reflection of the perfusion and blood pressure status within the core circulation. Pulse oximetry and end-tidal CO_2 give moment-to-moment data pertaining to pulmonary gas exchange, with abnormalities in either potentially affecting blood pressure. The placement of a pulmonary arterial catheter with fiberoptics allows measurement of mixed venous blood oxygen saturation (SvO_2) as well as continuous data to assess cardiac output, cardiac index, and pulmonary arterial pressures [26]. The invasive nature of catheter placement and the cost of the specialized catheter and monitoring system have limited their use in veterinary medicine.

Disorders of blood pressure

Large variations in ABP are common in critical illness and can be multifactorial. Many cardiac and vascular factors, as well as humoral and microcirculatory components, will affect the blood pressure. A normal blood pressure measurement does not guarantee adequate tissue perfusion in critical illness [27]. However, low blood pressure (*hypotension*) is a frequent and often rectifiable cause of poor tissue perfusion in this setting.

Blood pressure must also remain under a maximum value to avoid damage to tissues being perfused by the capillary beds. Tissues that are particularly sensitive to increased blood pressure (*hypertension*) include the ocular, cardiac, renal, and central nervous systems. Several small animal diseases (such as acute and chronic kidney disease, hyperthyroidism, diabetes mellitus, and pheochromocytoma) have been associated with hypertension. Because these diseases are frequently identified with the small animal in the ICU, ABP monitoring is of equal importance for detection of both hypotension and hypertension in this patient population.

Hypotension

Low blood pressure (hypotension) is defined as a SAP <80 mmHg or a MAP <60 mmHg in either dogs or cats [28]. Hypotension is estimated to occur in 24–81% of human ICU patients [29], and is anticipated to occur at a similar rate in dogs and cats. The hypotension seen in ICU patients may be a result of one or more of the following: (1) physiological characteristics of the illness, (2) severity of acute illness, and (3) medication administration [30]. Hypotension occurring within the first 24 hours of ICU admission has been associated with increased mortality in people, further emphasizing the importance of prompt recognition and treatment of hypotension in the emergency and critical care settings [31–33]. Similar findings have also been reported in critically ill cats, with 64% mortality observed in hypotensive cats compared to a 32% mortality in cats that remain normotensive during hospitalization [34].

The underlying cause of hypotension is often rooted in one or both of the following mechanisms: (1) decreased preload (caused by hypovolemia, obstructed venous return, decreased vasomotor tone or a combination) or (2) cardiac dysfunction (caused by cardiac disease, myocardial depression, arrhythmias or a combination) [28]. Although the initiating cause of hypotension can differ amongst patients, clinical signs of tissue hypoperfusion are most often similar. Specific treatment interventions vary depending on the inciting cause of hypotension, highlighting the value of an individualized approach to each animal. Serial ABP measurements are important when trending the severity of hypotension and assessing the appropriateness of therapeutic intervention.

Decreased preload

A decreased in preload (the volume of blood returning to the ventricles) can be caused by an absolute decrease in intravascular volume (hypovolemia), obstruction to venous return to the heart or a relative decrease in intravascular volume caused by decreased vasomotor tone (maldistribution of blood volume). Approximately 20–30% of the blood volume must be lost before hypotension from hypovolemia is clinically observed. Common causes of absolute decrease in intravascular volume in the ICU patient include hemorrhage, fluid loss through cutaneous evaporation (panting, fever), loss of fluid into third body fluid spaces (such as gastrointestinal tract, uterus, cavitary effusions), redistribution of blood flow away from the core,

and polyuria. Replacement of blood volume is required to resuscitate the ICU patient from any cause of hypovolemia.

Obstruction of the vena cava may not be evident on initial physical examination and is often only considered when the patient response to initial resuscitation efforts has proven inadequate. Causes of vena cava obstruction include pericardial disease (seen with tamponade, restrictive pericarditis), severe gastric distension (seen with gastric dilation-volvulus, aerophagia), increased intrathoracic pressure compressing the vena cava (seen with severe pneumothorax, positive pressure ventilation), or caval obstruction or thrombosis (seen with heartworm disease, coagulopathy). Relief of the obstruction is necessary along with intravascular volume support. Depending on the cause, procedures such as needle centesis or tube placement to decompress the pericardium, pleural space or stomach can improve venous return sufficiently to stabilize the patient during fluid resuscitation until definitive treatment can be accomplished.

Excessive vasodilation will decrease the SVR, which causes insufficient blood volume to return to the heart (relative hypovolemia). Common causes of decreased SVR in the ICU patient include drug administration, anesthetic agents, sepsis, anaphylaxis, acid–base disturbances, severe hyperthermia or hypothermia and electrolyte abnormalities. It is important to consider this as a potential contributor to hypotension as early as possible to facilitate adequate fluid volume replacement during resuscitation and to eliminate the inciting cause as quickly as possible. A list of common drugs associated with hypotension in the dog and cat is provided in Table 3.1.

A recent study in humans evaluated the prevalence of drug-induced hypotension in the ICU and found that within a 24-hour period, 23% of ICU patients had drug-induced hypotension [29]. Many of the drugs implicated in this study (propofol, fentanyl, metoprolol, lorazepam, hydralazine, and furosemide) are commonly utilized in the veterinary ICU setting. In the same study, 57% of the hypotensive events were associated with harm and 27% were considered preventable.

Hypotension is a commonly encountered complication during veterinary anesthesia and is estimated to occur in 7% of dogs and 8% of cats [35,36]. The measurement of SAP during the intraoperative period with management of hypotension has improved outcome and reduced postperative complications [35,37]. Intraoperative hypotension in veterinary patients has been defined as a SAP <87 ± 8 mmHg for surgical cases and <87 ± 6 mmHg for diagnostic cases, or MAP <62 ± 4 mmHg for both types of cases [38]. Arterial pressures reported to prompt treatment in these patients were SAP 85 ± 13 mmHg or MAP 61 ± 4 mmHg in surgical cases, and SAP 84 ± 11 mmHg or MAP 63 ± 8 mmHg in diagnostic cases requiring anesthesia [38].

Sepsis, anaphylaxis, and other SIRS-related disorders decrease SVR through the release of vasoactive substances (such as nitric oxide, histamine, prostacyclin, adenosine, platelet activating factor) that results in vasodilation and increased capillary permeability. This loss of vasomotor tone leads to maldistribution of blood flow, pooling of blood in the extremities, and a decrease in effective circulating volume. The combination of maldistribution of blood flow and hypovolemia from leakage of fluid from the capillaries causes hypotension.

A search for a site of onoing intravascular fluid loss with appropriate and rapid intervention is the first step in the resuscitation plan for hypotension from hypovolemia. Oxygen supplementation can be provided to enhance blood oxygen concentrations during resuscitation. Intravenous fluid therapy is the major component of the treatment plan (see Chapter 2). Fluids can be rapidly infused under pressure in the dog when the need for intravascular volume expansion is urgent. However, a careful incremental titration of fluid volume to reach the desired goals is required when there is a potential for ongoing hemorrhage, pulmonary or brain edema, oligoanuric renal failure or cardiac dysfunction, and in all cats.

A full blood volume is considered to be 80–90 mL/kg in dogs and 50–60 mL/kg in cats. Approximately one-quarter to one-third of this calculated amount of isotonic crystalloids can be rapidly infused as the initial IV fluid bolus when using crystalloids alone as the sole resuscitation fluid. Additional doses of isotonic crystalloids (10–30 mL/kg) can be titrated if hypotension persists. Colloids such as hydroxyethyl starch solutions (Hetastarch®, VetStarch®) may be considered with crystalloids to augment intravascular fluid retention, administered at 5–10 mL/kg IV rapidly in dogs and 5 mL/kg IV more slowly in cats; both can be repeated. The total amount of crystalloid (10–30 mL/kg) is reduced from the amount given when using crystalloids alone.

The use of hydroxyethyl starch has recently come under scrutiny for causing acute kidney injury (AKI) in humans, but it is unknown if these products have the potential to contribute to AKI in the veterinary setting. More data are needed before confirming a positive association in the dog and cat [39,40]. A maximum dose of 20 mL/kg/day in dogs of Hetastarch and 30 mL/kg/day of Vetstarch and 5–10 mL/kg/day in cats is suggested to minimize impact on coagulation [41]. Hypertonic saline (7.0–7.5% NaCl: 4–6 mL/kg IV) combined with a colloid is an option to aid in rapid intravascular volume resuscitation (see Chapter 2). In patients with decreased preload secondary to hemorrhage, blood product administration may also be required (see Chapter 10).

Hypothermia is an important component of shock in the cat. The rate of fluid infusion is reduced to maintenance rates (2–3 mL/kg/hour crystalloids) once the SBP is >60 mmHg and the cat is rapidly warmed to a body temperature >98°F (36.6°C). Crystalloids and colloids can then be titrated as needed to reach the desired goals of resuscitation while heat support is continued (see Chapter 17).

When fluid infusion alone has not been sufficient to correct hypotension, an assessment of cardiac contractility is warranted, most often assessed with echocardiography. If contractility is found to be sufficient, vasopressor agents may be required to increase vasomotor tone and normalize ABP, with the goal of improving tissue oxygenation. Drugs that can be given to support blood pressure are listed in Table 3.3 with their dose and mechanism of action. Since improved blood pressure readings may not equate with improved (organ) blood flow and subsequent delivery of oxygen, it is critical to use additional means (such as physical perfusion parameters, urine output, blood lactate, CVP) to monitor the perfusion of core organs (see Poiseuille's law – smaller radius reduces flow; Box 3.1). When treating anaphylaxis, aggressive IV fluid resuscitation and the administration of epinephrine (1:1000 concentration: 0.1–0.5 mL intramuscular or subcutaneous, repeat if necessary, in dogs and cats) is considered the treatment of choice for reversal of peracute signs of histamine-mediated cardiovascular effects.

Drug-induced hypotensive episodes can be initially managed by providing IV fluid infusion followed by discontinuation of the drug, decreased dosage or reversal of the offending drug. Blood pressure support during anesthesia is typically provided by IV fluid therapy using a combination of fluid types best suited to the patient. The anesthetic dose is reduced or a different anesthetic is administered and IV fluids are infused should hypotension occur. The surgeon can assess the distension of the vena cava, aorta, and other large vessels in an open abdomen during fluid resuscitation to determine whether intravascular volume has improved during resuscitation. Should moderate-to-severe hypotension persist during anesthesia, vasopressor agents or positive inotropes may also be required to maintain and adequate ABP and urine output (see Table 3.3).

Fluid resuscitation and other treatment modalities must be tailored to the individual needs of the patient, with concurrent hemodynamic monitoring throughout resuscitation [42]. Overzealous fluid administration can lead to widespread interstitial edema and fluid overload. Fluid overload has been shown to increase morbidity and mortality in people with deleterious effects on cardiac, pulmonary and renal function, gastrointestinal motility, tissue oxygenation, and wound healing [43]. The optimal balance between ABP goals and minimizing side-effects of fluids and drugs needs further investigation [44].

Cardiac dysfunction

Hypotension associated with cardiac dysfunction may be due to preexisting heart disease (such as valvular dysplasia, cardiomyopathy) or a transient condition associated with the underlying illness (poor contractility, cardiac arrhythmias). Reversible myocardial depression characterized by contractile dysfunction can occur in sepsis and other SIRS disorders. The mechanism of contractile dysfunction is suspected to be related to the proinflammatory mediators (such as cytokines, reactive oxygen species, nitric oxide) with secondary myocardial cellular effects (such as autonomic dysregulation, impaired myocardial cell calcium uptake and release) [45]. Approximately 60% of septic human patients were found to have left ventricular hypokinesia, potentially developing in the earliest stage of sepsis [46]. Approximately 15% of the deaths related to septic shock in humans are reported to occur secondary to myocardial depression [47].

Sepsis-related myocardial dysfunction has been reported in dogs [48,49]. Myocardial depression may be part of a larger picture relating to organ system dysfunction in critical illness. A large retrospective study of multiple organ dysfunction syndrome (MODS) in septic dogs found cardiovascular dysfunction (defined as hypotension sufficiently severe to require vasopressor treatment) in 17.5% of cases [50]. MODS, defined as dysfunction of at least two organ systems, was identified in 50% of the cases. Mortality rate increased as the number of dysfunctional organ systems increased and cardiovascular dysfunction independently increased the odds of death in this study.

The best treatment for myocardial dysfunction in sepsis or SIRS is proper management of the underlying inciting cause. The early

Table 3.3 Medications commonly used for increasing cardiac contractility and/or systemic vascular resistance.

	Clinical indication	Dose (intravenous)
Dobutamine	Decreased contractility	5–20 μg/kg/min
Dopamine	Decreased contractility; decreased vasomotor tone	5–20 μg/kg/min
Epinephrine	Decreased contractility; decreased vasomotor tone	0.05–1 μg/kg/min
Norepinephrine	Decreased vasomotor tone	0.1–2 μg/kg/min
Phenylephrine	Decreased vasomotor tone	0.5–5 μg/kg/min
Ephedrine	Decreased contractility, decreased vasomotor tone	0.1–0.25 mg/kg
Vasopressin	Decreased vasomotor tone	0.5–5 mU/kg/min

collection of blood and bodily fluids or tissues for culture and susceptibility testing in conjunction with adequate antibiotic care is critical in septic patients. Most patients will benefit from the administration of IV fluids with titration of the volume and rate of administration guided by assessment of parameters such as blood pressure, CVP, urine output, and blood lactate to indicate volume responsiveness. Poor cardiac performance can be demonstrated by echocardiography demonstrating a reduced left ventricular ejection fraction. Inotropic support is estimated to be required in only 10–20% of humans with sepsis and myocardial depression [51]. When inotropic support is needed to support cardiac output and improve hemodynamics, dobutamine (5–20 μg/kg/min IV by constant rate infusion (CRI)) is the first drug of choice. The ECG is monitored and arrhythmias treated that are deemed to affect cardiac or contribute to hypotension (see Chapter 11). Patients may have a poor response to beta-adrenergics due to myocardial depression.

An alternative drug used in humans is levosimendan, a calcium-sensitizing drug with inotropic and vasodilatory effects. A study comparing levosimendan to dobutamine in people in septic shock found levosimendan to have positive effects on both cardiovascular performance and regional perfusion [52]. Research using dogs found that levosimendan (10 μg/kg followed by 0.125–1.0 μg/kg/minute CRI) and fluid volume support with hydroxyethyl starch increased gastric mucosal oxygenation better than milrinone and dobutamine given with similar volume support [53]. Further studies are needed to evaluate the effect, benefits, and side-effects of levosimendan in dogs and cats.

Nonresponsive hypotension

Nonresponsive hypotension is diagnosed when the initial resuscitation efforts have failed to adequately improve the ABP and perfusion status of the patient. Cardiac function should be assessed and specific treatment provided as indicated to optimize cardiac performance (see Chapter 11).

One of the more common causes of nonresponsive hypotension is an inability to maintain appropriate volume within the intravascular space to effectively improve the preload to the heart. Conditions such as ongoing hemorrhage, vasodilation of blood vessels, increased capillary permeability, third body fluid spacing, polyuria, and inadequate fluid therapy planning can all contribute to insufficient vascular volume in spite of the amount of fluid infused. Monitoring the trends of change in the CVP can provide an indication of increases in pressure of the central veins resulting from fluid infusion. Targeting a CVP of 8–10 cmH$_2$O is reasonable when there is no evidence of ongoing hemorrhage or brain or lung edema in the patient. A fluid challenge can be given (5–10 mL/kg of colloid IV or 10–30 mL/kg of crystalloid if using alone) while monitoring for evidence of improvement in ABP and CVP in patients that are not intolerant of fluids. An improvement in ABP and CVP implies that intravascular volume is an issue and careful titration of additional fluids is indicated. A poor response to the initial fluid challenge may necessitate repeating the fluid challenge dose one additional time. Further lack of response directs a search for other contributing causes.

While monitoring the trend of change in the CVP is a readily accessible tool, the results may not directly equate with the preload status or volume responsiveness of the patient. Other methods for assessing intravascular volume status can be used, such as echocardiographic parameters (including vena cava diameter/collapse), and newer techniques such as Vigileo monitors and bioimpedance vector analysis may ultimately be of use in the future.

Systemic factors can also be responsible for the occurrence of nonresponsive hypotension. Hypoglycemia, severe acidemia or alkalemia, hypoxemia, hypercarbia, hypocarbia, cardiac arrhythmias, central nervous system disorders, medications, and electrolyte disorders are considered. Adverse effects of acute metabolic acidosis include decreased cardiac output, arterial dilation with hypotension, and predisposition to arrhythmias [54]. Severe hypoxemia (PaO$_2$ < 40 mmHg) may contribute to hypotension through local vasodilation of the tissue bed being perfused with hypoxic blood [55]. Many systemic factors can be identified through POC testing of arterial blood gas, blood glucose and electrolyte profile, repeating the physical and neurological examination and evaluating an ECG. Immediate therapeutic intervention is warranted when a potential contributing problem has been identified and is coupled with vigorous monitoring of ABP and CVP.

Poor ABP response to vasopressors may also be related to an endocrine condition known in humans as critical illness-related corticosteroid insufficiency (CIRCI; also called relative adrenal insufficiency). It has been described in critically ill humans with systemic inflammation that is causing tissue resistance to endogenous glucocorticoids [56]. Cortisol concentrations can be normal or high but still inadequate for a normal response to the physiological stress of illness [57]. The hallmark signs of CIRCI are hypotension refractory to fluid resuscitation and poor ABP response to vasopressor therapy. Although CIRCI is considered a transient condition, intervention with corticosteroids at physiological to supraphysiological doses (0.25–1 mg/kg IV q 24 h of prednisone equivalent) has been beneficial for effectively treating the hypotension of an affected patient. Evidence that dogs and cats experience CIRCI is provided within the veterinary literature [58–60], but the criteria for diagnosis as well as the most appropriate dose of corticosteroids are still uncertain at this time.

Hypertension

Systemic hypertension is a sustained elevation in ABP (≥150/95) and is generally categorized in veterinary medicine into three types related to cause. The first category is anxiety-induced hypertension (also termed "white coat" hypertension) caused by the autonomic response to excitement, stress or anxiety. At present, there is no justification for treating this specific type of hypertension in the dog and cat [15]. Idiopathic hypertension (also called *primary* or *essential hypertension*) is diagnosed in animals with high ABP occurring in the absence of an overt, clinically apparent disease known to cause hypertension. Secondary hypertension is the third type assigned to animals with high ABP and concurrent clinical disease, medications or other conditions known to cause hypertension. Renal disease, hyperthyroidism, pheochromocytoma, diabetes mellitus, hyperadrenocorticism, and hyperaldosteronism are diseases known to exacerbate secondary hypertension [61]. Less common diseases associated with hypertension include hepatic disease, polycythemia, chronic anemia, congestive heart failure, and neoplasia. Medications such as catecholamines, phenylpropanolamine, corticosteroids, and erythropoietin may also play a role in the development of secondary hypertension.

Hypertension can be detrimental to tissues, resulting in end-organ damage with significant morbidity. Tissues at highest risk of target organ damage (TOD) include the kidney (enhanced rate of decline in renal function), eye (retinopathy, choroidopathy), brain (encephalopathy, stroke), and heart and blood vessels (ventricular hypertrophy, gallop rhythm, arrhythmias, cardiac failure) [15]. The degree and duration of hypertension will determine the extent of

TOD, with acute ocular and neurological injury occurring at SAP ≥180 mmHg [61].

Diagnosis of hypertension should be based on reliable, repeatable measurements of ABP. It is important to rule out measurement artifact and stress-induced hypertension before definitively diagnosing a patient with idiopathic or secondary hypertension. Further categorization of hypertension is then performed based upon the risk of developing TOD. Risk of TOD is considered minimal when ABP <150/95 mmHg with this minimal risk category providing the targeted treatment goal for antihypertensive therapy. Mild risk is assigned when the ABP is 150–159/95–99 mmHg. Careful monitoring is the mainstay of antihypertensive treatment for this category of patient. Moderate risk is when ABP is 160–179/100–119 mmHg, with most animals in this category candidates for antihypertensive therapy. Severe risk is when ABP is ≥180/120 mmHg [15], demonstrated during at least two measurement sessions. Animals assigned to this category will receive antihypertensive therapy and appropriate disease-specific management of the underlying cause.

Immediate and more aggressive treatment can be required for patients in the severe risk category if the hypertension is causing rapid and progressive TOD (termed hypertensive emergencies), such as seen with hypertensive choriodopathy and encephalopathy. Those with severe hypertension that lack evidence of TOD are termed "hypertensive urgencies" [62]. If choroidopathy or encephalopathy is identified, emergency intervention using antihypertensive medications should be provided using a short-acting, intravenous antihypertensive agent titrated to the desired effect. Hypertensive urgencies are usually treated with oral antihypertensive agents [63,64].

Rapid-acting intravenous antihypertensive agents (Table 3.4) such as labetolol (0.25 mg/kg IV over 2 minutes, repeated up to 3.75 mg/kg total dose, then 25 μg/kg/min CRI), esmolol (50–75 μg/kg/min CRI), enalaprilat (0.2 mg/kg IV q 1–2 h as needed) or hydralazine (0.2 mg/kg IV or IM, q 2 h as needed) are preferred when available [15]. Newer injectable agents, such as fenoldopam and clevidipine, have been used with good success in hypertensive people but require further clinical investigation in veterinary medicine. The effects of rapid-acting, titratable drugs should be monitored using dABP measurement when possible. When injectable drugs are not available, oral drugs with a quick onset of action (amlodipine besylate 0.1–0.25 mg/kg q 24 h, up to 0.5 mg/kg q 24 h if needed) may be used.

Long-term management of hypertension includes addressing the underlying disease when applicable, avoidance of high dietary sodium chloride intake and pharmacological intervention. Angiotensin-converting enzyme inhibitors (ACEi), angiotensin receptor blockers, and aldosterone receptor blockers interfere with the renin-angiotensin-aldosterone hormonal system that promotes water retention and increased preload. The ACEi drugs also dilate the renal efferent arteriole and lower intraglomerular pressure, thereby decreasing proteinuria and glomerular filtration. In dogs, ACEi drugs (enalapril 0.5 mg/kg q 12–24 h dogs, q 24 h cats; benazepril 0.5 mg/kg q 12–24 h dogs, q 12 h cats) are considered first-line agents for treatment of hypertension, but are often avoided in patients with concurrent azotemia. Calcium channel blockers (CCB) are the first choice for antihypertensive therapy in cats and may be added as a second antihypertensive in dogs. The CCBs (amlodipine besylate 0.1–0.25 mg/kg q 24 h in dogs, 0.1–0.5 mg/kg in cats) are direct vasodilators that effectively lower ABP in animals with a relatively long duration of action. These drugs also help balance the effects of ACEi drugs on the kidney by decreasing afferent arteriole pressure and therefore stabilizing glomerular filtration.

Follow-up evaluations should be scheduled following the initiation of treatment for hypertension. In nonemergent cases, at least seven days should elapse before a medication dose is changed or a new antihypertensive medication is added [61]. Repeat ABP measurement, fundoscopic evaluation, and laboratory parameters (to include renal and electrolyte values, urinalysis) can help guide medication adjustments. Routine evaluations may then be scheduled every 1–4 months, depending on the underlying disease and stability of the documented hypertension.

Pheochromocytoma

Pheochromocytoma can induce severe hypertension, leading to TOD. Chromaffin cells from the adrenal medulla secrete an abnormally high amount of epinephrine, norepinephrine or both. Hypertension and arrhythmias are a life-threatening consequence, particularly in the perioperative period, with high mortality rates reported [62]. Treatment with phenoxybenzamine (0.6 mg/kg q 12 h PO) instituted several days to weeks prior to surgery for adrenalectomy has resulted in a significant decrease in mortality (48% mortality without phenoxybenzamine compared to 13% mortality with phenoxybenzamine) [62]. Phenoxybenzamine is given to reduce systemic vasoconstriction and the TOD caused by the circulating catecholamines. The goal is to restore normal vascular tone and therefore normal blood volume prior to the induction of anesthesia. During anesthesia for adrenalectomy in a dog with pheochromocytoma, the blood pressure should not be allowed to decline more than 25% lower than preoperative values to maintain adequate organ perfusion. Surgical manipulation of the adrenal tumor may cause tachyarrhythmias and hypertension. The administration of injectable vasodilating drugs as outlined for severe hypertension (see Table 3.4) may be required.

Table 3.4 Medications commonly used to treat hypertension.

Drug	Dose
Injectable medications	
Enalaprilat	0.2 mg/kg IV q 1–2 h
Esmolol	0.05–0.1 mg/kg 50–200 μg/kg/min CRI
Hydralazine	0.2 mg/kg IV q 2 h
Labetalol	0.25 mg/kg IV over 2 min, repeated to up 3.75 mg/kg total dose 25 μg/kg/min CRI
Phentolamine	0.02–0.1 mg/kg IV
Sodium nitroprusside	2–15 μg/kg/min CRI
Oral medications	
Amlodipine	0.1–0.25 mg/kg q 24 h dog 0.1–0.5 mg/kg q 24 h cat
Benazepril	0.5 mg/kg q 12–24 h
Enalapril	0.5 mg/kg q 12–24 h
Phenoxybenzamine	0.2–15 mg/kg q 12 h 10–20 days prior to surgery

References

1. Stepien RL, Rapoport GS. Clinical comparison of three methods to measure blood pressure in nonsedated dogs. J Am Vet Med Assoc. 1999;215:1623–8.
2. Brown S, Langford K, Tarver S. Effects of pharmacological agents on diurnal pattern of blood pressure, heart rate, and motor activity in cats. Am J Vet Res. 1997; 58:647–52.

3. Darovic GO. Arterial pressure monitoring. In: Hemodynamic Monitoring: Invasive and Noninvasive Clinical Application. Darovic GO, ed. Philadelphia: Saunders, 2002: pp 133–60.

4. Hall JE. Guyton and Hall Textbook of Medical Physiology. Philadelphia: Elsevier, 2011: pp 165–6, 319–21, 744–5.

5. Bodey AR, Michell AR. Epidemiological study of blood pressure in domestic dogs. J Small Anim Pract. 1996;37;116–25.

6. Flynn A, Mani BC, Mather PJ. Sepsis-induced cardiomyopathy: a review of pathophysiologic mechanisms. Heart Fail Rev. 2010;15(6):605–11.

7. Burkitt Creedon JM, Raffe MR. Fluid-filled hemodynamic monitoring systems. In: Advanced Monitoring and Procedures for Small Animal Emergency and Critical Care. Burkitt Creedon JM, Davis H, eds. Ames: John Wiley & Sons, 2012: pp 107–21.

8. Hamzaoui O, Monnet X, Teboul JL. Pulsus paradoxus. Eur Respir J. 2013;42: 1696–705.

9. Morgan BC, Martin WE, Hornbien TF, et al. Hemodynamic effects of intermittent positive pressure respiration. Anesthesiology 1966;27:584–90.

10. Perel A, Pizov R, Cotev S. Systolic blood pressure variation is a sensitive indicator of hypovolemia in ventilated dogs subjected to graded hemorrhage. Anesthesiology 1987;67:498–502.

11. Cooper E, Cooper S. Direct systemic arterial blood pressure monitoring. In: Advanced Monitoring and Procedures for Small Animal Emergency and Critical Care. Burkitt Creedon JM, Davis H, eds. Ames: John Wiley & Sons, 2012: pp.122–33.

12. 12.Cherpanath TG, Aarts LP, Groeneveld JA, et al. Defining fluid responsiveness: a guide to patient-tailored volume titration. J Cardiothor Vasc Anesth. 2014;28(3):745–54.

13. Michard F, Boussat S, Chemla D, et al. Relation between respiratory changes in arterial pulse pressure and fluid responsiveness in septic patients with acute circulatory failure. Am J Respir Crit Care Med. 2000;162:134–38.

14. Perel A, Pizov R, Cotev S. Respiratory variations in the arterial pressure during mechanical ventilation reflect volume status and fluid responsiveness. Intensive Care Med. 2014;40:798–807.

15. Brown S, Atkins C, Bagley R, et al. Guidelines for the identification, evaluation, and management of systemic hypertension in dogs and cats. J Vet Intern Med. 2007;21:542–58.

16. Chetboul V, Tissier R, Gouni V, et al. Comparison of Doppler ultrasonography and high-definition oscillometry for blood pressure measurements in healthy awake dogs. Am J Vet Res. 2010;71(7):766–72.

17. Sparkes AH, Caney SM, King MC, et al. Inter- and intraindividual variation in Doppler ultrasonic indirect blood pressure measurement in healthy cats. J Vet Intern Med. 1999;13:314–18.

18. Erhardt W, Henke J, Carr A, et al. Techniques. In: Essential Facts of Blood Pressure in Dogs and Cats. Egner B, Carr A, Brown S, eds. Guelph: Lifelearn Inc., 2007: pp 28–65.

19. Martel E, Egner B, Brown SA, et al. Comparison of high-definition oscillometry: a non-invasive technology for arterial blood pressure measurement with a direct invasive method using radio-telemetry in awake health cats. J Feline Med Surg. 2013;15(12):1104–13.

20. Allen J. Photoplethysmography and its application in clinical physiological measurement. Physiol Meas. 2007;28:R1–R39.

21. McGrath SP, Ryan KL, Wendelken SM, et al. Pulse oximeter plethysmographic waveform changes in awake, spontaneously breathing, hypovolemic volunteers. Anesth Analg. 2011;112:368–74.

22. Dyson SH. Indirect measurement of blood pressure using a pulse oximeter in isoflurane anesthetized dogs. J Vet Emerg Crit Care 2007;17(2):135–42.

23. Caulkett NA, Cantwell SL, Houston DM. A comparison of indirect blood pressure monitoring techniques in the anesthetized cat. Vet Surg. 1998;27:370–7.

24. Binns SH, Sisson DD, Buoscio DA, et al. Doppler ultrasonographic, oscillometric sphygmomanometric, and photoplethysmographic techniques for noninvasive blood pressure measurement in anesthetized cats. J Vet Intern Med. 1995;9:405–14.

25. Tuburu H, Watanabe H, Tanaka M, et al. Non-invasive measurement of systemic arterial pressure by Finapres in anesthetized dogs. Jpn J Vet Sci. 1990;52(2):427–30.

26. Cariou A, Monchi M, Dhainaut JF. Continuous cardiac output and mixed venous oxygen saturation monitoring. J Crit Care 1998;13(4):198–213.

27. Young BC, Prittie JE, Fox P, et al. Decreased central venous oxygen saturation despite normalization of heart rate and blood pressure post shock resuscitation in sick dogs. J Vet Emerg Crit Care 2014;24(2):154–61.

28. Waddell LS. Hypotension. In: Textbook of Veterinary Internal Medicine. Ettinger SJ, Feldman EC, eds. St Louis: Elsevier, 2010: pp 585–8.

29. Kane-Gill SL, LeBlanc JM, Dasta JF, et al. A multicenter study of the point prevalence of drug-induced hypotension in the ICU. Crit Care Med. 2014;42:2197–203.

30. Winchell RJ, Simons RK, Hoyt DB. Transient systolic hypotension. A serious problem in the management of head injury. Arch Surg. 1996;131:533–9.

31. Zenati MS, Billiar TR, Townsend RN, et al: A brief episode of hypotension increases mortality in critically ill trauma patients. J Trauma 2002; 53:232–6.

32. Dünser MW, Takala J, Ulmer H, et al. Arterial blood pressure during early sepsis and outcome. Intensive Care Med. 2009;35:1225–33.

33. Jones AE, Yiannibas V, Johnson C, et al. Emergency department hypotension predicts sudden unexpected in-hospital mortality: a prospective cohort study. Chest 2006;130(4):941–6.

34. Silverstein DC, Wininger FA, Shofer FS, et al. Relationship between Doppler blood pressure and survival or response to treatment in critically ill cats: 83 cases (2003–2004). J Am Vet Med Assoc. 2008;232(6):893–7.

35. Mazzaferro E, Wagner AE. Hypotension during anesthesia in dogs and cats: recognition, causes, and treatment. Compend Contin Educ Pract. 2001;23:728–37.

36. Gaynor JS, Dunlop CI, Wagner AE, et al. Complications and mortality associated with anesthesia in dogs and cats. J Am Anim Hosp Assoc. 1999;35:13–17.

37. Monk TG, Saini V, Weldon BC, et al. Anesthetic management and one-year mortality after noncardiac surgery. Anesth Analg. 2005;100:4–10.

38. Ruffato M, Novello L, Clark L. What is the definition of intraoperative hypotension in dogs? Results from a survey of diplomats of the ACVAA and ECVAA. Vet Anaesth Analg. 2015;42:55–64.

39. Perel P, Roberts I, Ker K. Colloids versus crystalloids for fluid resuscitation in critically ill patients. Cochrane Database Syst Rev. 2013;28:CD000567.

40. Bayer O, Reinhart K, Kohl M, et al. Effects of fluid resuscitation with synthetic colloids or crystalloids alone on shock reversal, fluid balance, and patient outcomes in patients with severe sepsis: a prospective sequential analysis. Crit Care Med. 2012;40:2543–51.

41. McBride D, Hosgood GL, Mansfield CS, Smart L. Effect of hydroxyethyl starch 130/0.4 and 200/0.5 solution on canine platelet function in vitro. Am J Vet Res. 2013;74(8):1133–7.

42. Butler AL. Goal-directed therapy in small animal critical illness. Vet Clin Small Anim. 2001;41:817–38.

43. Prowle JR, Echeverri JE, Ligabo EV, et al. Fluid balance and acute kidney injury. Nature Rev Nephrol. 2010;6:107–15.

44. Sevransky JE, Nour S, Susla GM, et al. Hemodynamic goals in randomized clinical trials in patients with sepsis: a systematic review of the literature. Crit Care 2007;11:R67.

45. Fernandez CJ, Cesar de Assuncao MS. Myocardial dysfunction in sepsis: unsolved puzzle. Crit Care Res Pract. 2012;896430.

46. Vieillard-Baron A, Caille V, Charron C, et al. Actual incidence of global left ventricular hypokinesia in adult septic shock. Crit Care Med. 2008;36(6):1701–6.

47. Parrillo JE. The cardiovascular pathophysiology of sepsis. Ann Rev Med. 1989;40:469–85.

48. Nelson OL, Thompson PA. Cardiovascular dysfunction in dogs associated with critical illnesses. J Am Anim Hosp Assoc. 2006;42(5):344–9.

49. Dickinson AE, Rozanski EA, Jush RE. Reversible myocardial depression associated with sepsis in a dog. J Vet Intern Med. 2007;21(5):1117-20.

50. Kenney EM, Rozanski EA, Rush JE, et al. Association between outcome and organ system dysfunction in dogs with sepsis: 114 cases (2003–2007). J Am Vet Med Assoc. 2010;236(1):83–7.

51. Rivers E, Nguyen B, Havstad S, et al. Early goal directed therapy in the treatment of severe sepsis and septic shock. N Engl J Med. 2001;345:1368–77.

52. Morelli S, DeCastro JL, Teboul J, et al. Effects of levosimendan on systemic and regional hemodynamics in septic myocardial depression. Intensive Care Med. 2003;31:638–44.

53. Schwarte LA, Picker O. Levosimendan is superior to milrinone and dobutamine in selectively increasing microvascular gastric mucosal oxygenation in dogs. Crit Care Med. 2005;33(1):135.

54. Kraut JA, Madias NE. Metabolic acidosis: pathophysiology, diagnosis, and management. Nat Rev Nephrol. 2010;6(5):274–85.

55. Heistad DD, Abboud FM. Circulatory adjustments to hypoxia. Circulation 1980;61:463–70.

56. Marik PE. Critical illness-related corticosteroid insufficiency. Chest 2009;135(1):181–93.

57. Martin LG. Critical illness-related corticosteroid insufficiency in small animals. Vet Clin Small Anim. 2001;41:767–82.

58. Burkitt JM, Haskins SC, Nelson RW, et al. Relative adrenal insufficiency in dogs with sepsis. J Vet Intern Med. 2007;21(2):226–31.

59. Martin LG, Groman RP, Fletcher DJ, et al. Pituitary-adrenal function in dogs with acute critical illness. J Am Vet Med Assoc. 2008;233(1):87–95.

60. Durkan S, de Laforcade A, Rozanski E. Suspected relative adrenal insufficiency in a critically ill cat. J Vet Emerg Crit Care 2007;17:197–201.

61. Stepien RL. Systemic hypertension. In: Kirk's Current Veterinary Therapy XV. Bonagura J, Twedt J, eds. St Louis: Elsevier, 2013: pp 726–30.

62. Herrera MA, Mehl PH, Kass PJ, et al. Predictive factors and the effect of phenoxybenzamine on outcome in dogs undergoing adrenalectomy for phenochromocytoma. J Vet Intern Med. 2008;22:1333.

63. Marik PE, Varon J. Hypertensive crises – challenges and management. Chest 2007;131:1949–62.

64. Varon J. Treatment of acute severe hypertension: current and newer agents. Drugs 2008;68(3):283–97.

Further reading

Burkitt Creedon JM, Raffe MR. Fluid-filled hemodynamic monitoring systems. In: Advanced Monitoring and Procedures for Small Animal Emergency and Critical Care. Burkitt Creedon JM, Davis H, eds. Ames: John Wiley & Sons, 2012: pp 107–21.

Cooper E, Cooper S. Direct systemic arterial blood pressure monitoring. In: Advanced Monitoring and Procedures for Small Animal Emergency and Critical Care. Burkitt Creedon JM, Davis H, eds. Ames: John Wiley & Sons, 2012: pp 122–33.

Egner B, Carr A, Brown S, eds. Essential Facts of Blood Pressure in Dogs and Cats. Babenhausen: VBS Vet Verlag, 2007.

Hopper K, Brown S. Hypertensive crisis. In: Small Animal Critical Care Medicine. Silverstein DC, Hopper K, eds. St Louis: Elsevier, 2015: pp 51–54.

Mazzaferro EM. Arterial catheterization. In: Small Animal Critical Care Medicine. Silverstein DC, Hopper K, eds. St Louis: Elsevier, 2015: pp 1040–3.

Waddell LS. Hypotension. In: Textbook of Veterinary Internal Medicine. Ettinger SJ, Feldman EC, eds. St Louis: Elsevier, 2010: pp 585–8.

Williamson JA, Leone S. Noninvasive arterial blood pressure monitoring. In: Advanced Monitoring and Procedures for Small Animal Emergency and Critical Care. Burkitt Creedon JM, Davis H, eds. Ames: John Wiley & Sons, 2012: pp 134–44.

CHAPTER 4

Albumin and colloid osmotic pressure

Adesola Odunayo

University of Tennessee, Knoxville, Tennessee

Introduction

Albumin has been found to be a nonspecific marker of critical illness [1]. The albumin level alone is of limited use in reaching a diagnosis for the patient. However, it has been found to be an important prognostic indicator of morbidity and mortality in critical veterinary and human patients. Unfortunately, the simple replacement of an albumin deficit has not been found to consistently improve survival. This suggests that the complex mechanisms underlying the alteration in serum albumin are of equal importance. A change in serum albumin will result in a corresponding change in the intravascular colloid osmotic pressure (COP). The COP has therefore also been demonstrated to be a prognostic indicator of pulmonary edema and mortality in human patients, with a low COP associated with an increased morbidity and mortality [2].

Albumin is the main protein of blood plasma, being small with a molecular weight of 65 000–69 000 daltons in the dog and cat. Box 4.1 provides the normal serum albumin concentration for those species. Highly water soluble, this elliptical shaped and flexible molecule has a strong net negative charge. It is made in the liver, with only 20–30% of the hepatocytes producing albumin at any one time. It is not stored, so cannot be released on demand. The primary factor controlling the rate of production is a change in the COP (also called oncotic pressure) and the osmolarity within the extravascular liver spaces [3]. Albumin synthesis is proportional to the hepatic interstitial COP. During maximal stimulus for production, the rate of synthesis increases only 2–3-fold. Albumin is catabolized in or adjacent to the vascular endothelium of tissues at a daily rate similar to the daily rate of production. Breakdown of albumin involves uptake into endocytotic vesicles after binding to endothelial surface membrane scavenger receptors. These receptors are widespread in the tissues [4]. The vesicles then fuse with lysosomes for degradation within the endothelial cells. Figure 4.1 depicts the major contributing factors responsible for the plasma albumin concentration.

Albumin is primarily an extravascular protein, with the largest quantity (grams) found in the interstitium (also known as the "albumin pool"). However, due to a wider distribution, the interstitium has a lower concentration (g/L) of albumin than the plasma. There is normal circulation of albumin between the intravascular space and the interstitial space through the lymphatic vessels. The movement of albumin through the capillary walls is called transcapillary escape, and is determined by the capillary, subglycocalyx, and interstitial free albumin concentrations, capillary permeability, solvent and solute movements, and electrical charge across the capillary wall [5]. Lymphatic flow is dependent upon interstitial fluid pressure, intrinsic lymphatic pumping, and external compression of the lymph vessels by muscle contraction, arterial pulsation, and body movement.

The role of albumin is complex and multifaceted, and includes:
- binding and transport
- maintenance of COP
- free radical scavenging
- platelet function inhibition and antithrombotic effects
- effects on vascular permeability [6,7].

Referred to as a molecular "taxi," albumin binds water, cations (such as calcium (Ca^{++}), copper (Cu^{++}) sodium (Na^+) and potassium (K^+)), fatty acids, hormones, bilirubin, thyroxine (T4), and drugs. Though it has a strong negative charge, it can bind weakly to both cations and anions. There are four discrete binding sites on one albumin molecule, with ligands competing at a single site or altering their affinity for a remote binding site [7]. Drugs that compete for binding at a single site can displace one another, affecting drug concentration and potency. The binding of a drug to albumin will greatly affect the delivery of the drug to tissue sites, and the metabolism and elimination of the drug.

Roughly 65–80% of the normal COP results from the presence of albumin, due to both its strong oncotic effect and negative charge. Colloid osmotic pressure is the force generated when two solutions with different concentrations of colloids (macromolecules, primarily albumin) are separated by a semipermeable membrane [8]. Sodium ions are noncovalently bound to albumin, contributing to the osmotic effect of that protein molecule; this is known as the Gibbs–Donnan effect [9]. The total oncotic pressure of an average capillary is about 21–25 mmHg in the dog and cat, with albumin contributing approximately 78% of this oncotic pressure. The remainder of intravascular COP is due to the concentration of globulins, fibrinogen, and hemoglobin, and, to a lesser degree, red blood cells (RBCs).

Classically, the mechanism of transvascular fluid exchange has been described by Starling forces [10] (Box.4.2), which include the capillary pore size (interendothelial cell space) and

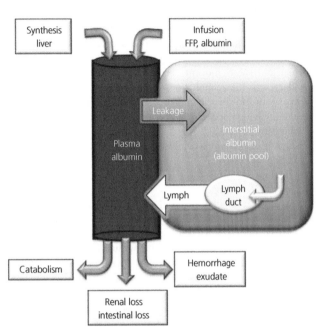

Figure 4.1 Mechanisms of albumin gain, loss, and distribution. The quantity of albumin in the plasma is provided through synthesis by the hepatocytes or by administration of exogenous albumin or fresh frozen plasma (FFP) which contains albumin. Albumin will leak through the endothelial glycocalyx layer when the interendothelial gaps permit and contribute to the interstitial concentration of albumin (also known as the "albumin pool"). Interstitial albumin will move into the blood through the lymphatics. Albumin loss from the body occurs through catabolism, renal or intestinal loss or loss through hemorrhage or exudation (such as burns, wounds, effusions). Source: modified from Margarson M, Soni N. Serum albumin: touchstone or totem? Anesthesia 1998:53,789–803.

Box 4.2 The Starling equation.

$J_v = K_f([P_c - P_i] - \sigma[\pi_c - \pi_i])$ where:
J_v is the net fluid movement between compartments
$[P_c - P_i] - \sigma[\pi_c - \pi_i]$ is the net driving force
P_c is the capillary hydrostatic pressure
P_i is the interstitial hydrostatic pressure
π_c is the capillary oncotic pressure
π_i is the interstitial oncotic pressure
K_f is the filtration coefficient – a proportionality constant
σ is the reflection coefficient

the hydrostatic pressure and oncotic pressure differences across the capillary endothelial barrier. The discovery of the endothelial glycocalyx layer (EGL) has led to the proposal of a revision of the Starling principle, often termed the glycocalyx model [11] (Figure 4.2). Some of the major differences between the original Starling principle and the glycocalyx model are listed in Table 4.1.

The EGL is a web of membrane-bound glycoproteins and proteoglycans positioned on the luminal side of the endothelial cells throughout the vasculature [12]. It has a net negative charge and acts as a macromolecular sieve [13]. It is semipermeable to anionic macromolecules, such as albumin, and when healthy, impermeable to RBCs and molecules greater than 70 000 daltons. The EGL regulates vascular permeability, influences blood cell-vessel wall interactions, affects rheology, and controls the vascular microenvironment [14]. Because it lies on top of the vascular endothelial cells, the EGL creates a subglycocalyx intercellular space that has its own COP established by albumin within that space. The oncotic forces, in this model, are only set up across this endothelial surface layer on the luminal aspect of the endothelial cell, not across the whole capillary wall [15].

While intravascular and subglycocalyx albumin is still a major component of COP and fluid movement, the interstitial albumin concentration does not affect transcapillary fluid movement in this model. Breaks within the interendothelial cell junctions constitute the primary pathway for transvascular fluid filtration from the capillary. Albumin has an oncotic role across the EGL and the COP difference opposes but does not reverse transcapillary flow. In this model, fluid does not enter the capillary from the interstitium (except in the intestines, brain, and kidneys) but instead by way of lymphatic deposition of fluid into the venous system. Figure 4.2 provides a schematic summary of the Starling forces and glycocalyx model of transcapillary fluid dynamics.

As a free radical scavenger, the sulfhydryl groups of albumin will scavenge reactive oxygen and nitrogen species, such as superoxide, hydroxyl, and peroxynitrite radicals. Albumin can also limit their production by binding free Cu^{++}, which is known as an accelerant in free radical production [16,17].

Many critical small animals patients have lost albumin as a consequence of their underlying disease but present to the ICU with a normal initial blood albumin value and COP. This can be due to dehydration as well as redistribution of albumin from the interstitial "albumin pool" into the blood through the lymphatics. This can delay the recognition of albumin and COP disorders until serious consequences have occurred. A marked decrease in the COP can eventually result in interstitial or pulmonary edema and arterial hypotension causing poor tissue perfusion [2,18,19]. The administration of crystalloid fluids can dilute blood albumin concentrations, raise capillary hydrostatic pressure, and lower intravascular COP, making therapy an important additional inciting factor. Albumin is also a negative acute-phase protein, meaning that hepatic production of albumin drops when systemic inflammation is present. The administration of various drugs can cause an increase or decrease in blood albumin (Table 4.2). It is important to identify and monitor patients that are likely to have a problem affecting albumin concentrations and the COP to minimize complications and maximize therapy.

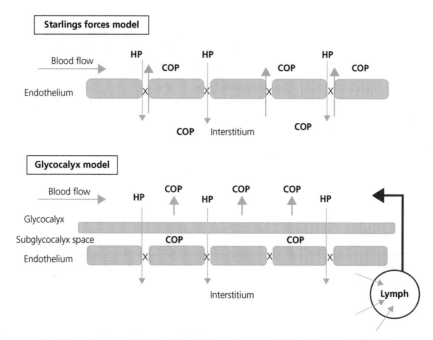

Figure 4.2 Schematic comparing the Starling forces model of capillary fluid movement to the glycocalyx model. The arrows represent the directional movement of water, with thicker arrows representing greater force or flow in the direction of the arrow under normal circumstances. Capillary hydrostatic pressure (HP) is a result of blood pressure, cardiac output, and intravascular fluid volume. The interstitial tissues have HP that opposes the capillary HP but does not reverse the fluid dynamics until there is a significant increase of interstitial pressure, such as with large quantities of interstitial edema. The HP plays a similar role in both models. The colloidal osmotic pressure (COP) is primarily generated by albumin in both models. The Starling model has the intravascular COP opposed by the interstitial COP. When plasma albumin concentration is normal, the driving force of COP retains fluid in the vasculature. When intravascular COP is higher than the interstitial COP, water will move from the interstitium into the intravascular space. The glycocalyx model shows that the COP force opposing the intravascular COP is due to the presence of albumin in the subglycocalyx space, with the amount of albumin in this space determined by the porosity of the glycocalyx "meshwork" and the charge of the glycocalyx layer. In both models, the size and type of molecule that leaves the capillary are dependent upon the reflection coefficient of the vessel, the type of interendothelial junction (shown as X), and the charge. In the glycocalyx model, fluid re-enters the vasculature through the lymphatics rather than directly from the interstitium.

Table 4.1 Differences between the original Starling principle and the glycocalyx model of capillary fluid dynamics.

Concept	Original Starling principle	Glycocalyx model
Composition of intravascular volume	Plasma and cellular elements	Glycocalyx, plasma, red cell distribution volume
Separation of intravascular from interstitial volume	Capillaries with high COP (proteins) within and ISF with lower COP (protein)	EGL semipermeable to anionic proteins with higher COP within and interendothelial clefts below with lower COP (proteins)
Site of fluid absorption	Along the capillary, magnified at venous end based on IV and ISF COP concentration difference	Continuous capillaries exhibit no absorption; fluid returned to vasculature via lymphatics
Important forces	Transendothelial (HP) pressure differences and plasma-interstitial COP difference	Transendothelial pressure difference and plasma-subglycocalyx COP difference; COP of ISF is not a direct determinant of transendothelial flow
Effect of raising COP within the capillary	Enhances absorption and shifts fluid from interstitial space to plasma	Reduced transcapillary flow but does not cause absorption
Effect of subnormal capillary pressure (HP)	Net transcapillary absorption increases plasma volume	Transcapillary flow approaches 0; any autotransfusion is acute and limited in quantity
Effect of supranormal capillary pressure (HP)	Net transcapillary filtration increases ISF volume	Transcapillary flow is proportional to transendothelial pressure differences (when COP difference is maximal)
Effect of infused colloid solution and isotonic crystalloid	Colloid distributed through plasma volume; crystalloid through the extracellular volume (IV and ISF)	Initially same as Starling's model. At supranormal HP, colloid preserves COP, raises HP, increases transcapillary flow. At supranormal HP isotonic crystalloid raises HP, lowers COP and increases transcapillary flow more than colloid. At subnormal HP, colloid increases plasma volume and crystalloids increase intravascular volume but transcapillary flow is low for both fluids

COP, colloid osmotic pressure; EGL, endothelial glycocalyx layer; HP, hydrostatic pressure; ISF, interstitial fluid; IV, intravascular.
Adapted from Woodcock TE, Woodcock TM. Revised Starling equation and the glycocalyx model of transvascular fluid exchange: an improved paradign for prescribinb intravenous fluid therapy. Br J Anaesth. 2012;108(3):384–94.

Table 4.2 Drugs and plasma albumin.

Drugs that increase plasma albumin concentrations	Drugs that decrease plasma albumin concentrations	Drugs that bind to albumin
Anabolic steroids	Crystalloid fluids	NSAIDS
Androgens	Synthetic colloid fluids	Sedatives
Growth hormone		Antiepileptics
Insulin		Digoxin
Albumin concentrates		Antibiotics
Fresh frozen plasma		Anticoagulants
Frozen plasma		Steroids
Whole blood		Furosemide
		Glucose
		Thyroxine
		Amino acids
		Vitamins
		Folate
		Vitamin D

NSAID, nonsteroidal antiinflammatory drug.

Diagnostic testing and monitoring

Diagnostic testing to identify disorders of albumin and the COP should begin with the patient history, physical examination, and the minimum laboratory database done by point of care (POC) cage-side testing. Additional clinicopathological testing, diagnostic imaging, and equipment-based monitoring can provide insight into the cause and consequences of alterations in these important parameters.

History and physical examination

The history begins with the signalment (age, sex, breed). Age-related changes in albumin values cause younger and geriatric animals to have a lower normal albumin concentration (see Box 4.1). Problems that can result in the loss of albumin may have a breed predilection, to include proteinuria in breeds such as Doberman Pinscher, Beagle, Collie, and Labrador Retriever; protein-losing enteropathy in breeds such as Yorkshire Terrier, Basenji, Soft-coated Wheaten Terrier; and liver disease in breeds such as Bedlington Terrier, Doberman Pinscher, and Labrador Retriever.

Past medical problems might identify gastrointestinal (GI) or urinary tract signs compatible with protein-losing disease. A complete review of the diet is done to find a nutritional source for albumin alterations. It is important to identify any possible exposure to drugs or toxins that could affect albumin concentrations or become potentially toxic due to changes in the albumin concentration. Table 4.2 provides a list of common drugs that are affected by albumin. The history might also reveal soft tissue swelling, labored breathing, polyuria, diarrhea, abdominal distension, and other clinical signs that can be related to alterations in blood albumin and COP (Table 4.3).

The physical examination incorporates the vital signs (temperature, pulse rate, respiratory rate, and effort) with the physical peripheral perfusion parameters (heart rate, mucous membrane color, pulse intensity, capillary refill time) to evaluate blood flow to the peripheral organs. Hypovolemia due to low COP can lead to poor perfusion, and eventually dehydration if fluid intake has been inadequate. Hydration is assessed with skin turgor, eye position within the orbit, and mucous membrane and corneal moisture (see Chapter 2).

Other physical findings indicative of hypoalbuminemia and a low intravascular COP can include cavitary effusions or tissue

Table 4.3 Organ systems that are affected by low COP and common clinical signs (from development of edema).

Organ system affected	Clinical signs
Cardiovascular system	Poor perfusion and arrhythmias; pericardial effusion with jugular vein distension
Gastrointestinal system	Vomiting, diarrhea, poor absorption of nutrients, weight loss, abdominal effusion
Respiratory system	Increased respiratory rate and effort, decreased lung sounds if effusion, wet lung sounds if pulmonary edema
Nervous system	Brain: mental depression, dementia, obtundation, stupor, coma. Spinal cord: ataxia, paresis or paralysis
Integument	Peripheral edema/weeping skin lesions
Eyes	Chemosis

edema. Abdominal effusions are common and can manifest as abdominal distension, reduced bowel sounds, and short or shallow breaths due to increased pressure on the diaphragm. Fluid waves might be felt during abdominal palpation or ballotment, but may require large volumes. Pleural fluid accumulation is less common from this cause but can produce an elevated respiratory rate and effort and muffled lungs sounds. Pulmonary edema may cause respiratory distress with a rapid, shallow breathing pattern and moist lung sounds heard on auscultation. Patients with evidence of heart disease (murmur, gallop sounds or arrhythmias) may have underlying heart pathology, which can exacerbate pulmonary edema due to fluid intolerance and low COP. Heart murmurs can also be heard due to severe alterations in blood rheology associated with anemia or low blood protein.

Edema of the intestines may result in poor GI function, altered normal borborygmi, vomiting or diarrhea. Peripheral edema is recognized first in body areas with thin skin, low muscle mass, and few fat stores, such as around the Achilles tendon or intermandibular space. Conjunctival edema (chemosis) is an early sign of fluid intolerance, followed quickly by subcutaneous fluid accumulation around the head and neck and the distal limbs. Other causes of interstitial edema or effusion such as increased hydrostatic pressure, right-sided heart failure, portal hypertension, neoplasia or vasculitis should also be considered as a possible cause. Assessment of the patient for improvement or resolution of clinical signs associated with alterations in albumin and COP (hypotension, edema, pleural effusion, ascites, and respiratory distress) is an important monitoring tool throughout resuscitation and definitive treatment.

Point of care testing

The minimum laboratory database blood samples should ideally be drawn prior to fluid resuscitation. The POC tests will include the packed cell volume (PCV), total protein (TP), blood glucose, blood urea nitrogen (BUN), blood gas analysis, electrolyte panel, coagulation profile (prothrombin time, activated partial thromboplastin time), platelet number estimation, and urinalysis.

A serum or plasma refractometer reading can provide a TP, which is a combination of albumin plus globulin and other blood proteins. A separate biochemical assay is required to determine the precise albumin and globulin concentration. An elevation in TP more commonly represents reduced plasma water but can be a consequence of an elevation in globulins. A low TP generally reflects a low albumin, with or without a loss of globulins, and can be found with dilution of blood with nonprotein-containing fluids, loss of protein from the vasculature or lack of blood protein production. Synthetic colloids are not demonstrated on the refractometer and will dilute the concentration of albumin and other proteins [1]. Refractometer readings should be interpreted in light of evaluation of other microhematocrit levels, including PCV, serum color, and buffy coat; this may provide further insight into the underlying disease process.

The BUN may be elevated with proteinuria from kidney disease or low with liver cirrhosis or failure, each a potential cause of hypoalbuminemia. Hyperglycemia can alter the glycocalyx layer of the vasculature, increasing the permeability of the glomerular capillary wall to albumin [20].

A large proportion of serum calcium is bound to albumin in the blood. Measuring the ionized portion of calcium will allow for a more accurate assessment of serum calcium concentrations.

Blood albumin concentrations can also affect the acid–base status of the patient. Albumin acts as a weak acid, with hypoalbuminemia therefore having an alkalinizing effect with an increase in the base excess. Increases in blood albumin are associated with an acidifying effect. Treatment for either acid–base derangement involves specific therapy for the underlying disease. See Chapter 7 for further information.

Platelet numbers may decline and coagulation times increase with disseminated intravascular coagulation (DIC), a common consequence of systemic inflammatory response syndrome (SIRS) diseases, to include sepsis. Increased vascular permeability leads to hypoalbuminemia. The transcapillary escape of albumin implies an interendothelial gap size of at least 69 000 daltons (size of albumin molecule). Antithrombin (AT), an important endogenous anticoagulant, has a smaller molecular weight (58 000 daltons) and will extravasate in a similar fashion. Loss of AT from the circulating blood can be a marker of a risk for thrombosis.

The urinalysis is evaluated for proteinuria as evidence of a protein-losing nephropathy and urine specific gravity (USG) as evidence of renal urine concentrating ability, which may indicate underlying renal disease. Administration of synthetic colloids may artificially raise urine specific gravity and should be considered when evaluating USG in critically ill animals. The urine sediment is examined for signs of a urinary tract infection as the cause of proteinuria or a focus of inflammation.

Clinicopathological testing

Blood for a complete blood count (CBC) and serum biochemical profile is drawn prior to fluid resuscitation and submitted for analysis. Leukocytosis and leukopenia can each be a consequence of systemic inflammation or sepsis.

The biochemical profile is evaluated for evidence of underlying diseases that cause disorders of albumin and COP. Table 4.4 provides a list of diseases that can cause changes in plasma albumin. The serum albumin concentration will be reported. Hyperalbuminemia is almost always associated with dehydration, but other causes must be considered. Hypoalbuminemia will be due to decreased production, transcapillary escape into tissues, albumin loss from the body, dilution by nonalbumin-containing fluids or a combination of these mechanisms. Hypercholesterolemia, hypoglycemia, decreased BUN and prolonged clotting times, with or without elevated liver enzymes, are strongly suggestive of severe liver disease as the cause of hypoalbuminemia.

Hypoalbuminemia is consistent with a low COP in patients that have *not* been treated with natural or synthetic colloids. The COP can be calculated using serum albumin or total protein values; however, this method has been found to provide an inaccurate assessment of COP in the critically ill patient [21–24]. The gold standard for assessing COP in human and veterinary patients is to directly measure the COP of plasma, serum or whole blood with the colloid osmometer, a bench-top membrane transducer instrument (Wescor Inc., Logan, UT). The normal value for measured COP in the dog is 21–25 mmHg and 23–25 mmHg in the cat [23,25].

Additional testing might be required to find the underlying cause of albumin alterations, such as serology for infectious pathogens, culture and susceptibility of urine or fluids, urine protein:creatinine ratio, drug concentrations, bile acids, and histopathology of intestinal biopsies. Analysis of fluid collected from thoracic or abdominal effusions will determine whether the fluid is a transudate (resulting from increased hydrostatic pressure and/or decreased COP) or exudate (resulting from inflammation) (see Table 4.5).

Table 4.4 Common disorders causing an alteration in serum albumin and colloid osmotic pressure.

Hypoalbuminemia	Hyperalbuminemia
Decreased production	**Decreased plasma water**
Hepatic disease	Adipsia
Acute inflammation	Dehydration from any cause
Sepsis	**Excessive production/poor**
Malnutrition	**catabolism**
Increased loss	Severe infection
Protein-losing enteropathy	Hepatitis
Protein-losing nephropathy	Overdose of cortisone
Hemorrhage	Chronic inflammatory disease
SIRS diseases	Congestive heart failure
Vasculitis	Kidney disease
Sepsis	Cancer (hepatic carcinoma)
Parvoviral enteritis	Hypoadrenocorticism
Hemorrhagic gastroenteritis	**Iatrogenic**
Burns	Albumin administration
Exudative wounds	Other drugs such as insulin
Trauma	
Decreased intake	
Malnutrition	
Anorexia	
Malabsorptive diseases	

SIRS, systemic inflammatory response syndrome.

Table 4.5 Differences in composition and characteristics between a transudate and an exudate.

Transudate	Exudate
Low cellularity	Intermediate to high cellularity
Watery component of plasma, often clear in appearance	Large molecules in solution (i.e. fibrinogen), often cloudy in appearance
Low protein content, <2.5 g/dL	High protein content, >2.9 g/dL
Unlikely to clot	More likely to clot
Low specific gravity, <1.012	High specific gravity, >1.020
Low albumin or low fluid/serum protein ratio, <0.5	High albumin or high fluid/serum protein ratio, >0.5

Diagnostic imaging

Diagnostic imaging begins with plain thoracic and abdominal radiographs. Thoracic radiographs are evaluated for pulmonary, cardiac or pleural space abnormalities. The presence of pleural fluid will direct centesis for diagnostic sampling and relief of pleural pressure. The presence of pulmonary edema can be a consequence of hypoalbuminemia and a low COP, heart disease, acute lung injury or acute respiratory distress syndrome. Abdominal radiographs can demonstrate organ size, positioning, and shape as well as the presence of abdominal effusion.

Ultrasound may provide a more detailed evaluation of organs for evidence of cysts, fluid, infiltrates, hemorrhage, edema or other anatomical abnormalities. The thoracic and abdominal focused assessment with sonography techniques (AFAST and TFAST) are useful in identifying free fluid; bedside ultrasound lung examination (VetBLUE) may also be useful to identify pulmonary edema or other pathology (see Chapter 10 (AFAST) and Chapter 8 (TFAST, VetBLUE)). The aspiration of abdominal or pleural fluid can be guided by ultrasound with the fluid evaluated by culture, cytology, and biochemistry as indicated. Endoscopic examination and mucosal biopsies of the stomach, upper duodenum, colon or rectum may be indicated when a protein-losing enteropathy is suspected. Advanced imaging such as a portovenogram, nuclear scintigraphy, computed tomography or nuclear magnetic resonance imaging may be indicated to better define the extent and nature of a suspected or confirmed abnormality.

Equipment-based monitoring

The selection of equipment-based monitoring tools will be guided by repeated physical examinations. Signs of poor perfusion, dehydration, peripheral edema, abdominal distension, and changes in breathing rate and effort can suggest fluid extravasation due to hypoalbuminemia and a lowered COP. The refractometer is used to easily follow the trends of change in total protein. The results can indicate a likely rise or fall in COP when crystalloids have been used as the sole resuscitation and maintenance fluid. However, direct measurement of the COP with a colloid osmometer is required after the administration of synthetic colloids since they are not measured by the refractometer. Monitoring blood pressure and pulse oximetry can provide an early indication of pulmonary complications attributable to hypoalbuminemia and a low COP and show progress during treatment. Monitoring the blood pressure, blood lactate, and urine output can provide insight into the tissue perfusion of core organs. The electrocardiogram can help with early detection of cardiac edema or ischemia. Careful patient assessment using the Rule of 20 (at least twice daily) is important to rapidly identify and manage potentially life-threatening complications arising from alterations in blood albumin and the intravascular COP.

Disorders of albumin and colloid osmotic pressure

Changes in serum albumin are the result of pathological events, not the cause of them. Critically ill patients often have one or more underlying disease processes that contribute to alterations in blood albumin and ultimately a significant change in COP (see Table 4.4). Both factors can have an important impact on the outcome of the patient. A high serum albumin is primarily a reflection of dehydration and is typically resolved through fluid therapy. However, low serum albumin and the resultant decrease in COP can be a component of any critical illness. The resulting complications of hypoalbuminemia must be strategically managed for an optimal therapeutic outcome.

Hypoalbuminemia and low COP

Hypoalbuminemia is to be anticipated as a complication of any critical illness. After a major insult, the serum albumin inevitably decreases and tends to increase slowly as the patient recovers. A clear association has been found between the albumin level and the severity of insult [26] but it is unclear whether there is a cause–effect relationship or whether it is just a marker of serious disease [27].

Hypoalbuminemia is associated with increased complications and reduced survival in critically ill humans, dogs, and cats [28–32]. Each 1.0 g/dL (10 g/L) decrease in serum albumin was associated with a 137% increase in the odds of death, an 89% increase in morbidity, and a 71% increase in length of hospital stay in humans [29].

Hypoalbuminemia in critical illness can result from mechanisms that include:

- loss through bleeding or wound seepage
- increased capillary permeability causing redistribution from the vasculature to the interstitial space or body cavity (third-spacing)
- dilution from intravenous fluids
- reduced albumin synthesis during critical illness
- malnutrition, kidney, GI or liver disease [33].

Loss of protein from the blood into the GI tract occurs due to mucosal disease with ulceration, obstruction of lymphatic flow, increased mucosal capillary permeability or a combination of these problems. Chapter 15 provides more information pertaining to the impact of GI disease in the critical patient.

Proteinuria occurs as the result of increased permeability of the glomerular filtration barrier, composed of the glomerular endothelial cell, the basement membrane, and the podocyte. Abnormalities in one or more of these components can result in proteinuria and albuminuria. The presence of protein in the renal tubule will stimulate inflammation and fibrinogenesis in the proximal tubular epithelial cells, contributing to the progression to end-stage renal disease [34]. Chapter 13 provides options for the diagnosis and treatment of proteinuria. The resultant hypoalbuminemia contributes to the morbidity and mortality in both GI and renal disorders.

The vascular endothelium is one of the earliest targets for inflammatory mediators in SIRS diseases and sepsis [35]. The EGL is damaged by TNF-alpha, IL-6, complement, and bacterial lipopolysaccharides. Cytokines, proteases, histamine, and heparinase released in inflammation further degrade the EGL. The transcapillary escape of albumin has been demonstrated in septic patients [36]. The loss of circulating albumin accompanies the loss of the glycocalyx, lowering the COP and increasing fluid extravasation [37]. Low intravascular COP in trauma patients correlated well to EGL degradation and thrombin loss, which subsequently affected vascular permeability and coagulation [38].

These changes can have a devastating impact on the intravascular fluid volume and oxygen delivery to the tissues [39]. Hypovolemia is an anticipated consequence and can lead to inadequate oxygen delivery, increased lactate production, decreased adenosine triphosphate (ATP) production, cell membrane breakdown, cellular death, organ failure, and death. Even a very minor intravascular volume deficit could lead to ischemia of splanchnic organs in the critical veterinary or human patient [40]. The onset and outcome of acute lung injury and acute respiratory distress syndrome are closely associated with hypoalbuminemia. The clinical signs resulting from low albumin are most frequently due to the accompanying decrease in intravascular COP. The signs can be subtle or quite dramatic. Common signs of low COP in critical patients are listed in Table 4.3 and determination of albumin deficit is noted in Box 4.3.

Treatment of hypoalbuminemia and colloid osmotic pressure

Treatment is initially directed toward immediate stabilization of life-threatening consequences attributable to the loss of albumin and COP. Cyanosis or airway compromise from severe pharyngeal or pulmonary tissue edema can require sedation, endotracheal intubation, and ventilation with 100% oxygen. Less severe respiratory distress can warrant oxygen supplementation, analgesics, diuretic administration (furosemide 2–4 mg/kg IV), and therapeutic thoracentesis (when pleural fluid is the cause of distress). Should a large quantity of abdominal fluid (ascites) or tissue edema in an enclosed portion of the body result in extreme pressure, there will be ischemia with damage to nerves and surrounding tissues. This is termed *compartmentalization syndrome* and requires immediate relief of the pressure by centesis (if free fluid), removal of any constricting bandage if present or surgical fasciotomy if there is no other method of decompression.

Stabilizing the intravascular fluid volume is critical whether the effects of hypoalbuminemia and low COP are severe or mild. This requires a meticulous fluid therapy plan to avoid compounding the extravasation of fluid into the tissues of vital organs (brain, heart, lungs) or interstitium (see Chapter 2). The decision to include natural or synthetic colloid solutions as part of the fluid therapy plan may help to minimize edema and reduce resuscitation time.

The main reasons for colloid administration in the veterinary small animal ICU are to increase (and maintain) COP in patients with low albumin and to provide rapid volume replacement during resuscitation from hypovolemia. A colloid solution contains high molecular weight molecules that are too large to freely pass through the capillary wall. Colloids remain in the intravascular compartment longer than crystalloids although this property can be lost when the capillary membrane permeability is severely altered in diseased states [41]. The higher the oncotic pressure of the colloid, the greater the initial volume expansion seen. Smaller volumes of colloids result in greater intravascular volume expansion compared to volume resuscitation with crystalloid solutions alone [41]. The size of the colloid macromolecules can become important during episodes of capillary leakage. When vascular permeability allows the transcapillary passage of albumin, the interendothelial spaces are at least 65 000–69 000 daltons in size. Administering a colloid

that is the size of albumin or smaller can result in transcapillary escape of these colloid molecules, as well.

Synthetic colloids do not influence measured plasma albumin concentration, but raise COP directly [1]. The effects of administered colloids on COP can be monitored using a colloid osmometer and by monitoring the clinical signs of the patient.

Numerous studies have examined the outcome of fluid therapy with crystalloids alone or with various colloid solutions (such as concentrated albumin, hydroxyethyl starch, dextran-70) in humans. While results have varied widely between studies, there has been no evidence that there is a better outcome for human patients treated with colloid solutions over those treated with only isotonic crystalloids [42–45]. However, the dose and time to reach the therapeutic target for fluid administration, the precise target for successful resuscitation, whether crystalloids were administered with the colloid solutions and the differences that might occur between the various colloid solutions have not been clearly defined for many of the studies. Chapter 2 provides recommendations and doses for the administration of crystalloids simultaneously with colloids to small animal critical patients.

Natural colloids

Natural colloids are derived from whole-blood donations and contain naturally occurring albumin. Natural colloids provide their COP primarily through albumin, and come in the form of albumin concentrate or plasma transfusions. Natural colloids directly supplement plasma albumin, thus maintaining or raising the COP. Table 4.6 provides the COP of the natural colloids and recommended initial dose.

Fresh frozen plasma (FFP) and frozen plasma (FP) are the natural colloids most commonly infused in veterinary medicine. They contain near normal concentrations of albumin as well as many procoagulants and natural anticoagulants, immunoglobulins, and acute-phase proteins. FFP and FP have a COP of ~17 mmHg [8], lower than most available synthetic colloids. The formula for estimating the albumin deficit is given in Box 4.3. A dose of 22 mL/kg of plasma is required to raise the serum albumin by 0.5 g/dL. This

Table 4.6 Colloid osmotic pressure and dose of natural colloids.

Product	COP(mmHg)	Dose/notes
Fresh frozen plasma	17	About 22 mL/kg will increase albumin by 0.5 g/dL, assuming no continued loss of albumin
Frozen plasma	17	As above
Whole blood	17	Administered when concurrent need for red blood cells
Human serum albumin (HSA), 5%	23.2	Dilute calculated dose for 25% HSA (see below) to a 5% solution
HSA, 25%	>200	5–7 mL/kg or using albumin deficit (see Box 4.3) initially give 1/4 to 1/3 the calculated dose and titrate at 2 mL/kg increments as needed. Give slowly, observing for allergic reaction. Risk of serious adverse reactions.
Canine albumin, 5%	21–25	17 mL/kg or to correct patient's albumin (Box 4.3)
Canine albumin, 16%		5 mL/kg Diluted with 0.9% saline to 5% solution or administered over 6 hours

---

Box 4.3 Determination of albumin deficit.

Albumin deficit = 10 × (2 mg/dL-patient's albumin) × weight (kg) × 0.3

means that a 20 kg dog would need close to 1 L of plasma to raise the albumin from 1.0 g/dL (10 g/L) to 2.0 g/dL (20 g/L). The volume required and cost can make this option prohibitive for specifically supplementing albumin. Adverse effects associated with the use of FFP and FP include transfusion-related lung injury, volume overload, transfusion reactions, and infection.

Fresh whole blood contains red blood cells, platelets, white blood cells, plasma proteins, and coagulation factors. After approximately 8–24 hours of storage, platelets and coagulation factors V and VIII are depleted and the unit is then labeled as stored whole blood. Whole blood has a COP that is similar to plasma [25], making it a poor choice for colloid supplementation, except when replacing blood loss in hemorrhaging patients. Chapter 10 provides indications and doses for administering whole blood and packed red cell products.

Human serum albumin (HSA) is a natural colloid with a molecular weight of 69 000 daltons, composed of purified human albumin. It is available for medical use and has been used to treat hypoalbuminemia in both canine and feline patients [46]. It is available in varying concentrations from 5% to 25%. The 25% HSA has a COP that is greater than 200 mmHg [47]. HSA has a long half-life and can be stored at room temperature. It can be given through a peripheral or central catheter, although a central catheter is preferred when using higher concentrations. Higher concentrations may be diluted with 0.9% NaCl to lower the concentration prior to administration [46].

The indications for HSA transfusions have included refractory hypotension or the supplementation of serum albumin, with priority given to preoperative patients. The use of HSA in veterinary patients is controversial and there are no defined guidelines for its use. The formula for calculating the albumin deficit in a patient is shown in Box 4.3. This formula takes both the serum and interstitial deficit into consideration and usually results in a large volume of HSA. It is common to initially give one-quarter to one-third of the calculated albumin deficit and then reassess the need for additional HSA. This has typically resulted in a volume of 5–7 mL/kg of 25% HSA as an initial dose. Generally, HSA should be given slowly (over 4–24 hours) except when used to treat hypotension (dose of 2 mL/kg given as a slow IV bolus) [48].

Because of the human origin of the protein, there is an increased risk of severe and potentially life-threatening allergic reactions. There is documented evidence of immediate life-threatening reactions, as well as delayed hypersensitivity reactions to HSA in healthy and hospitalized small animal patients [49–52]. Dogs and cats can develop anti-HSA antibodies [49]. Since it takes 3–5 days for antibodies to develop, the clinician can give multiple HSA transfusions within 3–5 days of the first transfusion, after which additional transfusions should not be given. Caution and careful

monitoring of veterinary patients are required during infusion and for weeks thereafter for a delayed hypersensitivity reaction. Signs of delayed reactions include polyarthritis, vasculitis, dermatitis, and/or glomerulonephritis [48]. Owners should also be instructed about the danger of repeating HSA transfusions in the future.

Lyophilized canine serum albumin (CSA) (Animal Blood Resources International, Stockbridge, MI) has recently become available for use in canine patients. The use of this product is not recommended in cats. The lyophilized product is stored at room temperature or refrigerated. It is stable for approximately 24 months post manufacturing. CSA is purchased as a 5.0 g bottle and the manufacturer recommends reconstitution with 0.9% NaCl to a 5% or 16% solution. The product must be used within six hours of reconstitution and given through a blood filter. The recommended dose is 5 mL/kg of the 16% solution and 17 mL/kg for the 5% solution (see Table 4.6). CSA should be administered slowly (over 4–8 hours), slower if administering the 16% solution. When used to resuscitate hypotensive patients, CSA may be given more quickly as a bolus infusion. It is proposed that dogs will be less likely to have a reaction to this allogeneic albumin, although this has yet to be validated. Immediate hypersensitivity reactions have not been observed nor have any delayed reactions been observed up to six weeks post infusion [53]. However, close monitoring for transfusion reactions during and after the transfusion is still warranted.

Synthetic colloids

Synthetic colloids are less expensive and have a long shelf-life compared to many of the natural colloid products. The family of hydroxyethyl starches (HES) is the most common type of synthetic colloid used in small animal veterinary ICUs. Other synthetic colloids include dextrans and gelatins. While the large molecular weight of synthetic colloids favors retention in the intravascular space, synthetic colloids are used cautiously in animals that have significant plasma exudation, such as with burns, snake envenomation, and severe vasculitis. These patients have an increased risk of colloid leakage into their interstitium due to very large gaps in the interendothelial spaces. A comparison of the common synthetic colloids is provided in Table 4.7. Controversies associated with potential side effects of synthetic colloids in human and veterinary patients warrant careful patient selection and cautious administration.

Hydroxyethyl starches

Hydroxyethyl starches contain modified polysaccharides of amylopectin with varying molecular weights [54]. Amylopectin is quickly hydrolyzed and has a half-life of about 20 minutes. HES are characterized by their molecular weight and may be grouped as high

Table 4.7 Comparison of synthetic colloids.

Synthetic colloid	Source	COP	MW	Molar substitution	C2:C6	Dose	Side-effects
Hetastarch, 6%*	Amylopectin	32	>450	0.7	4.5:1	Max 20 mL/kg	Impairs coagulation, possible renal effects (human)
Pentastarch, 6%*	Amylopectin	32	260	0.45	5:1	40 mL/kg	As above
Vetstarch, 6%	Amylopectin	37	70–130	0.4	9.1	20–50 mL/kg	As above
Dextran-40	Bacterial metabolism	168–191	40	n/a	n/a	20 mL/kg	Hypersensitivity, renal (not recc)
Dextran-70	Bacterial metabolism	56–68	70	n/a	n/a	20 mL/kg	Hypersensitivity, renal
Gelatin	Bovine collagen hydrolysis	26–29	12–50	n/a	n/a	Poorly reported	Anaphylaxis

COP, colloidal osmotic pressure; MW, molecular weight.
*The values vary depending on manufacturer.

6% Hydroxyethyl starch 650/0.5/13.4:1

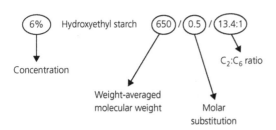

Figure 4.3 Schematic of interpretation of hydroxyethyl starch connotations, from left to right: concentration, type of colloid, weight-averaged molecular weight, molar substitution, and C_2:C_6 ratio.

molecular weight (>450 kD, e.g. Hetastarch®), medium molecular weight (~260 kD, e.g. Pentastarch®) and low molecular weight products (70–130 kD, e.g. Vetstarch®) [55]. The higher the degree of molar substitution, the more resistant to degradation and the longer the colloid remains in circulation [41]. A low molar substitution is between 0.45 and 0.58, while a high molar substitution is between 0.62 and 0.70. The C2:C6 ratio refers to the site of substitution on the initial glucose molecule. The higher the C2:C6 ratio, the longer is the persistence in blood due to its steric resistance to degradation by amylase. The abbreviations used to describe HES solutions and their connotations are provided in Figure 4.3. It is thought that HES products with a higher molecular weight, higher C2:C6 ratio and higher degree of substitution are more likely to persist longer in circulation, but may be associated with more adverse effects reported in humans [41]. HES solutions are metabolized by an amylase-dependent process and eventually undergo renal excretion [56].

A wide variety of HES solutions are readily available worldwide [47] and are commonly suspended in 0.9% NaCL or lactated Ringer's. They can be administered through a peripheral or central catheter and can be given simultaneously with other fluids. Compatibility of HES solutions with medications should be confirmed when administering through the same administration line. The efficacy of HES in raising the COP is best measured by a colloid osmometer as well as monitoring for resolution of clinical signs.

An increase in prothrombin time, partial thromboplastin time, platelet closure time, and decreased factor VIII activity has been reported in both human and veterinary patients receiving HES [55,57]. Hemodilution and reduced factor VIII and von Willebrand factor activity and impaired platelet function have been cited as the cause [55,58]. Significant clinical bleeding has not been reported in veterinary patients with the current dosage recommendations (see Table 4.6). However, careful attention to total daily dosage (<40 mL/kg/day) of HES and diligent surgical hemostasis are essential when using HES in patients with an increased risk of bleeding.

The HES solutions have been reported to be associated with an increase in acute kidney injury in critically ill human patients and an increased requirement for renal replacement therapy [59]. While the exact mechanism has not been defined, morphological abnormalities of the proximal tubular cells, or osmotic nephrosis, have been reported. The tubular lesions reflect the accumulation of proximal tubular lysosomes due to pinocytosis of exogenous osmotic solutes [60]. The tubular cells swell because they contain numerous lysosomes and endocytotic vacuoles. The oncotic forces of colloids used alone can decrease renal filtration pressure [61]. Both high and lower molecular weight/molar substitution HES formulations have been implicated in human patients [35–37,41]. The 10% HES 130/0.42 appears to be more proinflammatory and

cause more pronounced tubular damage than the 6% solution of a similar weight/molar substitution. Osmotic lesions in the kidney were also present but to a lesser degree after the sole administration of Ringer's lactate crystalloid, however [62]. In one retrospective study investigating the use of a 10% HES (pentastarch) solution in dogs, a comparative increase in AKI and mortality was seen. Further investigation using other HES solutions and concentrations is warranted [63].

The HES family of colloids has been used extensively in dogs and cats without clinical or clinicopathological evidence of kidney injury. While many of the reported studies in humans use the HES solution as the sole or primary component of fluid therapy, the use of HES in the dog and cat has been as an adjunct to crystalloid therapy. The 6% HES solution in the bag is actually much more dilute when given simultaneously with crystalloids for volume replacement (see Chapter 2) in the dog and cat. At this time, however, HES should be used with caution in animals with underlying kidney insufficiency and adequate crystalloids given to ensure adequate glomerular filtration and renal tubular flow.

Other reported complications of HES include accumulation and deposition in interstitial and reticuloendotheial systems. Such depositions have been associated with pruritus. Anaphylactoid reactions and increased serum amylase levels in human patients have been described as well [41]. To date, neither of these complications has been reported in the dog or cat after HES administration.

The first-generation and second-generation Hetastarch (0.7 molar substitution) solutions come in a variety of formulations. Commonly available forms include HES 6%/670/0.75 and HES 6%/450/0.7. Patients that benefit from fluid resuscitation with Hetastarch may also be continued on a CRI of hetastarch with crystalloids for maintenance of COP. Hetastarch will last longer in the intravascular space compared to crystalloids (24 hours compared to 60 minutes).

Pentastarch (0.5 molar substitution) has a lower average molecular weight than hetastarch (~260 kD vs 450 kD). These characteristics lead to a shorter half-life, faster renal elimination, and a less significant effect on coagulation [55]. 6% Pentastarch can be administered at the same dose as 6% Hetastarch, with a recommended maximum daily dose of 40 mL/kg/day.

Tetrastarch (0.4 molar substitution) is a third-generation HES developed to improve the safety and pharmacological properties of previous HES generations. The reduction in molecular weight and molar substitution has led to solutions with shorter half-lives and fewer side-effects. In human patients, tetrastarch solutions have been found to have a lesser effect on coagulation and are less likely to accumulate. One veterinary study showed that *in vitro* dilution of canine blood with a tetrastarch solution led to hypocoagulable changes on thromboelastography [64]. This change was thought to be secondary to a dose-dependent alteration in fibrinogen concentration and an inhibition of platelet function [64].

Dextrans

Dextrans contain glucose polymers of differing lengths produced by bacteria grown on sucrose media [47]. The most common forms of dextran solutions available are dextran- 40 and dextran-70, with molecular weights of 40 000 daltons and 70 000 daltons, respectively. Dextran-70 has a COP of 62 mmHg, while dextran-40 has a COP of 40 mmHg. Both dextran solutions initially produce intravascular volume expansion due to the increased COP, but their effect is temporary [47]. About 40% of dextran-40 and 70% of dextran-70 remain in circulation 12 hours after a dose is given [41].

The dose for the dextran solutions is similar to other synthetic colloids (see Table 4.6). Adverse effects of dextran solutions include coagulopathies due to their effects on fibrin clot formation, reduced factor VIII activity, and hemodilution [65]. They have also been reported to cause severe hypersensitivity reactions in human patients. Dextrans have been associated with increased risk of acute kidney injury. Dextran-40 has a high kidney excretion rate due to its low molecular weight and is thought to lodge in the renal tubules, causing tubular injury [66,67].

Due to their negative side-effects and the availability of newer colloids, dextrans are not commonly used in veterinary patients. Their use should be accompanied by the same precautions as when using HES in patients with a coagulopathy or kidney disease.

Gelatins

Gelatins are prepared by hydrolysis of bovine collagen. The protein is formed when connective tissues of animals are boiled and a jelly forms when cooled [41]. Several modified gelatin products are now available including polygeline, plasmagel, plasmion, and gelifundol. The molecular weights range from 12 000 to 50 000 daltons with an average of 35 000 daltons. Gelatins are rapidly excreted by the kidneys and lead to about 70–80% volume expansion although their duration of action is shorter than HES or dextrans. In human patients, the daily dose of gelatins is not limited, as opposed to other synthetic colloids [68]. While gelatins can cause coagulation abnormalities, they are thought to cause minimal perioperative bleeding in human patients [68]. They have very little to no effect on renal function since their small size allows for rapid excretion. Gelatins are associated with a higher incidence of anaphylactoid reactions, however. They are primarily used in the United Kingdom and have not been approved by the United States Food and Drug Administration.

Hyperalbuminemia

High albumin (hyperalbuminemia) is most commonly caused by dehydration. Other reported causes include severe infection, hepatitis, overdose of cortisone, chronic inflammatory diseases, congestive heart failure, kidney disease, and cancer. In these disorders, high albumin is a symptom of dysfunction within the body associated with impaired immunity leading to an elevation of proteins. In some cases of retinol (vitamin A) deficiency in humans, the albumin level can be elevated to high normal values. Infusion of natural colloid solutions with a high concentration of albumin or the administration of drugs that cause an increase in albumin (see Table 4.2) can lead to iatrogenic hyperalbuminemia. Hyperalbuminemia has been reported with hepatic carcinoma and hypoadrenocorticism in the dog [69,70]. Treatment requires adequate intravascular volume replacement with crystalloid solutions and the diagnosis and treatment of the inciting disorder.

References

1. Whicher J, Spence C. When is serum albumin worth measuring? Ann Clin Biochem. 1987;24:572–80.
2. Rackow E, Fein I, Leppo J. Colloid osmotic pressure as a prognostic indicator of pulmonary edema and mortality in the critically ill. Chest 1977;72:709–13.
3. Pietrangelo A, Panduro A, Chowdhury JR, Shafritz DA. Albumin gene expression is down-regulated by albumin or macromolecule infusion in the rat. J Clin Invest. 1992;89:1755.
4. Schnitzer J, Bravo J. High affinity binding, endocytosis, and degradation of conformationally modified albumins. Potential role of gp30 and gp18 as novel scavenger receptors. J Biol Chem. 1993;268:7562–70.
5. Parving H, Gyntelberg F. Transcapillary escape rate of albumin and plasma volume in essential hypertension. Circ Res. 1973;32:643–52.
6. Mazzaferro EM, Rudloff E, Kirby R. The role of albumin replacement in the critically ill veterinary patient. J Vet Emerg Crit Care 2002;12:113–24.
7. Margarson M, Soni N. Serum albumin: touchstone or totem? Anaesthesia 1998;53:789–803.
8. Chan DL, Freeman LM, Rozanski EA, Rush JE. Colloid osmotic pressure of parenteral nutrition components and intravenous fluids. J Vet Emerg Crit Care 2001;11:269–73.
9. Stewart RH. Editorial: the case for measuring plasma colloid osmotic pressure. J Vet Intern Med. 2000;14:473–4.
10. Starling EH. On the absorption of fluids from the connective tissue spaces. J Physiol. 1896;19:312–26.
11. Levick JR, Michel CC. Microvascular fluid exchange and the revised Starling principle. Cardiovasc Res. 2010;27:198–210.
12. Clough G. Relationship between microvascular permeability and ultrastructure. Progress Biophys Molec Biol. 1991;55:47–69.
13. Van den Berg BM, Nieuwdorp M, Stroes E, Vink H. Glycocalyx and endothelial (dys) function: from mice to men. Pharmacol Rep. 2006;58:75–80.
14. Becker BF, Chappell D, Jacob M. Endothelial glycocalyx and coronary vascular permeability: the fringe benefit. Basic Res Cardiol. 2010;105:687–701.
15. Alphonsus C, Rodseth R. The endothelial glycocalyx: a review of the vascular barrier. Anaesthesia 2014;69:777–84.
16. Halliwell B. Albumin – an important extracellular antioxidant? Biochem Pharmacol. 1988;37:569–71.
17. Strubelt O, Younes M, Li Y. Protection by albumin against ischaemia-and hypoxia-induced hepatic injury. Pharmacol Toxicol. 1994;75:280–4.
18. Morissette M. Colloid osmotic pressure: its measurement and clinical value. Can Med Assoc J. 1977;116:897.
19. Jones PA, Bain FT, Byars TD, David JB, Boston RC. Effect of hydroxyethyl starch infusion on colloid oncotic pressure in hypoproteinemic horses. J Am Vet Med Assoc. 2001;218:1130–5.
20. Jeansson M, Haraldsson B. Morphological and functional evidence for an important role of the endothelial cell glycocalyx in the glomerular barrier. Am J Physiol-Renal Physiol. 2006;290:F111–F16.
21. Thomas L, Brown S. Relationship between colloid osmotic pressure and plasma protein concentration in cattle, horses, dogs, and cats. Am J Vet Res. 1992;53:2241–4.
22. Brown S, Dusza K, Boehmer J. Comparison of measured and calculated values for colloid osmotic pressure in hospitalized animals. Am J Vet Res. 1994;55:910–15.
23. Rudloff E, Kirby R. Colloid osmometry. Clin Tech Small Anim Pract. 2000;15:119–25.
24. Barclay S, Bennett D. The direct measurement of plasma colloid osmotic pressure is superior to colloid osmotic pressure derived from albumin or total protein. Intensive Care Med. 1987;13:114–18.
25. Odunayo A, Kerl ME. Comparison of whole blood and plasma colloid osmotic pressure in healthy dogs. J Vet Emerg Crit Care 2011;21:236–41.
26. Gibbs J, Cull W, Henderson W, Daley J, Hur K, Khuri SF. Preoperative serum albumin level as a predictor of operative mortality and morbidity: results from the National VA Surgical Risk Study. Arch Surg. 1999;134:36–42.
27. Vincent J-L, Russell JA, Jacob M, et al. Albumin administration in the acutely ill: what is new and where next? Crit Care 2014;18:231.
28. Hoeboer SH, Oudemans-van Straaten HM, Groeneveld AJ. Albumin rather than C-reactive protein may be valuable in predicting and monitoring the severity and course of acute respiratory distress syndrome in critically ill patients with or at risk for the syndrome after new onset fever. BMC Pulmon Med. 2015;15:22.
29. Vincent J-L, Dubois M-J, Navickis RJ, Wilkes MM. Hypoalbuminemia in acute illness: is there a rationale for intervention? A meta-analysis of cohort studies and controlled trials. Ann Surg. 2003;237:319.
30. Lee YJ, Chan JW, Hsu WL, Lin KW, Chang CC. Prognostic factors and a prognostic index for cats with acute kidney injury. J Vet Int Med. 2012;26:500–5.
31. Allenspach K, Wieland B, Gröne A, Gaschen F. Chronic enteropathies in dogs: evaluation of risk factors for negative outcome. J Vet Intern Med. 2007;21:700–8.
32. Ralphs SC, Jessen CR, Lipowitz AJ. Risk factors for leakage following intestinal anastomosis in dogs and cats: 115 cases (1991–2000). J Am Vet Med Assoc. 2003;223:73–7.
33. Moshage H, Janssen J, Franssen J, Hafkenscheid J, Yap S. Study of the molecular mechanism of decreased liver synthesis of albumin in inflammation. J Clin Invest. 1987;79:1635.

34. Abbate M, Zoja C, Remuzzi G. How does proteinuria cause progressive renal damage? J Am Soc Nephrol. 2006;17:2974–84.

35. Becker BF, Chappell D, Bruegger D, Annecke T, Jacob M. Therapeutic strategies targeting the endothelial glycocalyx: acute deficits, but great potential. Cardiovasc Res. 2010;87:300–10.

36. Bent-Hansen L. Whole body capillary exchange of albumin. Acta Physiol Scand. 1991;603(Suppl):5.

37. Jacob M, Bruegger D, Rehm M, Welsch U, Conzen P, Becker BF. Contrasting effects of colloid and crystalloid resuscitation fluids on cardiac vascular permeability. Anesthesiology 2006;104:1223–31.

38. Rahbar E, Cardenas JC, Baimukanova G, et al. Endothelial glycocalyx shedding and vascular permeability in severely injured trauma patients. J Transl Med. 2015;13:117.

39. Bumpus SE, Haskins SC, Kass PH. Effect of synthetic colloids on refractometric readings of total solids. J Vet Emerg Crit Care 1998;8:21–6.

40. Price HL, Deutsch S, Marshall BE, Stephen GW, Behar MG, Neufeld GR. Hemodynamic and metabolic effects of hemorrhage in man, with particular reference to the splanchnic circulation. Circ Res. 1966;18:469–74.

41. Mitra S, Khandelwal P. Are all colloids the same? How to select the right colloid? Indian J Anaesth. 2009;53:592.

42. Perel P, Roberts I, Ker K. Colloids versus crystalloids for fluid resuscitation in critically ill patients. Cochrane Database Syst Rev. 2013;2:CD000567.

43. Van der Heijden M, Verheij J, van Nieuw Amerongen GP, Groeneveld ABJ. Crystalloid or colloid fluid loading and pulmonary permeability, edema, and injury in septic and nonseptic critically ill patients with hypovolemia. Crit Care Med. 2009;37:1275–81.

44. Schortgen F, Girou E, Deye N, Brochard L. The risk associated with hyperoncotic colloids in patients with shock. Intens Care Med. 2008;34:2157–68.

45. Finfer S, Norton R, Bellomo R, Boyce N, French J, Myburgh J. The SAFE study: saline vs. albumin for fluid resuscitation in the critically ill. Vox Sang. 2004;87:123–31.

46. Viganó F, Perissinotto L, Bosco VR. Administration of 5% human serum albumin in critically ill small animal patients with hypoalbuminemia: 418 dogs and 170 cats (1994–2008). J Vet Emerg Crit Care 2010;20:237–43.

47. Roberts JS, Bratton SL. Colloid volume expanders. Drugs 1998;55:621–30.

48. Mathews KA, Barry M. The use of 25% human serum albumin: outcome and efficacy in raising serum albumin and systemic blood pressure in critically ill dogs and cats. J Vet Emerg Crit Care 2005;15:110–18.

49. Cohn LA, Kerl ME, Lenox CE, Livingston RS, Dodam JR. Response of healthy dogs to infusions of human serum albumin. Am J Vet Res. 2007;68:657–63.

50. Francis AH, Martin LG, Haldorson GJ, et al. Adverse reactions suggestive of type III hypersensitivity in six healthy dogs given human albumin. J Am Vet Med Assoc. 2007;230:873–9.

51. Trow AV, Rozanski EA, Chan DL. Evaluation of use of human albumin in critically ill dogs: 73 cases (2003–2006). J Am Vet Med Assoc. 2008;233:607–12.

52. Mathews KA. The therapeutic use of 25% human serum albumin in critically ill dogs and cats. Vet Clin North Am Small Anim Pract. 2008;38:595–605.

53. Craft EM, Powell LL. The use of canine-specific albumin in dogs with septic peritonitis. J Vet Emerg Crit Care 2012;22:631–9.

54. Chan DL. Colloids: current recommendations. Vet Clin North Am Small Anim Pract. 2008;38:587–93.

55. Strauss RG, Pennell BJ, Stump DC. A randomized, blinded trial comparing the hemostatic effects of pentastarch versus hetastarch. Transfusion 2002;42:27–36.

56. Yacboi A, Stoll RG, Sum CY, et al. Pharmacokinetics of hydroxyethyl starch in normal subjects. J Clin Pharmacol. 1982;22:206–12.

57. Smart L, Jandrey KE, Kass PH, Wierenga JR, Tablin F. The effect of Hetastarch (670/0.75) in vivo on platelet closure time in the dog. J Vet Emerg Crit Care 2009;19:444–9.

58. Langer R, Jordan U, Wölfle A, Henrich H. Action of hydroxyethyl starch (HES) on the activity of plasmatic clotting factors. Clin Hemorheol Microcirc. 1998;18:103–16.

59. Wiedermann CJ, Dunzendorfer S, Gaioni LU, Zaraca F, Joannidis M. Hyperoncotic colloids and acute kidney injury: a meta-analysis of randomized trials. Crit Care 2010;14:R191.

60. Dickenmann M, Oettl T, Mihatsch MJ. Osmotic nephrosis: acute kidney injury with accumulation of proximal tubular lysosomes due to administration of exogenous solutes. Am J Kid Dis. 2008;51:491–503.

61. Moran M, Kapsner C. Acute renal failure associated with elevated plasma oncotic pressure. N Engl J Med. 1987;317:150–3.

62. Hüter L, Simon T-P, Weinmann L, et al. Hydroxyethylstarch impairs renal function and induces interstitial proliferation, macrophage infiltration and tubular damage in an isolated renal perfusion model. Crit Care 2009;13:R23.

63. Hayes G, Benedicenti L, Matthews K. Retrospective cohort study on the incidence of acute kidney injury and death following hydroxyethyl starch (HES 10% 205/0.5/5:1) administration in dogs (2007–2010). J Vet Emerg Crit Care 2016;26:35–40.

64. Falco S, Bruno B, Maurella C, et al. In vitro evaluation of canine hemostasis following dilution with hydroxyethyl starch (130/0.4) via thromboelastometry. J Vet Emerg Crit Care 2012;22:640–5.

65. Glowaski MM, Moon-Massat PF, Erb HN, Barr SC. Effects of oxypolygelatin and dextran 70 on hemostatic variables in dogs. Vet Anaesth Analg. 2003;30:202–10.

66. Ferraboli R, Malheiro PS, Abdulkader RC, Yu L, Sabbaga E, Burdmann EA. Anuric acute renal failure caused by dextran 40 administration. Renal Fail. 1997;19:303–6.

67. Mailloux L, Swartz CD, Capizzi R, et al. Acute renal failure after administration of low-molecular-weight dextran. N Engl J Med. 1967;277:1113–18.

68. Van der Linden P, Ickx BE. The effects of colloid solutions on hemostasis. Can J Anaesth. 2006;53:S30–S39.

69. Cooper ES, Wellman ML, Carsillo ME. Hyperalbuminemia associated with hepatocellular carcinoma in a dog. Vet Clin Pathol. 2009;38:516–20.

70. Saito M, Olby NJ, Obledo L, Gookin JL. Muscle cramps in two standard poodles with hypoadrenocorticism. J Am Anim Hosp Assoc. 2002;38:437–43.

CHAPTER 5

Glucose

Natara Loose
Brooklyn, New York

Introduction

Glucose is required for energy production by every cell of the body, making it vital to the ongoing function and repair of all cells. Life-sustaining activities such as heart rate and rhythm, vasomotor tone, respiration, and neurological and immune functions depend on having glucose available to the cells. In addition to energy production, glucose makes an important contribution to serum osmolarity, influencing fluid distribution throughout the body. Therefore, every patient in the intensive care unit is at risk for experiencing life-threatening complications associated with alterations in blood glucose.

The reported normal range for blood glucose is 67–168 mg/dL (3.71–9.32 mmol/L) in cats and 62–172 mg/dL (3.44–9.55 mmol/L) in dogs [1]. Box 5.1 provides conversion factors for changing mg/dL to mmol/L for glucose. Hypoglycemia is defined as a blood glucose concentration of <60 mg/dL (<3.33 mmol/L) for both species [2]. The definition of hyperglycemia varies between dogs and cats. For dogs, values greater than 120 mg/dL (6.66 mmol/L) indicate hyperglycemia [3]. Stress hyperglycemia has been shown to cause values as high as 613 mg/dL (34 mmol/L) in cats [4]. In general, fasting levels >140 mg/dL (7.77 mmol/L) should be considered as hyperglycemia in both the dog and cat.

Following ingestion of a meal, glucose is extracted from the blood by the liver, brain, skeletal muscle, red blood cells, fat cells, and skin. The endocrine and autonomic nervous systems control moment-to-moment regulation of blood glucose [5]. The hormones responsible for endogenous glucose production are numerous and include insulin, glucagon, cortisol, and catecholamines (Table 5.1). Glucose is released on demand into the blood by the breakdown of endogenous glycogen stores, primarily by the liver. The pancreas responds to alterations in blood glucose by releasing either insulin or glucagon which signal the liver to either release or to store glucose, respectively (Figure 5.1). Glycogenolysis and gluconeogenesis contribute equally to the basal rate of hepatic glucose production. When insulin concentrations are low, hepatic glucose output rises.

Since glucose cannot readily diffuse through most cell membranes, assistance from facilitated glucose transporter (GLUT) molecules and insulin is required for entry. The glucose transporters form an aqueous pore through which glucose can move into the cell more easily. The rate of glucose entry at these sites is proportional to the blood glucose levels. Glucose enters hepatic and pancreatic beta-cells by GLUT-facilitated diffusion and does not require insulin at these sites. Once within the cell, the glucose is phosphorylated and trapped. While the liver does not require insulin to facilitate glucose uptake, it does need insulin to regulate glucose output [6].

Within the pancreatic beta-cells, glycolysis results in ATP production, providing the energy to release insulin into the blood by exocytosis. Insulin then reduces blood glucose levels by accelerating transport of glucose into insulin-sensitive cells, facilitating glucose conversion to glycogen, promoting fat formation, and suppressing endogenous (primarily hepatic) glucose production.

The majority of glucose uptake in peripheral tissue occurs in muscle, where it is used immediately for energy or stored as glycogen [7]. Adipose tissue contributes significantly to glucose homeostasis by regulating the release of free fatty acids that increase gluconeogenesis [8]. The kidneys play an important role in glucose homeostasis through gluconeogenesis and eliminating excess glucose in the urine [9].

The main consumer of glucose is the brain, accounting for approximately 50% of glucose use in the fasting phase [8]. Brain cells have high metabolic activity with neurons needing energy for depolarization, axonal and dendritic transport, and structural renovation of brain tissue [10]. Glucose enters the brain tissue by GLUT-facilitated diffusion. The brain's energy metabolism depends almost exclusively on the constant supply of glucose. The glucose supply required for normal brain function remains steady even during blood flow fluctuations [11].

Hypoglycemia stimulates the pancreatic alpha-cells to produce glucagon (see Figure 5.1, Table 5.1). This hormone increases glucose levels by accelerating glycogenolysis and promoting gluconeogenesis. In response to the elevation in blood glucose, serum insulin levels rise, which then inhibit glucagon release and suppress hepatic glucose production.

The complicated and critical role that glucose and the glucose regulatory hormones play in the function of every organ in the body makes blood glucose concentration one of the most important variables in critical illness. Discovering fluctuations in blood glucose can afford insight into the metabolic activity of the patient while providing direction for therapeutic intervention and minimizing complications. The evaluation of diagnostic and monitoring data will aid in the early detection of glucose abnormalities

Monitoring and Intervention for the Critically Ill Small Animal: The Rule of 20, First Edition. Edited by Rebecca Kirby and Andrew Linklater.
© 2017 John Wiley & Sons, Inc. Published 2017 by John Wiley & Sons, Inc.

and in the detection of any potential underlying systemic disorder contributing to the illness.

Monitoring methods

The patient history and physical parameters provide valuable information for assessing the urgency and frequency of blood glucose monitoring. The determination of blood glucose levels can be rapid and accurate by using cage-side point of care (POC) testing. Further clinicopathological testing and diagnostic imaging may be necessary to identify an underlying cause. Potentially life-threatening consequences of glucose alterations (such as seizures, tremors, coma) should be rapidly stabilized prior to initiating extensive diagnostic testing.

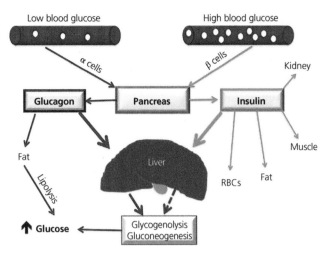

Figure 5.1 The endocrine response to low and high blood glucose. Green arrows, mechanisms to reduce blood glucose: sites of glucose uptake and storage by cells after insulin release; insulin not required for uptake by liver and brain; insulin promotes glucose storage as glycogen in the liver; red arrow, inhibition of activity; blue lines, mechanisms to increase blood glucose.

Box 5.1 Glucose unit conversion factors.

1 mg/dL = 0.0555 mmol/L
1 mmol/L = 18.018 mg/dL

Table 5.1 Hormones that regulate blood glucose.

Hormone	Site of production	Glucose-related action	Effect on blood glucose
Insulin	Pancreatic beta-cells	Enhances glucose entry into cells; storage of glucose as glycogen or fatty acids Suppresses breakdown of proteins and fats to amino acids and free fatty acids (antilipolytic), suppresses insulin secretion Regulates glucose release from hepatic cells	⬇
Glucagon	Pancreatic alpha-cells	Release of glucose from glycogen; promotes glucose production from amino acids and fatty acids	⬆
Amylin	Pancreatic beta-cells	Secreted with insulin; slows the rate of postprandial blood glucose appearance; promotes gastric emptying; promotes satiety	⬇
Somatostatin	Pancreatic delta-cells	Local suppression of glucagon release from alpha-cells; suppresses release of insulin, gastrin and secretin	⬇
Incretins GIP GLP-1	Gastrointestinal tract	Postprandial: enhance insulin release and inhibit glucagon release; reduced gastric emptying to slow nutrient absorption	⬇
Epinephrine	Adrenal gland	Release of glucose from glycogen; release of fatty acids from fat cells	⬆
Cortisol	Adrenal gland	Antagonizes insulin; promotes gluconeogenesis	⬆
Adrenocorticotropic hormone	Anterior pituitary gland	Promotes release of cortisol and release of fatty acids from fat cells	⬆
Growth hormone	Anterior pituitary gland	Stimulation of lipolysis in fat; decreased glucose uptake by muscle; increased hepatic gluconeogenesis	⬆
Thyroxine	Thyroid gland	Release of glucose from glycogen; enhanced absorption of sugars from gastrointestinal tract	⬆

History and physical exam

The signalment (age, sex, breed), initial history, and physical examination are assessed for evidence of problems associated with alterations in blood glucose. Historical findings compatible with or suggestive of hypoglycemia and hyperglycemia can be found in Table 5.2. Young dogs and cats, toy breed dogs, and hunting dogs may have a propensity for hypoglycemia. Cats frequently experience transient hyperglycemia due to stress. The current diet and appetite of the patient can become significant when related to blood glucose. Past medical problems could reveal clinical signs of underlying problems that will manifest as an alteration in blood glucose. Exposure to drugs or toxins known to be associated with changes in blood glucose (Table 5.3) should be identified.

Clinical signs will be influenced by the degree and rapidity of onset of glucose alterations. The level of consciousness, cardiovascular status, muscle strength and tone, urine production, and state of hydration are of particular interest when evaluating the physical examination related to blood glucose. The body condition score may demonstrate cachexia or obesity, both related to alterations in blood gluocse. A list of physical signs common to acute and chronic glucose disorders is provided in Table 5.2. Hospitalized critical patients are to be examined at least twice daily for new, worsening or changing physical signs compatible with abnormalities in blood glucose.

Typically, hypoglycemia is more consistent in showing overt clinical signs than hyperglycemia. Depressed mentation, tremors, seizures, and hypotension (weak or absent pulses, pale mucous membrane color) can be life-threatening signs of acute and severe hypoglycemia. With chronic, gradual hypoglycemia, the clinical signs are often more vague. Foul- or sweet-smelling breath (ketosis), depressed mentation or a plantigrade or palmigrade stance (Figure 5.2) can be signs of severe and chronic hyperglycemia.

Minimum database

The packed cell volume (PCV), total protein (TP), blood glucose, blood urea nitrogen (BUN), serum electrolytes, blood gas analysis, and coagulation profile (platelet estimate, prothrombin time, partial thromboplastin time) are considered crucial components of the minimum laboratory database for any critical animal. The PCV and TP can reflect anemia or hemoconcentration, each significant when assessing blood glucose results. A low BUN can direct investigation for liver disease, a known cause of hypoglycemia. The presence of a metabolic acidosis directs assessment of the electrolyte status and a search for blood and urine ketones. Hypokalemia and hypernatremia are important electrolyte changes that can occur with severe or chronic hyperglycemia. Hyperkalemia with hyponatremia can be a

result of hypoadrenocorticism, a cause of hypoglycemia. Alterations in coagulation must be identified and can occur secondary to diseases such as hyperadrenocorticism, hypothyroidism, and renal disease, known to be associated with glucose disorders.

Point of care testing

Blood glucose testing becomes a priority for any patient displaying signs of severe hypoglycemia, such as ataxia, collapse, altered consciousness, depressed mentation, seizures, muscle tremors or twitching, and coma. However, any patient admitted to the hospital should have at least one blood glucose test performed daily. Additional measurements are indicated for those patients with

Table 5.3 Drugs and toxins reported to affect blood glucose. This is a representation of agents and not intended to be a complete listing of all drugs and toxins affecting blood glucose.

Hyperglycemia	Hypoglycemia
Corticosteroids	Acetohexamide
Octreotide	Amprenavir
Beta-blockers	Chloramphenicol
Epinephrine	Chlorpromazine
Thiazide diuretics	Chlorpropamide
Niacin	Cibenzoline
Pentamidine	Clove
Protease inhibitors	Ethanol
L-asparaginase	Ethionamide
Acute amphetamine ingestion	Fluorodeoxyglucose
Zyprexa (olanzapine) and	Gatifloxacin
Cymbalta (duloxetine)	Ginseng
Dexmedetomidine	Glibenclamide
	Gliclazide
	Glimepiride
	Glipizide
	Gliquidone
	Insulin
	Insulin-like growth factor
	Pentamidine
	Perazine
	Pipothiazine
	Quinine
	Somatostatin
	Sulfamethoxazole
	Temafloxacin
	Tolazamide
	Tolbutamide
	Trimethoprim
	Xylitol

Table 5.2 Common historical and physical findings with hyperglycemia and hypoglycemia in the dog and cat.

Historical findings	Acute physical findings	Chronic physical findings
Hypoglycemia		
Toy breed, decreased appetite, gastrointestinal signs, neurological changes, exposure to toxins, medications (insulin), history of liver disease, prolonged fever, prolonged tremors or seizures	Ataxia, weakness, tachyarrhythmias, bradyarrhythmias, hypertension, nonresponsive hypotension, altered mentation, tremors, muscle fasciculations, seizures, blindness, coma, death	Lethargy, altered appetite, weakness, paresis, hypotension, bradycardia
Hyperglycemia		
Polyuria, polydipsia, polyphagia, severe stress	Dehydration, weight loss, polyuria, polydipsia, polyphagia, weakness, peripheral neuropathy, altered mentation, stupor, coma, death	Weight loss and muscle wasting, plantigrade stance, cataracts

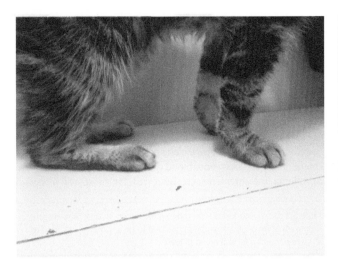

Figure 5.2 Plantigrade and palmigrade stance: clinical signs associated with chronic hyperglycemia. With therapy, this patient returned to normal neurological function and gait.

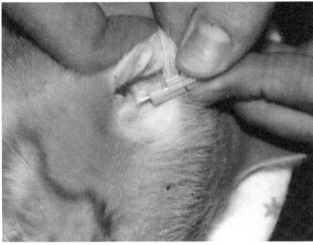

(a)

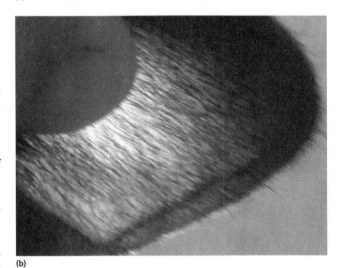

(b)

Figure 5.3 (a) A lancet can be used on the tragus of the ear to collect a drop of blood from the cat. (b) The lateral ear vein provides an additional source for collecting a drop of blood by lancet in the cat.

identified glucose disorders, on dextrose supplementation, receiving parenteral nutrition or requiring insulin therapy. More frequent or continuous monitoring may be indicated depending on the underlying disease and patient physical condition. A single blood glucose measurement may not be an accurate representation of the blood glucose status over time. Therefore, the interpretation of any single result should be made in light of how the condition of the patient has changed over time.

All hospitals should have a rapid, in-hospital method for quantitating blood glucose. While visual assessment of glucose test strips provides a quick estimation, POC testing is more accurate and cost-effective with portable blood glucose meters (PBGMs); the accuracy of the results from these POC glucose monitors has been investigated [12]. It is important to employ the manufacturer's guidelines, proper instrument care, and appropriate sample collection and handling. User error has been cited as one of the most common reasons for inaccurate results from PBGMs. Human glucometers have consistently underestimated actual glucose concentrations in the blood of dog and cats [13]. The human glucometers rely on universal distribution of glucose between plasma to whole blood. Unfortunately, that glucose distribution in whole blood is more variable in dogs and cats [13].

Veterinary-specific PBGMs are commercially available which have been tested and approved for analyzing canine and feline whole-blood glucose from miniscule quantities of blood. Test results are immediate, with many models showing results in <6 seconds. The use, accuracy, and efficacy have been reported for the AlphaTRAK® (Abbott Laboratories, Abbott Park, IL) and GlucoPet® (Animal Diabetes Management, Janesville, WI) veterinary PBGMs [14–18]. The GlucoPet requires 1 μL for testing and the AlphaTRAK only 0.3 μ for accurate results. The g-pet® (Woodley Equipment Copany, Horwich, UK), i-pet® (UltiCare Inc., St Paul, MN), and GlucoPet have been shown to have comparable results to the AlphaTRAK [14–18]. The use of a lancet minimizes the volume of blood drawn and reduces the risk of anemia from repeated blood collection in smaller patients. The use of the marginal ear vein technique (Figure 5.3) has been shown to be effective and safe, and to provide blood glucose values comparable to a peripheral vein in healthy cats and cats with diabetes mellitus [19].

The results from whole-blood testing by PBGMs can differ from serum biochemistry blood glucose results, depending upon the patient hematocrit. A false elevation in blood glucose can be reported in dogs with anemia and a false decline in blood glucose in dogs with elevated packed cell volumes [20,21] using veterinary PBGMs. Results from PBGMs should be assessed in light of the patient hematocrit to avoid missing a true hypoglycemia in an anemic patient.

Point of care measurement of blood beta-hydroxybutyrate is available to diagnose ketonemia. The POC Precision Xtra® ketone meter (Abbott, Alameda, CA) was found to be a valid tool for the measurement of beta-hydroxybutyrate in diabetic cats, with values <2.55 mmol/L excluding ketoacidosis [22].

Interstitial glucose monitors

Continuous glucose monitoring (CGM) is possible with interstitial glucose monitors (Figure 5.4). The CGMs measure the concentration of glucose in the interstitial space. Real-time continuous glucose evaluation can provide important data in critically ill animals [23,24].

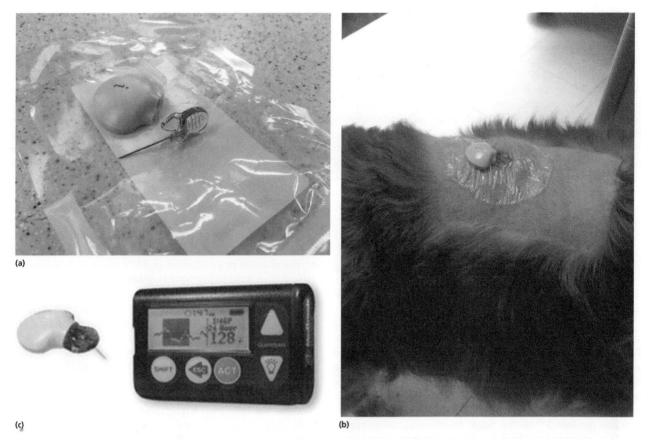

(a)

(c)

(b)

Figure 5.4 Continuous interstitial blood glucose monitoring system. (a) The sensor (needle) with transmitter. (b) The sensor and transmitter attached to the patient. (c) The real-time interstitial glucometer with graphic (glucose curve) display. Information from the system can be wirelessly transmitted to the receiver to collect and download data. Most systems require several calibration points, often every 12 hours. *Source*: photos courtesy of Dr Tyler Klose (a, b) and Medtronic (c).

Evaluation of CGMs in multiple veterinary populations has found the results to correlate well with serum reference laboratory results. These devices have been shown to provide early detection of hypoglycemia and demonstrate more accurate glucose trends over the course of treatment in diabetic animals compared to intermittent PBGM collection [25,26]. The use of CGMs in the ICU can also reduce the need for repeated blood collection, thereby improving patient comfort and potentially decreasing morbidity and mortality through prompt recognition and resolution of hyperglycemia or hypoglycemia.

The CGM devices consist of a portable recording device and a flexible glucose sensor electrode. Once placed in the subcutaneous tissues, glucose is measured at set intervals, which may be as little as every 10 seconds. An average value is generated and recorded at regular intervals (such as every 5 minutes). Studies in the cat have shown that dorsal neck placement of the probe may be superior to lateral chest wall and lateral knee fold placement for accuracy of glucose measurement [27]. The electrodes have a single patient use and must be replaced at recommended intervals. Calibration of the unit, which requires collecting whole-blood glucose, is required at least once during each 24-hour period. As the technology advances, veterinary-specific models with real-time measurements may become available.

Initial clinicopathological tests

The complete blood count (CBC), serum biochemical profile and urinalysis are important to identify disorders known to be associated with alterations in blood glucose. Neutrophilia with a left shift or leukopenia may direct diagnostic efforts to sepsis as a cause of hypoglycemia. A stress leukogram (neutrophila, eosinopenia, lymphopenia) may be consistent with a stress hyperglycemia.

The serum biochemical profile is used to assess for potential underlying metabolic conditions that can be associated with glucose disorders. The concentration of liver enzymes, albumin, cholesterol, and glucose can suggest the presence of liver disease, a cause of hypoglycemia. An elevated alkaline phosphatase is often present in hyperadrenocorticism, known to be associated with hyperglycemia. The BUN and creatinine are evaluated as a reflection of renal function, since the kidney is important in glucose homeostasis. Pancreatitis is recognized as a cause of diabetes mellitus with elevated pancreatic enzymes supporting the diagnosis, though additional testing and imaging are warranted.

The urinalysis can provide a significant amount of information in patients with glucose disorders. The urine specific gravity reflects renal function, with concentrated urine anticipated with dehydration from glycosuria in a normal kidney. Urine biochemical tests will detect the presence of glycosuria, ketonuria, proteinuria, and inflammatory cells, each a potential consequence of hyperglycemia. Urinary tract infection is a common consequence of glycosuria and can be diagnosed by microscopic examination of urine sediment for white blood cells and bacteria and urine culture.

Additional clinicopathological testing

Additional clinicopathological testing is often required to definitely diagnose underlying disorders causing alterations in blood glucose. Evaluation of the resting cortisol and adrenocorticotropic hormone (ACTH) stimulation may reveal hyper- or hypoadrenocortical disease. A diagnosis of pancreatitis requires assessment of pancreatic lipase immunoreactivity and abdominal imaging. Fasting and postprandial bile acids and blood ammonia levels might be indicated to identify hepatic contributions to a glucose disorder.

The assessment of plasma insulin concentrations compared to plasma glucose will aid in the diagnosis of insulinoma. A number of ratios have been utilized to aid in the diagnosis of an insulinoma (e.g. insulin:glucose ratio, amended insulin:glucose ratio). The most commonly utilized index is the amended insulin:glucose ratio which is calculated by the following equation:

$$\text{Amended insulin:glucose ratio} =$$
$$\text{plasma insulin}\left(\mu U/mL\right) \times 100 / \left(\text{plasma glucose}\left(mg/dL\right) - 30\right)$$

The insulin:glucose ratio must be assessed in conjunction with the historical and physical findings [28].

Fructosamine and glycosylated hemoglobin are two glycated proteins which can be quantitated in the serum for monitoring diabetic dogs and cats [29,30]. The two proteins reflect the mean blood glucose over a period of time. The levels are proportional to the blood glucose concentration and are not affected by stress. The bonding of glucose to proteins produces fructosamines. A single fructosamine measurement indicates the average glucose concentration over the previous 2–3 weeks. Single fructosamine measurements should be interpreted in light of clinical signs of diabetes, body weight, and blood glucose concentration. In general, the closer the fructosamine concentration is to the reference range for healthy dogs and cats, the better the glycemic control.

When blood glucose levels are high, glucose molecules attach to the hemoglobin in red blood cells. The hemoglobin molecule is permanently glycosylated. The glycosylated hemoglobin level is proportional to the average blood glucose concentration over the previous four weeks to three months.

Diagnostic imaging

Diagnostic imaging may be indicated to further characterize an underlying cause of a glucose disorder. Plain and contrast radiography can be used to demonstrate the size, shape, and location of internal organs and rapidly identify lesions suggestive of neoplasia. The presence of peritoneal or pleural effusions may be compatible with sepsis, a neoplastic process or liver failure, each potentially causing alterations in blood glucose. Studies have shown that the finding of a lower abdominal fluid glucose compared to the peripheral blood glucose is supportive of septic peritonitis (see Chapter 15).

In addition to these findings, abdominal ultrasound can demonstrate less obvious changes in individual organ size and structure, neoplastic lesions, vasculature, and compartmentalized fluid. Ultrasound examination of the adrenal glands can identify adrenal tumors that cause hyperadrenocorticism and hyperglycemia or smaller adrenal glands, which can support the presence of hypoadrenocorticism causing hypoglycemia [31]. A skilled ultrasonographer may identify portovascular anomalies. When a definitive diagnosis of a persistent glucose disorder is not possible by plain radiographs or ultrasound, advanced imaging such as a portovenogram, nuclear scintigraphy, computed tomography, or nuclear magnetic imaging may be indicated.

Disorders of glucose

Variability in blood glucose levels during critical illness can have a deleterious impact on complications, length of hospital stay, and mortality in ICU patients. Acute hypoglycemia has been known to cause life-threatening changes in brain function and vasomotor tone. Hyperglycemia affects fluid balance, brain function, and susceptibility to infection. The evaluation of blood glucose concentration by PBGMs enables rapid detection of glucose disorders. Therapeutic intervention for complications caused by hypoglycemia or hyperglycemia may be necessary prior to making the definitive diagnosis of the underlying disease state.

Hypoglycemia

Hypoglycemia presents the most immediate life-threatening glucose disorder in the critical patient. It can be a direct result of the primary pathology, a consequence of the increased energy demands of critical illness or a side-effect of medications administered (see Table 5.3). Symptoms attributable to hypoglycemia (see Table 5.2) in the critical patient are dependent upon the rate of change (acute or chronic) and the magnitude of change in blood glucose. Whipple's triad has been used as a tool to make the definitive diagnosis of hypoglycemia when the diagnosis is uncertain and consists of (1) symptoms known to be caused by hypoglycemia, (2) low blood glucose at the time the symptoms occurred, and (3) reversal or improvement of symptoms or problems when blood glucose is returned to normal.

When left untreated, hypoglycemia can result in permanent brain damage and eventually death. Neuroglycopenia causes dysfunction of cerebral Na-K-ATPase pumps and calcium channels. Subsequent cellular swelling and membrane disruption further augment neuronal excitotoxicity, leading to a series of events that risk permanent neuronal death [32].

The neurological symptoms of hypoglycemia could be overlooked due to similarity to preexisting signs of the underlying critical illness or the presence of sedation. Close and reliable monitoring of the glycemic level is crucial for rapidly detecting and treating hypoglycemia.

A mild decline in blood glucose concentration (blood glucose between 65 and 80 mg/dL (3.6–4.4 mmol/L) causes inhibition of insulin secretion from the pancreatic beta-cells. This results in decreased use of glucose by peripheral insulin-dependent tissues and removal of the blockade on hepatic gluconeogenesis. Should the blood glucose fall below 65 mg/dL (3.57 mmol/L), glucagon secretion rises, contributing to an increase in blood glucose concentration.

At this time the brain senses the drop in blood glucose and triggers a central sympathetic response (Figure 5.5). Metabolically, these compensatory mechanisms lead to increased glucose production through glycogenolysis initially and then gluconeogenesis, decreased muscle glucose oxidation and storage and increased release and use of alternate fuels, primarily free fatty acids. The free fatty acids are converted by the liver into ketone bodies, which can be used by the brain as an energy source. The restoration of plasma glucose to normoglycemia diminishes central sympathetic outflow.

Should hypoglycemia persist, growth hormone and cortisol release contribute to an increase in blood glucose. Cortisol enhances the mobilization of amino acids from proteins in many tissues and enhances the ability of the liver to convert these amino acids into glucose and glycogen by activating gluconeogenesis. The acute metabolic effects of growth hormone (see Table 5.1) oppose the normal

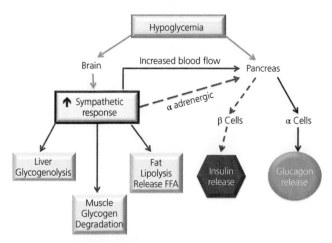

Figure 5.5 The effects of hypoglycemia on the brain and pancreas. Hypoglycemia stimulates an increase in the sympathetic response from the brain, resulting in increased hepatic glycogenolysis, muscle glycogen degradations, and lipolysis with the release of free fatty acids. The sympathetic-mediated increase in blood flow to the pancreas stimulates the alpha-cells to release glucagon and inhibits beta-cell release of insulin. There is also direct suppression of the beta-cells by the alpha-adrenergic sympathetic response. α, alpha; β, beta; FFA, free fatty acids.

effects of insulin on peripheral tissues and have been called the anti-insulin action of growth hormone [33].

Clinical signs

In acute or chronic presentations, clinical signs are typically influenced by both the rate and magnitude of onset of hypoglycemia. Blood glucose values typically need to be <64.8–68.4 mg/dL (3.5–3.79 mmol/L) to cause any clinical signs specifically attributable to hypoglycemia [2]. Depressed mentation, tremors, seizures, and hypotension (weak or absent pulses, pale mucous membrane color) can be life-threatening signs of acute and severe hypoglycemia. When hypoglycemia is acute, the patient is likely to manifest the classic neurological signs [10,34,35]. With chronic, gradual hypoglycemia, the clinical signs are often more vague. Table 5.2 lists the historical and physical examination findings typical of acute and chronic hypoglycemia.

The etiology of hypoglycemia can be divided into three broad categories: (1) decreased glucose production, (2) increased glucose consumption, or (3) increased glucose loss. Common causes of hypoglycemia in the dog and cat are listed in Table 5.4, with a summary of the mechanism(s) causing the low glucose. In addition to the comments below, diagnostic and initial therapeutic interventions for common causes of hypoglycemia are presented in Table 5.5.

Therapy

The initial goal of therapy is to supplement glucose to a level adequate to eliminate detrimental clinical signs. The method of treatment is guided by the severity of clinical signs and the suspected underlying cause of hypoglycemia.

The presence of critical clinical signs such as dementia, seizures, coma, tremors, hypotension, and generalized weakness warrants immediate correction of hypoglycemia with intravenous (IV) glucose (also labeled as dextrose) supplementation. Intravenous or intraosseous access is required and 0.5 g/kg of dextrose as a 25% dextrose solution is administered.

Persistent or refractory hypoglycemia may necessitate adding dextrose to the IV fluids. The goal is to administer the lowest

Table 5.4 Differential diagnosis for causes of hypoglycemia in the dog and cat.

Disorder	Mechanism of hypoglycemia
Artifactual hypoglycemia	Improper handling of samples
Decreased glucose production	
Hypoadrenocorticism	Cortisol deficiency
Liver disease, hepatoportal	Failure of gluconeogenesis, insufficient hepatic glycogen stores
Glycogen storage disease	Hepatic enzyme deficiency
Toy breed, puppy hypoglycemia	Alanine deficiency, limited hepatic glycogen stores, decreased muscle mass, lack of adipose tissue, impaired gluconeogenesis
Long-term starvation	Decreased intake of components for glucose production
Increased glucose consumption	
Sepsis	Hypoxic injury to hepatic cells, utilization of glucose by bacteria, increased tissue utilization of glucose, other mechanisms
Toxicosis	Xylitol, other medications (see Table 5.3)
Insulinoma	Insulin-secreting pancreatic beta-cells neoplasm
Other neoplasia	Insulin-like factors, liver metastasis, glucose utilization by large tumors
Polycythemia, high white blood cell counts	Increased utilization by red blood cells or white blood cells
Insulin overdose	Hyperinsulinism
Increased glucose loss	
Renal disease	Renal tubular problem causing glycosuria

Source: adapted from Koenig A. Hypoglycemia. In: Small Animal Critical Care Medicine, 2nd edn. Silverstein DC, Hopper K, eds. St Louis: Elsevier Saunders, 2015: pp 352–6.

concentration of dextrose that will maintain the blood glucose concentration between 80 and 100 mg/dL (4.44–5.55 mmol/L). Up to 7.5% dextrose can be given through a peripheral vein. When a higher concentration is required, central venous access is necessary to avoid phlebitis [37]. Since glucose will cause an intracellular shifting of serum potassium, monitoring blood potassium levels is necessary during glucose infusion. Potassium supplementation is provided in the IV crystalloids as outlined in Box 5.2 below. When a patient does not respond to glucose supplementation or requires increasing amounts of glucose for stabilization, investigation for causes such as insulinoma, septicemia or organ ischemia should be initiated.

Table 5.6 provides the amount of dextrose to add to the IV fluids to create the targeted dextrose percentage concentration. The addition of dextrose to IV fluids will increase the osmolarity of the solution, which can influence patient fluid balance. Because glucose cannot freely diffuse across a cell membrane, the added dextrose will cause the movement of water into the fluid compartment containing the higher concentration of glucose or dextrose. If the patient already has an abnormally high osmolarity (hypernatremia, elevated BUN), the addition of dextrose can amplify the negative effects of a high osmolarity. Should the patient be dehydrated, the higher amount of dextrose in IV fluids can further amplify dehydration of the tissues by pulling fluid from the interstitial space into the intravascular space.

Table 5.5 Diagnotic testing and possible treatment plans for common causes of hypoglycemia in critical small animal patients.

Disease	Diagnostics	Treatment plan
Hypoadrenocorticism	Baseline cortisol ACTH stimulation test Pre, 1 µg/kg cortisyn IV, 1 hour post	Dexamethasone NaP IV 0.1–0.3 mg/kg DOCP 2 mg/kg (only if indicated) Prednisone 0.5–1 mg/kg/day PO
Hepatopathy	Ultrasound (hepatic size, vascular anomalies) Blood ammonia level Ammonia level Bile acids (pre/post-prandial) Scintigraphy/MRI	Surgical correction (portovenous anomaly) Nutritional support based on needs Nutriceuticals Antibiotic coverage
Toxin	Thorough history	Activate charcoal depending on need Supportive care
Neoplasia	Ultrasound Thoracic radiographs/CT scan Amended Insulin:glucose ratio	Surgical removal of neoplasia Chemotherapy Glucagon CRI (insulinoma)
Renal insult	Urinanalysis for glucosuria Ultrasound Urine culture/susceptibility & MIC Dietary history (Fanconi's syndrome)	Removal of nutritional influence if any Renal diet
Septicemia	Complete blood count Serum chemistry Abdominal ultrasound Abdominal radiographs Thoracic radiographs and/or CT scan Urine culture/susceptibility & MIC Blood culture/susceptibility & MIC Fluid analysis Blood pressure monitoring	Antibiotic coverage guided by diagnostics Surgical intervention when appropriate Fluid supportive care (see Chapter 2) Nutritional support (see Chapter 16)

Table 5.6 Amount of dextrose to create desired percentage supplementation in IV fluids.

% Dextrose solution	mL of 50% dextrose	mL of isotonic fluids
1.25	25	975
2.50	50	950
5	100	900
7.50	150	750
10	200	800

Glucose or dextrose supplementation can be provided orally for at-home emergencies by rubbing a solution containing a high glucose concentration (honey, corn syrup, or commercial oral glucose preparations) on mucous membranes when the animal is unable to swallow. However, oral administration is not the mainstay for emergency management of hypoglycemia and is more important for long-term maintenance therapy, if required. Oral administration is metabolically more effective when the intestinal tract is functioning appropriately. It is recommended that patients be transitioned onto enteral supplementation of glucose, ideally through their diet. The use of feeding tubes (esophagostomy, nasogastric, jejunostomy, or gastrostomy tubes) may facilitate feeding and oral glucose supplementation in the critical patient.

Neurological signs such as seizures, tremors, facial twitching or coma can persist even after normoglycemia has been achieved. Brain edema and ischemia are potential residual effects of hypoglycemia that could necessitate therapy to reduce edema and protect the brain tissues. Benzodiazepines, levetiracetam, phenobarbital, and propofol can be used individually or in combination for the control of residual seizures, facial twitching, and neurogenic tremors. The selection of a specific drug is dependent on the suspected underlying disease process and neurological status of the patient (see treatment of cerebral edema and seizures in Chapter 12).

Insulinoma

Insulinoma is suspected in middle-aged or older dogs with clinical signs of hypoglycemia (such as weakness, tremors, lethargy, depression, seizures or collapse). The diagnosis relies on the measurement of normal or high serum insulin (normal 5–20 IU/mL) in the presence of a blood glucose concentration less than 60 mg/dL (<3.33 mmol/L). If the serum insulin is below detectable limits when the dog is hypoglycemic, the presence of an insulinoma is unlikely. Appropriately timed collection, storage, and transport of blood insulin levels is essential for accurate measurement. If a borderline result is obtained, a repeat measurement should be made. In the case of nondiagnostic results, detection of an insulin peak is more likely if at least four glucose and insulin measurements are made during a 24-hour period [37].

A high percentage of dextrose is often required to maintain the blood glucose within an acceptable range when treating animals with insulinoma. Dextrose supplementation must be titrated cautiously since hyperglycemia can amplify insulin release from the tumor cells, resulting in a persistent or rebound hypoglycemia.

The administration of glucagon may be required for glycemic stability. Glucagon induces glycogenolysis and increases hepatic glucose metabolism, which requires sufficient glycogen stores and adequate liver function. Cirrhosis, fulminant hepatic failure, portosystemic shunts, neonatal hepatopathy, or glycogen storage disease are not likely to have the desired glucose response from glucagon administration. Glucagon is given at a recommended dose of 50 ng/kg IV. Continuous rate infusions (5–40 ng/kg/min IV) of glucagon titrated to effect may be required to stabilize patients with an insulinoma [38,39].

Continued medical management with glucocorticosteroids (starting at 0.25 mg/kg q 12 h) to increase gluconeogenesis and decrease cellular uptake of glucose [40] may be indicated. Other drug options for medical management of an insulinoma include diazoxide (starting at 5 mg/kg q 12 h) to inhibit pancreatic insulin secretion and inhibit tissue glucose uptake [40], octreotide acetate (somatostatin: 1–2 μg/kg subcutaneously q 8–12 h) to inhibit secretion of insulin and glucagon [41] or streptozotocin (500 mg/m²) which is an alkylating agent, taken up by GLUT2 trasnporters on pancreatic beta-cells [42,43]. Imaging and surgical intervention may be required for diagnosis and definitive treatment; one study demonstrated an improved outcome for dogs with insulinoma which were treated surgically [44].

Hyperglycemia

Symptoms of hyperglycemia in the critical patient are dependent upon the rate and magnitude of elevation in blood glucose, and are listed in Tables 5.2 and 5.7. Mild forms of hyperglycemia may be subtle. As the hyperglycemia becomes prolonged, polyuria, polyphagia, polydipsia, and peripheral neuropathy (see Figure 5.2) can develop. These signs can be common with disorders such as diabetes mellitus, agromegaly, hyperadrenocorticism, and chronic stress. A nondiabetic form of hyperglycemia is found secondary to illness and has been named diabetes of injury or stress hyperglycemia [45]. In addition, nondiabetic hyperglycemia can be associated with various drugs, toxins, and common analgesics (see Table 5.3).

Numerous studies have proven the negative outcomes associated with hyperglycemia in various disease states. Reduced neutrophil and phagocytic activity, hypercoagulability, increased proinflammatory cytokine production, vascular injury, and impaired complement activity are important systemic detrimental effects [46–54]. Prolonged untreated hyperglycemia leads to organ failure (see Table 5.7) and eventually death.

Tight glycemic control (TGC) has been a topic of considerable debate and is advocated in human medical, coronary, and surgical ICUs to improve survival. However, there is evidence that both supports and refutes the benefits of TGC.

Diabetes mellitus and stress-induced hyperglycemia are two of the more common causes of hyperglycemia in the critically ill small animal patient. Early recognition and treatment of hyperglycemic disorders are necessary to minimize complications and improve survival.

Stress-induced hyperglycemia

Acute illness or injury may result in hyperglycemia, insulin resistance, and glucose intolerance. This is collectively termed *stress hyperglycemia* or *diabetes of injury*. The neuroendocrine response to stress plays a significant role in the pathophysiology and deleterious consequences of stress hyperglycemia (Figure 5.6). Adverse complications including immune disorders, oxidative stress, susceptibility to infection, and endothelial dysfunction have been reported in humans with this syndrome [55–57]. A strong association has been

Table 5.7 Effects of hyperglycemia on body systems.

Organ or system affected	Pathophysiology	Manifestation	Clinical signs
Osmolarity	High Osmolarity initially causes fluid shift out of cells; with time, cells produce idiogenic osmols to equilibrate osmolality across cell membrane	Cell volume reduction; cellular dysfunction	Mental depression, seizures, stupor, coma, respiratory distress
Fluid balance	Glucose-induced diuresis with reduced water intake, intracellular osmolar shifting of fluids	Dehydration and increased blood viscosity; decreased perfusion of organs	Dehydration; organ dysfunction
Immune system	Neutrophil, phagocytic, complement activity; proinflammatory cytokine production	Systemic infections, systemic inflammatory response, urinary bladder infections	Fever, systemic illness, weakness, evidence of SIRS
Vasculature	Overproduction of superoxide radicals by endothelial cell electron transport chain causing endothelial cell dysfunction and cell death	Increased capillary permeability; exposure of subendothelial collagen; changes in vascular tone	Hypertension, peripheral edema, proteinuria,
Hypertension	Changes in vascular structure and function	Reduced blood flow to critical organs causing structural damage and dysfunction: kidneys, myocardium, retinas	Acute blindness; arrhythmias, altered mentation, weakness
Myocardium	Acute glucose extraction; lactate production; later reduced glucose uptake; production of reactive oxygen species; microvascular disease		
Renal	Glycosuria, potentially glomerular pathology	Polyuria, proteinuria	Polyuria, polydipsia, dehydration
Coagulation	Vascular damage and inflammatory mediators stimulating coagulation	Thrombosis of vessels, arrhythmias, hypoxemia	Cold limbs, sudden focal pain, labored breathing, weakness
Brain	Osmolar shifting of intracellular fluid, impaired recovery of brain cell membrane function and energy metabolism after hypoxia	Depressed mentation, stupor, coma	Depressed mentation, stupor, coma
Peripheral nerves	Microvascular injury; production of glycosylated proteins within nerve cell; activation of protein kinase C in nerve	Delayed nerve conduction	Weakness, falling, plantigrade or palmigrade stance
Eyes	Microvascular changes	Retinal detachment or hemorrhage, cataracts	Sudden blindness, cloudy lens

SIRS, systemic inflammatory response syndrome.

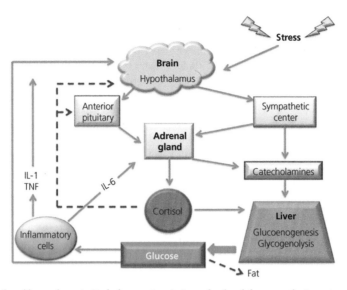

Figure 5.6 Mechanisms of stress-induced hyperglycemia. Both the anterior pituitary gland and the sympathetic center are stimulated by stress impacting the hypothalamus of the brain. The adrenal glands are stimulated to produce cortisol and epinephrine. The sympathetic stimulation results in the release of norepinephrine and further stimulates the adrenal gland. The result is an elevated blood glucose arising from hormonal stimulation of hepatic gluconeogenesis and glycogenolysis. Hyperglycemia provides a stimulus for the activation of inflammatory cells, with the resultant cytokine release further stimulating the central stress response. Green lines indicate stimulation; red dashed lines indicate inhibition.

found between stress hyperglycemia and poor clinical outcomes, including mortality, morbidity, length of stay, occurrence of infections, and other complications in human ICU patients.

The negative impact that hyperglycemia has on critical patients [58–61] prompted human ICUs to administer insulin to maintain TGC of their patients [62–65]. The optimal glucose level, the accuracy of measurements, the resources required to attain TGC, and the impact of TGC across the heterogeneous ICU population provide points of controversy in human medicine. The process of TGC requires the staff to adhere to established protocols for insulin administration and diligent monitoring for hypoglycemia. Subsequent data has demonstrated increased risks of hypoglycemia, with the consequences of hypoglycemia potentially outweighing the benefits of TGC [66–68]. A modified range of glycemic control was adapted after the NICE-SUGAR study in people that showed improved morbidity and decreased mortality with permissive mild hyperglycemia of <180 mg/dL (<9.99 mmol/L) compared to the previous tight standards of 81–108 mg/dL (4.49–5.99 mmol/L) [69].

The frequency and impact of stress-induced hyperglycemia in dogs and cats in the veterinary ICU are unknown at this time, and there is little to no research available on TGC in veterinary patients. Not all hyperglycemia needs immediate treatment. Stress hyperglycemia can resolve within a few hours, requiring close monitoring to establish a positive trend. Mild hyperglycemia related to sepsis should be closely monitored. A reasonable goal is to monitor and maintain the patient blood glucose between 80 and 180 mg/dL (4.4–9.9 mmol/L) to minimize complications associated with hyperglycemia and avoid hypoglycemia associated with insulin administration.

Diabetes mellitus

Diabetes mellitus is a metabolic disease causing high blood sugar over a prolonged period of time. Clinical signs do not develop until hyperglycemia reaches a concentration that results in glycosuria, typically blood glucose of 180–220 mg/dL (9.99–12.21 mmol/L) in

dogs and 220–270 mg/dL (12.21–14.98 mmol/L) in cats [71]. The disease is commonly divided into two types, depending on the origin of the condition. Type 1 diabetes (also called insulin-dependent diabetes or primary diabetes) results from loss of functional pancreatic beta-cells, causing the loss of normal insulin production and secretion. Glucagon production and release from the alpha-cells is typically preserved. This is the most common form of diabetes found in the dog. Insulin deficiency is severe and glucose and ketone production rise. The administration of exogenous insulin is a key component to successful therapy of type 1 diabetes.

Type 2 diabetes (also called insulin-resistant or secondary diabetes) is due to abnormal cellular uptake or abnormal utilization of glucose in response to insulin. Eventually, insufficient secretion of insulin occurs as well. Type 2 diabetes is found more often in the cat than the dog, with most cats being insulin dependent by the time symptoms are diagnosed. Secondary or type 2 diabetes may be caused by conditions such as pancreatitis, use of steroid medications or estrus hormones, acromegaly, pregnancy, hyperadrenocorticism, and obesity. Insulin resistance evolving during weight gain is often reversible after weight loss in the cat [71].

Systemic consequences

The hyperglycemia of diabetes mellitus has detrimental and multisystemic consequences (see Table 5.7). Changes in serum osmolarity and electrolytes can result in dangerous alterations in brain and muscle function in the critical diabetic patient. Glucose cannot freely diffuse across a cell membrane and acts as an effective osmole. Serum osmolarity can be measured and when not available, serum sodium, potassium, glucose, and BUN are used to calculate osmolarity by the following equation [72]:

$$\text{Osmolarity}\left(\text{mg}/\text{dL}\right) = 2\left(\text{Na}^+ + \text{K}^+\right) + \text{Glucose}/18 + \text{BUN}/2.8 \text{ or}$$

$$\text{Osmolarity}\left(\text{mmol}/\text{L}\right) = 2\left(\text{Na}^+\right) + \text{Glucose}/18 + \text{BUN}/2.8$$

Normal osmolarity in the dog and cat is 290–310 mOsm/L. Since urea freely passes cell membranes, it is an ineffective osmole. This makes sodium and glucose the most important natural contributors to serum osmolality (and tonicity), and both can be altered in the animal with diabetes mellitus.

A schematic illustration of fluid shifts and the compensatory cellular response to extravascular changes in osmolarity are presented in Figure 5.7. Most cell membranes are freely permeable to water, causing cells to shrink or swell in response to changes in extracellular fluid tonicity. This is generally undesirable since most cells need a constant volume to maintain function. However, brain cells are capable of increasing their intracellular osmolarity (and tonicity) by producing solutes (idiogenic osmoles or osmolytes) from cellular metabolism. These substances include taurine, glycine,

glutamine, sorbitol, and inositol. An increase in these idiogenic osmoles can occur within hours after an acute hypertonic challenge. The idiogenic osmoles cannot freely cross the cell membrane and must be removed by cellular metabolism. A sudden drop in interstitial osmolarity will cause a sudden and possibly dramatic shift of the osmolar gradient. The gradient then favors water movement into the cell with subsequent cell swelling. Clinical signs of brain cell swelling can range from mild depression to seizures, tremors, stupor, coma, and death.

The hyperglycemia of diabetes mellitus will affect serum electrolyte concentrations. Total body hypokalemia is anticipated due to the loss of potassium through polyuria and, potentially, vomiting. Insulin therapy will cause a transient shifting of extracellular potassium into the cells and lower blood potassium concentrations.

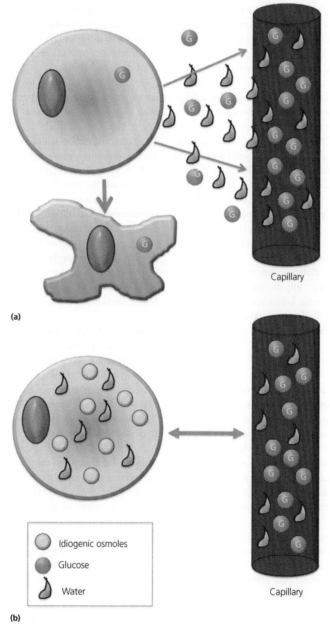

(a)

(b)

Idiogenic osmoles

Glucose

Water

Capillary

Figure 5.7 (a) Initially the high blood glucose causes increases in interstitial glucose concentrations and creates an osmolar gradient between the cell, interstitium, and the blood, favoring movement of water from the cell into the blood. This results in loss of intracellular volume. (b) The brain attempts to counteract this osmotic gradient by forming idiogenic osmoles. However, as the surrounding hyperosmolality increases, water will eventually leave the cells. The resulting cellular changes include shrinking of the oligodendroglial cytoplasm, decreased oligodendroglial processes about the vessels, vacuolation of endothelial cells, and increased neuronal density.

Persistent or low potassium can lead to life-threatening paresis or paralysis of cardiac and respiratory muscles.

Disorders of serum sodium concentrations can be catastrophic in the diabetic patient and must be identified and appropriately managed. Hypernatremia can occur due to glycosuria causing the loss of water in excess of sodium. Compensatory water intake declines as the animal becomes ill, resulting in significant hypernatremia and the resultant changes in serum osmolarity. Clinical manifestations of hypernatremia can be subtle, consisting of lethargy, weakness, and neuromuscular excitability. With more severe elevations, seizures and coma may occur. See Chapter 6 for further discussion on electrolytes.

Hyponatremia can also be found in the diabetic patient. While the actual total body sodium concentration may be normal, the serum value is often reduced due to the presence of high blood glucose. The hyperglycemia causes a shift of water into the intravascular space, leading to dilution of the sodium concentration. This is often called pseudohyponatremia (also seen with high serum protein concentrations and lipemia). True hyonatremia can also occur if water intake becomes excessive, surpassing the amount of water lost through polyuria. Clinical signs of hyponatremia include nausea and vomiting, lethargy, fatigue, loss of appetite, muscle weakness, ventroflexion of the neck, spasms or cramps, seizures, and decreased consciousness or coma.

The alterations in immune function and high glucose concentrations in the blood and urine predispose animals with diabetes to infections. Urinary tract, skin, and dental infections place these patients at risk for sepsis and other complications. Insulin resistance can be a consequence and will make stabilization of blood glucose difficult. Monitoring for the presence of occult urinary tract infections, gingivitis, skin disease, and pneumonia is critical in the diabetic patient, with meticulous care taken to ensure aseptic technique when performing any invasive procedures.

The systemic consequences of diabetes can contribute to the development of two potentially life-threatening metabolic syndromes in the dog and cat: diabetic ketoacidosis and hyperosmolar hyperglycemic syndromes. Early recognition of a diabetic crisis is essential with intensive therapy and monitoring required for a successful outcome.

Diabetic ketoacidosis syndrome

Diabetic ketoacidosis is characterized by high blood and urine glucose and ketone concentrations, acidemia, and dehydration. Prolonged stress results in the production and release of stress hormones (such as cortisol, glucagon, growth hormone, epinephrine, norepinephrine). These hormones accelerate lipolysis, resulting in the production of ketoacids (acetoacetic acid, beta-hydroxybutyric acid) [73,74]. The breakdown of acetoacetic acid produces acetone and carbon dioxide. These are exhaled and cause a smell to the breath similar to nail polish remover or paint thinner.

Severe acidosis can cause depressed cardiac contractility and cardiac output, vasodilation, impaired cellular energy production, insulin resistance, and impaired leukocyte function. In addition to urinary losses from polyuria and volume contraction, an obligate loss of potassium occurs with the excretion of the negatively charged ketone beta-hydroxybutyrate by the kidneys. A reported mortality rate of up to 30% in dogs [75] with ketoacidosis syndrome makes the therapy of these patients a challenge. It is important to search for the underlying stress factor(s) initiating the ketoacidosis, with infection, heat cycle, pregnancy, pancreatitis,

hyperadrenocorticism, hyperthyroidism, and medications administered being possible causes.

Hyperosmolar hyperglycemic syndromes

When hyperosmolar hyperglycemic syndrome is associated with type 2 diabetes, there is enough insulin present to prevent significant ketone production. This form is called hyperosmolar nonketotic diabetes. However, ketosis may be present (called hyperosmolar ketotic syndrome), but at a reduced level to that occurring in the animal with diabetic ketoacidosis syndrome. The blood glucose elevations are dramatic ($\geq$600 mg/dL; $\geq$33.3 mmol/L) in both syndromes, causing an increased extracellular osmolarity and severe fluid loss through polyuria. Depressed mentation and severe dehydration are hallmarks of both hyperosmolar hyperglycemic syndromes. Hypotension and stupor or coma can occur as potentially life-threatening consequences.

In a retrospective study of dogs with the hyperosmolar hyperglycemic state, those with ketosis were found to have a higher incidence of acute pancreatitis, lower venous blood pH, higher white blood cell count, and shorter duration of clinical signs when compared to hyperosmolar nonketotic dogs. Hyperosmolar nonketotic dogs had higher osmolarity and higher BUN and creatinine concentrations than dogs with hyperosmolar ketosis [76].

Diagnosis of diabetic crisis

Past medical problems might reveal health problems potentiating a diabetic crisis. It is important to look for underlying problems such as hyperadrenocorticism, pyometra, prostatitis, urinary tract infections, pancreatitis, deep-seated infections or inflammation, growth hormone abnormalities, thyroid abnormalities, and pheochromocytoma. The findings of metabolic acidosis and ketones in the blood and urine make the diagnosis of diabetic ketoacidosis syndrome. Severe hyperglycemia (>600 mg/dL; 33.3 mmol/L) with few or no ketones in the blood in the dehydrated animal with depressed mentation or altered consciousness supports the diagnosis of hyperosmolar hyperglycemic syndromes.

Treatment of hyperglycemic crisis

Careful therapeutic planning and diligent patient monitoring are mandatory for a successful outcome. The mortality rate can be high, with 38% of the animals in a study of dogs with hyperosmolar hyperglycemic syndromes not surviving to discharge; however, the majority were euthanized [76]. General treatment guidelines for stabilizing the patient in a diabetic crisis (diabetic ketoacidosis and hyperosmolar hyperglycemic syndrome) are provided in Box 5.2.

It is critical to lower the blood glucose and to correct serum sodium slowly to allow equilibration of fluid between the intra- and extracellular compartments to occur without causing cellular edema. The choice of crystalloids to infuse will depend upon the electrolyte status of the patient. Normal saline and an isotonic balanced maintenance solution (such as Plasmalyte-A®, Normosol-R®, lactated Ringer's) are examples of typical initial fluid choices. The use of hydroxyethyl starch with crystalloids can be of benefit for resuscitation of perfusion deficits and during rehydration and maintenance. The administered colloid can favor the retention of fluid within the blood vessels and potentially reduce extravasation of crystalloids. Rehydration will occur over hours, with the time span dependent upon which crisis syndrome is present (see Table 5.7)

The presence of harmful ketoacids necessitates the initiation of insulin therapy to stop ketone production in the animal with

Box 5.2 General guidelines for stabilizing the small animal in a hyperglycemic crisis.

1. **Identify diabetic ketoacidosis or hyperglycemic hyperosmolar syndromes**
   Calculate osmolarity. Identify: hypernatremia, hyponatremia, hypokalemia, hypophosphatemia, metabolic acidosis, ketoacids.
2. **Draw and submit samples for clinicopathological testing**
   CBC, biochemical profile, urine for culture, and possibly ACTH stimulation test, T3, T4 as indicated.
3. **Assess and support perfusion and hydration – avoid rapid shifts in IV hydrostatic pressure and osmolarity**
   Place an IV or IO catheter. Estimate perfusion and hydration status– assess blood pressure, perfusion parameters.
   Resuscitate hypotension using crystalloids and ± hydroxyethyl starch colloid (minimizes extravascular fluid shifts). Resuscitation volumes (bolus over
   10 minutes when patient is in shock (dogs): 10–30 mL/kg crystalloids, 5–10 mL/kg hydroxyethyl starch in dogs; 10 mL/kg crystalloids, 5 mL/kg
   hydroxyethyl starch in cats, then warming. Titrate additional crystalloids (5–10 mL/kg) and colloid (5 mL/kg) to low normal resuscitation end points.
   See Chapter 2 for more information.
   Establish rehydration crystalloid fluid rate accounting for residual dehydration, metabolic needs and polyuria.
   Consider CRI of hydroxyethyl starch (0.6–0.8 mL/kg/h) with crystalloids to support intravascular COP.
   Conscious ketoacidosis patient: begin rehydration over 2–4 h before insulin infusion is started.
   Moribund or unconscious hyperosmolar patient: rehydrate over 6–24 h before insulin infusion is initiated.
4. **Repeat glucose, Na, K, blood gas values once hydrated; more frequently for hyperosmolar patient**
5. **Supplement potassium** if hypokalemia is present and prior to initiation of CRI insulin therapy
   Make sure animal is producing urine first

SERUM POTASSIUM	K+ ADDED TO 250 ML FLUIDS
Less than 2.0 mEq/L	20 mEq/250 mL
2.0–2.5 mEq/L	15 mEq/250 mL
2.5–3.0 mEq/L	10 mEq/250 mL
3.0–3.5 mEq/L	7 mEq/250 mL

   If potassium is normal, supplement fluids with 7 mEq/250 mL once insulin infusion is initiated.
6. **Begin CRI infusion of regular insulin (+/- long-acting insulin):** CRIs requires a separate IV fluid bag, infusion line and fluid pump from IV fluid
   therapy; insulin is reported to stick to plastic so 50 mL of fluid should be run through line.
   Ketoacidosis: dog: 2 units/kg/day; cat: 1 unit/kg/day
   Hyperglycemic hyperosmolar syndromes: 0.25–0.5 units/kg/day dog and cat
7. **Monitor** blood glucose q 2–4 h or continuously, Na, K, blood gases q 4–6 h, fluid ins and outs q 4–6 h, perfusion parameters q 1–6 h, mentation q
   1–4 h, TPR q 4–8 h, urine sediment for casts q 2–8 h, body weight q 24 h on same scale.
8. **Consider further investigation for underlying disease**
   Imaging, urine culture, testing for endocrine disease, etc.
9. **Alter insulin CRI infusion or fluids** as follows:

BLOOD GLUCOSE	TREATMENT CHANGES
>400 mg/dL	Continue as above. If glucose is not declining after 2–3 rechecks, increase insulin by 1 unit/kg/day
250–400 mg/dL	Continue as initially planned
200–250 mg/dL	Change fluids to 2.5% dextrose in half-strength lactated Ringer's
150–200 mg/dL	Change fluids to 2.5% dextrose in half-strength lactated Ringer's and stop insulin infusion
100–150 mg/dL	Stop insulin infusion and put on 5% dextrose in half-strength lactated Ringer's
<100 mg/dL	Stop insulin infusion, put on 5% dextrose in half-strength lactated Ringer's and bolus 0.1–0.25 g/kg 50% dextrose (0.5–1 mL/kg)

Begin maintenance insulin when: Eating, ketones production has stopped, mentation has returned, blood glucose is maintained below 200 mg/dl
   on IV infusion.

ketoacidosis earlier compared to the patient with a hyperosmolar hyperglycemic syndrome. Regular insulin is administered intravenously by constant rate infusion (CRI; see Box 5.2) or by intermittent intramuscular (IM) injection. Lispro insulin given as a CRI has been shown to be an acceptable alternative to regular insulin given by CRI in the dog [77]. Guidelines for adjustments of insulin administration and fluid composition for CRI insulin administration are based on blood glucose levels and are provided in Box 5.2.

An IM regular insulin protocol has been described as a substitute for the CRI regular insulin protocol [78]. Regular insulin is given at 0.1 U/kg IM as an initial dose, followed by 0.05 U/kg IM every 1–2 hours until glucose is <300 mg/dL (16.65 mmol/L). The IM injections are then continued every 4–6 hours. A protocol giving glargine IM in cats with diabetic ketoacidosis has provided an alternative to regular insulin or may be initiated along with continuous infusions of regular insulin [79,80]. Most cats required a combination of IM glargine (1–2 units per cat) combined with subcutaneous glargine (1–3 units per cat) as required at intervals for the IM injection of two or more hours and the subcutaneous injection every 12 hours.

Adjustments in insulin dosage, timing, and fluid composition (glucose supplementation) must be made based on the blood glucose concentrations. Serum glucose blood levels should be checked every 1–2 hours initially, and every 4–6 hours once the glucose has been stabilized, or real-time continuous glucose monitoring may be utilized.

Complications should be anticipated with patient assessment using the Rule of 20 twice daily during the stabilization process. Anticipated complications include hypoglycemia, acidosis, hypokalemia, hyper- or hyponatremia, acute renal failure, infections, hypophosphatemia, thromboemboli, and decline in mentation or level of consciousness. Cerebral edema can develop if hyperglycemia or hypernatremia is decreased too rapidly, causing brain cell swelling, making monitoring of serum osmolarity essential; it is important to not alter patients that may be chronically hyperosmolar by more than 0.5–1 mEq/h (81). Signs of severe and sudden changes in osmolarity can include

hypotension, cardiac arrhythmias, tremors, facial twitching, seizures, stupor, coma, and sudden death. Hypophosphatemia can occur after initiation of insulin therapy and feeding in patients with diabetic ketoacidosis. The increased demand for energy production causes a shift of phosphorus from the extracellular fluid into the cell. Most commonly, there are no clinical signs, but hemolytic anemia can occur if severe hypophosphatemia is untreated. In situations where phosphate supplementation is deemed necessary, the recommended dose is 0.01–0.03 mmol/kg/h of phosphate followed by repeat serum phosphorus determinations every six hours.

Maintenance insulin therapy in the ICU

Maintenance insulin therapy is required after the diabetic crisis has been stabilized or when the patient has been on insulin therapy at home. There are many types of insulin available, with the selection based on the onset and duration of action of the insulin, time to peak concentration, and patient response to treatment. A list of available types of insulin and their manufacturer is provided in Table 5.8. The insulin vial should be refrigerated after opening and handled carefully to avoid shaking the insulin, which could alter its potency and absorption.

The initial insulin type used for maintenance in the dog is typically NPH or lente, and in the cat is PZI or glargine. Glargine (0.3 units/kg subcutaneously, twice daily) has been reported to be a

Table 5.8 Types of insulin commonly used in dogs and cats.

Insulin type	Brand/ manufacturer	Onset time	Peak time	Duration	Comment
Rapid acting Lispro Aspart	Humalog® Eli LillyNovoLog® Novo Nordisk	10–20 min 10–20 min	1.5–2.5 h 1.5–2.5 h	4–5 h 4–5 h	Lispro has been shown to be interchangeable with regular insulin as a CRI in dogs when treating diabetes ketoacidosis – no obvious advantage over regular insulin in dogs and cats
Short acting Regular	Humulin R® Eli Lilly Novolin R® Novo Nordisk	30–45 min 30–60 min	2–4 h 2–3 h	5–7 h 4–6 h	Can be given 30–45 min before meals if hyperglycemia postprandial; used as CRI or IM to stabilize diabetic ketoacidosis and hyperosmolar hyperglycemia syndromes
Intermediate acting NPH Lente	Humulin N® Eli Lilly Novolin N® Novo Nordisk Caninsulin® Intervet/Schering Plough	1–3 h 1–1.5 h <1 h	4–9 h 6–8 h 4–8 h	14–20 h 12–16 h 12–24 h	Duration of NPH often too short for use in cats; must be given twice daily in dogs Considered ideal for the dog since pork insulin source
Intermediate and short acting mixtures (NPH/regular)	Humulin® 50/50 Humulin® 70/30 Humalog Mix® 75/25 Humalog Mix® 50/50 Eli LillyNovolin® 70/30 Novolog Mix® 70/30 Novo Nordisk	Varies with mixture mixture 30 min	Varies with mixture mixture 2–12 h	Varies with mixture mixture 24 h	Can be used in dogs with problems of postprandial hyperglycemia
Long-acting minimal peak Glargine PZI	Lantus® Aventis Novo Nordisk Prozinc® Boehringer Ingelheim	2 h 1 h	6 h 8–10 h	18–26 h 18–24 h	Cats: glucose ≥360 mg/dL (≥19.98 mmol/L) = 0.5 U/kg q12h; glucose ≤360 mg/dL (≤19.98 mmol/L) = 0.25 U/kg Dogs: 0.1–0.2 U/kg q12h; cats same as glargine. Effective in cats, most requiring twice daily dosing

CRI, constant rate of infusion; IM, intramuscular; NPH, neutral protein Hagedorn.

peakless insulin that successfully regulates diabetic dogs fed a diet high in insoluble fiber [82] and it has been associated with reversion of diabetes mellitus in newly diagnosed cats [83]. Most dogs with diabetes mellitus are clinically regulated with twice daily insulin injections, with hypoglycemia common in dogs receiving insulin only once daily [84]. The initial subcutaneous twice-daily dosing range for the dog is reported as between 0.25 and 0.7 unit/kg, given after the meal [85,86]. The recommended initial twice-daily dose for the cat is 0.25 units/kg subcutaneously (not to exceed 2 units per cat during the adjustment period, 3–4 weeks). Dosage should be based on ideal body weight and always rounded down when appropriate [87]. It is ideal, however, to administer the same type of insulin that the animal received at home if previously diagnosed as a diabetic. Since the quantity and type of food and the timing of feeding can be disrupted in the critically ill patient, diligent monitoring for hypoglycemia or hyperglycemia is imperative.

The *ideal* goal of insulin therapy is to maintain the blood glucose concentration between 90 and 270 mg/dL (5–15 mmol/L) in dogs and 90 and 306 mg/dL (5–17 mmol/L) in cats throughout the day and night. Typically, the highest blood glucose concentrations should occur at the time of each insulin injection [88].

It generally takes several weeks to establish an acceptable insulin dosage protocol in newly diagnosed patients. Blood glucose levels should be interpreted along with the history and physical exam findings; a generally accepted starting point is to have blood glucose 150–250 mg/dL within one hour of insulin administration [29]. Persistent clinical signs of diabetes, high serum fructosamine and/ or inadequate response on a blood glucose curve support an insulin dosage that is too low.

Difficulties encountered in regulating blood glucose with insulin should be investigated by performing a glucose curve. Blood glucose is determined immediately before insulin administration and then measured every 60–120 minutes for 12 hours (if insulin given q 12 h) or for 24 hours (if insulin given once daily) [29]. The information is plotted on a graph with the x-axis providing the time in hours from glucose administration and blood glucose concentration indicated on the y-axis. Guidelines for adjustments in either dosage or timing can be derived from assessment of the plotted glucose curve (Figure 5.8). By measuring blood glucose concentrations throughout the day, the clinician will be able to determine if the insulin is effective in lowering the blood glucose concentration, identify the blood glucose nadir, estimate the duration of insulin effect, and determine the average blood glucose concentration for the time period of the glucose curve. It is best to have the average blood glucose concentration <270 mg/dL (<15 mmol/L) during the time period of the glucose curve [29]. Interstitial real-time or at-home monitoring is likely to improve diabetic control.

Hypoglycemia is fairly common in diabetic dogs and cats receiving insulin therapy but may not cause symptoms due to the release of stress hormones that will increase blood glucose. Glucose may increase to over 400 mg/dL (Somogyi phenomenon) and remain increased for hours to days. This can be demonstrated on a 24-hour glucose curve. An adjustment in insulin dosage or timing is made as indicated by the patient glucose history, feeding schedule, and findings from the glucose curve.

Hypoglycemia occurs when this Somogyi mechanism is blunted, more commonly occurring in newly diagnosed diabetics, cats with transient diabetes, animals with large increases in dose of insulin, patients on twice-daily long-acting insulin, with increased activity and with decreased caloric consumption [29]. New diabetic cats can revert to a nondiabetic state as the result of some endogenous insulin production or resolution of an underlying disease causing insulin resistance.

Insulin resistance has classically been defined as poor or lack of glycemic control at >1.5 U/kg/dose in the dog and cat and most animals can be controlled on a <1 U/kg/dose [29]. Common conditions associated with transient insulin resistance are listed in Box 5.3. With insulin resistance, glucose curves may show little to no response to insulin or a response may be noted but excessive amounts of insulin required. Identification and treatment of any underlying disorder associated with insulin resistance are essential for successful glycemic control.

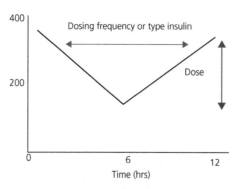

Figure 5.8 The glucose curve. The initial sample is taken just prior to insulin administration and serves as the value at time 0. Blood glucose levels are taken every 1–2 hours for 12 hours, or may be collected with a continuous interstitial monitor. The glucose values are plotted on the y-axis and the time from administration on the x-axis. The dip in the curve is the "nadir" or peak insulin time and glucose value. How the graph moves vertically is dependent upon the insulin dosage, and how it moves horizonatally depends upon the dosing frequency or type of insulin.

Box 5.3 Common conditions associated with insulin resistance in dogs and cats.

- Insulin underdose
- Antiinsulin antibodies
- Bacterial infections: oral, urinary tract, pulmonary
- Pancreatitis
- Hyperadrenocorticism
- Drugs: glucocorticoids, progestins, beta-blockers
- Hyperthyroidism (cat)
- Stress (cat)
- Obesity
- Chronic inflammation
- Acromegaly (cat)
- Hypothyroidism (dog)
- Renal disease
- Liver disease
- Cardiac disease
- Glucagonoma
- Pheochromocytoma
- Exocrine pancreatic insufficiency
- Hyperlipidemia
- Neoplasia
- Inappropriate storage, admininstration and handling of insulin
- Ineffective or inappropriate dose, type or frequency of administration

References

1. Silverstein DC, Hopper K, eds. Small Animal Critical Care Medicine, 2nd edn. St Louis: Elsevier Saunders, 2015.
2. Koenig A. Hypoglycemia. In: Small Animal Critical Care Medicine, 2nd edn. Silverstein DC, Hopper K, eds. St Louis: Elsevier Saunders, 2015: p 353.
3. Torre DM, deLaforcade AM, Chan DL. Incidence and clinical relevance of hyperglycemia in critically ill dogs. J Vet Intern Med. 2007;21(3):971–5.
4. De Oliveira JC, Ludemann CR, Barella LF, et al. Anesthetic-induced transient hyperglycemia and insulin resistance do not depend on the sympathoadrenal axis. Minerva Endocrinologica 2013;38(4):379–88.
5. Guyton AC, Hall JE, eds. Insulin, glucagon and diabetes mellitus. In: Textbook of Medical Physiology, 10th edn. St Louis: WB Saunders, 2000: pp 884–97.
6. Guyton AC, Hall JE, eds. Metabolism of carbohydrates, and formation of adenosine triphosphate. In: Textbook of Medical Physiology, 10th edn. St Louis: WB Saunders, 2000: pp 772–80.
7. Guyton AC, Hall JE, eds. Textbook of Physiology, 11th edn. Philadelphia: Elsevier, 2006.
8. Defronzo RA. Diabetes: pathogenesis of type 2 diabetes mellitus. Med Clin North Am. 2004;88:787–835.
9. Wright EM, Hirayama BA, Loo DF. Active sugar transport in health and disease. J Int Med. 2007;261(1):32–43.
10. Loose NL, Rudloff E, Kirby R. Hypoglycemia and its effects on the brain. J Vet Emerg Crit Care 18(3);2008:223–34.
11. Gejl M, Gjedde A. Brain glucose metabolism. Available at: http://www.diapedia.org/metabolism-insulin-and-other-hormones/5105374816/brain-glucose-metabolism (accessed 18 May 2016).
12. Cohn LA, McCaw DL, Tate D, Johnson J. Assessment of five portable blood glucose meters, a point-of-care analyzer, and color test strips for measuring blood glucose concentration in dogs. J Am Vet Med Assoc. 2000;216(2):198–202.
13. Surman S, Fleeman L. Continuous glucose monitoring in small animals. Vet Clin North Am Small Anim Pract. 2013;43(2):381–406.
14. Johnson BM, Fry MM, Flatland B, Kirk CA. Comparison of a human portable blood glucose meter, veterinary portable blood glucose meter, and automated chemistry analyzer for measurement of blood glucose concentrations in dogs. J Am Vet Med Assoc. 2009;235(11):1309–13.
15. Paul AE, Shiel RE, Juvet F, et al. Effect of hematocrit on accuracy of two point-of-care glucometers for use in dogs. Am J Vet Res. 2011;72(9):1204–8.
16. Burkitt Creedon JM, Davis HL. Advanced Monitoring and Procedures in Small Animal Emergency and Critical Care. Ames: Wiley-Blackwell, 2012.
17. Acierno MJ, Schnellbacher R, Tully TN. Measuring the level of agreement between a veterinary and a human point-of-care glucometer and a laboratory blood analyzer in Hispaniolan Amazon parrots (Amazona ventralis). J Avian Med Surg. 2012;26(4):221–4.
18. Acierno MJ, Mitchell MA, Schuster PJ, et al. Evaluation of the agreement among three handheld blood glucose meters and a laboratory blood analyzer for measurement of blood glucose concentration in Hispaniolan Amazon parrots (Amazona ventralis). Am J Vet Res. 2009;70(2):172–5.
19. Thompson MD, Taylor SM, Adams VJ, et al. Comparison of glucose concentrations in blood samples obtained with a marginal ear vein nick technique versus from a peripheral vein in healthy cats and cats with diabetes mellitus. J Am Vet Med Assoc. 2002;221(3):389–92.
20. Paul AE, Shiel RE, Juvet F, et al. Effect of hematocrit on accuracy of two point-of-care glucometers for use in dogs. Am J Vet Res. 2011;72(9):1204–8.
21. Mann EA, Mora AG, Pidcoke HF, et al. Glycemic control in the burn intensive care unit: focus on the role of anemia in glucose measurement. J Diabetes Sci Technol. 2009;1(3):1219–29.
22. Zeugswetter FK, Rebuzzi L. Point-of-care β-hydroxybutyrate measurement for the diagnosis of feline diabetic ketoacidemia. J Small Anim Pract. 2012;53(6):328–31.
23. Reineke EL, Fletcher DJ, King LJ, Drobatz KJ. Accuracy of a continuous glucose monitoring system in dogs and cats with diabetic ketoacidosis. J Vet Emerg Crit Care 2010;20(3):303–12.
24. Affenzeller N, Thalhammer JF, Willmann M. Home-based subcutaneous continuous glucose monitoring in 10 diabetic dogs. Vet Rec. 2011;169(8): 206.
25. Hug SA, Riond B, Schwarzwald CC. Evaluation of a continuous glucose monitoring system compared with an in-house standard laboratory assay and a handheld point-of-care glucometer in critically ill neonatal foals. J Vet Emerg Crit Care 2013;23(4):408–15.
26. Dietiker-Moretti S, Muller C, Sieber-Ruckstuhl N, etal. Comparison of a continous glucose monitoring system with a portable blood glucose meter to determine insulin dose in cats with diabetes mellitus. J Vet Intern Med. 2011;25(5):1084–8.
27. Hafner M, Lutz TA, Reusch CE, Zini C. Evaluation of sensor sites for continuous glucose monitoring in cats with diabetes mellitus. J Feline Med Surg. 2013;15(2):117–23.
28. Feldman EC, Nelson RW, eds. Canine and Feline Endocrinology and Reproduction, 3rd edn. St Louis: Saunders, 2004: pp 629–32.
29. Feldman EC, Nelson RW, eds. Canine diabetes mellitus/Feline diabetes mellitus. In: Canine and Feline Endocrinology and Reproduction, 3rd edn. St Louis: Saunders, 2004: pp 486–538, 539–79 respectively.
30. Reusch, CE, Leihs MR, Hoyer M, Vochezer R. A new parameter for diagnosis and metabolic control in diabetic dogs and cats. J Vet Intern Med. 1993;7(3):177–82.
31. Hoerauf A, Reusch C. Ultrasonographic evaluation of adrenal glands in six dogs with hypoadrenocorticism. J Am Anim Hosp Assoc. 1999;35(3):214–18.
32. Mergenthaler P, Lindauer U, Dienel G, Meisel A. Sugar for the brain: the role of glucose in physiological and pathological brain function. Trends Neurosci. 2013;36(10):587–97.
33. Barrett EJ. Endocrine regulation of growth and body mass. In: Medical Physiology, 2nd edn. Boron WF, Boulpaep EL, eds. Philadephia: Saunders Elsevier, 2012: p 1032.
34. Clark, AL, Best CJ, Fischer SJ. Even silent hypoglycemia induces cardiac arrhythmias. Diabetes 2014;63:1457–9.
35. LeRoith D. Glucose counterregulatory hormones: physiology, pathophysiology, and relevance to clinical hypoglycemia. In: Diabetes Mellitus: A Fundamental and Clinical Text, 3rd edn. LeRoith D, Olefsky J, Taylor S, eds. Philadelphia: Lippincott Williams and Wilkins, 2004.
36. Turnwald GH, Troy GC. Disorders of glucose homeostasis in neonatal and juvenile dogs: hypoglycemia: part II. Clinical aspects. Compend Contin Educ Pract Vet. 1984;6(2):115–23.
37. Koenig A. Hypoglycemia. In: Small Animal Critical Care Medicine, 2nd edn. Silverstein DC, Hopper K, eds. St Louis: Elsevier Saunders, 2015: pp 352–6.
38. Fisher JR, Smith SA, Harkin K. Glucagon constant-rate infusion: a novel strategy for the management of hyperinsulinemic-hypoglycemic crisis in the dog. J Am Anim Hosp Assoc. 2000;36:27–32.
39. Goutal CM, Brugmann BL, Ryan KA. Insulinoma in dogs: a review. J Am Anim Hosp Assoc. 2012;48(3):151–63.
40. Kintzer PP. Insulinoma and other gastrointestinal tract tumours In: BSAVA Manual of Canine and Feline Endocrinology. Mooney CT, Peterson ME, eds. Gloucester: British Small Animal Veterinary Association, 2012; pp 148–55.
41. Maton PN. The use of the long-acting somatostatin analogue, octreotide acetate, in patients with islet cell tumors. Gastroenterol Clin North Am. 1989;18:897–922.
42. Northrup NC, Rassnick KM, Gieger TL, et al. Prospective evaluation of biweekly streptozotocin in 19 dogs with insulinoma. J Vet Intern Med. 2013;27(3):483–90.
43. Moore AS, Nelson RW, Henry CJ, et al. Streptozotocin for treatment of pancreatic islet cell tumors in dogs: 17 cases (1989–1999). J Am Vet Med Assoc. 2002;221(6):811–18.
44. Tobin, RL, Nelson RW, Lucroy MD, et al. Outcome of surgical versus medical treatment of dogs with beta cell neoplasia: 39 cases (1990–1997). J Am Vet Med Assoc. 1999;215(2):226–30.
45. Vanhorebeek I, van den Berghe G. Diabetes of injury: novel insights. Endocrinol Metab Clin North Am. 2006;35(4):859–72.
46. Mann EA, Mora AG, Pidcoke HF, et al. Glycemic control in the burn intensive care unit: focus on the role of anemia in glucose measurement. J Diabetes Sci Technol. 2009;1(3):1319–29.
47. Goutal CM, Keir I, Kenney S, et al. Evaluation of acute congestive heart failure in dogs and cats: 145 cases (2007–2008). J Vet Emerg Crit Care 2010;20(3):330–7.
48. Lazzeri C, Valente S, Gensini GF. Hyperglycemia in acute heart failure: an opportunity to intervene? Curr Heart Fail Rep. 2014;11(3):231–5.
49. Torre DM, deLaforcade AM, Chan DL. Incidence and clinical relevance of hyperglycemia in critically ill dogs. J Vet Intern Med. 2007;21(5):971–5.
50. Li WA, Moore-Langston S, Chakraborty T, et al. Hyperglycemia in stroke and possible treatments. Neurol Res. 2013;35(5):479–91.
51. Sande A, West C. Traumatic brain injury: a review of pathophysiology and management. J Vet Emerg Crit Care 2010;20(2):177–90.
52. Hopper K, Borchers A, Epstein S. Acid base, electrolyte, glucose, and lactate values during cardiopulmonary resuscitation in dogs and cats. J Vet Emerg Crit Care 2014;24(2):208–14.
53. Maton BL, Smarick S. Updates in the American Heart Association guidelines for cardiopulmonary resuscitation and potential applications to veterinary patients. J Vet Emerg Crit Care 2012;22(2):148–59.
54. Smith R, Lin JC, Adelson PD. Relationship between hyperglycemia and outcome in children with severe traumatic brain injury. Pediatr Crit Care Med. 2012;13(1):85–91.
55. Paul E, Bellomo R, Kansagar D, et al. Stress hyperglycemia: an essential survival response! Crit Care 2013;17:305.
56. Freeman M, Wolf F, Helfand M. Intensive insulin therapy in hospitalized patients: a systematic review. Ann Intern Med. 2011;154:268–82.
57. Marik PE, Preiser JC. Towards understanding tight glycemic control in the ICU: a systemic review and meta-analysis. Chest 2010;137:544–51.

58. Badawi O, Waite MD, Fuhrman SA, Zuckerman IH. Association between intensive care unit-acquired dysglycemia and in-hospital mortality. Crit Care Med. 2012;40:3180–8.

59. Bruno A, Levine SR, Frankel MR, et al. Admission glucose level and clinical outcomes in the NINDS rt-PA Stroke Trial. Neurology 2002;59:669–74.

60. Capes SE, Hunt D, Malmberg K, Gerstein HC. Stress hyperglycaemia and increased risk of death after myocardial infarction in patients with and without diabetes: a systematic overview. Lancet 2000;355:773–8.

61. Dungan K, Braithwaite SS, Preiser JC. Stress hyperglycemia. Lancet 2009;373:1798–807.

62. Van den Berghe G, Wouters PJ, Bouillon R, et al.Outcome benefit of intensive insulin therapy in the critically ill: insulin dose versus glycemic control. Crit Care Med. 2003;31(2):359–66.

63. Meyfroidt G, Ingels C, van den Berghe G. Glycemic control in the ICU. N Engl J Med. 2011;364(13):1280.

64. Van Herpe T, Vanhonsebrouck K, Mesotten D, et al. Glycemic control in the pediatric intensive care unit of Leuven: two years of experience. J Diabetes Sci Technol. 2012;6(1):15–21.

65. Hermans G, Schetz M, van den Berghe G. Tight glucose control in critically ill adults. J Am Med Assoc. 2008;300(23):2725.

66. Kalfon P, Giraudeau B, Ichai C, et al. Tight computerized versus conventional glucose control in the ICU: a randomized controlled trial. Intensive Care Med. 2014;40(2):171–81.

67. Gartemann J, Caffrey E, Hadker N, et al. Nurse workload in implementing a tight glycaemic control protocol in a UK hospital: a pilot time-in-motion study.Nurs Crit Care. 2012;17(6):279–84.

68. Anabtawi A, Hurst M, Titi M, et al. Incidence of hypoglycemia with tight glycemic control protocols: a comparative study. Diabetes Technol Ther. 2010;12(8):635–9.

69. Finfer S, Chittock DR, Su SY, et al. Intensive versus conventional glucose control in critically ill patients. N Engl J Med. 2009;360(13):1283–97.

70. Nelson RW, Reusch CE. Classification and etiology of diabetes in dogs and cats. J Endocrinol. 2014;222:T1–T9.

71. Biourge V, Nelson RW, Feldman EC, et al. Effect of weight gain and subsequent weight loss on glucose tolerance and insulin response in healthy cats. J Vet Intern Med. 1997;11:86–91.

72. Dugger DT, Epstein SE, Hopper K, Mellema MS. A comparison of the clinical utility of several published formulae for estimated osmolality of canine serum. J Vet Emerg Crit Care 2014;24(2):188–93.

73. Feldman EC, Nelson RW. Canine and Feline Endocrinology and Reproduction, 3rd edn. St Louis: Elsevier, 2004: pp 581–615.

74. Kerl ME. Diabetic ketoacidosis: pathophysiology and clinical laboratory presentation. Compend Contin Educ Pract Vet. 2001;23:220–9.

75. Hume DZ, Drobatz KJ, Hess RS. Outcome of dogs with diabetic ketoacidosis: 127 dogs (1993–2003). J Vet Intern Med. 2006;20(3):547–55.

76. Trotman TK1, Drobatz KJ, Hess RS. Retrospective evaluation of hyperosmolar hyperglycemia in 66 dogs (1993–2008). J Vet Emerg Crit Care 2013;23(5):557–64.

77. Sears KW, Drobatz K, Hess RS. Use of lispro insulin for treatment of dogs with diabetes ketoacidosis. J Vet Intern Med. 2009;23(3):696.

78. Chastain CB, Nichols CE. Low-dose intramuscular insulin therapy for diabetic ketoacidosis in dogs. J Am Vet Med Assoc. 1981;178(6):561–4.

79. Marshall, RD, Rand JS, Gunew M, Menrath V. Intramuscular glargine with or without concurrent subcutaneous administration for treatment of feline diabetic ketoacidosis. J Vet Emerg Crit Care 2013;23(3):286–90.

80. Gallagher B, Mahony OM, Rozanski EA, et al. A pilot study comparing a protocol using intermittent administration of glargine and regular insulin to a continuous rate infusion of regular insulin in cats with naturally occurring diabetic ketoacidosis. J Vet Emerg Crit Care 2015;25(2):234–9.

81. Burkitt Creedon JM. Sodium disorders. In: Small Animal Critical Care Medicine, 2nd edn. Silverstein CD, Hopper K, eds. St Louis: Elsevier Saunders, 2015: p 265.

82. Hess RS, Drobatz,KJ. Glargine insulin for treatment of naturally occurring diabetes mellitus in dogs. J Am Vet Med Assoc. 2013;243(8):1154–61.

83. Marshall RD, Rand JS, Morton JM. Treatment of newly diagnosed diabetic cats with glargine insulin improves glycaemic control and results in higher probability of remission than protamine zinc and lente insulins J Feline Med Surg. 2009;11(8):683–91.

84. Hess RS, Ward CR. Effect of insulin on glycemic response in dogs with diabetes mellitus: 221 cases (1993–1998). J Am Vet Med Assoc. 2000;216(2):217–21.

85. Broussard JD, Wallace MS. Insulin treatment of diabetes mellitus in the dog and cat. In: Kirk's Current Veterinary Therapy XII Small Animal Practice. Bonagura J, ed. Philadelphia: Saunders, 1995: pp 393–8.

86. Fleeman LM, Rand JS. Management of canine diabetes. Vet Clin North Am Small Anim Pract. 2001;31:855–80.

87. Rucinsky R, Cook A, Haley S, et al. 2010 AAHA Diabetes Management Guidelines for Dogs and Cats. J Am Anim Hosp Assoc. 2010;46:215–24.

88. Nelson RW. Blood glucose curves: when, why and how. New Zealand Veterinary Nursing Association Proceedings. Available at: http://www.nzvna.org.nz/site/nzvna/files/Quizzes/Blood%20Glucose%20Curves%20When%20Why%20and%20How.pdf (accessed 18 May 2016).

CHAPTER 6

Electrolytes

Linda Barton[1] and Rebecca Kirby[2]

[1] BluePearl Specialty and Emergency Medicine for Pets, Renton, Washington

[2] (Formerly) Animal Emergency Center, Gainesville, Florida

Introduction

Electrolytes are substances that dissociate into charged particles (ions) in solution and acquire the capacity to conduct electricity. It is the gain or loss of electrons that creates a negative or positive charge, respectively. Positive ions, known as cations, often attract negative ions, known as anions, and form an ionic bond. These bonds can be found in many biological compounds such as acids, bases, and salts. However, these ionic bonds will break when added to water.

Sodium (Na), potassium (K), chloride (Cl), calcium (Ca), magnesium (Mg), and phosphorus (P) are the electrolytes that play a critical role in maintaining normal cellular functions. These ions will regulate or affect two important physiological functions: the flow of water molecules and the electrical charge across the cell membrane. Electrolytes are constantly lost from the body through the urine and gastrointestinal secretions. Therefore, the regulation and preservation of normal concentrations of these important electrolytes can be crucial for supporting life-sustaining functions, such as cardiac performance, vascular tone, brain function, neuromuscular activity, and fluid balance.

Electrolytes (ions) cannot diffuse passively across cell membranes. Their concentrations are therefore regulated by facilitated diffusion and active transport. Facilitated diffusion occurs through protein-based channels, which allow passage of the solute along a concentration gradient. In active transport, energy from adenosine triphosphate (ATP) changes the shape of membrane proteins that move ions against a concentration gradient [1].

The flow of water molecules across cell membranes is primarily dependent upon the concentration of Na, and to a lesser extent the K concentration. The extracellular fluid (ECF) compartment volume is maintained by Na salts and the intracellular fluid (ICF) compartment by K salts. Because the cell membrane is freely permeable to water but not to ions, the ECF and ICF spaces will strive to establish an osmotic equilibrium. Water will flow from the compartment of lower osmolarity to the compartment with a higher osmolarity until the osmotic pressures are equalized across the cell membrane. This state is not a true equilibrium but rather a steady state achieved by active transport by the Na/K pump and other interrelated channels and transporters [1]. An increase in osmolarity of the ECF can result in cellular dehydration and conversely a decrease in ECF osmolarity can result in cellular overhydration.

The electrical charge across the cell membrane is a function of Na, K, Cl, Ca, and Mg. The action potential or nerve impulse is a transient alteration of the transmembrane voltage across an excitable membrane in an excitable cell (such as a neuron or myocyte). This is generated by the activity of voltage-gated ion channels embedded in the cell membrane. An action potential develops when the threshold of the cell membrane potential is reached. Pulse-like waves of voltage travel along the axons of neurons and myocytes (Figure 6.1) and result in electrical activity such as nerve impulses, muscle contraction, and cardiac conduction.

Each major cation (Na, K, Ca, Mg) and anion (Cl, P) has an individual and specific role to play in the function and homeostasis of every cell in the body. The charge, location, and concentration of each electrolyte contribute to the role it plays in a cell and can affect the function and concentration of other electrolytes.

Specific functions of electrolytes

Sodium is the major cation in ECF and thus the major contributor to extracellular (including plasma) osmolarity. The plasma osmolarity is maintained within narrow limits by balancing water intake with water losses. Small elevations in the plasma osmolarity are sensed by osmoreceptors in the hypothalamus. Thirst and water excretion are both altered in response to the secretion of antidiuretic hormone (ADH, also called arginine vasopressin). The secretion of ADH occurs in response to increased plasma osmolarity or decreased effective circulating volume. The ADH binds with vasopressin (V_2) receptors in the distal tubules and collecting ducts of the kidneys, stimulating the activation of renal epithelial Na channels. The resultant Na resorption contributes to the corticomedullary osmotic gradient that is necessary for maximum water absorption. This allows free water resorption, hence lowering sodium and increasing vascular volume [2]. In addition to the role that Na plays in fluid balance, the transmission of Na into and out of the cell is a critical part of many cellular functions. The transmembrane movement of Na is particularly important in the generation of electrical signals or currents in the brain, spinal cord, peripheral nervous system, myocardium, and muscles.

Potassium is the major intracellular cation, playing an important role in neuromuscular transmission as well as other vital cell functions. The resting cell membrane potential is dependent upon a higher intracellular to extracellular ratio of K. The K concentration must be tightly regulated. Both insulin and beta-adrenergic catecholamines will increase cellular K uptake by stimulating cell membrane Na/K–ATPase.

The kidneys are primarily responsible for maintaining the total body K, matching excretion with intake. Under most homeostatic

Monitoring and Intervention for the Critically Ill Small Animal: The Rule of 20, First Edition. Edited by Rebecca Kirby and Andrew Linklater.

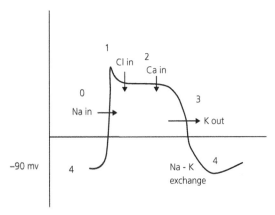

Figure 6.1 Pulse-like waves across the cell membrane of the cardiac myocyte are a result of shifting of electrolytes and initiate the action potential. Phase 0 causes depolarization. Rapid sodium (Na) channels are stimulated to open, flooding the cell with positive Na ions. This causes a positively directed change in the transmembrane potential. Depolarization of one cell triggers the Na channels in surrounding cells to open as well, causing the depolarization wave front to propagate cell by cell throughout the heart. Phase 1 is the initial stage of repolarization. The voltage is rapidly lowered by the movement of chloride (Cl⁻) ions into the cell. Phase 2 (the plateau stage) is where the rate of repolarization is slowed by the influx of calcium (Ca) ions into the cell. The Ca ions enter the cell more slowly than the Na ions and help prevent the cell from repolarizing too quickly, thus extending the refractory period. This mechanism helps regulate the rate at which cardiac tissue can depolarize. Phase 3 is the later stage of repolarization where intracellular potassium (K) leaves the cell in an effort to restore the resting membrane potential (−90 millivolts (mv)). Once repolarization is complete, the cell will be able to respond to a new stimulus. Phase 4 occurs after repolarization is complete and restores the Na and K balance to the original intracellular and extracellular concentrations.

conditions, K delivery to the distal nephron remains small and is fairly constant. By contrast, the rate of K secretion by the distal nephron varies and is regulated according to physiological needs. Aldosterone will upregulate the basolateral Na/K pump in the principal cells in the distal renal tubule, creating a concentration gradient for the resorption of Na and the secretion of K [3]. Aldosterone synthesis is stimulated by increased concentrations of K, as well as angiotensin II, adrenocorticotropic hormone (ACTH), acidosis, and atrial stretch receptors.

Calcium, as calcium phosphate, acts as supporting material in bones, with 99% percent of the total body Ca residing in the bones and teeth. The remaining 1% of the Ca performs important life-sustaining cellular functions. Calcium is involved in maintaining the stability of fibrin, the transmission of nerve impulses, the flow of fluid through cell membranes, and the contraction and relaxation of muscle. In addition, the Ca ion is one of the most widespread second messengers for cellular signal transduction, particularly those related to neuromuscular function and cardiac conduction. Endothelial Ca ions regulate the production of nitric oxide and the stimulation of K channels to efflux K, causing hyperpolarization and vascular smooth muscle relaxation [4].

The cytoplasmic concentration of Ca ions is a consequence of Ca ion passage through the cell membrane by way of Ca-binding proteins or voltage-gated calcium channels. Calcium ions can also be released into the cytoplasm from intracellular Ca stores, such as the endoplasmic or sarcoplasmic reticulum and mitochondria. However, excessive intracellular calcium may damage the cell or even cause it to undergo apoptosis, or death by necrosis. Therefore,

the quantity of intracellular calcium must be tightly regulated. Extrusion of Ca from the cell is facilitated by transport proteins such as the Na/Ca exchanger and Ca/ATPase plasma exchanger.

Ionized calcium is hormonally regulated and normally maintained within narrow limits by the actions of parathyroid hormone (PTH), calcitonin, and vitamin D. Low calcium levels trigger PTH release, which promotes bone mineral dissolution and increased renal reabsorption of Ca. PTH also increases renal hydroxylation of inactive vitamin D to calcitriol, which increases gastrointestinal absorption of dietary calcium. Increased serum calcium and calcitriol levels inhibit PTH secretion. Calcitonin is released from the thyroid gland in response to high Ca concentration. As opposed to PTH, calcitonin inhibits bone resorption of Ca and renal reabsorption of Ca and P.

Magnesium is the second most abundant intracellular cation, with most of the total body Mg found in bone and skeletal muscle. In addition, Mg is a co-factor to more than 300 enzyme-driven biochemical reactions occurring in the body [5]. Magnesium influences the activity of enzymes by:
- binding to ligands such as ATP in ATP-requiring enzymes
- binding to the active site of the enzyme (such as pyruvate kinase)
- causing a conformational change during the catalytic process (such as Na/K-ATPase)
- promoting the aggregation of multienzyme complexes (such as aldehyde dehydrogenase)
- a mixture of the above mechanisms [6].

Intracellular Mg will block Ca and K channels, regulating Ca and K entry into the cell [7,8]. By competing with Ca for membrane binding sites and by stimulating Ca sequestration by sarcoplasmic reticulum, Mg helps to maintain a low resting intracellular Ca ion concentration. Magnesium has a key role in many other important biological processes such as cellular energy metabolism, cell replication, and protein synthesis.

The electrical properties of membranes and their permeability characteristics are also affected by magnesium. It affects myocardial contractility by influencing the intracellular Ca concentration and the electrical activity of myocardial cells. Magnesium affects the movement of ions such as Na, K, and Ca across the sarcolemmal membrane of the myocardial conduction system [9]. It may also affect the vascular smooth muscle tone.

Intracellular Mg is maintained within narrow concentration limits except in extreme situations such as hypoxia or prolonged Mg depletion. Very little is known about the mechanisms involved in the regulation of intracellular Mg [10]. Most Mg is bound to anionic compounds such as ATP, ADP, citrate, proteins, RNA, and DNA or is sequestered within mitochondria and endoplasmic reticulum. The kidney plays a major role in Mg homeostasis and the maintenance of plasma Mg concentration. Most of the filtered Mg (65%) is resorbed in the ascending loop of Henle [10]. The plasma Mg concentration is a major determinant of urinary magnesium excretion. Several hormones including PTH, ADH, calcitonin, glucagon, and insulin have been shown to affect Mg reabsorption [11,12].

Chloride is the most abundant anion in the extracellular fluid and the second most important contributor to plasma tonicity. Chloride is distributed primarily to the ECF compartment and can diffuse easily across vascular endothelial membranes. Chloride transport is closely linked to Na movement. This anion helps to regulate osmotic pressure differences between fluid compartments, having an important role in maintaining proper hydration and balancing cations in the ECF to maintain electrical neutrality.

Renewed interest in the physicochemical approach to acid–base analysis (Stewart approach and semiquantitative acid–base analysis) has refocused attention on Cl as a major determinant of acid–base status (see Chapter 7). The Cl shift within the blood helps to move bicarbonate ions out of the red blood cells and into the plasma for transport. In the gastric mucosa, chlorine and hydrogen combine to form hydrochloric acid.

The kidney excretes chloride, where the paths of secretion and reabsorption of Cl ions follow the paths of Na ions. Aldosterone therefore plays an indirect role in Cl regulation.

Phosphorus is the major intracellular anion, with most of the P located in the bone. Less than 1% of the total body P is located within the ECF and ICF spaces. The intracellular organic phosphate is an important constituent of nucleic acids, phospholipids, enzymatic phosphoproteins, and nucleotide co-factors for enzymes and proteins. Cytosolic phosphate regulates intracellular reactions such as glucose transport, lactate production, and ATP synthesis [13]. Phosphorus also acts as both a urinary and a body buffer. Urinary phosphate constitutes the majority of titratable acidity. Phosphorus shifts into cells in response to alkalemia. Similar to Ca homeostasis, PTH, calcitonin, and vitamin D regulate phosphate intestinal absorption, deposition, and resorption from bone and renal excretion. In response to low serum phosphate concentration, calcitriol increases gastrointestinal P absorption and the kidneys decrease phosphate excretion. Elevated serum PTH levels promote rapid renal phosphate excretion.

Electrolyte abnormalities in the critically ill small animal patient are both common and complex. The severity of Na and K disturbances remains a significant predictor of mortality in human ICUs [14].

Critical illness causes major stress on all the regulatory functions of the body, including those responsible for normal electrolyte balance. The stress of sepsis, acute renal failure, impaired perfusion, multiple organ dysfunction syndrome and the administration of vasoactive agents all affect the neuroendocrine system that controls serum electrolyte balance. Many therapies directed at maintaining vital organ function directly or indirectly affect these regulatory systems. Assessment of the patient electrolyte status can be further complicated by the infusion of electrolyte-containing fluids and parenteral and enteral nutrition. Appropriate and timely diagnostic and monitoring procedures are required for early intervention and to improve patient outcome.

Diagnostic and monitoring procedures

The electrolyte status of the ICU patient will have an impact on every body system, with emphasis on the neurological, muscular, renal, cardiovascular, gastrointestinal, acid–base, and hematological functions. The underlying diseases, as well as the therapeutic interventions, place every ICU patient at risk for electrolyte disorders. Often one electrolyte abnormality can lead to abnormalities with the other electrolytes. Important information helping to recognize a problem, define the cause, and identify the effects of electrolyte disorders can be obtained through the history, physical examination, point of care (POC) testing, clinicopathological testing, diagnostic imaging, and monitoring tools.

History and physical examination

The history will begin with the signalment (age, sex, breed). Breed-associated problems that can affect the electrolytes should be considered, such as pseudohyperkalemia found in Shar Pei, Akita, Japanese Shiba Inu and Korean Jindo [15] or Addison's disease

(causing hyperkalemia, hyponatremia) in the Standard Poodle and Bearded Collie. Female dogs are affected by hypoadrenocorticism twice as often as males. The past medical history may identify diseases such as diabetes mellitus, hyper- and hypoadrenocorticism, hyper- and hypothyroidism, renal disease, and various cardiovascular diseases that can manifest with acute and chronic electrolyte disorders (Tables 6.1, 6.2, and 6.3). A history of polyuria and polydipsia, gastrointestinal (GI) disturbance, neuromuscular

Table 6.1 Common disorders of sodium and potassium in the small animal ICU patient.

Hypernatremia	Hyperkalemia
Free water loss	**Impaired renal excretion**
Fever	Prerenal azotemia
Heat stroke	Thrombosis
Adipsia	Renal azotemia (acute, severe)
Primary hypodypsia	Postrenal azotemia
Diabetes insipidus	Uroabdomen
Central	**Reduced aldosterone level or**
Renal	**response**
Water loss > Na	Hypoadrenocorticism
Diuretics	**Massive tissue injury**
Intrinsic renal disease	Systemic thrombosis
Post obstructive diuresis	Tumor lysis syndrome
Nasogastric suction	Post cardiac arrest
Osmotic cathartics	Severe heat stroke
Cutaneous burns	Rhabdomyolysis
Na gain > water	**Acute metabolic acidosis**
Salt ingestion	Diabetic ketoacidosis
Sea water ingestion	Lactic acidosis
Sodium bicarbonate	Post cardiac arrest
Hypertonic saline	**Release from intracellular stores**
Hyperalimentation	Hereditary disorders (such as Akitas)
Sodium phosphate enema	**Pseudohyperkalemia**
Reset osmostat	
Primary hyperaldosteronism	
Essential hypernatremia	

Hyponatremia	Hypokalemia
Impaired water excretion	**Transcellular shift (ECF → ICF)**
Hypoadrenocorticism	Acute metabolic alkalosis
Diuretic therapy	Acute correction of acidosis
Loss through bodily fluids	Insulin
Vomiting	Glucose
Diarrhea	B$_2$-agonists (albuterol overdose)
Third body fluid space Na loss	Refeeding syndrome
Pancreatitis	**Reduced intake**
Cutaneous burns	Inadequate K in parenteral fluids
Hormonal dysregulation	**Increased loss**
SIADH	Renal failure
Hypothyroidism (myxedema coma)	Diuretic therapy
	Osmotic diuresis
Water overload	Post obstructive diuresis
Hypotonic fluid administration	Renal tubular acidosis
Congestive heart failure	Primary hyperaldosteronism
Severe liver disease	Hyperadrenocorticism
Nephrotic syndrome	Hypomagnesemia
Advanced renal failure	**Gastrointestinal loss**
Primary (psychogenic) polydipsia	Vomiting
	Nasogastric suction
	Diarrhea

ECF, extracellular fluid; ICF, intracellular fluid; SIADH, syndrome of inappropriate ADH secretion.

Table 6.2 Common disorders of ionized calcium and magnesium in the small animal ICU patient.

Hypercalcemia	Hypermagnesemia
Young growing animals	Renal insufficiency
Malignancy	Excessive Mg infusion or intake
Renal failure	Hypothyroidism
Hypervitaminosis D	Hypoadrenocorticism
Iatrogenic	Milk alkali syndrome
Cholecalciferol rodenticides	Shift of K from ICF to ECF
Toxic plant ingestion	Massive cell lysis
Antipsoriasis creams	
Oral vitamin D supplementation	
Granulomatous disease	
Primary hyperparathyroidism	
Hypoadrenocorticism	
Idiopathic (cats)	
Osteolytic diseases	
Calcium administration	
Lipemia	

Hypocalcemia	Hypomagnesemia
Primary hypoparathyroidism	Gastrointestinal loss
Secondary hypoparathyroidism	Chronic diarrhea
Neck surgery or trauma	Steatorrhea
Parathyroidectomy, thyroidectomy	Renal loss
Hypomagnesemia	Loop diuretics
Hypermagnesemia	Thiazides
Pancreatitis	Parathyroidectomy
Rhabdomyolysis	Diabetic ketoacidosis
Renal failure	Hyperaldosteronism
Eclampsia	Hyperthyroidism
Poor dietary intake	Nephrotoxins
Excessive P intake	Eclampsia
Intestinal malabsorption	
Ethylene glycol toxicity	
Phosphate-containing enemas	
IV phosphate supplementation	
Sepsis	
Laboratory error	
Hypoalbuminemia (total Ca)	
Citrate toxicity	
Hypovitaminosis D	
Chelation with EDTA (transfusion)	
Nutritional secondary hyperparathyroidism	

ECF, extracellular fluid; ICF, intracellular fluid.

Table 6.3 Common disorders of corrected chloride and phosphorus in the small animal ICU patient.

Hyperchloremia	Hyperphosphatemia
Pseudohyperchloremia	**Age of sample (release from RBCs)**
Lipemic samples (colorimetric methods)	**Young growing animals**
Potassium bromide therapy	**Renal**
Excessive loss of Na relative to Cl	Acute or chronic renal failure
Diarrhea	Pre- and postrenal azotemia
Excessive gain of Cl relative to Na	**High phosphorus intake**
0.9% NaCl fluids	Dietary, poor-quality protein
Hypertonic saline	Phosphate enemas
Renal retention	**Vitamin D toxicity**
Renal failure	**Hypoparathyroidism**
Renal tubular acidosis	**Intracellular release of P**
Drug induced	Tissue trauma
Spironolactone	Tissue necrosis
Acetazolamide	Tumor lysis syndrome
	Hemolysis
	Rhabdomyolysis

Hypochloremia	Hypophosphatemia
Pseudohypochloremia	**Inadequate intake**
lipemic samples (titrimetric methods)	Dietary deficiency
	Malabsorption
Excessive loss of Cl relative to Na	**Hypovitaminosis D**
	Translocation from ECF to ICF
Gastric fluid losses	Alkalosis
Loop diuretics	Glucose
Thiazide diuretics	Insulin
Chronic respiratory acidosis	Bicarbonate
High Na intake compared to Cl	**Renal**
Bicarbonate	Renal tubular defects
Penicillins	Diuretics
	Eclampsia

ECF, extracellular fluid; ICF, intracellular fluid; RBC, red blood cell.

changes (such as muscle weakness, fatigue, muscle tremors or twitches), seizure activity, change in mentation or behavioral changes, generalized weakness or difficulty breathing can suggest a cause or effect of an electrolyte problem. Historical problems such as high salt intake, protracted vomiting or diarrhea, severe hyperthermia, adipsia or hypodipsia, rapid ventilation, chronic nasal discharge or urinary obstruction should direct evaluation of serum Na. A list of prescribed and over-the-counter medications is important to identify any drugs that can have an impact on the electrolyte status.

Physical and neurological examination findings that can be associated with electrolyte alterations in the ICU patient are summarized in Table 6.4. The severity of these clinical signs is often attributable to the magnitude and rapidity of the development of the disorder. Since electrolytes are critical for the flow of water and electrical charges across cell membranes, life-threatening electro-lyte problems will frequently be associated with fluid imbalances, or neuromuscular, vascular, cardiac or neurological abnormalities.

The temperature, pulse rate and intensity, oral mucous membrane color, and capillary refill time provide a reasonable assessment of peripheral tissue perfusion and intravascular fluid balance. Skin turgor, mucous membrane and corneal moisture, and eye position within the orbit are used to estimate the hydration status (extravascular fluid balance) of the patient. An abnormal heart rate, pulse deficits, alterations in pulse intensity, and signs of poor perfusion can result from electrolyte abnormalities causing cardiovascular dysfunction.

The presence of dementia, seizures, coma or tremors can be a neurological consequence of abnormal electrical impulses associated with electrolyte problems. Changes in muscle strength and tone (such as generalized weakness, ventral flexion of the head and neck, weak ventilator muscles) and motor activity may reflect electrolyte-induced neuromuscular abnormalities.

Point of care testing

A minimum database is provided through POC in-hospital testing and should include the packed cell volume (PCV), total protein (TP), blood glucose, blood urea nitrogen (BUN) electrolyte panel (Na, K, ionized Ca, Mg, Cl, P), blood lactate, acid–base status, coagulation profile, and urinalysis. A low PCV could be due to hypophosphatemia and red blood cell (RBC) lysis. Assessing the PCV and TP together might reflect overhydration or dehydration,

Table 6.4 Common clinical signs associated with an excess or deficiency of the major electrolytes (Na, K, Ca, Mg, Cl, and P).

Electrolyte change	Considered abnormal	Clinical Signs
Hyponatremia	Dog <140 mEq/L Cat <142 mEq/L	Nonspecific central nervous system abnormalities: lethargy, weakness, ataxia, seizure, coma, death
Hypernatremia	Dog >155 mEq/L Cat >162 mEq/L	Nonspecific central nervous system abnormalities: lethargy, weakness, ataxia, seizure, coma, death
Corrected hypochloremia	Dog <107 mEq/L Cat <117 mEq/L	Signs are nonspecific and more likely related to the underlying disease process or changes in acid-base status
Corrected hyperchloremia	Dog >113 mEq/L Cat >123 mEq/L	Signs are nonspecific and more likely related to the underlying disease process or changes in acid base status
Hypokalemia	Dog, cat <3.5 mEq/L	Muscle weakness (skeletal muscle), ventroflexion of the neck (cats), rhabdomyolysis (severe), impaired ventilation (when severe), gastrointestinal ileus/atony, arrhythmias
Hyperkalemia	Dog, cat >5.5 mEq/L	Signs are attributable to the underlying disorder and brady- or tachyarrhythmias may be immediately life threatening resulting in signs of poor cardiac output; muscle fasciculations, gastrointestinal signs and polydypsia may also occur
Hypocalcemia ionized	Dog <5 mg/dL <1.2 mmol/L Cat <4.5 mg/dL <1.1 mmol/L	Behavioral changes, abnormal/stiff gait, panting, facial rubbing, muscle spasm/fasciculation, tetany, and seizures. Hyperthermia (secondary to increased muscle activity), anorexia, vomiting, and diarrhea have also been reported. In human patients, laryngospasm or bronchospasm have been reported. Cardiac changes including hypotension, bradycardia, arrhythmias, and poor Ca-mediated drug response
Hypercalcemia ionized	Dog >11.5 mg/dL >1.5 mmol/L Cat >10.5 mg/dL >1.4 mmol/L	Polyuria, polydipsia, anorexia, dehydration, lethargy, weakness, hypertension, seizures, and acute renal failure. Mineralization of soft tissues is possible when Ca (mg/dL) × P (mg/dL) product is >60
Hypophosphatemia	Dog, cat <2.4 mg/dL (0.775 mmol/L)	Muscle weakness, rhabdomyolysis, hemolysis, impaired platelet and white blood cell function
Hyperphosphatemia	Dog, cat >6.0 mg/dL (>1.92 mmol/L)	No primary clinical signs, but signs associated with hypocalcemia or renal failure may be noted
Hypomagnesemia	Dog <0.7 mmol/L (<1.7 mg/dL) Cat <0.41 mmol/L (<1.0 mg/dL)	Hypomagnesemia is commonly associated with other electrolyte abnormalities, including hypokalemia, hyponatremia, hypocalcemia, and hypophosphatemia. Signs ascribed to hypomagnesemia include cardiac arrhythmias, muscle weakness, muscle fasciculations, altered mentation, esophageal motility disorders, respiratory muscle paralysis, dysphagia, dyspnea, ataxia, seizures, and coma
Hypermagnesemia	Dog >1.2 mmol/L (>2.92 mg/dL) Cat >1.25 mmol/L (>3.04 mg/dL)	Concomitant hypocalcemia, hyperkalemia, or uremia may exaggerate the symptoms. Patients demonstrated vomiting, bradycardia, hypotension, decreased mentation, hypothermia, weakness with generalized flaccid muscle tone with absent patellar and palpebral reflexes

each a potential cause or effect of a Na disorder. Alterations in blood glucose can be associated with changes in the plasma K concentration. Each electrolyte will play a role in the acid–base status of the patient, necessitating that the blood gas results be assessed in conjunction with the electrolyte panel results (see semiquantitative acid–base analysis in Chapter 7).

Elevations in the BUN in conjunction with abnormal urine concentration, proteinuria, and cast formation can be an indication of renal disease, which can alter the excretion of all the electrolytes. Urine electrolytes, such as urine Na and Cl, have been reported to be helpful in discerning prerenal azotemia (low urine Na) from acute renal tubular damage (high urine Na), which can occur secondary to nephrotoxins or ischemia [16].

The results from the blood or serum electrolyte panel will provide the most important evidence of electrolyte disorders, but do not necessarily reflect the changes in total body (including intracellular and interstitial) electrolyte quantities. Normal electrolyte concentration will vary slightly among laboratories. A variety of techniques using ion-specific electrodes can be utilized to measure serum electrolytes. Collection of blood samples into the correct

blood collection tube is essential since the type of anticoagulant can falsely decrease or elevate electrolyte values.

Blood or serum Mg concentrations will not reflect the important intracellular Mg concentration. Knowledge of the underlying disorder and any clinical signs attributable to an abnormal Mg concentration plays an important role in making the diagnosis of a Mg disorder.

Serum Ca exists in three forms: 55% is ionized (physiologically active form), 35% is protein bound (primarily albumin and to a lesser extent globulin), and 10% is complexed to anions (citrate, bicarbonate, phosphate, or lactate). It is important to quantitate the active ionized Ca rather than the total Ca (which includes all three forms). Calcium is an important factor in blood coagulation, with alterations in ionized Ca a viable cause of both hypo- and hypercoagulable states.

Serum Cl should be evaluated relative to the serum Na concentration. Proportional changes in Na and Cl reflect changes in water balance. Nonparallel changes in Cl relative to Na identify clinical disorders of Cl that affect acid–base balance (see Chapter 7). To account for changes in water balance, measured serum Cl should be corrected for changes in serum Na by the formula in Box 6.1. Normal corrected Cl is approximately 107–113 mEq/L in dogs and

Box 6.1 Correction of serum chloride for changes in water balance.

$$Cl^-_{corrected} = Cl^-_{measured} \times \left(Na^+_{normal} / Na^+_{measured} \right)$$

117–123 mEq/L in cats but can vary with different laboratories and analyzers. Chloride is most commonly measured by potentiometry using an ion-specific electrode. With this method, bromide, cyanide, and other halides are measured as Cl. Pseudohyperchloremia will occur in patients treated with potassium bromide.

Clinicopathological testing

A complete blood count and serum biochemical profile will provide data pertaining to possible contributions of the internal organs to electrolyte abnormalities. An elevation in serum creatinine and BUN (along with the urinalysis) directs further investigation for kidney disease as the cause of fluid imbalance and abnormal serum electrolyte concentrations. Problems such as liver disease, pancreatitis or hypoadrenocorticism might be found as a cause of hypovolemia as well as altered electrolyte concentrations.

Underlying problems known to be associated with electrolyte disorders are listed in Tables 6.1, 6.2, and 6.3. Additional testing is often required and could include fecal examination, serology for inciting pathogens (cause of SIRS-related diseases), adrenal function testing (for hypoadrenocorticism, hyperadrenocorticism, or pheochromocytoma), thyroid panels, and diagnostic imaging. Fecal examination for parasites might find a cause for diarrhea and the resultant electrolyte changes. Pseudo-hypoadrenocorticism (hyperkalemia and hyponatremia) is reported to occur with whipworm infections [17].

Diagnostic imaging

Survey thoracic and abdominal radiographs provide the initial diagnostic imaging data once the patient has been stabilized. Abdominal and thoracic ultrasound provides a more in-depth assessment of organ structure and an evaluation of the size and structure of the adrenal glands, a possible source of electrolyte changes.

The electrocardiogram (ECG) will provide a waveform image of the electrical activity of the cardiac conduction system which is generated by the electrolytes. Hyperkalemia will cause changes in the ECG. However, these changes are not predictive of the magnitude of the plasma K alterations, especially in cats (Figure 6.2). An example of ECG changes associated with hyperkalemia is shown in Figure 6.3. ECG changes are also seen with Ca disorders. The ECG hallmark of hypocalcemia is the prolongation of the QT interval due to lengthening of the ST segment. The exact opposite holds true for hypercalcemia [18]. Hypercalcemia produces a quicker ventricular repolarization and therefore shorter QT interval.

Monitoring methods

The physical and neurological examination should be repeated at least twice daily for early detection of clinical signs of an electrolyte alteration before life-threatening consequences occur. The electrolyte panel is assessed at least daily, or more frequently depending upon the urgency of the anticipated or diagnosed electrolyte disorder. Assessment of the fluid balance should be ongoing and can incorporate monitoring of body weight, central venous pressure (CVP), arterial blood pressure, echocardiography (diameter of vena cava or aorta), urine output, and blood lactate. The ECG is monitored for evidence of electrolyte-related conduction disturbances and to assess the efficacy of any therapeutic interventions.

Electrolyte disorders

Abnormalities in Na, K, Ca, Mg, Cl, and P concentrations can have serious consequences in the small animal ICU patient. The electrolyte disorder can occur as a direct result of the underlying problem, a consequence of the clinical signs associated with the underlying disease (such as vomiting, diarrhea, polyuria) or a complication of treatment (such as fluid therapy, drug administration).

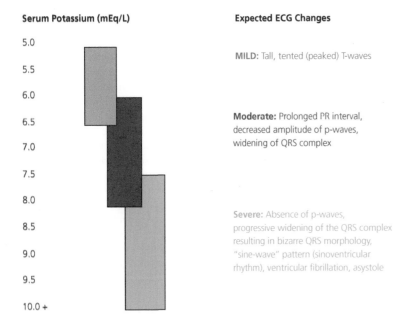

Serum Potassium (mEq/L)

5.0
5.5
6.0
6.5
7.0
7.5
8.0
8.5
9.0
9.5
10.0 +

Expected ECG Changes

MILD: Tall, tented (peaked) T-waves

Moderate: Prolonged PR interval, decreased amplitude of p-waves, widening of QRS complex

Severe: Absence of p-waves, progressive widening of the QRS complex resulting in bizarre QRS morphology, "sine-wave" pattern (sinoventricular rhythm), ventricular fibrillation, asystole

Figure 6.2 Potassium levels and associated common electrocardiogram changes.

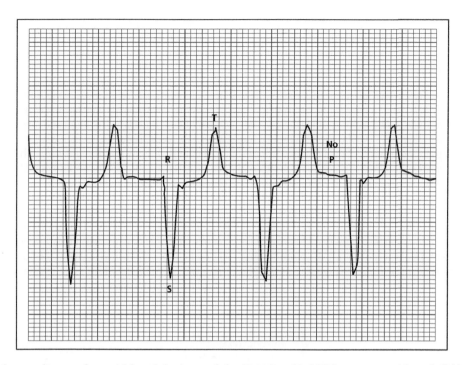

Figure 6.3 Example electrocardiogram of a cat with hyperkalemia, recorded at 50 mm/sec; this ECG demonstrates atrial standstill (absence of P waves) with supraventricular escape beats (associated regular QRS and T waves present) at a rate of 140 bpm.

Sodium disorders

Blood Na concentration reflects the ratio of Na to water in the ECF and accounts for most of the osmotic particles in the serum. Normal serum Na is 139–154 mEq/L or mmol/L in the dog and 145–158 mEq/L or mmol/L in the cat. Note that the quantity of Na expressed in mEq/L is equivalent to the same quantity in mmol/L. Abnormalities in serum Na concentration are caused most commonly by changes in water balance. Total body water is estimated to be 60% of lean body weight. The distribution of this water is one-third extracellular (intravascular and interstitial) and two-thirds intracellular.

The flow of water in and out of cells, particularly brain cells, is primarily responsible for the symptoms of both hyponatremia and hypernatremia. Clinical signs of Na disorders are nonspecific and may be difficult to separate from the clinical signs of the underlying disease. Central nervous system signs are most common with alterations in Na and can range from lethargy and weakness to ataxia, seizures, coma, and death. The severity of neurological dysfunction is related to the rapidity of onset and the degree of deviation from "normal."

The most life-threatening consequence of Na disorders and their treatment is the excessive movement of water into or out of the brain cells in response to the osmotic shift that Na disorders cause in the interstitium and blood. A high interstitial Na (hypernatremia) will draw water out of the cells, causing cell shrinkage. In response to this, the cells will make idiogenic osmoles or osmolytes (taurine, glysine, glutamine, sorbitol, and inositol) to generate an intracellular osmolarity that is now similar to the extracellular hyperosmolarity.

In contrast, a low interstitial Na (hyponatremia) will cause water to move from the interstitium into the cells where the osmolality is higher. This can lead to dangerous cell swelling and cerebral edema. The key to surviving a Na disorder is to manage clinical signs and restore the osmolar balance slowly.

Hypernatremia

Hypernatremia is defined as a serum sodium concentration >155 mEq/L (>155 mmol/L) in dogs and >162 mEq/L (>162 mmol/L) in cats (see Table 6.4). One or more of the following mechanisms will be responsible for this hyperosmolar Na-water imbalance: (1) Na gain greater than water gain, often due to the administration of hypertonic sodium-containing solutions (such as hypertonic saline, sodium bicarbonate or hypertonic parenteral nutrition); (2) water loss greater than Na loss (such as osmotic diuresis, diuretics, gastrointestinal secretions); and (3) loss of solute-free water (such as diabetes insipidus, adipsia, fever) (see Table 6.1).

Normally, hypernatremia stimulates the thirst mechanism and renal water conservation through the action of ADH. In patients with intact thirst mechanisms and the ability to drink, serum Na levels can remain more normal despite possible ongoing water losses. However, several factors can contribute to the onset of hypernatremia in the ICU patient, including the inability to drink (such as orders for nil per os, vomiting, mental impairment, inability to swallow), impaired renal ability to resorb water (such as nephrogenic diabetes insipidus, renal medullary washout, glucosuria) and the administration of IV fluids and medications that affect water or Na concentrations (such as diuretics, Na-containing fluids and drugs). Persistently elevated serum Na (>155 mEq/L or >155 mmol/L) in association with protracted hypotension portends a dismal prognosis in hospitalized hypernatremic human patients [19].

Possible causes of hypernatremia in the small animal ICU patient are listed in Table 6.1. Hypernatremia has been generally classified as hypovolemic (inadequate water intake or loss of water over Na), euvolemic (diabetes insipidus), and hypervolemic (intake of hypertonic fluids, hyperaldosteronism, salt poisoning). The more common causes are attributable to a relative lack of free water.

Early symptoms of hypernatremia include lethargy and weakness, progressing to muscular rigidity, seizures, and coma. Untreated hypernatraemia (170–190 mmol/L) resulted in brain lesions demonstrating myelinolysis and cellular necrosis in rats and rabbits [20]. Normalization of the hypernatraemia over 4–24 hours resulted in cerebral edema, due primarily to failure of brain amino acids and idiogenic osmoles to dissipate as plasma Na is decreased to normal.

Therapy for hypernatremia is first directed at correcting any concurrent perfusion deficits, and subsequently, correcting the serum Na with hypotonic fluids. An algorithm to guide the lowering of serum Na is presented in Figure 6.4. A four-step plan for making the necessary calculations for the quantity of fluid required to lower the serum Na to the desired concentration is presented in Box 6.2 with sample calculations. The replacement method outlined estimates the Na-lowering effect of possible choices of IV fluid formulations on the patient serum Na [21]. An advantage of this method is that Na values are known rather than estimated. Box 6.2 also lists the Na content of common fluid infusates. These formulas serve as a guideline, with frequent monitoring of serum Na and adjustments in fluid infusion made to meet the specific needs of the individual patient.

Patients with hypernatremia and volume depletion require fluid resuscitation with high Na replacement fluids to prevent rapid water movement into the brain cells. Isotonic saline remains the initial fluid treatment of choice. The titration of hydroxyethyl starch (synthetic colloid) at 5 mL/kg increments to low normal resuscitation endpoints can be given with the isotonic saline. The colloid provides intravascular volume resuscitation with minimal extravasation of fluid into the interstitium and no subsequent intracellular water gain (see Chapter 2).

The infused fluids are administered with the goal of correcting the high Na at a rate of 0.5–1 mEq/hour. Hypotonic fluids can be administered to lower the serum Na once perfusion has been corrected (see Box 6.2). When hypernatremia has developed rapidly (over hours), the Na can be lowered at the more rapid rate (1.0 mEq/L/hour or 1.0 mmol/L/hour). If the hypernatremia is more chronic, it should be corrected at the slower rate (0.5 mEq/L/hour or 0.5 mmol/L/hour). Maintenance fluids are required simultaneously to replace ongoing fluid losses and the Na content of these fluids added to the calculations.

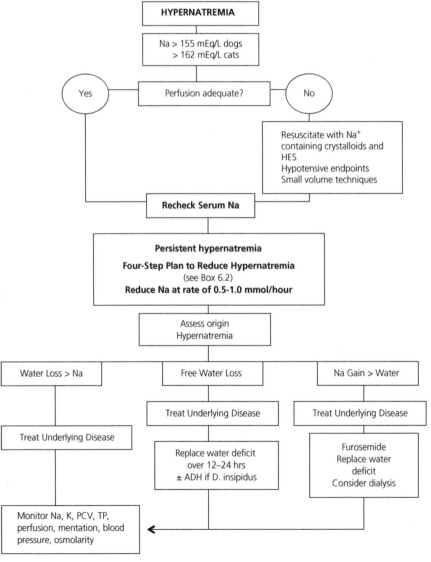

Figure 6.4 Decision-making algorithm for management of hypernatremia.

<table>
<tr><td>

Box 6.2 Example of four-step plan to correct hypernatremia by calculating fluid dose.

Example patient: 20 kg dog with serum Na$^+$ = 180 mmol/L with normal perfusion.

Step 1. Determine the amount to reduce serum Na:
  Patient Na$^+$ – normal Na = Na (mmol/L) decrease needed
  180 mmol/L – 155 mmol/L = 25 mmol/L decrease needed

Step 2. Calculate the effect of 1 L of fluid infusate on patient Na$^+$.
  Change in serum Na from infusing 1 L of selected infusate =
    (infusate Na – serum Na)/(kg BW × 0.6) +1
  5% dextrose in water (D5W) = 0 mmol/L Na$^+$
  Change in serum Na =(0 – 180)/(20 × 0.6) + 1 = –13.8 mmol/L

Step 3. Calculate fluid dose.
  (Na reduction desired)/(reduction of 1 L of infusate)
  (25 mmol/L)/(13.8 mmol/L reduction by 1 L D5W) = 1.8 L D5W
    required

Step 4. Rate of administration.
  Reduce Na by 0.5–1 mmol/L/h (based upon chronicity and severity of
    clinical signs)
  25 mmol/L deficit/0.5–1 mmol/L/h → 25–50 h delivery time
  1.8 L/25–50 h = 36–72 mL/h rate

Notes
Na levels are measured every 4–12 h
The fluid plan should include replacement of ongoing losses

Na content of common infusates:
  5% dextrose in water (D5W): 0 mmol/L
  0.45% sodium chloride: 77 mmol/L
  LRS: 130 mmol/L
  0.9% sodium chloride: 154 mmol/L
  Plasmalyte®, Normosol®: 140 mmol/L

</td></tr>
</table>

Enteral replacement of free water by oral access to water or through an enteral feeding tube can be a safe alternative to intravascular hypotonic fluid replacement. Oral intake must be limited judiciously until hypernatremia slowly resolves.

In patients with hypervolemia and hypernatremia and impaired renal excretion of Na (such as renal failure), the addition of a loop diuretic (such as furosemide) with the hypotonic fluid infusions will increase renal Na excretion. Fluid loss during loop diuretic therapy must be restored with the administration of fluid that is hypotonic compared to the urine. Hypernatremia in the setting of volume overload (such as heart failure and pulmonary edema) may require dialysis for correction.

Once hypernatremia is corrected, efforts are directed at treating the underlying cause of the condition. Such efforts may include free access to water and better control of diabetes insipidus. In addition, correction of hypokalemia and hypercalcemia as etiologies for nephrogenic diabetes insipidus may be required. Vasopressin (desmopressin acetate, 2–8 μg per dog or cat SC or 2–10 drops of nasal formulation per dog or cat) can be used for the treatment of central diabetes insipidus.

Hyponatremia

Hyponatremia is defined as a serum Na concentration <140 mEq/L (<140 mmol/L) in dogs and <149 mEq/L (<149 mmol/L) in cats. Hyponatremia can be associated with low (hypotonic), normal (isotonic) or high (hypertonic) plasma osmolality. Table 6.1 lists causes of hyponatremia. The therapeutic approach to the hyponatremic patient should include identification and treatment of the underlying cause and possibly therapy targeted to increase the serum sodium level. With the exception of concurrent hyponatremia and renal failure, clinically significant hyponatremia is associated with hypotonicity. Normotonic and hypertonic hyponatremia are occasionally seen. In these two conditions, therapy should be directed against the primary abnormality rather than the decreased serum sodium.

Hypertonic hyponatremia can occur when there is an increase in effective osmoles other than Na in the ECF (such as glucose or mannitol). There is a shift of water from the ICF to the ECF, causing a "translocational hyponatremia." Patients with hypertonic hyponatremia have a normal body sodium concentration but a dilutional drop in the measured serum sodium due to movement of water. Hyperglycemia produces a drop in serum Na of 1.6 mEq/L (1.6 mmol/L) for each 100 mg/dL (5.5 mmol/L) of serum glucose greater than 100 mg/dL. This relationship is nonlinear, with greater reduction in serum Na concentration when the blood glucose is >440 mg/dL (24.4 mmol/L). A change in Na of 2.4 mEq/L (2.4 mmol/L) for each 100 mg/dL (5.5 mmol/L) increase in glucose over 100 mg/dL has been reported as a more accurate correction factor when glucose is greater than 440 mg/dL (24.4 mmol/L) [22].

When flame photometry is used to measure the Na concentration, severe elevations in serum lipids (such as triglycerides) and proteins (such as from multiple myeloma) can cause the Na concentration to be reported as reduced. However, the actual plasma Na and water concentrations are unchanged. This is termed "pseudohyponatremia" and is the most common cause of normotonic hyponatremia. The more current methods of measuring blood Na using ion-selective electrodes have virtually eliminated this laboratory artifact [23]. Patients with renal failure and hyponatremia will have a normal or even elevated measured serum osmolality due to the increased BUN concentration. However, their effective osmolality will be low and they should be treated as patients with hypotonic hyponatremia.

Hypotonic hyponatremia is the most common form of clinically significant hyponatremia and can occur by two mechanisms: impaired renal water excretion with normal water intake or, less commonly, water intake in excess of renal excretion and other losses of water. Water excretion by the kidneys depends on the diluting ability of the nephron. Dilution of urine normally occurs through the reabsorption of solutes from the filtrate by the Na-K-2Cl transporter in the thick ascending loop of Henle, the Na-Cl transporter in the distal convoluted tubule, and the absence of ADH action at the collecting tubule. Dysfunction in any of these steps limits the ability of the kidney to dilute urine, with water retention and hyponatremia a potential consequence.

During hypotonic hyponatremia, water moves into brain cells (primarily astrocytes and other glial cells) in response to the osmotic gradient, causing cerebral edema [24,25]. In response, inherent brain volume regulation mechanisms are activated to counteract the potentially harmful volume changes within the brain cells [26].

The first response is an immediate displacement of ICF into the cerebral spinal fluid, and subsequently into the systemic circulation. During the first three hours of hypotonicity, the extrusion of intracellular inorganic ions (such as Na, K, and Cl$^-$) and water reduces cellular swelling in the brain. This occurs through Na-K-ATPase and cellular channels such as K channels and the volume-sensitive Cl channels, accounting for 65% of the observed brain volume regulation [27,28]. A second response consists of the loss of small organic osmolytes, in particular amino acids (glutamate, taurine, glycine) and myoinositol through osmolyte and anion channels. The efflux of organic osmolytes is sustained as long as hyponatremia persists, becoming an essential adaptive mechanism during chronic hyponatremia [25].

During acute, severe hypotonic hyponatremia, the rapid accumulation of intracellular water in the brain can surpass the ability of the compensatory volume regulation mechanisms. As a result, severe neurological signs will be evident, potentially leading to brain herniation or death. However, in chronic hyponatremia (imbalance present ≥48 hours), the loss of both electrolytes and organic osmolytes represents a very efficient mechanism to regulate the brain volume. Therefore, in chronic hyponatremia, brain edema is minimized and neurological symptoms may be absent or mild. However, several of the organic osmolytes lost during volume regulation, in particular glutamate, are neuroactive and could produce transient neurological abnormalities, such as increased seizure activity and decreased synaptic release of excitatory neurotransmitters [29].

Hypotonic hyponatremia represents an excess of water in relation to existing sodium stores, which can be decreased (hypovolemia, decreased extracellular volume (ECV)), normal (normovolemic, normal ECV), or increased (hypervolemic, increased ECV). Further classification of patients with hypotonic hyponatremia by their ECV status aids in therapy. With the exception of renal failure, most conditions causing hypotonic hyponatremia are characterized by high plasma concentrations of ADH despite the presence of hypotonicity. Increased ADH levels are the result of physiological stimulation (volume depletion) or secondary to an inappropriate secretion of ADH (SIADH). In a minority of cases, hyponatremia is caused by excessive water intake, with a normal excretory capacity.

Animals with hypotonic hyponatremia and hypovolemia (decreased ECV) have lost sodium in excess of water. Common causes of loss include renal (hypoadrenocorticism, diuretic use), gastrointestinal (vomiting, diarrhea, repeated NG suctioning) and third space fluid losses (pleural, peritoneal effusions). Clinically, solute loss most often occurs in a fluid that is isotonic or hypotonic to plasma. Isotonic or hypotonic fluid loss will not directly lower sodium concentration. Hyponatremia develops due to the body's physiological response to volume depletion (nonosmotic vasopressin release and increased renal water reabsorption) causing decreased water excretion. Additionally, thirst is stimulated and the attempt to replace volume depletion by drinking water contributes to the hyponatremia. Resuscitation with a high-sodium replacement fluid will typically correct the volume depletion and terminate the volume-mediated release of ADH.

The most common cause of normvolemic hypotonic hyponatremia in humans is the syndrome of inappropriate ADH secretion (SIADH) which has been reported to occur in dogs with or without associated conditions [30]. Antidiuretic hormone (ADH, vasopressin) is secreted in spite of the absence of a physiological stimulus for secretion. The SIADH syndrome in humans has been attributed to a number of drugs, neoplasia, pulmonary disease, and CNS disorders. Normovolemic hypotonic hyponatremia has also been reported in dogs with psychogenic polydipsia, administration of hypotonic fluids and severe hypothyroidism causing myxedema coma [31].

Hypervolemic hypotonic hyponatremia can occur and is most commonly seen with congestive heart failure, severe liver disease, and in patients with the nephrotic syndrome. Sodium and water retention is stimulated by subnormal atrial stretch that is perceived by the brain as a decrease in circulating volume. In patients with the nephrotic syndrome, a primary intrarenal mechanism for Na and water retention has been proposed [32]. Dilutional hypontremia (a form of hypervolemic hypotonic hyponatremia) can occur when water intake exceeds the renal excretion of free water due to advanced renal failure.

The therapeutic approach to the small animal ICU patient with hypotonic hyponatremia will include resuscitation of any volume deficits with high Na intravenous fluids, identification and treatment of the underlying cause and possibly therapy targeted to increase the serum Na concentration very slowly. An algorithm to guide decision making during the treatment of hyponatremia is presented in Figure 6.5. If large quantities of fluids are required for resuscitation of perfusion deficits in these patients, hydroxyethyl starch (colloid) can be titrated (5 mL/kg IV increments) as needed to reach low normal resuscitation endpoints. The colloid can expand the intravascular volume and pressure with minimal extravasation of water into the interstitial space. Hypoadrenocorticism is treated with IV glucocorticosteroids and the infusion of normal saline.

Correction of serum Na at a rate faster than brain cells can restore the extruded osmolytes can lead to brain dehydration and trigger osmotic demyelination (ODS). Although rare, ODS can develop one to several days after aggressive treatment of hyponatremia, and can cause irreversible brain damage. The ODS is characterized by astrocyte apoptosis followed by the induction of inflammatory responses, such as proinflammatory cytokine production and microglia activation, eventually resulting in demyelination [33]. The diagnosis of ODS is clinical in patients with neurological symptoms after a recent overly rapid correction of hyponatremia. It can be confirmed by the presence of typical lesions at magnetic resonance imaging [34].

Therapy for hypotonic hyponatremia should be instituted at a rate that balances the risk of hyponatremia with the risk of too rapid correction and ODS. This is guided primarily by the presence of neurological symptoms and by the duration of the hyponatremia (ODS more likely with chronic hyponatremia). Aggressive correction of Na is not indicated in any asymptomatic patient. If overcorrection occurs, therapeutic relowering of serum Na could be considered, especially in patients at high risk of ODS. Relowering of serum Na can be achieved by administering desmopressin (desmopressin acetate 2–8 μg per dog or cat or 2–10 drops of nasal formulation per dog or cat) or by infusion of 5% dextrose in water (see Box 6.2).

In general, therapy for hypotonic hyponatremia consists of Na administration to patients that are hypovolemic and water restriction in patients that are normovolemic or hypervolemic. In hypovolemic patients, normal saline (Na 154 mEq or mmol per 1000 mL) will provide additional sodium. The secretion of ADH will be suppressed following correction of hypovolemia, resulting in the production of dilute urine and excretion of the excess water. The correction of concomitant hypokalemia may cause a more rapid increase of serum Na because the Na-K-ATPase extrudes Na as K enters the cell to restore depleted intracellular K storage, thus increasing the correction rate of hyponatremia. The quantity of K supplemented must be considered when determining the desired amount of Na to be supplemented.

Hypertonic saline administration may be required in patients with severe hypotonic hyponatremia (<110 meq/L) or in symptomatic patients. The formulas presented in Box 6.3 can be used to estimate the amount of hypertonic saline required to reach the desired serum Na concentration (125–130 mEq/L or 125–130 mmol/L). The Na concentration in maintenance and hypertonic saline solutions is provided in Box 6.3. The Na concentration of maintenance fluids must be considered in the calculations. It must be remembered that all of the Na infused will remain in the ECF and has a greater volume effect than the exact amount infused due to the osmotic movement of water in response to the infused Na.

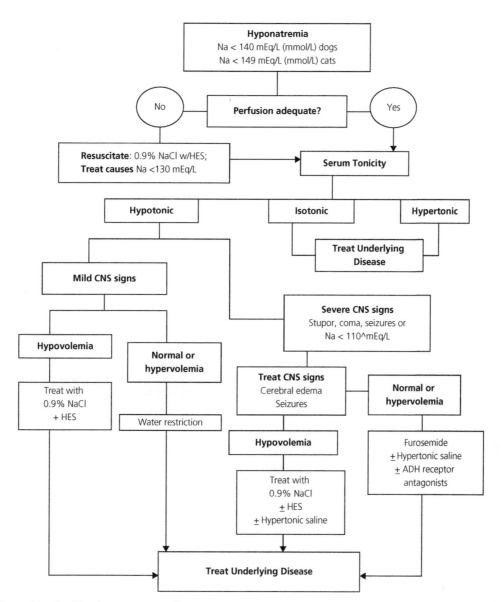

Figure 6.5 Decision-making algorithm for management of hyponatremia.

In patients with severe neurological signs, the serum Na can be increased by 1–2 mEq/L/h (1–2 mmol/L/h) for the first few hours but should not exceed 8 mEq/L/h (8 mmol/L/h) over 24 hours [35].

Studies in experimental animals suggest that the rate of correction over the first 24 hours is more important than the maximum rate in any given hour or several hour period [36]. The patient should be carefully monitored with frequent evaluation of the serum Na concentration. Recommended indications for stopping the infusion of hypertonic saline include the cessation of life-threatening manifestations, moderation of other symptoms, or the achievement of the targeted serum Na concentration of 125–130 mEq/L (125–130 mmol/L). The full correction of the serum Na is not necessary, and as neurological symptoms subside, a more conservative approach should be prescribed.

In normovolemic and hypervolemic patients, therapy is typically aimed at water removal. In mild or asymptomatic patients water restriction is indicated. In patients with more severe, symptomatic hyponatremia, the serum Na concentration can be increased more rapidly with the administration of a loop diuretic (such as furosemide 1–2 mL/kg IV) while administering Na-containing fluids (isotonic or hypertonic saline as indicated).

The response to isotonic saline is different in SIADH. The Na balance is normal in SIADH since it is regulated by aldosterone and atrial natriuretic peptide, not ADH. Thus, the administered Na will be excreted in the urine, while some of the water may be retained, leading to possible worsening of the hyponatremia. Treatment of SIADH begins with fluid restriction and correction of any identified inciting cause (such as discontinuing causative drug, treating traumatic brain injury) [37]. If fluid must be given or the serum Na concentration must be raised quickly because of symptoms, isotonic saline has a limited role in correction of the hyponatremia and hypertonic saline may then be required. Careful monitoring is required to prevent overly rapid correction.

Concurrent use of a loop diuretic may be beneficial in patients with SIADH since, by inhibiting NaCl reabsorption in the thick ascending limb of the loop of Henle, it interferes with the countercurrent mechanism and induces a state of ADH resistance and more dilute urine is excreted. Demeclocycline (an antibiotic) induces ADH resistance and

Box 6.3 Example of four-step plan to correct hyponatremia by calculating fluid dose.

Patient: 20 kg dog with serum Na⁺ = 110 mmol/L* with normal perfusion

Step 1. Determine the amount to increase serum Na+.

Desired Na⁺ − patient Na⁺ = Na⁺ mmol/L decrease needed
(125 mmol/L) − (110 mmol/L) = 15 mmol/L Na⁺ increase needed

Step 2. Calculate the effect of 1 L of fluid infusate on patient Na+.

Change in serum sodium from infusing 1 L of selected fluid infusate:
= (infusate Na⁺ − serum Na⁺)/(kg BW × 0.6) + 1
3% hypertonic saline = 513 mmol/L Na⁺
Change in serum sodium from infusing 1 L 3% HTS = (513 − 110)/
(20 kg × 0.6) + 1 = 31 mmol/L

Step 3. Fluid dose.

Na⁺ addition desired ÷ addition by 1 L of the desired infusate
15 mmol/L ÷ 31 mmol/L addition from 1 L 3% HTS = **0.484 L of 3% HTS needed**

Step 4. Rate of administration.

Increase Na⁺ = 0.25 mmol/L/h (6 mmol/L/day)
15 mmol/L deficit = **60 h delivery time**
Based upon chronicity and severity of clinical signs, the 484 mL of 3% NaCl would be delivered over 60 hours (8 mL/h)
Na⁺ content in additional fluids must be figured into amount of Na⁺ infused, not to exceed the 4–8 mmol/L/day
Sodium is monitored every 2–6 hours initially
The fluid plan should include replacement of ongoing fluid losses with Na⁺ added to above calculations

Na⁺ content of common infusates:

Ringer's lactate solution: 130 mmol/L
0.9% sodium chloride in water (0.9NS): 154 mmol/L
Plasmalyte-A® and Normosol-R®: 140 mmol/L
3% sodium chloride in water: 513 mmol/L
5% sodium chloride in water: 856 mmol/L
* mmol/L = mEq/L

has been used to limit water retention chronically. Arginine vasopressin (V2) receptor antagonists (such as conivaptan, tolvaptan) capable of blocking the effect of excessive ADH and secondary water retention have been used successfully in human medicine [38]. Conivaptan and tolvaptan have been found to be safe and effective V1 and V2 receptor antagonists in the dog but await clinical trials [39,40].

Potassium disorders

Potassium is located primarily in the ICF. Changes in serum K can reflect either changes in total body stores or transcellular shifts between the ICF and ECF. Because the effects of K on cell membrane potential are determined by the ratio of intracellular to extracellular K, transcellular shifts are more likely to produce clinical signs than are changes in whole-body K levels.

Normal serum K values for the dog are 3.6–5.5 mEq/L or mmol/L and for the cat 3.4–5.6 mEq/L or mmol/L (see Table 6.4). Measuring K in serum not separated from blood cells immediately will produce an artifactual increase in K. In the dog, the clotting mechanism releases K, likely from platelets. For accuracy, plasma K values should be measured in heparinized plasma and separated from RBCs within 30 minutes of sampling. Fluctuations in the ECF K concentration do not necessarily reflect the total body K level.

Acute changes in blood pH will affect potassium concentration by causing translocation of K between the ICF and ECF. Acidosis can increase the ECF concentration of K by an exchange of K ions from the ICF for hydrogen ions in the ECF. In contrast, alkalosis can decrease the ECF concentration of K by an exchange of hydrogen from the ICF for K ions in the ECF. This ion exchange is a normal buffering process in the body (see Chapter 7). A predictable change in K based on the measured change in pH has previously been reported. However, a number of experimental studies have shown this response to be variable [41]. Acute mineral acidosis is the only acid–base disorder expected to cause any clinically revelant change in serum K concentration.

Alterations in serum K can cause life-threatening complications associated with ventilation, cardiac contractility and rhythm, blood pressure, and neuromuscular functions. Early recognition and intervention of a K disorder can be of critical importance for a favorable outcome in the small animal ICU patient.

Hyperkalemia

Hyperkalemia is diagnosed when the serum K is greater than 5.55 mEq/L (5.55 mmol/L) in the dog and cat, though reference ranges can vary. Life-threatening complications are likely when the serum K is >7.5 mEq/L (>7.5 mmol/L). Pseudohyperkalemia can occur as a post blood collection artifact caused by release of K from platelets in thrombocytosis and hemolysis in Akitas and other breeds with high red blood cell K.

Causes of hyperkalemia seen in the ICU small animal patient are listed in Table 6.1. The more common pathophysiological mechanisms causing hyperkalemia in the small animal ICU patient include: (1) a decrease in the glomerular filtration rate, (2) the failure to excrete urine from the body, and (3) a lack of or ineffective aldosterone concentrations or responsiveness. Hyperkalemia has been reported in veterinary patients that have experienced massive tissue breakdown, acute tumor lysis syndrome, reperfusion of tissues in cats with aortic thromboembolism and immediately after return of spontaneous circulation in patients suffering cardiopulmonary arrest [42]. Under these circumstances, hyperkalemia is expected to be transient if renal function and urine outflow are normal. Hyperkalemia has also been associated with pleural and peritoneal effusions in cats [43].

The most significant clinical effects of hyperkalemia are due to alterations in the transmembrane resting potential in cardiac and neuromuscular cells. Hyperkalemia decreases the resting potential, making the cell relatively hyperexcitable. However, if the resting potential decreases to less than the threshold potential, the cell is unable to repolarize after a depolarization and becomes nonexcitable. Changes in neuromuscular excitability are dependent upon a variety of other factors, including the extracellular Ca concentration and blood pH.

The electrocardiogram changes associated with increasing serum potassium levels have been described and are illustrated in Figures 6.2 and 6.3. However, the ECG changes do not necessarily correlate with the magnitude of the change in the plasma K concentration, especially in cats [44]. The presence of compatible ECG changes reflects the functional consequences of hyperkalemia and warrants specific therapy for hyperkalemia as well as treatment of the underlying disease process.

Options for treatment of hyperkalemia include administration of calcium gluconate to antagonize the effects on cell membrane excitability, lowering serum K by causing a transcellular shift of K into cells with insulin, sodium bicarbonate or beta-agonists, or by removing excess K from the body with exchange resins or renal replacement therapy. Table 6.5 provides a list of agents with doses and indication for the use of these agents in the dog and cat. Fluid therapy with K-free (0.9% NaCl) or low K-containing fluids (such as LRS, Norm-R®, Plasmalyte-A®) will dilute

Table 6.5 Therapeutic options for patients with hyperkalemia.

Mechanism of action	Agent	Dose	Onset of action	Duration of action	Complications
Membrane stabilization	10% calcium gluconate	0.5–1.5 mL/kg slowly IV with ECG monitoring	Immediate	30–60 minutes	Hypercalcemia, bradyarrhythmias
Transcellular shift ECF→ICF	Regular insulin	0.5 units/kg with coadministration of 2 g of dextrose/unit of insulin	15–30 minutes	4–6 hours	Hypoglycemia, hyperglycemia (Somogyi effect or concurrent dextrose administration)
	Sodium bicarbonate	1–2 mEq/kg IV over 10–15 minutes	30–60 minutes	Several hours	Metabolic alkalosis, paradoxical CNS acidosis
	Beta-agonist				
	Terbutaline	0.01 mg/kg slow IV	30 minutes	2 hours	Tachycardia
	Albuterol	1–3 puffs	30 minutes	2 hours	Tachycardia
Remove excess potassium	Furosemide	2–4 mg/kg IV	15 minutes	2–3 hours	Volume depletion
	Cation exchange resin (Kayexalate)	Orally: 20 g with 100 ml 20% sorbitol. Retention enema: 50 g in 100–200 mL water	1–2 hours	Several hours	Volume overload, intestinal necrosis
	Renal replacement (PD, CRRT, IHD)	N/A	Depends on modality		Availability, cost
Avoiding iatrogenic administration of potassium	Use of fluids without potassium (i.e. 0.9% NaCl)	Dependent upon clinical perfusion and hydration parameters			Fluid intolerance

CNS, central nervous system; CRRT, continuous renal replacement therapy; ECF, extracellular fluid; ECG, electrocardiogram; ICF, intracellular fluid; IHD, intermittent hemodialysis; PD, peritoneal dialysis.

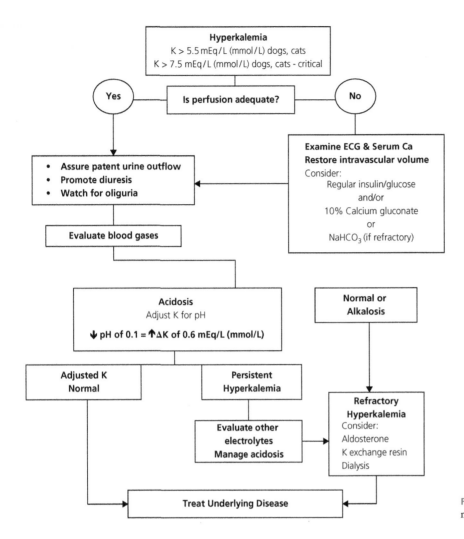

Figure 6.6 Decision-making algorithm for management of hyperkalemia.

the potassium in the ECF, improve renal perfusion, and enhance urinary excretion of potassium.

When the underlying cause of the hyperkalemia can be rapidly corrected (such as urethral obstruction, hypoadrenocorticism), the pharmacological shifting of K into the ICF will provide adequate control of serum K levels until renal excretion can be reestablished. Techniques to remove K from the body (such as dialysis, continuous renal replacement therapy, hemoperfusion techniques, or K exchange resins) will be needed in patients with acute or late-stage chronic renal failure when the underlying problem cannot be rapidly corrected. An algorithm to guide the decision-making process during the treatment of hyperkalemia is presented in Figure 6.6.

Hypokalemia

Hypokalemia occurs when potassium concentrations are <3.5 mEq/L (3.5 mmol/L) and can become critical when <2.5 mEq/L (2.5 mmol/L).

Causes of hypokalemia seen in the ICU small animal patient are listed in Table 6.1. The more common pathophysiological mechanisms causing hypokalemia include increased K loss through the kidneys or GI tract, or a transcellular shift of K into cells. Hypokalemia strictly from decreased dietary intake is unlikely, but can occur in anorectic animals receiving inadequate K supplementation through their intravenous fluids or nutritional support. Chronic fluid therapy causing medullary washout, diuretic therapy,

insulin therapy, and medications that cause vomiting can be reasons for hypokalemia associated with therapy in the ICU patient. In uncontrolled diabetes mellitus, transcellular movement of K is caused by hypertonicity and insulin deficiency. Despite normal or mild decreases in serum K values at presentation, severe hypokalemia can develop with correction of the metabolic acidosis and administration of insulin.

Hypokalemia increases the resting potential and results in a relatively hyperpolarized cell. Clinical signs of hypokelamia may therefore involve the skeletal, muscular, GI, respiratory, and renal systems (see Table 6.4). Hypokalemia causes skeletal muscle weakness and at serum levels <2.0 mEq/L (<2.0 mmol/L) can result in rhabdomyolysis. Cats often exhibit ventroflexion of the head and neck (Figure 6.7). Weakness of the respiratory muscles can impair ventilation and may lead to respiratory acidosis, hypoxemia or respiratory arrest.

Dysfunction of smooth muscles of the GI tract is reported to cause constipation, paralytic ileus, and gastric atony in human patients but is not well documented in veterinary medicine. Cardiac arrhythmias, to include atrial and ventricular tachyarrhythmias, atrioventricular dissociation and ventricular fibrillation, have been reported in association with hypokalemia in dogs and cats. Hypokalemia increases the arrhythmogenic potential of digoxin and causes the myocardium to become refractory to the effects of class 1 antiarrhythmic agents. Hypokalemia can also impair renal tubular cell functions, resulting in polyuria and polydipsia.

Magnesium depletion often co-exists with K depletion as a result of drug therapy or disease processes. The ability to correct hypokalemia is impaired when Mg deficiency is present, particularly when the serum Mg concentration is <0.5 mmol/L

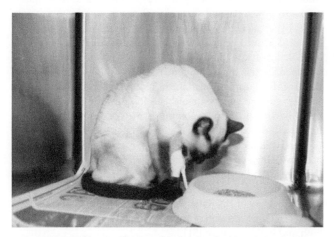

Figure 6.7 Cat with ventroflexion of the head and neck associated with hypokalemia.

(<1.21 mg/dL). Concurrent Mg repletion aids in the correction of the hypokalemia [45].

Treatment of hypokalemia involves K administration and prevention of ongoing losses. An algorithm to guide the decision-making processes when treating hypokalemia is presented in Figure 6.8. In the nonemergent setting, oral potassium gluconate can be titrated to effect. Intravenous administration of K as an additive to fluid therapy is more common in hospitalized patients, primarily with potassium chloride (2 mEq of K per mL, 2 mmol of K per mL). Any intravenous K supplementation must be diluted to prevent fatal arrhythmias from rapid changes in extracellular K. Potassium phosphate (4.36 mEq of K per mL, 4.36 mmol of K per mL) can be used in patients with concurrent P depletion. A sliding scale for K supplementation is noted in Box 6.4. Potassium concentrations exceeding 40 mEq/L may produce pain at the infusion site and sclerosis of smaller vessels. However, central venous infusion of K at high concentrations should be avoided to prevent depolarization of the conduction tissues, potentially leading to cardiac arrest.

When hypokalemia is causing impaired ventilation (insufficient contraction of ventilator muscles) or potentially fatal cardiac arrhythmias, a more concentrated dose of diluted potassium chloride can be administered over 20–30 minutes. The dose can be calculated by multiplying the estimate of ECF volume (body weight

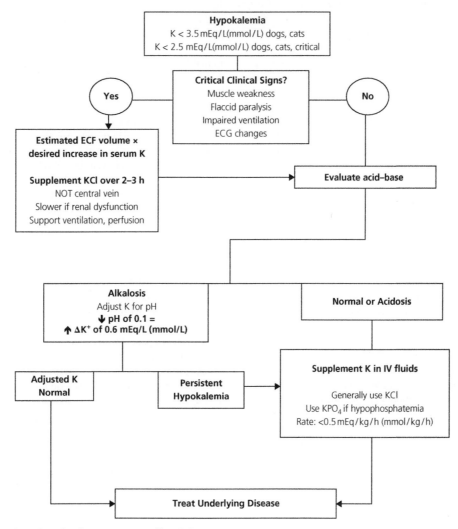

Figure 6.8 Decision-making algorithm for management of hypokalemia.

Box 6.4 Sliding scale for potassium supplementation of intravenous maintenance fluids.

Serum potassium (mEq/L or mmol/L)	mEq/LK to add 1 liter
≤ 2.0	20
2.1–2.5	15
2.5–3.0	10
3.0–3.5	5

in kg × 0.2) by the desired increase in serum K [46]. Glucose-containing solutions are not to be used as a diluent for the potassium chloride when the goal is to more rapidly increase the serum K to ameliorate clinical signs. Glucose stimulates the release of insulin causing a shift of K into cells. The treatment of hypokalemia must be closely monitored with an ECG, blood gas for acid–base status and electrolyte panels.

Calcium disorders

Calcium plays a critical role in every cell of the body, with the intracellular concentration tightly regulated by membrane channels, pumps, and transport proteins. The additional effects of Ca on transmembrane electrical potentials makes Ca disorders a critical priority in the small animal ICU patient.

Normal serum total Ca values are 8.9–11.4 mg/dL (2.2–3.0 mmol/L) in the dog and 8.2–10.8 mg/dL (2.0–2.7 mmol/L) in the cat (see Table 6.4). However, it is the ionized fraction of Ca that is physiologically active, homeostatically regulated and best correlated with clinical signs. Formulas have been proposed to mathematically correct total Ca values for alterations in serum albumin levels. However, these formulas have been shown to be poor predictors of measured ionized Ca. Normal serum values for ionized Ca are 1.2–1.5 mmol/L (5.0–6.0 mg/dL) in the dog and 1.1–1.4 mmol/L (4.5–5.5 mg/dL) in the cat.

Point of care testing requires that blood samples be collected and handled anaerobically for accurate measurement of ionized Ca. Changes in sample pH caused by decreased pCO_2 will change the measured value of ionized Ca. Reference laboratories can correct Ca measurements in samples exposed to air using species-specific mathematical formulas [47]. Incorrect ratio of blood to heparin can also cause a preanalytical error. An *in vitro* study investigating the effect of heparin dilution on canine blood samples demonstrated that the measurement of the ionized Ca concentration was most affected compared to other analytes tested [48].

Hypercalcemia

Hypercalcemia is commonly defined as a serum total Ca concentration >11.5 mg/dL (2.87 mmol/L) for dogs and >10.5 mg/dL (2.62 mmol/L) for cats, with laboratory variations possible. Ionized serum calcium concentrations ≥1.5 mmol/L (6.01 mg/dL) in dogs and ≥1.4 mmol/L (5.61 mg/dL) in cats are considered as hypercalcemia. High blood calcium concentrations are a result of calcium entering the vascular space faster than it can be excreted or sequestered.

Ca^{2+} ions can damage cells if they enter in excessive numbers, such as in the case of excitotoxicity or overexcitation of neural circuits, after insults such as brain trauma. Calcium also acts as one of the primary regulators of osmotic stress (osmotic shock).

Hypercalcemia has a negative chronotropic effect and a positive inotropic effect in the heart. Abnormal heart rhythms can result, with ECG findings of a short QT interval. The high levels of Ca decrease the neuron membrane permeability to Na, thus decreasing the transmembrane excitability. Hypotonicity of smooth and striated muscle results, explaining the fatigue, muscle weakness, low tone, and sluggish reflexes in muscle groups seen with hypercalcemia. In the gut this causes constipation. Hypercalcaemia can also increase gastrin production, leading to increased gastric acidity.

Hypercalcemia can cause tubular damage and vasoconstriction of the renal afferent artiole, leading to acute renal failure. Hypercalcemia can also cause nephrogenic diabetes insipidus by inhibiting vasopressin action at the V2 receptor in the collecting duct, causing impaired renal concentrating ability, leading to increased Na excretion and volume depletion [49,50]. A furosemide-like effect can occur with high serum Ca inhibiting secretory K channel activity in the thick ascending limb of Henle. Hypercalcemia is also associated with an increased urinary excretion of both Ca and Mg due to greater delivery of Na, water, Ca, and Mg to the loop of Henle and high peritubular concentrations of Ca inhibiting the reabsorption of both ions in this segment [51].

In addition, renal dysfunction can occur as a result of Ca precipitation in the kidney, manifested as nephrocalcinosis. Calcium deposits may also develop in other tissues, such as the vasculature, cardiac valves, and cornea [52]. Patients with a total Ca × P product >50 are at risk of tissue calcification.

Possible causes of ionized hypercalcemia diagnosed in the small animal ICU patient are listed in Table 6.2. Neoplastic cells can produce a PTH-related protein (PTHrP) that binds with PTH receptors to cause hypercalcemia. Lymphosarcoma, anal sac apocrine gland adenocarcinoma, multiple myeloma, thyroid carcinoma, GI or vaginal squamous cell carcinoma are the types of neoplasia most commonly associated with hypercalcemia in the dog. In the cat, humoral hypercalcemia of malignancy is most commonly associated with squamous cell carcinoma. Cats may also have an idiopathic hypercalcemia that does not result in clinical signs; however, this is a diagnosis of exclusion and all other causes must be ruled out. Acidifying diets may be associated with the development of this disease in cats [53].

Common clinical manifestations of hypercalcemia include polyuria, polydipsia, anorexia, dehydration, lethargy, weakness, hypertension, seizures, and acute renal failure (see Table 6.4). While definitive therapy of hypercalcemia is the correction of the underlying cause, patients exhibiting signs of dehydration, azotemia, cardiac arrhythmia, weakness or other neurological dysfunction require aggressive supportive therapy while the underlying cause is diagnosed and treated. An algorithm to guide the decision-making processes when treating a patient with hypercalcemia is presented in Figure 6.9.

Perfusion and hydration deficits are correct with 0.9% NaCl, which promotes calciuresis. Pharmacological options for promoting Ca redistribution or excretion are listed in Table 6.6 with doses, mechanism of action and indications. Diagnosis and treatment of the causative disorder are essential.

Hypocalcemia

Hypocalcemia is defined as a total Ca concentration <9.0 mg/dL (2.25 mmol/L) in dogs and <8.0 mg/dL (2.0 mmol/L) in cats. Values for ionized Ca defining hypocalcemia are <1.2 mmol/L (4.81 mg/dL) in dogs and <1.1 mmol/L (4.41 mg/dL) in cats. If ionized hyocalcemia is identified, serum Mg and P levels should also be evaluated. Samples should be saved for plasma PTH and vitamin D levels, as well.

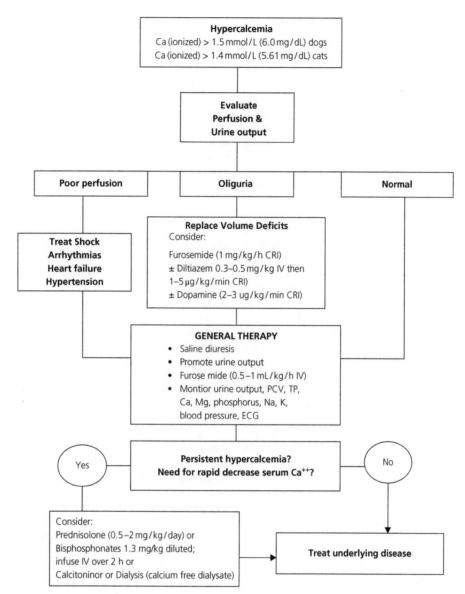

Hypercalcemia
Ca (ionized) > 1.5 mmol / L (6.0 mg / dL) dogs
Ca (ionized) > 1.4 mmol / L (5.61 mg / dL) cats

Evaluate
Perfusion &
Urine output

Poor perfusion   **Oliguria**   **Normal**

Treat Shock
Arrhythmias
Heart failure
Hypertension

Replace Volume Deficits
Consider:

Furosemide (1 mg / kg / h CRI)
± Diltiazem 0.3–0.5 mg / kg IV then
1–5 µg / kg / min CRI)
± Dopamine (2–3 ug / kg / min CRI)

GENERAL THERAPY
• Saline diuresis
• Promote urine output
• Furose mide (0.5–1 mL / kg / h IV)
• Montior urine output, PCV, TP,
  Ca, Mg, phosphorus, Na, K,
  blood pressure, ECG

Yes   **Persistent hypercalcemia?**
        Need for rapid decrease serum Ca⁺⁺?   No

Consider:
Prednisolone (0.5–2 mg / kg / day) or
Bisphosphonates 1.3 mg/kg diluted;
infuse IV over 2 h or
Calcitoninor or Dialysis (calcium free dialysate)

Treat underlying disease

Figure 6.9 Decision-making algorithm for management of hypercalcemia.

Table 6.6 Therapeutic options for treating hypercalcemia.

Drug class	Example/dose	Mechanism	Notes
IV fluids	Calcium free fluids (i.e. 0.9% NaCl), replace rehydration, diuresis rate	Diuresis	LRS contains Ca and is not recommended
Loop diuretic	Furosemide, 1–2 mg/kg IV, PO or continuous infusion	Inhibit calcium resorption in the thick ascending limb of Henle	Hypokalemia and metabolic alkalosis
Glucocorticoids	Prednisone, 0.5–1 mg/kg PO q 24 h or 25 mg/m² PO q 24 h	Decrease osteoclastic bone resorption, inhibit osteoclast activating factor, block prostaglandin synthesis and antagonize vitamin D action, treat underlying neoplasia	Beginning this medication prior to making the diagnosis may make diagnosis of neoplasia challenging or impossible
Bisphosphonates	Pamidronate: 1.3 mg/kg diluted in 0.9% saline and delivered as a 2 h IV infusion.	Reduce osteoclast activity and function	Pamidronate 1.3 mg/kg dilute in 0.9% saline and delivered as 2 h infusion, may repeat in 1–3 weeks
Calcitonin	Calcitonin 4–6 IU/kg subcutaneously q 8 h	Inhibits osteoclast bone resorption, reducing tubular resorption of electrolytes	Young animals may be more sensitive to the drug

IV, intravenous; LRS, lactated Ringer's solution; PO, per os.

Hypocalcemia occurs when Ca is lost from the ECF faster than it can be replaced by absorption from the intestine or mobilized from the bone. Since Ca blocks Na channels and inhibits depolarization of nerve and muscle fibers, diminished Ca lowers the threshold for depolarization [54]. Hypocalcemia causes neuromuscular irritability and tetany. Alkalemia induces tetany due to a decrease in ionized Ca, whereas acidemia is protective. This pathophysiology is important in patients with renal failure who have hypocalcemia because rapid correction of acidemia or development of alkalemia can both trigger tetany.

Common causes of ionized hypocalcemia in the small animal ICU patient are listed in Table 6.2. Acute illness may lead to hypocalcemia for multiple reasons. In one study, the three most common factors identified in human patients with hypocalcemia associated with acute illness were hypomagnesemia, acute renal failure, and transfusions. In gram-negative sepsis in humans, there is a reduction in total and ionized serum Ca. The mechanism for this remains unknown but it appears to be associated with multiple factors, including elevated levels of cytokines (such as interleukin-6, interleukin-1, TNF-alpha), hypoparathyroidism, and vitamin D deficiency or resistance. Mortality rates are increased in humans with sepsis and hypocalcemia, compared with patients who are normocalcemic [55]. However, there is no clear evidence that treating critically ill patients with supplemental Ca alters outcomes [56].

Less is known about the incidence and clinical significance of ionized hypocalcemia in veterinary patients. In a study of 141 dogs admitted to the ICU, ionized hypocalcemia at admission was associated with longer duration of hospitalization but not outcome [57]. Severity and duration of ionized hypocalcemia were associated with increased mortality and longer hospitalization in a study of 58 septic dogs [58].

The clinical signs of hypocalcemia vary widely, from asymptomatic to life-threatening situations. Depending on the cause, unrecognized or poorly treated hypocalcemic emergencies can lead to significant morbidity or death. The symptoms in humans can be recalled by the proposed mnemonic "CATS go numb" – Convulsions, Arrhythmias, Tetany and numbness/paresthesias – which is applicable to the dog and cat. The severity of clinical signs correlates with the magnitude and rapidity of the decrease in Ca and is generally related to neuronal irritability. The clinical signs of hypocalcemia in the dog and cat are listed in Table 6.4.

Life-threatening complications can be a consequence of the cardiac effects or the secondary effects of prolonged neuromuscular excitability (such as hypoglycemia, hyperthermia, SIRS). Hypocalcemia will have a positive chronotropic effect and a negative inotropic effect on the heart, resulting in tachycardia and poor cardiac output. The ECG changes include intermittent prolongation of the QT interval, indicative of electrical instability. Torsades de pointes is a potential consequence, requiring immediate intervention.

Treatment requires emergency intervention of hypocalcemic tetany and any life-threatening arrhythmias, followed by support of secondary complications and the diagnosis and management of the underlying disease process. An algorithm to guide the decision-making processes when treating hypocalcemia is provided in Figure 6.10. Acute, symptomatic hypocalcemia necessitates intravenous Ca therapy. It is important to calculate the dosage of Ca based on elemental (available) calcium, because different products vary in the amount of calcium available. The dosage of elemental Ca for hypocalcemia is 5–15 mg/kg/h (0.12–0.37 mmol/kg/h). Calcium

gluconate, 10%, contains 9.3 mg of elemental Ca/mL (0.23 mmol/mL). Calcium chloride, 27%, contains 27.2 mg of elemental calcium/mL (0.68 mmol/mL). Thus, for 10% calcium gluconate, the dosage is 0.5–1.5 mL/kg/h IV, and for 27% calcium chloride the dosage is 0.22–0.66 mL/kg/h IV [59]. Calcium gluconate, as a 10% solution, is recommended because, unlike calcium chloride, calcium gluconate extravasation is not caustic. In addition, large animal calcium gluconate products may have a higher concentration (23% compared to 10%), requiring careful calculation of the drug dose when used in small animals.

Rapid IV administration of Ca can cause bradycardia, prolonged PR intervals, wide QRS or short QT interval. Monitoring of the ECG is required during the IV administration. If arrhythmias are noted, Ca administration should be discontinued and the Ca and other electrolyte values rechecked. Supportive care for the systemic effects of severe tetany, seizure or arrhythmias will be required. Subacute or long-term Ca supplementation may be necessary for some animals, depending on the underlying etiology. Oral calcium carbonate, lactate chloride or gluconate or calcitriol may be necessary. Weaning newborns and feeding appropriate diets is essential for postpartum animals with puerperal hypocalcemia. Hypocalcemia not resulting in immediate clinical signs may warrant treatment of the underlying condition only.

Hyperphosphatemia may cause hypocalcemia as a result of Ca precipitation, inhibiting bone reabsorption and suppression of renal hydroxylation of vitamin D. The administration of Ca to patients with an elevation of serum P may increase Ca precipitation and cause further tissue damage. When hypocalcemia is present with hyperphosphatemia, the patient is treated by lowering the serum P level.

Magnesium disorders

Magnesium is the second most abundant intracellular cation. Accurate assessment of the intracellular Mg status through serum Mg values can therefore be challenging. Low serum Mg reflects a total body Mg deficit. Normal serum Mg in the dog is 0.7–1.0 mmol/L (1.7–2.4 mg/dL) and in the cat is 0.41–1.02 mmol/L (1.0–2.5 mg/dL). However, Mg deficiency can occur with normal serum values. The importance of Mg during energy production and enzymatic processes within the cells makes it a critical cation in the small animal ICU patient. It plays a vital role in the maintenance of normal brain neurotransmission, vascular tone, skeletal muscle activity, and cardiac conduction and contractility.

Hypermagnesemia

Hypermagnesemia is considered when serum Mg is ≥1.2 mmol/L (>2.92 mg/dL) in dogs and ≥1.25 mmol/L (>3.04 mg/dL) in cats. Hypermagnesemia is rare in the dog and cat because of the ability of the kidney to rapidly increase Mg excretion. The two most common causes of hypermagnesemia are renal failure and excessive administration of Mg-containing drugs or fluids. The administration of normal doses of Mg-containing drugs can result in hypermagnesemia in animals with renal failure.

Symptoms of hypermagnesemia are not usually apparent until the serum Mg level is >1.97 mmol/L (4.8 mg/dL) [13]. Concomitant hypocalcemia, hyperkalemia, or uremia may exaggerate the symptoms. Iatrogenic parenteral Mg overdose has been reported in veterinary patients. Due to miscalculation, the patients received excessive amounts of IV Mg, resulting in ionized Mg levels 6–8 times above the normal reference range. The animals (one cat, one dog) demonstrated vomiting, bradycardia, hypotension, decreased

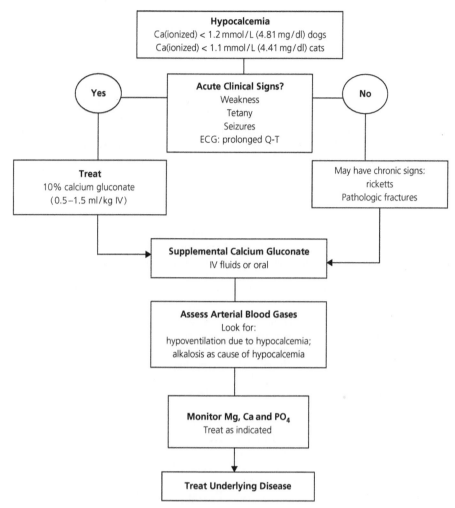

Hypocalcemia
Ca(ionized) < 1.2 mmol/L (4.81 mg/dl) dogs
Ca(ionized) < 1.1 mmol/L (4.41 mg/dl) cats

Yes

Acute Clinical Signs?
Weakness
Tetany
Seizures
ECG: prolonged Q-T

No

Treat
10% calcium gluconate
(0.5–1.5 ml/kg IV)

May have chronic signs:
ricketts
Pathologic fractures

Supplemental Calcium Gluconate
IV fluids or oral

Assess Arterial Blood Gases
Look for:
hypoventilation due to hypocalcemia;
alkalosis as cause of hypocalcemia

Monitor Mg, Ca and PO$_4$
Treat as indicated

Treat Underlying Disease

Figure 6.10 Decision-making algorithm for management of hypercalcemia.

mentation, hypothermia and weakness with generalized flaccid muscle tone with absent patellar and palpebral reflexes [60].

Specific therapy is not required for mild elevations in Mg. Severe, symptomatic hypermagnesemia should be treated by discontinuation of any exogenous source of Mg, as well as therapy to increase renal excretion such as diuresis with 0.9% NaCl and furosemide (1–2 mg/kg IV). Renal replacement therapy may be required in patients with renal failure. Cardiac dysfunction can be reversed with IV Ca gluconate (5–15 mg/kg (0.12–0.37 mmol/kg)) titrated to effect [61]. The ECG must be monitored and supportive care provided to counteract hypotension, hypothermia, and any CNS signs.

Hypomagnesemia

Hypomagnesemia is suspected when the serum Mg concentration is <0.7 mmol/L (<1.7 mg/dL) in the dog and <0.41 mmol/L (<1.0 mg/dL) in the cat. Hypomagnesemia is commonly associated with other electrolyte abnormalities, including hypokalemia, hyponatremia, hypocalcemia, and hypophosphatemia.

Magnesium depletion has been identified as a common electrolyte abnormalitiy in both critically ill human and veterinary patients. Hypomagnesemia is reported in up to 60% of critically ill human patients [62,63], 54% of critically ill dogs [64], and 23% of critically ill cats [65]. Hypomagnesemia is associated with prolonged

hospitalization in critically ill dogs and both longer hospitalization and increased mortality in cats [65]. Hospitalized patients are at risk of Mg deficiency from prolonged anorexia and administration of Mg-deficient intravenous fluids. This is often in combination with excessive losses of Mg, increased renal Mg excretion or the redistribution of Mg from extracellular to intracellular fluid. Common causes of hypomagnesemia in the small animal ICU patient are listed in Table 6.2.

Clinical signs ascribed to hypomagnesemia include cardiac arrhythmias, muscle weakness, muscle fasiculations, altered mentation, esophageal motility disorders, respiratory muscle paralysis, dysphagia, dyspnea, ataxia, seizures, and coma (see Table 6.4). Chronic hypomagnesemia may result in decreased release of PTH from the parathyroid gland, causing end-organ resistance to PTH and Ca deficiency. Magnesium depletion reduces the intracellular K concentration and causes renal K wasting. Hypomagnesemia may lead to refractory hypokalemia.

Magnesium should be monitored in critically ill dogs and cats. Magnesium-containing fluids (such as Plasmalyte-A©) are recommended for high-risk patients (such as patients with diabetic ketoacidosis).

Magnesium supplementation is recommended in patients with decreased serum Mg levels. Additionally, Mg deficiency should be suspected and treated in patients with refractory hypokalemia and hypocalcemia despite normal serum Mg values. Magnesium should be administered cautiously in patients with renal failure.

Intravenous administration of magnesium sulfate ($MgSO_4$; comes as 50% (500 mg/mL; 4.06 mEq/mL) solution) or magnesium chloride is recommended for symptomatic hypomagnesemia as a CRI at 0.75–1.0 mEq/kg/day (9.2–12.3 mg/kg/day or 0.375–0.5 mmol/kg/day IV). As repletion occurs, the dose can be lowered to 0.3–0.5 mEq/kg/day (3.7–6.1 mg/kg/day or 0.15–0.25 mmol/kg/day). Care should be taken to reduce K supplementation once parenteral Mg is started since hyperkalemia can occur. Oral Mg supplementation (1–2 mEq/kg/day or 12.3–14.6 mg/kg/day PO or 0.5–1.0 mmol/kg/day) may be adequate in patients with mild, asymptomatic Mg deficiency. The major side-effect of oral administration is diarrhea.

Chloride disorders

Chloride is the most abundant extracellular anion. This anion helps to regulate osmotic pressure differences between fluid compartments, having an important role in maintaining proper hydration and balancing cations in the ECF to maintain electrical neutrality. The movement of Cl is closely linked to the transport of Na. Measured serum Cl should be corrected for changes in serum Na by the formula in Box 6.1. The corrected Cl values are used to diagnose hyperchloremia and hypochloremia. Clinical signs specific to changes in corrected chloride have not been reported. The clinical signs seen in patients with Cl disorders are related to their underlying disease process or changes in acid–base status.

Hyperchloremia

Hyperchloremia is diagnosed when the corrected Cl is >113 mEq/L (>113 mmol/L) in the dog and >123 mEq/L (>123 mmol/L) in the cat. Hyperchloremia causes a decrease in strong ion difference and a hyperchloremic acidosis (see Chapter 7). There is a growing body of evidence, in both animal and human patients, showing adverse effects of hyperchloremic acidosis. Studies have demonstrated decreased renal and splanchnic blood flow, altered hemostasis and decreased survival in sepsis associated with the administration of chloride-rich fluids [66]. In a study of 760 human ICU patients, the implementation of a chloride-restrictive fluid strategy was associated with a significant decrease in the incidence of AKI and use of renal replacement therapy [67].

Animal studies suggest that hyperchloremia causes renal vasoconstriction. In a canine model, it was shown that renal blood flow and glomerular filtration rate are regulated by plasma Cl [68]. Hyperchloremia produces a progressive renal vasoconstriction by inhibiting the intrarenal release of renin and angiotensin II, and a decrease in glomerular filtration rate and renal blood flow that was independent of renal innervation. The Cl-induced vasoconstriction appeared to be specific for the renal vessels. A study in rabbits showed that plasma Cl levels directly affect renal afferent arteriolar tone through Ca-activated Cl channels in the afferent arteriolar smooth muscle [69].

Thromboelastography indicates more effects on coagulation and platelet function with 0.9% NaCl when compared with a balanced salt solution [70]. Saline may also result in the release of more inflammatory markers [71].

The common causes of hyperchloremia in the small animal ICU patient are listed in Table 6.3. Hyperchloremia may be due to excessive loss of Na relative to Cl or conditions causing renal Cl retention. In hospitalized patients, the administration of Cl-rich fluids is a common cause of hyperchloremic acidosis. The correction of acid–base disturbances will require concurrent correction of Cl levels. Normal saline, colloids suspended in saline, hypertonic saline, and balanced electrolyte solutions supplemented with KCl contain supraphysiological concentrations of Cl.

Therapy for a hyperchloremia involves management of the underlying disease process, avoiding the administration of Cl-rich fluids (such as 0.9% NaCl, hypertonic saline, KCl supplementation) and normalizing renal function. Restoring perfusion and hydration with a balanced isotonic crystalloid solution can promote glomerular filtration and renal excretion of Cl while improving blood flow and tissue oxygenation.

Hypochloremia

Hypochloremia is diagnosed when the corrected Cl is <107 mEq/L (<107 mmol/L) in the dog and <117 mEq/L (<117 mmol/L) in the cat. Hypochloremia causes an increase in strong ion difference and a hypochloremic alkalosis (see Chapter 7).

The more common causes of corrected hypochloremia in cats and dogs (see Table 6.3) are vomiting of stomach contents and therapy with loop or thiazide diuretics, caused by loss of chloride in excess of sodium from the GI tract and kidneys, respectively. Renal chloride wasting resulting in hypochloremia is the expected compensatory response to chronic respiratory acidosis. Hypochloremia may be seen in patients receiving therapy with agents high in Na relative to Cl such as sodium bicarbonate and high-dose sodium penicillin.

Treatment of patients with corrected hypochloremia should be directed at the underlying cause and replacement of the Cl deficit. Administration of a higher Cl-containing fluid such as 0.9% NaCl is recommended for hypochloremic patients requiring volume expansion. The depletion of K is common during hypochloremia, often requiring K supplementation of the fluids (see Box 6.4).

Phosphorus disorders

Normal serum P values are 2.5–6.0 mg/dL (1.0–2.0 mmol/L) in the dog and 2.4–8.2 mg/dL (1.3–2.4 mmol/L) in the cat. Hemolysis occurring during or after blood sample collection results in release of intracellular P from RBCs and therefore gives erroneously high serum P concentrations. Therefore, hemolytic blood samples should not be used to determine the serum or plasma P concentration.

Phosphorus is used in the structural proteins of cell walls, bone, and other tissues and in active metabolic enzymes and pathways. It is one of the major components of the ATP molecule for energy storage. As a consequence, membrane-associated ion pumps, as well as receptor–ion channel interactions, involve P. In addition, the synthesis, storage, and release of local and systemic hormones that regulate cardiac output and vascular resistance require P. In vascular tissue, P is a vital co-factor for Ca and Mg in the activation of contractile proteins of cardiovascular muscle. Functionally, the primary roles of these three ionic species in vascular cell physiology are highly integrated. The extracellular and intracellular shifting of P mirrors that of K with acidosis and alkalosis and insulin-mediated glucose uptake or insulin deficiency.

Serum concentrations of phosphorus are regulated primarily by the renal tubules responding to PTH stimulation, which decreases the tubular resorption of P. Vitamin D enhances P absorption from the intestine and resorption from bone. Since the P level is related with protein intake, the nutritional status should be evaluated in the patient with a P disorder.

Hyperphosphatemia

Hyperphosphatemia is diagnosed when serum P is >6.0 mg/dL (>1.92 mmol/L) in dogs and cats, though values may vary with different laboratories. Hyperphosphatemia can be caused by increased intestinal absorption, decreased urinary excretion or a rapid intracellular-to-extracellular shifting of P (see Table 6.3). Increased intestinal absorption of P is unlikely to cause a sustained hyperphosphatemia in patients with normal renal function. Transient hyperphosphatemia has been reported in cats and small dogs following the administration of phosphate-containing enemas and in patients ingesting toxic amounts of cholecalciferol rodenticides. Increased amounts of P are released in patients with rhabdomyolysis, hemolysis, and during treatment of hemolymphatic malignancies. Hypoparathyroidism can result in the reabsorption of P in the absence of PTH. The most common cause of persistent hyperphosphatemia in veterinary patients is renal failure.

Acute hyperphosphatemia usually does not cause symptoms unless phosphate complexes with Ca causing soft tissue mineralization or signs of hypocalcemia. Chronic elevation in serum P triggers PTH release due to decreased ionized Ca and decreased serum calcitriol. This induces secondary hyperparathyroidism and increases bone turnover.

Management of hyperphosphatemia targets correction of the underlying cause when possible. Phosphorus-restricted diets may be sufficient to control hyperphosphatemia in early chronic renal failure, but the addition of oral phosphate binders (such as aluminum hydroxide) is usually necessary in more advanced stages of the disease. Oral phosphate binders are only effective in patients that can tolerate enteral nutrition, as they bind enterally delivered or ingested phosphate. Intravenous fluids to promote renal phosphate excretion should be considered when initiating chemotherapy in patients with lymphosarcoma suspected of having a large tumor burden.

Hypophosphatemia

Hypophosphatemia is diagnosed when the serum P is <2.4 mg/dL (0.775 mmol/L) in dogs and cats. It can be a result of decreased intestinal absorption, increased urinary excretion or an extracellular-to-intracellular shift of P. Phosphate depletion is associated with a significant increase in urinary Mg excretion and may cause hypomagnesaemia.

Common causes of hypophosphatemia in the small animal ICU patient are listed in Table 6.3. In critically ill patients, hypophosphatemia most often results from translocation from the ECF to ICF. Phosphorus moves into cells in patients with respiratory alkalosis, with insulin administration in the treatment of diabetes ketoacidosis, and refeeding syndrome in malnourished patients.

Clinical signs of hypophosphatemia are generally seen only in patients with moderate-to-severe hypophosphatemia (<2.0 mg/dL or <0.646 mmol/L) and include muscle weakness, pain associated with rhabdomyolysis, hemolysis, and impaired platelet and white blood cell function. Neurological disorders such as coma, seizures, and confusion are reported in human patients.

Phosphate supplementation is recommended for symptomatic patients or asymptomatic patients judged to be at risk of progressive decline in serum P (such as during treatment of diabetes ketoacidosis). Oral repletion is considered safer than intravenous supplementation, but may be impractical in many critically ill patients. Phosphorus administered intravenously can complex Ca and result in soft tissue mineralization [13]. The product of Ca × P should not exceed 70 mg/dL (5.6 mmol/L) to avoid tissue calcification. Intravenously, P is most often replaced using potassium phosphate (9.28 mg/mL (3 mmol/mL) of P and 4.4 mEq/mL (4.4 mmol/mL) of K as a CRI dosed at 0.01–0.09 mmol/kg/h). Serum P should be monitored every 8–24 hours. Less commonly, sodium phosphate (9.28 mg/mL (3 mmol/mL) of P and 4 mEq/mL (4 mmol/ml) of Na) may be administered. Vitamin D supplementation is indicated in patients with vitamin D deficiency.

References

1. Aronson PS, Boron WF, Boulpaep EL. Transport of solutes and water. In: Medical Physiology, 2nd edn. Boron WF, Boulpaep EL, eds. Philadelphia: Elsevier, 2009: pp 109–35.
2. Stockand JD. Vasopressin regulation of renal sodium excretion. Kidney Int. 2010;78(9):849–56.
3. Stokes JB. Mineralocorticoid effect on K permeability of the rabbit cortical collecting tubule. Kidney Int. 1985;28:640–5.
4. Garland CJ, Hiley CR, Dora KA. EDHF: spreading the influence of the endothelium. Br J Pharmacol. 2011;164(3):839–52.
5. Swaminathan R. Magnesium metabolism and its disorders. Clin Biochem Rev. 2003;24(2):47–66.
6. Ryan MF. The role of magnesium in clinical biochemistry: an overview. Ann Clin Biochem. 1991;28:19–26.
7. Horie M, Irisawa H, Noma A. Voltage-dependent magnesium block of adenosine-triphosphate-sensitive potassium channel in guinea-pig ventricular cells. J Physiol. 1987;387:251–72.
8. Agus ZS, Kelepouris E, Dukes I, Morad M. Cytosolic magnesium modulates calcium channel activity in mammalian ventricular cells. Am J Physiol. 1989;256(2 Pt 1):C452–5.
9. Noronha JL, Matuschak GM. Magnesium in critical illness: metabolism, assessment, and treatment. Intensive Care Med. 2002;28:667–79.
10. De Rouffignac C, Quamme G. Renal magnesium handling and its hormonal control. Physiol Rev. 1994;74:305–22.
11. Dai LJ, Ritchie G, Kerstan D, Kang HS, Cole DE, Quamme GA. Magnesium transport in the renal distal convoluted tubule. Physiol Rev. 2001;81:51–84.
12. Vetter T, Lohse MJ. Magnesium and the parathyroid. Curr Opin Nephrol Hypertens. 2002;11:403–10.
13. Chang WW, Radin B, McCurdy MT. Calcium, magnesium and phosphate abnormalities in the emergency department. Emerg Med Clin North Am. 2014;32(2):349–66.
14. Mousavi SJ, Shahabi, SJ. Mostafapour E, et al. Comparison of the serum electrolyte levels among patients died and survived in the intensive care unit. Tanaffos 2012;11(4):36–42.
15. Battison A. Apparent pseudohyperkalemia in a Chinese Shar Pei dog. Vet Clin Pathol. 2007;36(1):89–93.
16. Waldrop JE. Urinary electrolytes, solutes, and osmolality. Vet Clin North Am Small Anim Pract. 2008;38(3):503–12.
17. Graves TK, Schall WD, Refsal K, et al. Basal and ACTH-stimulated plasma aldosterone concentrations are normal or increased in dogs with trichuriasis-associated pseudohypoadrenocorticism. J Vet Intern Med. 1994;8:287–9.
18. RuDusky BM. ECG abnormalities associated with hypocalcemia. Chest 2001;119(2):668–9.
19. Mandal AK, Saklayen MG, Hillman NM, Markert RJ. Predictive factors for high mortality in hypernatremic patients. Am J Emerg Med. 1997;15(2):130–2.
20. Ayus JC, Armstrong DL, Arieff AI. Effects of hypernatraemia in the central nervous system and its therapy in rats and rabbits. J Physiol. 1996;492(1):243–55.
21. Adrogue HJ, Madias NE. Hypernatremia. N Engl J Med. 2000;342(20):1493–9.
22. Hillier TA, Abbott RD, Barrett EJ. Hyponatremia: evaluating the correction factor for hyperglycemia. Am J Med. 1999;106(4):399–403.
23. Aw TC, Kiechle FL. Pseudohyponatremia. Am J Emerg Med. 1985;3(3):236–9.
24. Guillani C, Peri A. Effects of hyponatremia on the brain. J Clin Med. 2014;3(4):1163–77.
25. Ayus C, Achinger SG, Arieff A. Brain cell volume regulation in hyponatremia: role of sex, age, vasopressin, and hypoxia. Am J Physiol Renal Physiol. 2008;295(3):F619–24.
26. Kimelberg HK. Water homeostasis in the brain: basic concepts. Neuroscience 2004;129(4):851–60.
27. Pasantes-Morales H, Franco R, Ordaz B, Ochoa LD. Mechanisms counteracting swelling in brain cells during hyponatremia. Arch Med Res. 2002;33(3):237–44.
28 28.Fisher SK, Heacock AM, Keep RF, Foster DJ. Receptor regulation of osmolyte homeostasis in neural cells. J Physiol. 2010;588(18):3355–64.

29. Verbalis JG. Brain volume regulation in response to changes in osmolality. Neuroscience 2010;168(4):862–70.

30. DiBartola SP. Disorders of sodium and water: hypernatremia and hyponatremia. In: Fluid, Electrolyte and Acid-Base Disorders in Small Animal Practice, 4th edn. DiBartola SP, ed. St Louis: Elsevier Saunders, 2012: pp 61–75.

31. Atkinson K, Aubert I. Myxedema coma leading to respiratory depression in a dog. Can Vet J. 2004;45(4):318–20.

32. Brown E, Markandu ND, Roulston JE, et al. Is the renin-angiotensin-aldosterone system involved in the retention of the nephrotic syndrome? Nephron 1982;32:102–7.

33. Gankam Kengne F, Nicaise C, Soupart A, et al. Astrocytes are an early target in osmotic demyelination syndrome. J Am Soc Nephrol. 2011;22(11):1834–45.

34. Miller GM, Baker HL Jr, Okazaki H, Whisnant J. Central pontine and extrapontine myelinolysis and its imitators: MR findings. Radiology 1988;168(3):795–802.

35. Adrogue HJ, Madias NE. Hyponatremia. N Engl J Med. 2000;342(21):1581–9.

36. Soupart A, Penninckx R, Crenier L, et al. Prevention of brain demyelination in rats after excessive correction of chronic hyponatremia by serum sodium lowering. Kidney Int. 1994;45(1):193–200.

37. Gross P. Clinical management of SIADH. Ther Adv Endocrinol Metab. 2012;3(2):61–73.

38. Velez JC, Dopson SJ, Sanders DS, Delay TA, Arthur JM. Intravenous conivaptan for the treatment of hyponatraemia caused by the syndrome of inappropriate secretion of antidiuretic hormone in hospitalized patients: a single-centre experience. Nephrol Dial Transplant. 2010;25(5):1524–31.

39. Oi A, Morishita K, Awogi T, et al. Nonclinical safety profile of tolvaptan. Cardiovasc Drugs Ther. 2011;25(Suppl 1):S1–9.

40. Yatsu T, Tomura Y, Tahara A, et al. Pharmacological profile of YM087, a novel nonpeptide dual vasopressin V1A and V2 receptor antagonist, in dogs. Eur J Pharmacol. 1997 26;321(2):225–30.

41. Adrogue HJ, Madias NE. Changes in plasma potassium concentration during acute acid base disturbances. J Clin Invest. 1981;71:456.

42. Hopper K, Borchers A, Epstein SE. Acid base, electrolyte, glucose, and lactate values during cardiopulmonary resuscitation in dogs and cats. J Vet Emerg Crit Care 2014;24(2):208–14.

43. Thompson MD, Carr AP. Hyponatremia and hyperkalemia associated with chylous pleural and peritoneal effusion in a cat. Can Vet J. 2001;43(8):610–13.

44. Tag TL, Day TK. Electrocardiographic assessment of hyperkalemia in dogs and cats. J Vet Emerg Crit Care 2008;18(1):61–7.

45. Gennari FJ. Hypokalemia. N Engl J Med. 1998;339(7):451–8.

46. Oh MS, Carroll HJ. Electrolyte and acid-base disturbances. In: The Pharmacologic Approach to the Critically Ill Patient, 3rd edn. Chernow B, ed. Baltimore: Williams and Wilkins, 1994.

47. Schenck PA, Chew DJ, Nagode LA, Rosol TJ. Disorders of calcium: hypercalcemia and hypocalcemia. In: Fluid, Electrolyte and Acid-Base Disorders in Small Animal Practice, 4th edn. DiBartola SP, ed. St Louis: Elsevier Saunders, 2012: pp 132–5.

48. Hopper K, Rezende ML, Haskins SC. Assessment of the effect of dilution of blood samples with sodium heparin on blood gas, electrolyte, and lactate measurements in dogs. Am J Vet Res; 2005;66(4):656–60.

49. Beall DP, Henslee HB, Webb H, Scofield R. Milk-alkali syndrome, a historical review and description of the modern version of the syndrome. Am J Med Sci. 2006;331(5):233–42.

50. Riccardi D, Brown EM. Physiology and pathophysiology of the calcium-sensing receptor in the kidney. Am J Physiol Renal Physiol. 2011;298:F485–99.

51. Swaminathan R. Magnesium metabolism and its disorders. Clin Biochem Rev. 2003;24(2):47–66.

52. Medarov BI. Milk-alkali syndrome. Mayo Clin Proc. 2009;84:261–7.

53. Midkiff AM, Chew DJ, Randolph JF, Center SA, DiBartola SP. Idiopathic hypercalcemia in cats. J Vet Intern Med. 2000;14(6):619–26.

54. Armstrong CM, Cota G. Calcium block of Na channels and its effect on closing rate. Proc Natl Acad Sci USA 1999;96(7):4154–57.

55. Steele T, Kolamunnage-Dona R, Downey C, et al. Assessment and clinical course of hypocalcemia in critical illness. Crit Care 2013;17(3):R106.

56. Forsythe RM, Wessel CB, Billiar TR, Angus DC, Rosengart MR. Parenteral calcium for intensive care unit patients. Cochrane Database Syst Rev. 2008;8(4): CD006163.

57. Holowaychuk MK, Hansen BD, DeFrancesco TC, et al. Ionized hypocalcmeia in critically ill dogs. J Vet Intern Med. 2009;23(3):509–13.

58. Luschini MA, Fletcher DJ, Schoeffler GL Incidence of ionized hypocalcemia in septic dogs and its association with morbitity and mortality: 58 cases (2006–2007). J Vet Emerg Crit Care 2010;20(4):406–12.

59. Hall JA. Puerperal hypocalcemia in small animals. In: The Merck Veterinary Manual. Whitehouse Station: Merck, 2015.

60. Jackson CB, Drobatz KJ. Iatrogenic magnesium overdose: 2 case reports. J Vet Emerg Crit Care 2004;14(2):115–23.

61. Dhupi N. Magnesium therapy. In: Current Veterinary Therapy XII. Kirk RW, ed. Philadelphia: WB Saunders, 1995: pp 132–3.

62. Chernow B, Bamberger S, Stoiko M, Vadnais M. Hypomagnesemia in patients in postoperative intensive care. Chest 1989;95:391–7.

63. Humphrey S, Kirby R, Rudloff E. Magnesium physiology in veterinary critical care. J Vet Emerg Crit Care 2015;25(2):210–25.

64. Martin LG, Matteson VL, Wingfield, WE, et al. Abnormalities of serum magnesium in critically ill dogs: incidence and implications. J Vet Emerg Crit Care 1994;4(1):15–20.

65. Toll J, Erb H, Birnbaum N, Schermerhorn T. Prevalence and incidence of serum magnesium abnormalities in hospitalized cats. J Vet Intern Med. 2002;16(3):217–21.

66. Yunos NM, Bellomo R, Story D, Kellum J. Bench-to-bedside review: chloride in critical illness. Crit Care 2010;14(4):226.

67. Yunos NM, Bellomo R, Hegarty C, et al. Association between a chloride-liberal vs chloride-restrictive intravenous fluid administration strategy and kidney injury in critically ill adults. JAMA. 2012;308(15):1566–72.

68. Wilcox CS. Regulation of renal blood flow by plasma chloride. J Clin Invest. 1983;71:726–35.

69. Hansen PB, Jensen BL, Skott O. Chloride regulates afferent arteriolar contraction in response to depolarization. Hypertension 1998;32:1066–70.

70. Boldt J, Wolf M, Mengistu A. A new plasma-adapted hydroxyethylstarch preparation: in vitro coagulation studies using thrombelastography and whole blood aggregometry. Anesth Analg. 2007;104(2):425–30.

71. Kellum JA, Song M, Almasri E. Hyperchloremic acidosis increases circulating inflammatory molecules in experimental sepsis. Chest 2006;130(4):962–7.

CHAPTER 7

Acid–base status

Ryan Wheeler[1] and Jan Kovacic[1,2]
[1] Four Seasons Animal Hospital, Lafayette, California
[2] Horizon Veterinary Services, Lafayette, California

Introduction

The acid–base status of critically ill patients is a complex interplay of multiple dysfunctional organs, depleted buffer systems, mixed acid–base disorders, and conflicting homeostatic mechanisms. It is often complicated by iatrogenic problems associated with imprecise fluid therapy, unforeseen effects from medications, and unanticipated complications when the treatment for one acid–base disturbance ends up creating another.

Every acute, life-threatening illness or injury will eventually cause changes in acid–base status, sometimes within minutes of the inciting cause. Every chronic illness that becomes life threatening will eventually change acid–base balance. Therefore, acid–base monitoring should be viewed as a window into serious illness. Finding alterations in acid–base status provides an alert that the patient and their problems may be more serious than anticipated. The goal is to unmask the components of the acid–base disturbance as early as possible and specifically treat the underlying cause.

Acidosis is the term for acidifying events and alkalosis is the term for alkalinizing events. The terms acidemia and alkalemia have been used to describe the acid or alkali status of the blood. However, these terms, as previously defined, are not entirely accurate nor descriptive of the true acid–base status of the blood. A patient with a blood pH <7.4 has been termed "acidemic." However, the neutral pH of an aqueous solution at the body temperature of 37 °C is 6.8, so the pH of blood is almost never on the acid side of neutral. At best, the term *acidemia* should be used for an increase in blood acidity and *alkalemia* for a decrease in blood acidity [1–3]. Terms commonly used when discussing acid–base status are provided in Box 7.1.

There are multiple homeostatic mechanisms, chemical and physiological, intra- and extracellular, that control the hydrogen ion concentration ($[H^+]$) of body fluid compartments. A normal $[H^+]$ of 40 nmol/L is reported as pH = 7.4, and the range compatible with life is 15–158 nmol/L (pH = 6.8–7.8). Acidity increases with an increase in $[H^+]$, but the pH value goes down. Buffer systems of weak acids and their conjugate bases help to control hydrogen activity through their relative affinity for protons. Peripheral chemoreceptors in the aortic and carotid bodies sense $[H^+]$ and trigger renal and pulmonary mechanisms to normalize pH. Central chemoreceptors in the medullary respiratory center of the brain also sense changes in the partial pressure of carbon dioxide in plasma (PCO_2) independent of changes in pH, a critical step in the rapid ventilatory response to metabolic changes that alter $[H^+]$. The kidney is equipped to respond to changes in the plasma $[H^+]$, bicarbonate (HCO_3^-), sodium (Na^+), potassium (K^+), chloride (Cl^-), CO_2, angiotensin, and aldosterone, all of which affect $[H^+]$. The liver is a net producer or consumer of H^+ depending on diet, metabolism, volume status, perfusion, medications, toxins, and fluids. Even the skeletal system plays a role in acid–base balance by contributing calcium carbonate as a buffer [4].

More important is the H^+ environment in which most of the body's work is done – the intracellular space. Intracellular pH is close to neutral (6.8–7.1) and can be acidic (pH <6.8) without serious deleterious effects on the cells. Intracellular pH is also more tightly controlled than extracellular pH. For example, lymphocytes are able to maintain an almost constant intracellular pH = 7.1 ± 0.06 when exposed to a blood pH = 6.8–7.4 [5]. The cells have some defense against extracellular pH changes, making cellular metabolism relatively resistant to changes in blood pH. Unfortunately, there is currently no technology available in the clinical setting to measure intracellular pH.

The critical importance of acid–base balance lies in the fact that extremes in $[H^+]$ can be reached within minutes due to cardiopulmonary arrest, shock, trauma, hypo- or hyperventilation, or toxins, and within hours due to almost any serious medical condition. The pH and $[H^+]$ reported as lethal are listed in Table 7.1. Extreme changes in $[H^+]$ cause loss of function of membrane channels, especially in critical cardiac, brain, and nerve cells, alter the structural and functional integrity of proteins causing changes in enzyme function, and disrupt K^+ balance between intra- and extracellular fluid [3,6,7]. In addition, patient therapy can play a role in creating critical acid–base disturbances, usually due to the unanticipated deleterious effects of drug and fluid therapy. For this reason, when treating critical patients, acid–base monitoring is essential.

The mantra of critical care medicine is "treat the underlying cause." Never is this more important than in the clinical application of acid–base physiology. Rarely is an acidemia or alkalemia so severe that the objective is to treat the disturbance without regard to etiology. The real value in acid–base analysis is to discover the multiple compensating and counterbalancing causes that are common in critical patient care. Therefore, the goal of therapy is not to treat the acidemia or alkalemia *per se*. Physiological compensation or the counter-balancing effects of mixed disorders (acidosis + alkalosis) may even make a serious disorder appear less severe than it really is. It is important to uncover and treat the underlying causes which may be extreme even if the acidemia or alkalemia is not. Fortunately, we have many tools to use in this process.

Monitoring and Intervention for the Critically Ill Small Animal: The Rule of 20, First Edition. Edited by Rebecca Kirby and Andrew Linklater.
© 2017 John Wiley & Sons, Inc. Published 2017 by John Wiley & Sons, Inc.

Box 7.1 Acid–base definitions.

- Acidemia – an increase in hydrogen ion activity in the blood
- Alkalemia – a decrease in hydrogen ion activity in the blood
- Acidosis – a physiological or pathological process that creates an increase in hydrogen ion activity
- Alkalosis – a physiological or pathological process that creates a decrease in hydrogen ion activity
- pH – the negative logarithm of the hydrogen ion concentration extrapolated from the measurement of hydrogen ion activity in blood
- HCO_3^- – bicarbonate is the anion resulting from the dissociation of carbonic acid, H_2CO_3. It is calculated from the patient's pH and the dissociation constant for carbonic acid:

$$H_2CO_3 \longleftrightarrow H^+ + HCO_3^-$$
$$\text{carbonic acid} \quad \text{hydrogen ion} \quad \text{bicarbonate}$$

- Base Excess (BE) – a calculation in mEq/L of the amount of H^+ ions required to return the pH of the blood to normal (7.4) under standard conditions ($PCO_2 = 40\,mmHg$, temperature 37 °C, and saturated with oxygen)
- PCO_2 – a measurement of the partial pressure of carbon dioxide dissolved in the blood
- Anion Gap (AG) – a calculation of the difference between the measured cations and anions in the blood. In reality, there is no "gap" as cations always equal anions; the difference is that they are not all measured.

$$AG = \left(\left[Na^+ \right] + \left[K^+ \right] \right) - \left(\left[Cl^- \right] + \left[HCO_3^- \right] \right)$$

Box 7.2 Traditional and nontraditional acid base formulas.

Traditional

Henderson-Hasselbalch equation:

$$pH = \log_{10} \left(\frac{\left[HCO_3^- \right]}{\left[H_2CO_3 \right]} \right)$$

Carbonic anhydrase (CA) equation:

$$H_2O + CO_2 \xleftrightarrow{\text{carbonic anhydrase}} H_2CO_3 \longleftrightarrow H^+ + HCO_3^-$$

Nontraditional

Strong ion difference (SID) – a calculation of the difference between the measured strong cations and anions in the blood. Strong ions are those that are completely dissociated within the range of body pH.

Simple formula:

$$SID = \left[Na^+ \right] + \left[K^+ \right] - \left[Cl^- \right]$$

Extended formula:

$$SID = \left[Na^+ \right] + \left[K^+ \right] + \left[Ca^{++} \right] + \left[Mg^{++} \right] - \left[Cl^- \right] - \left[Lactate^- \right] - \left[Ketoacids^- \right]$$

ATOT – the total plasma concentration of the weak nonvolatile acids; the sum of the concentrations of inorganic phosphate, albumin, and other serum proteins:

$$ATOT = \left(\left[Phos \right] + \left[albumin \right] \right) + \left[\text{other plasma proteins} \right]$$

Table 7.1 Range of pH and H^+ compatible with life.

	pH	[H^+] nmol/L	[H^+] mmol/L	[H^+] mEq/L
Lethal	6.8	158	0.000158	0.000158
Normal	7.4	40	0.000040	0.000040
Lethal	7.8	15	0.000015	0.000015

Methods of acid–base analysis

The primary goal is to identify and quantify the effect made by each agent known to cause changes in acid–base balance, within the limits of our current understanding and of available analyzer technology. The two most popular descriptions of acid–base physiology are the Henderson–Hasselbalch (HH) approach, also termed the "traditional" approach, and the Stewart strong ion approach, also termed "nontraditional." Common biochemical formulas used to define each method are provided in Box 7.2 and Table 7.2. The HH approach provides a simple means for identifying respiratory or metabolic acidosis or alkalosis, and whether appropriate compensatory mechanisms are present (Box 7.3 and Table 7.3); however, this method is incomplete in evaluation of independent variables. The biggest problem with each of these approaches is that, except for PCO_2, the endpoints of their analysis reflect a summation of multiple physiological or pathological processes without isolating or quantifying the effect of any individual causative agent. Many of the major concerns and inadequacies of the traditional and nontraditional methods of acid–base assessment are outlined in Table 7.2.

Acid–base analysis became clinically useful when researchers expanded on HH and Stewart acid–base physiology to describe a semiquantitative approach that yields the approximate contribution of measurable agents (independent variables) known to cause acid–base disturbances [8–11]. Through experimental evidence, formulas were derived that permit the calculation of the contribution that each agent makes to metabolic acid–base status as reflected in base excess (BE). These formulas vary from species to species. The calculations are inherently approximations, hence the term "semiquantitative." This approach allows the clinician to (1) identify each contributing factor, (2) isolate cause effect, (3) target interventions on normalizing each contributing factor, (4) support the homeostatic mechanisms that will help to normalize each factor, and (5) avoid therapies that can interfere with normalization or create acid–base disturbances on their own.

The sum of the effects of the measured agents, if different from the total BE, reveals that the difference is due to agents yet unidentified and unmeasured. This directs supplemental testing that can help identify, if not quantify, the unidentified factors altering acid–base balance. In veterinary medicine, there is evidence that this semiquantitative acid–base (SQAB) approach is more clinically useful than either the HH or Stewart methodology [12–14].

The agents that create change in acid–base status all play critical roles in cellular function – membrane structure, membrane integrity, membrane potentials, enzyme structure, enzyme kinetics, electron transport, proton motive force, channels, transporters, energy metabolism, hormone interactions, second messengers, cell signaling, neuromuscular function, neuron function, and the like. Disruptions in these functions often become life threatening even before they create a significant acidemia or alkalemia, and even when acidemia or alkalemia is not significant because of counterbalancing disturbances or therapies. This is the primary reason why acid–base disorders are treated early and why therapy is directed at the underlying cause.

Table 7.2 Comparison and Clinical Limitations of Traditional (HH) and Non-Traditional (Stewart) Acid-Base Analysis.

Parameter	Traditional	Non-Traditional	Notes
Terms used	• pH (calculated from H+ activity) • HCO3 (calculated) • Base Excess (calculated) • PCO₂ (measured) • Anion Gap (calculated)	• pH (calculated from H+ activity) • SID (calculated) • ATOT (calculated) • PCO₂ (measured) • Strong Ion Gap (calculated)	• These calculations are used to describe the physiology of acid-base chemistry but fail to isolate cause and effect which are needed for clinical decisions

Acid-Base diagnoses	• Respiratory acidosis
	• Respiratory alkalosis
	• Metabolic acidosis
	  ○ High anion gap
	  ○ Normal anion gap
	• Metabolic alkalosis
		• Respiratory acidosis
		• Respiratory alkalosis
		• Metabolic acidosis
		Decreased SID
		Increased A_{TOT}
		• Metabolic alkalosis
		Increased SID
		Decreased A_{TOT}
			• These diagnoses are physiologically descriptive but fail to isolate the effect of the individual agents causing the change in acid-base status.
			• There is little information in these diagnoses to guide specific therapies.

pH	• pH = Negative logarithm$_{10}$ of [H+] [H+] is controlled by acid buffering, i.e. bicarbonate & carbonic acid, alveolar ventilation (PCO₂) and balance between renal excretion and reabsorption of H+ and HCO₃⁻	• [H+] and [HCO₃] are dependent on (not the cause of) changes in acid-base status. [4,10]	• HH Equation: $pH = \log_{10}\left(\dfrac{[HCO_3^-]}{H_2CO_3}\right)$ • Carbonic anhydrase equation: $H_2O + CO_2 \xrightleftharpoons[\text{carbonic anhydrase}]{\text{carbonic anhydrase}} H_2CO_3 \longrightarrow H^+ + HCO_3^-$
HCO₃⁻	• HCO₃⁻ plays a role in determining pH • [Cl] is not accepted as a direct cause of acidemia	• [HCO₃] is determined by the pH, i.e. the dissociation of carbonic acid (H₂CO₃) based on its dissociation constant (pKa). • [Cl⁻] is one of the variables that drives changes in pH and [HCO₃]	• [HCO₃] usefulness is compromised because it sums the effect of numerous agents, both metabolic and respiratory, without isolating the specific effect of any. • [Cl⁻] may fail to be recognized as a driver of changes in [H+] and [HCO₃]
Base Excess (BE)	• BE is the amount of strong acid or base needed to restore whole blood in vitro to pH = 7.4 • BE reflects hemoglobin buffering.	• Same as HH	• BE sums the effect of all agents driving changes in acid-base status but fails to isolate cause and effect of any individual agent. • Standard BE more accurately reflects hemoglobin buffering because it considers both blood and interstitial fluid.
Anion Gap (AG)	• Needed to account for the role of electrolytes (specifically Cl⁻) in acid-base physiology	• Not applicable	• AG = ([Na+]+[K+]−[Cl]+[HCO₃]) • AG sums the effect of all unmeasured anions and cations but fails to isolate cause and effect of any of them.

(Continued)

Table 7.2 (Continued)

Parameter	Traditional	Non-Traditional	Notes
Strong Ion Difference (SID)	• Not applicable	$SID=[Na^+]+[K^+]+[Ca^{++}]+[Mg^{++}] - [Cl] - [lactate] - [ketoacids]$	• Changes with species. • Sums multiple effects without isolating any specific effect • Has not proven to be more useful than HH
ATOT	• Not applicable	• $A_{TOT} = [PO_4^-]+[Albumin]+[other plasma proteins]$ • Total plasma concentration of weak nonvolatile acids	• Sums multiple effects without isolating any specific effect
pCO$_2$ and Compensation	• The ability of ventilation to retain or eliminate CO_2 and increase or decrease carbonic acid levels represents the respiratory control of H^+ activity. • Calculation for the physiological component of both metabolic and respiratory changes still apply (see Table 7.3) • Respiratory compensation for metabolic changes can be very effective and can return pH to normal range. [4, 10]	• Same as HH • Metabolic "compensation" occurs over several days through alterations in the excretion of acid load through kidneys. [18,28]	• Respiratory "compensation" occurs within minutes to hours when CO_2 lowers through hyperventilation in response to metabolic acidosis or when CO_2 increases through hypoventilation in response to metabolic alkalosis • Compensation can be harmful - profound alteration in PCO_2 can affect cerebral blood flow, intracranial volume and intracranial pressure • Compensatory hyper and hypoventilation should still be recognized as disturbances (respiratory alkalosis and respiratory acidosis, respectively) to alert potential serious consequences. [18,42]

Box 7.3 Traditional approach to acid–base analysis.

1. Evaluate pH (acidemia or alkalemia)
2. Evaluate the respiratory component: PCO_2 as increased, normal or decreased
3. Evaluate the metabolic component (HCO_3, TCO_2 or BE): acidosis (low HCO_3 or more negative BE) or alkalosis (high HCO_3 or more positive BE)
4. Decide the primary process which led to metabolic or respiratory acidosis or alkalosis
5. Evaluate if compensatory process is appropriate (see Table 7.3)
6. Examine anion gap (AG) = $Na^+ + K^+ - HCO_3^- - Cl^-$; an increase in the AG may indicate the presence of ketoacids, uremic acids, lactate, ethylene glycol or other toxins

Box 7.4 The semiquantitative acid–base profile (SQAB).

Blood Gas

pH
PCO_2
HCO_3^-
BE

Electrolytes

Na^+
K^+
Cl^-

Serum biochemistry tests

Phosphorus
Albumin (proteins)
Lactate

Supplemental tests

Glucose, beta-hydroxybutyrate, blood urea nitrogen, creatinine, sulfate, urate, ALT, SAP, bilirubin, toxic acids, urine electrolytes, urine osmolality

ALT, alanine aminotransferase; SAP, serum alkaline phosphatase.

Table 7.3 Expected compensation for metabolic and respiratory acidosis and alkalosis with intact physiological mechanisms.

Metabolic acidosis	↓ HCO_3^- of 1 mEq/L results in a	↓ in PCO_2 of 0.70 mmHg
Metabolic alkalosis	↑ HCO_3^- of 1 mEq/L results in an	↑ in PCO_2 of 0.70 mmHg
Respiratory acidosis		
– acute	↑ PCO_2 of 1 mmHg results in an	↑ in HCO_3^- of 0.15 mEq/L
– chronic	↑ PCO_2 of 1 mmHg results in an	↑ in HCO_3^- of 0.35 mEq/L
Respiratory alkalosis		
– acute	↓ PCO_2 of 1 mmHg results in a	↓ in HCO_3^- of 0.25 mEq/L
– chronic	↓ PCO_2 of 1 mmHg results in a	↓ in HCO_3^- of 0.55 mEq/L

Source: adapted from DiBartola S. Introduction to acid–base disorders. In: Fluid, Electrolyte, and Acid–base Disorders in Small Animal Practice, 4th edn. St Louis: Saunders, 2012: pp 231–52.

Initial diagnostics and monitoring

Important contributions to the underlying factors contributing to acid–base disorders can be derived from the initial history, physical examination, minimum database, and clinicopathological testing. A specific SQAB profile can be created to expedite analysis of the acid–base status of the patient (Box 7.4). Diagnostic imaging can be necessary to further define the causal disorder.

History and physical examination

Signalment (age, sex, breed), past medical history, drug therapy, noted alterations in drinking, urination, defecation, vomiting, weight loss, respiratory changes, behavior and mentation, and possible toxic exposures are all important when collecting a history. Historical information may provide insight into the nature of the acid–base disturbance.

A list of physical examination findings associated with acidemia and alkalemia is provided in Table 7.4 and covers the entire spectrum of serious illness. It is important to remember that this association does not imply that the acidemia or alkalemia is the direct biochemical cause of these signs. Continuous monitoring of physical parameters such as temperature, pulse rate, pulse quality, heart rate and rhythm, respiratory rate, respiratory effort, mentation, mucous membrane color, and capillary refill time is essential for early detection of problems resulting from or causing changes in acid–base balance.

Table 7.4 Clinical signs associated with acidosis and alkalosis.

Clinical signs seen with acidosis	Clinical signs see with alkalosis
Respiratory	Respiratory
Hyperventilation	Hypoventilation
Brady- or tachypnea	Brady- or tachypnea
Cardiovascular	Cardiovascular
Poor perfusion	Poor perfusion
Abnormal blood pressure	Abnormal blood pressure
Brady- or tachycardia	Brady- or tachycardia
Decreased cardiac contractility	Altered cardiac contractility
ECG ST changes	ECG ST changes
Dysrhythmias	Dysrhythmias
Coronary vasodilation	Coronary vasodilation
Cerebral vasodilation	Cerebral vasoconstriction
Systemic vasodilation	Systemic vasoconstriction or dilation
Neurological	Neurological
Altered mentation	Altered mentation
Cognitive dysfunction	Cognitive dysfunction
Blunted cranial nerve reflexes	Blunted cranial nerve reflexes
Abnormal musculoskeletal reflexes	Abnormal musculoskeletal reflexes
Stupor, coma, death	Stupor, coma, death
Hemolymphatic	Hemolymphatic
Altered O_2-hemoglobin affinity	Altered O_2-hemoglobin affinity
Coagulation disorders	Coagulation disorders
Genitourinary	Genitourinary
Anuria, oliguria, polyuria	Anuria, oliguria, polyuria
Gastrointestinal	Gastrointestinal
Anorexia	Anorexia
Vomiting	Vomiting
Diarrhea	Diarrhea
Altered GI motility	Altered GI motility
Musculoskeletal	Musculoskeletal
Muscle weakness	Muscle weakness
Myoclonus	Myoclonus
Endocrine/metabolic	Endocrine/metabolic
Protein alterations	Protein alterations
Hormone dysfunction	Hormone dysfunction
Enzyme dysfunction	Enzyme dysfunction

ECG, electrocardiogram; GI, gastrointestinal.

Point of care testing

The minimum database consists of packed cell volume (PCV), total proteins (TP), blood glucose, blood urea nitrogen (BUN), electrolytes, and blood gas analysis. The PCV is important in determining the contribution that hemoglobin makes to the assessment of pH. The remainder of the database will contribute to the SQAB profile (see Box 7.4). A complete blood count, serum biochemistry, and urinalysis provide important data for identifying factors potentially contributing to acid–base disorders.

There are no analyzers that will assay all of the necessary SQAB analytes from one sample. Therefore, an important step for SQAB analysis is to equip the ICU with the point of care (POC) analyzers (blood gas, electrolyte, biochemistry) that can provide SQAB profile results rapidly and efficiently. Point of care analyzers should be selected that use minimal sample size and provide rapid sample processing. It is important to use a brand of analyzer that has been validated in animals and for which reference ranges for the species being studied have been provided.

Data is only useful if it is free from errors in sampling or laboratory technique, and if it is obtained often enough to reflect important changes in a patient's condition. The frequency of testing intervals should be based on the severity of illness, the presence of unstable trends in monitored parameters, and the presence of known or anticipated etiologies that cause rapid changes in acid–base status. It is important to: (1) draw blood samples only in the frequency and quantity needed, to prevent significant patient blood loss, (2) use lyophilized or minimal volume of anticoagulant to prevent dilution of the sample, and (3) run the tests with minimal delay from time of sample collection.

Diagnostic imaging

Diagnostic imaging will typically include plain thoracic and abdominal radiographs. Assessment of the lungs and pulmonary vasculature can aid in the assessment of respiratory acid–base changes. Should the lungs appear normal, changes in PCO_2 may reflect physiological compensation for metabolic acid–base disturbances. Normal lungs also suggest that the patient will probably be able to expire any additional CO_2 that is produced (such as after bicarbonate administration). Imaging of the heart may support the presence of heart disease, which could be a contributor to the acid–base disturbance or to a lack of response to therapy. A small vena cava and cardiac silhouette may indicate a hypovolemic state.

Ultrasound is used in evaluation of the heart, vessels, gastrointestinal tract, pancreas, spleen, liver, kidneys, and bladder. Abnormalities could support an underlying cause or demonstrate a serious consequence of an acid–base disorder.

Equipment-based monitoring

In seriously ill patients, change in acid–base balance can be continuous and dynamic. The life-threatening potential of the causes and effects of acid–base disorders necessitates POC testing and intensive monitoring. Monitoring intensity can be decreased when: (1) response to therapy is predictable and appropriate, (2) repeated results stabilize into favorable trends, and (3) the patient's overall condition (not just acid–base status) is improving.

Blood pressure is monitored to detect alterations in cardiac output and peripheral vascular resistance, each potentially a cause or result of acid–base disturbances (see Chapter 3). End-tidal CO_2 monitoring ($ETCO_2$) provides a continuous reflection of the PCO_2 in the blood (see Chapter 8). This can provide a direct indication of respiratory acidosis or alkalosis, whether it is physiological (compensatory) or pathological. During early recovery from cardiopulmonary arrest, a rise in $ETCO_2$ helps to confirm return to spontaneous circulation, restoration of oxidative metabolism, and clearance of acidity in the tissues as CO_2 is transported to the lungs for excretion.

Pulse oximetry (see Chapter 8) measures the oxygen saturation of hemoglobin (SpO_2), a major component of oxygen delivery (DO_2) and of the maintenance of oxidative metabolism. A significant decrease in SpO_2 and DO_2 can lead directly to anaerobic metabolism and severe lactic acidosis. It can also lead indirectly to a full spectrum of acid–base changes due to complete disruption of cellular physiology. Continuous electrocardiographic monitoring (see Chapter 11) can demonstrate changes in heart rate, rhythm, and electrical activity, which could cause acid–base abnormalities or result from changes in acid–base status. If a dysrhythmia disrupts cardiac output, the alteration in DO_2 can create global problems down to the cellular level.

The ability to continuously monitor many of the parameters of acid–base analysis (PO_2, PCO_2, glucose, electrolytes, lactate) is under development using subcutaneous probes that measure these analytes in interstitial fluid or intravascular probes that analyze blood. The technology is costly and of limited use at this time since many of the important parameters needed for complete acid–base analysis are not reported. Currently, the most useful continuous monitoring is $ETCO_2$ during anesthesia, ventilator therapy, or during treatment and recovery of cardiopulmonary arrest.

Disorders of acid–base balance

The use of SQAB analysis offers a better understanding of the factors contributing to acid–base disturbances. Because the sickest patients often have multiple disturbances, the therapeutic response can be more precise and less likely to create or exacerbate other problems. With this improved understanding, acidemia or alkalemia *per se* is rarely treated; instead, treatment is directed at the underlying cause(s). Currently, cautious attempts to treat acidemia or alkalemia directly are reserved for when efforts to treat the underlying causes have failed. Contributions from Na^+, K^+, Cl^-, phosphate, proteins (albumin), and lactate are recognized through the SQAB analysis, with each becoming a potential therapeutic target. When a new therapy has been initiated, frequent monitoring is necessary to insure that the desired and predicted effect is confirmed. When a response to therapy is not as predicted, a search for additional causes ensues. Often, homeostatic mechanisms have priority over acid–base balance, such as the maintenance of effective circulating volume.

Disorders of pH, HCO_3^-, and BE

As in all systems of acid–base analysis, pH is the final summation of all acid–base disturbances, metabolic and respiratory. Base excess and $[HCO_3^-]$ are parameters that sum the effects of all metabolic disturbances. Using the SQAB method, the standard BE is compared with the sum of the individual metabolic effects to unmask acid–base effects from unmeasured anions or cations. Since it is not a causative agent of acid–base change, $[HCO_3^-]$ is of little importance. It is included to compare the SQAB profile to HH analysis.

The plasma $[H^+]$ in dogs and cats is approximately 40 nmol/L, with cats normally slightly more acidic than dogs. In comparison, K^+ is 100 000 times more concentrated than H^+ in plasma; Na^+ and Cl^- are

3 000 000 times more concentrated. One of the variables that alters hydrogen ion activity, and therefore pH, is temperature. Aqueous solutions are neutral when hydrogen ion equals hydroxyl ion, $H^+ = OH^-$. This occurs at pH = 7.0 when the temperature of the solution is 25 °C. However, at body temperature (37 °C), neutral pH = 6.8. Hydrogen ion activity increases with increased temperature and the pH is lower [1,15].

The pH range compatible with life (6.8–7.8; see Table 7.1) represents a 10-fold difference in H^+, a wider range than is tolerated with other important ionic species. However, because normal [H^+] is so small (40 nmol/L), this range represents a change in H^+ of only 0.000143 mEq/L. It is remarkable that the body can sense and adjust to such minute changes in H^+ and that clinicians can successfully intervene, without doing more harm than good, when homeostatic mechanisms are overwhelmed by illness or injury.

There is accumulating evidence that increased extracellular H^+ may be well tolerated and may even have a protective effect in some clinical situations. Permissive hypercapnia in the management of acute respiratory distress syndrome (ARDS) is a ventilator strategy that is considered to be beneficial to the patient when compared to the damage to the lung that may occur with greater tidal volumes and inspiratory pressures [16]. Acidemia may improve outcomes in ARDS patients and there is evidence that buffering respiratory acidosis may exacerbate the condition.

Animal studies have demonstrated that acidemia can protect myocardial and hepatic cells during hypoxia [17]. A lower pH increases the release of oxygen from hemoglobin, thereby increasing oxygen extraction by the tissues. In exercising athletes (with lactic acidosis and pH as low as 7.0), this mechanism can account for up to 60% of the oxygen available to the tissues. Experimental levels of arterial PCO_2 up to 1 atmosphere (750 mmHg) and intracellular brain pH of 6.2 have been tolerated in rats for 15 minutes without neurological impairment [17–19]. Acidemia has been found to attenuate inflammatory processes, including leukocyte superoxide formation, apoptosis of nerve cells, phospholipase A2 activity, expression of cell adhesion complexes, and xanthine oxidase activity [16,20,21].

Studies have shown, however, that the body reacts differently depending on the source of substances creating the acidemia. Cardiac myocytes show a faster increase in intracellular [H^+] caused by increased PCO_2 compared to hydrochloric acid (HCl), a fixed acid. This increased acidity does decrease myocardial contractility, but it also decreases myocardial oxygen consumption that may have a short-term protective effect. When brain acidosis is a result of CO_2 rather than HCl, there is less free radical production and less lipid peroxidation. Acidosis caused by CO_2, compared to acidosis from HCl, has an inhibitory effect on lactate production in the tissues [16,18,20,21].

At this early stage of our understanding of alkalemia and acidemia, the take-home message is that alkalemia may be far more harmful than a comparable acidemia, and that a change in H^+ activity is almost always less important than the underlying cause of the change.

Disorders of CO_2

An increase in PCO_2 >44 mmHg (hypercapnia) is also termed hypoventilation and creates a respiratory acidosis, with low pH, high H^+, and a compensatory *increase* in HCO_3^-. The development of respiratory acidosis can be classified as acute or chronic, which will subsequently influence the degree of metabolic compensation that has been demonstrated in dogs and cats (see Table 7.3) [22].

Respiratory acidosis may result from any disease process that can affect neuromuscular control of ventilation, loss of small or large airway integrity, or alveolar gas exchange. Common causes include large airway obstruction, respiratory center depression, increased CO_2 production, impaired alveolar ventilation, restrictive extrapulmonary disorders, parenchymal and small airway diseases, improper mechanical ventilation, and obesity. Clinical signs of respiratory acidosis may be more indicative of the underlying disease process than of the hypercapnia itself. These are typically more severe in patients with acute disorders (such as congestive heart failure, pneumonia) than in those with chronic, compensated respiratory disorders. Hypercapnia can also trigger cardiovascular changes such as tachycardia and vasodilation. Vasodilation can be of clinical significance in patients with intracranial disease; the increase in intracranial volume can cause a dramatic increase in intracranial pressure. Altered mentation is known to occur when PCO_2 is significantly elevated.

Treatment of respiratory acidosis is aimed at the underlying cause. Oxygen therapy is indicated in the treatment of hypoxemia caused by hypoventilation. In cases of airway obstruction, sedation, oxygen therapy, and airway management may be necessary to allow adequate ventilation. In some instances, mechanical ventilation may be required until the underlying disease process is corrected. Treatment with sodium bicarbonate or other alkalizing agents should be undertaken with extreme caution because, without mechanical ventilation, the patient may not be able to remove the CO_2 that is produced when these agents are metabolized [3,23–25].

A decrease in PCO_2 <36 mmHg (hypocapnia) is also termed hyperventilation and creates a respiratory alkalosis, with high pH, low H^+ and a compensatory *decrease* in HCO_3^-. The development of respiratory alkalosis can be classified as acute or chronic, which will subsequently influence the degree of metabolic compensation that may be expected (see Table 7.3) [24]. Respiratory alkalosis may result from any disease process that can increase alveolar ventilation above what is necessary to expire the CO_2 produced through normal metabolic processes. Common causes include hypoxemia, pulmonary parenchymal disease independent of hypoxemia, centrally mediated hyperventilation, overzealous mechanical ventilation, or situations that induce pain, fear, or anxiety. Treatment is aimed at addressing the underlying cause, and may include sedation, pain medications, and diuretics. Oxygen should be provided when hypoxemia contributes to respiratory alkalosis [24–26].

Disorders of Na^+ or free water

Sodium is the major extracellular cation and exists in the ionic form in body fluids at any pH. The contribution that Na^+ makes to the SQAB analysis is expressed in the formulas shown in Box 7.5.

Because water follows Na^+, hyponatremia is either a decrease in [Na^+] relative to body water or an increase in free water relative to [Na^+]. One explanation for the acid–base effect of hyponatremia is that free water is acidic relative to normal body pH, so increases in free water (decreases in [Na^+]) will have an acidifying effect. This is termed a dilutional acidosis The precise mechanisms by which a relative increase in free water or a decrease in [Na^+] contributes to acidemia have not been elaborated at the biochemical level. However, clinically, it is known that a low [Na^+] is acidifying, causing a change in BE of −0.25 mEq/L for every 1 mEq/L decline in [Na^+] below normal in dogs, and −0.22 mEq/L for every 1 mEq/L decline in cats [3,27–29].

Hyponatremic acidosis is caused by diseases or clinical conditions that can increase free water or reduce Na^+ concentrations.

Box 7.5 Semiquantitative acid–base calculations.

1. **The Na⁺/free water effect:**

    Contribution to BE in dogs = 0.25 x (Patient's Na⁺ − Normal Na⁺)
    Contribution to BE in cats = 0.22 x (Patient's Na⁺ − Normal Na⁺)

2. **The Cl⁻ effect:**
First correct for free water effect:

$$\text{Patient corrected Cl}^- = \text{Patient Cl}^- \times \frac{\text{Normal}\left[\text{Na}^+\right]}{\text{Patient}\left[\text{Na}^+\right]}$$

Then calculate the Cl⁻ effect:

    Contribution to BE = Normal Cl⁻ − Patient corrected Cl⁻

3. **The phosphate effect:**

    Contribution to BE = 0.6 x (Normal PO₄⁻ − Patient PO₄⁻)

4. **The albumin or total protein effect:**

    Contribution to BE = 3.0 x (Normal protein − Patient protein)
    Contribution to BE = 3.7 x (Normal albumin − Patient albumin)

5. **The lactate effect:**

    Contribution to BE = −1 x (Patient Lactate⁻)

6. **The sum of measured effects:**
The sum of the above calculations is the total effect on base excess due to the measured effectors of metabolic (nonrespiratory) acid–base change.

7. **The unmeasured cation and anion effect:**
The effect on base excess due to unmeasured cations and anions is the difference between the BE reported by the analyzer and the sum of the above calculations for the measured cations and anions:

    UX = UC⁺ − UA⁻ = BE − [Sum]

Where [Sum] = Na⁺ effect + Cl⁻ effect + protein effect + phosphate effect + lactate effect.

    If UX is a large number, there may be unmeasured anions or cations impacting acid–base.

IMPORTANT TOOL: The Acid–Base Calculator: www.ncstatevets.org/eccresources/, developed by B. Hanson, North Carolina State College of Veterinary Medicine

Common etiologies are Na⁺ loss from vomiting or diarrhea, third space Na⁺ loss, nephrotic syndrome, hypoadrenocorticism, congestive heart failure, psychogenic polydipsia, diuretic administration, hypotonic fluid use, and the syndrome of inappropriate antidiuretic hormone (SIADH). Pseudohyponatremia can occur with high plasma glucose or mannitol concentrations.

Treatment is directed at correcting the true underlying cause and normalizing renal function so that Na⁺ balance can be restored. In most cases, immediate corrections are made with intravenous fluids designed to both normalize total body water, total body Na⁺, and their relative concentrations. Care should be taken not to correct severe hyponatremia (≤130 mEq/L) too rapidly; the rate of correction should not exceed 1–2 mEq/L/h. Correcting hyponatremia too quickly can lead to central pontine myelinolysis within 2–5 days. Care should also be taken that fluids do not contain excess Cl⁻, which can create a hyperchloremic metabolic acidosis and exacerbate the acidemia [27,30–37].

Hypernatremia is either an increase in [Na⁺] relative to body water or a decrease in free water relative to [Na⁺]. One explanation for the acid–base effect of hypernatremia is that since free water is acidic relative to normal body pH, decreases in free water (increases in Na⁺) will have an alkalinizing effect. This is termed a concentration or contraction alkalosis. The precise mechanisms by which a relative decrease in free water or an increase in [Na⁺] contributes to

alkalemia have not been elaborated at the biochemical level. However, clinically, it is known that a high [Na⁺] is alkalinizing, causing a change in BE of +0.25 mEq/L for every 1 mEq/L increase in [Na⁺] above normal in dogs, and +0.22 mEq/L for every 1 mEq/L increase in cats [27–29].

Hypernatremic alkalosis is caused by diseases or clinical conditions that can decrease free water or increase sodium concentration. Common etiologies are vomiting, renal failure, postobstructive diuresis, diabetes insipidus, water deprivation, sodium bicarbonate administration, use of other medications complexed with Na⁺, and hypertonic fluid use.

Treatment is directed at correcting the true underlying cause, restricting Na⁺ intake if necessary, and normalizing renal function so that Na⁺ balance can be restored. In most cases, immediate corrections are made with intravenous fluids designed to normalize total body water, total body Na⁺, and their relative concentrations. Care should be taken not to correct severe hypernatremia (≥170 mEq/L) too rapidly; the rate of correction should not exceed 0.5–1 mEq/L/h [3,27]. Correcting hypernatremia too quickly can lead to cellular swelling and cerebral edema.

Disorders of Cl⁻ (corrected)

Chloride is the only major strong anion that is in high concentration in extracellular fluid. The inverse relationship between [Cl⁻] and [HCO₃⁻] has long been known and is the basis for the terms "chloride responsive" and "nonchloride responsive" metabolic acidosis. The [Cl⁻] may change independently of [Na⁺], but it will also be altered by changes in free water in a manner parallel with [Na⁺]. The free water-associated changes and their influence on acid–base status are calculated in the Na⁺ equation. Therefore, to isolate independent changes in [Cl⁻], the measured [Cl⁻] must be corrected for this free water change (see Box 7.5) [27,28,38,39].

The precise mechanisms by which a change in [Cl⁻] contributes to alkalemia or acidemia have not been elaborated at the biochemical level. However, clinically, it is known that a low chloride concentration is alkalinizing, causing a change in BE of +1 mEq/L for every 1 mEq/L decline in [Cl⁻] below normal. A high chloride concentration is acidifying, causing a change in BE of -1 for every 1 mEq/L increase in [Cl⁻] above normal [3,8,9].

Treatment is directed at correcting the true underlying cause, restricting Cl⁻ intake if necessary, and normalizing renal function so that Cl⁻ balance can be restored. In most cases, immediate corrections are made with intravenous fluids designed to normalize [Cl⁻] in blood and extracellular fluid (ECF). However, many drugs and fluids (such as KCl, normal saline), when administered over time, contain enough Cl⁻ to create a clinically significant increase in Cl⁻. It can take days for the kidneys to correct the hyperchloremia, assuming that the renal mechanisms of Cl⁻ excretion are intact. This process of iatrogenic hyperchloremic metabolic acidosis is termed "chloride creep." The contribution of the Cl⁻ effect to SQAB analysis is shown in the formulas in Box 7.5.

Disorders of phosphate

The terms "PO₄⁻," "phosphate," "phosphorus," and "inorganic phosphorus" are commonly used interchangeably. The contribution that phosphate makes to the SQAB analysis is exhibited in the formulas in Box 7.5. A decline in phosphate concentration has an alkalinizing effect, but because phosphate levels are normally low, a decrease in phosphate is considered to be life threatening before it creates a dramatic change in [H⁺]. Hypophosphatemia may be caused by malnutrition, nutritional disorders, excess renal excretion, or hemodilution. Treatment is directed at careful intravenous phosphate replacement and treating the underlying cause [8,27,29,39].

Elevations in serum phosphate have an acidifying effect. The traditional explanation is that phosphate acts not only as a buffer but also as an acid at physiological pH; hence increases in serum phosphate concentration are acidifying. The Stewart explanation is that the normal phosphate level of 5 mg/dL contributes approximately 2.9 mEq/L of net negative charge to plasma. An increase in negative charge from an increase in phosphate is balanced by an increase in [H^+] and a decrease in [HCO_3^-], an acidifying event. Clinically, it is known that a high phosphate concentration is acidifying, causing a change in BE of -0.6 mEq/L for every 1 mEq/L increase in [PO_4^-] above normal [8,27,29,39].

Hyperphosphatemia is associated with renal failure, urinary tract obstruction or disruption, cell lysis, or medications such as intravenous phosphates, phosphate urinary acidifiers, and phosphate enemas. Treatment is directed at the underlying disease or removing the offending therapeutic agent. Hemodialysis and peritoneal dialysis are both effective at reducing serum phosphate concentration [8,27,39].

Disorders of protein or albumin

Hypoproteinemia is common in critically ill patients. The traditional explanation for this acid–base effect is that at physiological pH, plasma proteins (primarily albumin) act as weak acids. Consequently, decreases in plasma protein will have an alkalinizing effect. The Stewart explanation is that at physiological pH, proteins exert a net negative charge that in canine plasma totals about 16 mEq/L. If the protein level of plasma decreases, the decrease in negative charge is offset by a decrease in [H^+] and an increase in [HCO_3^-]. This is an alkalinizing event [8,27–29].

A decrease in plasma proteins may be caused by dilution following an increase in body water, loss due to vascular leak states (such as protein-losing nephropathy, protein-losing enteropathy, or systemic inflammation), or decreased synthesis due to hepatic disease or reprioritization. The result of a decrease in plasma protein is to increase the BE, although recent evidence suggests that this inverse relationship may not be as linear as the formula suggests. Treatment for hypoproteinemic metabolic alkalosis is directed at the underlying cause of the protein dilution, deficit, or loss [8,27–29].

Increases in serum protein are associated with an acidifying effect. The traditional explanation is that at physiological pH, plasma proteins (primarily albumin) act as weak acids [2,40]. Consequently, increases in plasma protein will have an acidifying effect. The Stewart explanation is that at physiological pH, proteins exert a net negative charge that in canine plasma totals about 16 mEq/L. If the protein level of plasma increases, the increase in negative charge is offset by an increase in [H^+]and a decrease in [HCO_3^-] concentration. This is an acidifying event [8,27–29].

An increase in plasma proteins is associated with dehydration, inflammation, excess albumin administration, or neoplasia such as multiple myeloma [8,27–29]. Treatment of hyperproteinemic metabolic acidosis involves specific therapy for the underlying disease and, in extreme cases, plasmapheresis. The impact that protein (or albumin) has on the semiquantitative approach is noted in Box 7.5.

Disorders of lactate

When DO_2 does not meet oxygen demand, oxidative phosphorylation through the Krebs cycle ceases and pyruvate is converted to lactate. Lactate is a marker for anaerobic metabolism [14,23,27].

The pKa for lactic acid is 3.9, so it is completely dissociated within the range of body pH and is therefore a strong anion. As with Cl⁻ anion, lactate⁻ anion is acidifying and each mEq/L increase changes BE by -1 mEq/L.

When lactate anion is delivered with a strong cation other than a hydrogen ion, such as Na^+ in lactated Ringer's solution (LRS), its acidifying effect is balanced by the alkalinizing effect of the strong cation and there is no immediate change in acid–base status [14,23,27,39]. When the lactate is metabolized more rapidly than the Na^+ is excreted, the influence of the increased Na^+ predominates, giving LRS a net alkalinizing effect. In patients that have severe impairment of lactate metabolism (such as severe liver dysfunction), the lactate can persist and have the opposite, acidifying effect. The contribution of lactate to BE is shown by the formula in Box 7.5.

Disorders of unmeasured cations and anions

Acid–base changes commonly occur in plasma due to substances that are not routinely measured. This is revealed when the sum of the BE effects calculated for the measured factors (Na^+, Cl^-, protein, phosphate, and lactate) does not equal the BE as reported by the analyzer. If a significant inequality exists between the total BE and sum of the calculated effects, there are two possible explanations. One is that the calculations are imprecise because they use the average normal value for each parameter (the mean within the reference range) instead of the normal value for the patient (which is rarely known). The second but also very common explanation is that the sample blood contains unmeasured cations (UX^+) and/or unmeasured anions (UX^-). The difference between UX^+ and UX^- is reflected in the difference between summed measured effects and the reported BE (see Box 7.5) [33,41].

Almost all of the unmeasured ions determined to be clinically important are anions. Therefore, the sum of these unmeasured species (UX^+ - UX^-) is commonly termed "unmeasured anions" (UX). These include diabetic ketoacids, toxic acids (ethylene glycol, alcohols, salicylate), and the acids of renal failure other than phosphate [8].

The acid–base calculator

The equations listed in Box 7.5 are used to calculate contributions to BE as part of the SQAB analysis. This process can be time-consuming and problematic due to the need to track multiple parameters and the complexity of adding and subtracting positive and negative values. The use of an acid–base calculator is recommended, a good example can be accessed at: http://www.ncstatevets.org/eccresources/. The site can assist in providing a more precise acid–base analysis, along with interpretation of the respiratory components of any acid–base disorder. The calculator performs HH, Stewart, and semiquantitative analysis with the added benefit of permitting each user to input the normal reference ranges for their in-house laboratory analyzers.

The steps for SQAB analysis are summarized in Box 7.6. It is up to the clinician to determine the frequency of SQAB profile testing based on the volatility of the patient's condition and the aggressiveness of therapy. It is important to increase frequency of testing when the patient's response to therapy is not as predicted.

Supplemental tests

When the clinician finds that a significant contribution to the change in BE may be due to unmeasured anions and/or cations, there is a battery of supplemental tests that will help to isolate the

Box 7.6 Steps for SQAB analysis.

1. Use point of care analyzers for small sample size and rapid processing and reporting.
2. Run the SQAB profile:
   Blood gas: pH, PCO_2, HCO_3^-, BE
   Electrolytes: Na^+, Cl^-, K^+
   Biochemistry: phosphorus, albumin (protein), lactate
3. Calculate the contribution to BE of each analyte in the SQAB profile using the acid–base calculator: www.ncstatevets.org/eccresources/.
4. Perform supplemental tests based on calculated unmeasured ion levels and on clinical assessment of the patient.
   Supplemental tests: glucose, beta-hydroxybutyrate, BUN, creatinine, sulfate, urate, ALT, SAP, bilirubin, toxic acids, urine electrolyes, urine osmolality
5. Determine treatment plan.
   Primary survey: Determine life-threatening analytes
   Resuscitation: Stabilize life-threatening disturbances
   Secondary survey: Diagnostic tests for definitive diagnosis
   Definitive care: Treat the underlying cause(s)
6. Repeat SQAB profile and supplemental tests to determine:
   • response to the treatment plan in a predictable manner
   • that therapy is not creating disturbances in acid–base balance
   • that other clinical problems are not emerging.

ALT, alanine aminotransferase; BE, base excess; BUN, blood urea nitrogen; SAP, serum alkaline phosphatase.

causative factors. Substances such as glucose, ketones, urate, liver enzymes, sulfate, and toxins should each be considered as a potential source of unmeasured cations or anions (see Box 7.4).

Glucose and ketones (beta-hydroxybutyrate)

Diabetic ketoacidosis is a common acid–base disturbance associated with diabetes mellitus in dogs and cats. Many critical care analyzers measure blood glucose concentration (BG). Although this analyte is not used in SQAB analysis calculations, an elevation in BG increases the suspicion for diabetes mellitus and prompts a test for urine and/or blood ketones. Test strips are available for beta-hydroxybutyrate and the color change is semiquantitative. Point of care analyzers are available to quantify beta-hydroxybutyrate levels in plasma and computerized acid–base calculators may include this parameter in the BE calculations. The nitroprusside in urine test strips semiquantitatively test for acetoacetate, not for beta-hydroxybutyrate.

BUN, creatinine, sulfate, urate

Uremic acidosis is a well-known clinical problem associated with renal failure. In a review of the existing knowledge regarding uremic toxins, 88 substances were identified. Twenty-one of these solutes were in plasma concentrations more than 10 times normal, with seven acids ranging from 22 to 334 times normal [42].

Phosphate, sulfate, and urate are reported to be among the important retention solutes affecting acid–base levels. Elevations in phosphate concentration are commonly associated with renal failure and its contribution to the change in BE is part of SQAB analysis. In the future, advances in analyzer technology are likely to expand assays of causative agents by measuring more uremic toxins and calculating their contributions to acid–base imbalance.

Phosphorus is not always elevated in renal failure but other uremic toxins may be elevated. This makes the assessment of BUN and creatinine important when unmeasured anions are present and renal disease is a potential contributor. An increase in these analytes suggests that uremic toxins are contributing to the UX.

ALT, SAP, and bilirubin

The liver is a net producer or consumer of H^+ depending on diet, metabolism, volume status, perfusion, medications, toxins, and fluids. Tests for hepatocellular injury and liver function are important supplemental tests when an acid–base disturbance is present and the clinician is looking for the underlying cause. When albumin concentration is low or lactate levels are elevated, these tests can help determine if these abnormalities may be linked to loss of liver function. Albumin and lactate are analytes measured in the SQAB profile, but other contributions to acid–base disturbances related to liver function are not and must be inferred from other tests.

Toxins

There are a number of toxin panels available through reference and hospital laboratories that make it possible to search for causative agents when unmeasured ions are known to be a major contributor to changes in BE. As technology improves, the identification of these toxins can be done using POC testing. Ethylene glycol is a common toxin in veterinary medicine and patient recovery is dependent on its timely identification. Semiquantitative analysis of the profound acid–base disturbance will reveal a large contribution from unmeasured ions, directing supplemental testing for renal function and renal toxins.

Urine parameters

Although not a direct indicator of acid–base status in plasma, urine parameters (electrolytes, pH, and osmolality) can be helpful in identifying etiologies for acid–base disturbances in veterinary patients when used to supplement the SQAB quantitative analysis. Disorders in perfusion, renal function, and other underlying disease processes [43–45] can be reflected in alterations in the excretion of electrolytes and acids. However, critical care patients are not "normal," making the interpretation of urine electrolytes more difficult in these patients. Table 7.5 presents a list of frequently measured urine parameters and their clinical application for patient management and acid–base analysis.

The urinary excretion of electrolytes can be expressed as a concentration (mEq/L or mmol/L), as total over a period of time (mEq/hour or day), or as a fraction of that filtered by the glomerulus (%). Urine $[Na^+]$ can be a reflection of volume status, antidiuretic hormone activity, renin-angiotensin-aldosterone, natriuretic peptides, and other renal hormones. Table 7.6 presents clinical conditions with possible etiologies based on different electrolyte concentrations.

Urine $[Cl^-]$ should be low with hypochloremic metabolic alkalosis but normal in other causes of metabolic alkalosis. It may be elevated by the elevated excretion of ammonium ($NH4^+$, a nonresorbable cation) in chronic metabolic acidosis. Paradoxical aciduria occurs when there is a need for Na^+ conservation and yet there is a depletion of exchange electrolytes in the renal tubules (Cl^- and K^+). In the ascending loop where NaCl reabsorption is strong, if Cl^- is depleted (as occurs with gastric losses of HCl and ensuing alkalosis), HCO_3 will be reabsorbed to maintain electroneutrality, resulting in more acidic urine and increasing alkalosis.

If K^+ is depleted in the distal tubules where aldosterone promotes Na^+-K^+ exchange, H^+ will be swapped with the Na^+, leading to more acidic urine and more alkaline blood. As long as the drive for Na^+ absorption continues due to dehydration or Na^+ depletion or sequestration, this continues as a vicious cycle leading to greater alkalosis and maintaining electrolyte depletions. Restoring hydration and normonatremia is critical to resolving the cycle [43,44].

Table 7.5 Clinical applications of urine electrolytes, osmolality, and other analytes.

Analyte	Application
Na+	**To assess volume status**
	Differential diagnosis of hyponatremia
	Differential diagnosis of AKI
	To assess salt intake in patients with hypertension
	To evaluate calcium and uric acid excretion in stone-formers
	To calculate electrolyte-free water clearance
Cl⁻	**Differential diagnosis of metabolic alkalosis**
K⁺	Differential diagnosis of hypokalemia
	To calculate electrolyte-free water reabsorption
	To calculate transtubular K⁺ gradient
Urine osmolality	**Differential diagnosis of hyponatremia**
	Differential diagnosis of polyuria
	Differential diagnosis of AKI
Urine anion gap	**To distinguish between distal renal tubular acidosis and diarrhea as cause of primary hyperchloremic metabolic acidosis**
Electrolyte-free water clearance	**To assess the amount of water excretion (without solutes) in the management of hypo- and hypernatremia**
Creatinine	**To calculate fractional excretion of Na+ and renal failure index**
	To assess the adequacy of 24-h urine collection

Bold items are applications that relate to acid–base status.
AKI, acute kidney injury.
Source: adapted from Reddi AS. Fluid, Electrolyte, and Acid–Base Disorders. New York: Springer Science & Business Media, 2014.

The urine anion gap (UAG) is calculated using urine Na⁺, urine K⁺, urine ammonium, and urine Cl⁻. Normal UAG is approximately zero, with other cations and anions in low concentration. There is normally very little calcium and magnesium in urine. There is no HCO_3^- in urine if the pH is <6.5. Other anions such as phosphate, sulfate, and organic anions are also in low concentration. Since urine ammonium is not typically measured, the normal average urine ammonium level (50 mmol/L) is substituted in the formula:

$$U_{AG} = \left(U_{[Na+]} + U_{[K+]} + U_{[NH4^+]} - U_{[Cl-]} \right)$$

or

$$U_{AG} = \left(U_{[Na+]} + U_{[K+]} + 50 - U_{[Cl-]} \right)$$

Using this equation, a calculated UAG <0 most likely reflects an increase in urine ammonium. UAG >0 suggests an increase in urinary concentrations of HCO_3^-, phosphate, sulfate, albumin, lactate, ketoacids, drugs such as salicylates or penicillins, or defects in ammonium production [43,44,46].

Osmolality is defined as the number of solute particles per kilogram of solvent. The major determinants of extracellular and intracellular fluid osmolality are Na⁺ and K⁺ respectively, whereas urine osmolality (UOSM) reflects a more heterogeneous mixture of solutes. Urine solutes include urea, Na⁺, K⁺, ammonium (NH_4), Cl⁻, and other anions. Urine osmolality is calculated by the formula:

$$U_{OSM} = 2 \times U_{[Na+]} + U_{[K+]} + U_{[urea]} / 2.8 + U_{[glucose]} / 18$$

Normal UOSM can range widely between 800 and 2500 mOsm/kg in the dog and 600 and 3000 mOsm/kg in the cat. Table 7.7 lists the expected urine osmolality under various clinical conditions. The clinical importance of measuring UOSM is most obvious in

Table 7.6 Use of urine electrolytes to interpret the etiology of selected clinical conditions.

Condition	Electrolyte (mEq/L)	Possible etiologies
Hypovolemia	Na⁺ (0–20)	Extrarenal loss of Na⁺
	Na⁺ (>20)	Renal salt wasting
		Adrenal insufficiency
		Diuretic use or osmotic diuresis
Acute kidney injury	Na⁺ (0–20)	Prerenal azotemia
	Na⁺ (>20)	Acute tubular necrosis (ATN)
	FENa (<1%)	Prerenal azotemia
	FENa (>2%)	ATN due to contrast agent
		Rhabdomyolysis
		ATN
		Diuretic use
Hyponatremia	Na+ (0–20)	Hypovolemia
		Edematous disorders
		Water intoxication
	Na+ (>20)	SIADH
		Cerebral salt wasting (CSW)
		Adrenal insufficiency
	↑FEUA (>10%)	SIADH and CSW
	↑FEPO4 (>20%)	CSW
Metabolic alkalosis	Cl⁻ (0–10)	Cl⁻ responsive alkalosis
	Cl⁻ (>20)	Cl⁻ resistant alkalosis
Hypokalemia	K⁺ (0–10)	Extrarenal loss of K⁺
	K⁺ (>20)	Renal loss of K⁺
UAG	Positive (from 0 to + 50)	Distal renal tubular acidosis
	Negative (from 0 to − 50)	Diarrhea

SIADH, syndrome of inappropriate ADH; UAG, urine anion gap.
Source: adapted from Reddi AS. Fluid, Electrolyte, and Acid–Base Disorders. New York: Springer Science & Business Media, 2014.

Table 7.7 Expected urine osmolality in various clinical conditions.

Condition	~Osmolality (mOsm/kg)	Comment
Normal	50–1200	Normal urine dilution and concentration
AKI – prerenal azotemia	>400	Increased water reabsorption by nephrons
AKI – acute tubular necrosis	<400	Injured tubules cannot reabsorb water
SIADH	>200	Excess water reabsorption by distal nephron
Osmotic diuresis	>300	Usually UOsm > POsm, excretion of excess osmoles
Central diabetes insipidus (DI)	≤100	Lack of ADH
Nephrogenic DI	<300	ADH resistance
Psychogenic polydipsia	~50	Decreased medullary hypertonicity
Hydrochlorothiazide therapy	>200	Inability to dilute urine
Furosemide therapy	~300	Isosthenuria, inability to concentrate and dilute urine

ADH, antidiuretic hormone; AKI, acute kidney injury; SIADH, syndrome of inappropriate ADH.
Source: adapted from Reddi AS. Fluid, Electrolyte, and Acid–Base Disorders. New York: Springer Science & Business Media, 2014.

differentiating prerenal and renal causes of azotemia. An increase in unmeasured cations and/or anions will be reflected in the urine osmolal gap, if these species are excreted by the kidney. The urinary osmolal gap is the difference between the measured and the calculated osmolality. The typical urine osmolal gap is 100 mOsm/kg. The normal osmolal gap is primarily due to ammonium salts. Elevated values may represent increased concentrations of ammonium, calcium, magnesium, HCO_3^-, phosphate, sulfate, albumin, lactate, ketoacids, and certain drugs (e.g. salicylates, penicillins) [43].

Urine pH is a measure of the acidification processes of the distal nephron. It should normally vary in the direction of the pH of the plasma. In metabolic acidosis the urine pH should be low. An acid urine pH in the presence of systemic alkalemia can occur secondary to volume depletion with Na^+ retention and H^+ excretion. Alkaline urine in the face of systemic metabolic acidosis may indicate proximal or distal renal tubular acidosis or carbonic anhydrase therapy. Urine pH or H^+ is not a good indicator of the total amount of acid excreted. Most acid excretion is in the form of phosphoric acid or ammonium.

References

1. Berend K. Acid–base pathophysiology after 130 years: confusing, irrational and controversial. J Nephrol. 2013;26:254–65.
2. Corey H, Kellum J, Wooten W. Stewart's acid–base theory: equation, implementation and mechanism. Trends Comp Bioch Physiol. 2009;14:35–54.
3. DiBartola S. Introduction to acid–base disorders. In: Fluid, Electrolyte, and Acid–base Disorders in Small Animal Practice, 4th edn. DiBartola S, ed. St Louis: Saunders, 2012: pp 231–52.
4. Guyton A. Textbook of Medical Physiology, 12th edn. St Louis: Saunders, 2010: pp 463–72.
5. Deutsch C, Taylor JS, Wilson DF. Regulation of intracellular pH by human peripheral blood lymphocytes as measured by ^{19}F NMR. Proc Natl Acad Sci USA 1982;79(24):7944–8.
6. Haskins SC, Pascoe PJ, Ilkiw JE, et al. Reference cardiopulmonary values in normal dogs. Compar Med. 2005;55:146–61.
7. Richey MT, McGarth CJ, Portillo E, Scott M, Claypool L. Effect of sample handling on venous PCO2, pH, bicarbonate, and base excess measured with point-of-care-analyzer. J Vet Emerg Crit Care 2004;14:253–8.
8. Constable PD. Clinical assessment of acid–base status: comparison of the Henderson–Hasselbalch and strong ion approaches. Vet Clin Pathol. 2000;29:115–28.
9. Fencl V, Jabor A, Kazda A, et al. Diagnosis of metabolic acid–base disturbances in critically ill patients. Am J Resp Crit Care Med. 2000;162:2246–51.
10. Figge J, Rossing TH, Fencl V. The role of serum proteins in acid–base equilibria. J Lab Clin Med. 1991;117:453–67.
11. McCullough S, Constable P. Calculation of the total plasma concentration of non-volatile weak acids and the effective dissociation constant of non-volatile buffers in plasma for use in the strong ion approach to acid–base balance in cats. Am J Vet Res. 2003;64(8):1047–51.
12. Hopper K, Epstein S, Kass P, Mellema M. Evaluation of acid–base disorders in dogs and cats presenting to an emergency room. Part 1: Comparison of three methods of acid–base analysis. J Vet Emerg Crit Care 2014;24:493–501.
13. Hopper K, Epstein S, Kass P, Mellema M. Evaluation of acid–base disorders in dogs and cats presenting to an emergency room. Part 2: Comparison of anion gap, strong ion gap, and semiquantitative analysis. J Vet Emerg Crit Care 2014;24:502–8.
14. Hopper K, Haskins SC. A case base review of a simplified quantitative approach to acid–base analysis. J Vet Emerg Crit Care 2008;17:467.
15. Gehlbach B, Schmidt G. Bench-to-bedside review: treating acid–base abnormalities in the intensive care unit – the role of buffers. Crit Care 2004;8:259–65.
16. Croinin D, Chonghaile M, Higgins B, Laffey J. Bench-to-bedside review: permissive hypercapnia. Crit Care 2005;9:51–9.
17. Wu S, Wu C, Kang B, Li M, Chu S, Huang K. Hypercapnic acidosis attenuates reperfusion injury in isolated and perfused rat lungs. Crit Care Med. 2012;40(2):553–9.
18. Xu F, Uh J, Brier M, et al. The influence of carbon dioxide on brain activity and metabolism in conscious humans. J Cereb Blood Flow Metab. 2011;31:58–67.
19. Xu Y, Cohen Y, Chang LH, James TL. Tolerance of low cerebral intracellular pH in rats during hyperbaric hypercapnia. Stroke 1991;22(10):1303–8.
20. Contreras M, Ansari B, Curley G, et al. Hypercapnic acidosis attenuates ventilation-induced lung injury by a nuclear factor-kβ dependent mechanism. Crit Care Med. 2012;40(9):2622–30.
21. Curley G, Kavanagh B, Laffey J. Hypocapnia and the injured brain: more harm than benefit. Crit Care Med. 2010;38(5):1348–59.
22. Berend K, deVries A, Gans R. Physiologic approach to acid–base disturbances. N Engl J Med. 2014;371:1434–45.
23. Hackett T. Tachypnea and hypoxemia. In: Small Animal Critical Care Medicine. Silverstein D, Hopper K, eds. St Louis: Saunders, 2009: pp 249–53.
24. Johnson RA, de Morais HA. Respiratory acid–base disorders. In: Fluid, Electrolyte, and Acid–base Disorders in Small Animal Practice, 4th edn. DiBartola S, ed. St Louis: Saunders, 2012: pp 287–301.
25. Morning AA. Practical acid–base in veterinary medicine. Vet Clin North Am Small Anim Pract. 2013;43:1273–86.
26. Kovacic J. Lactic acidosis. In: Small Animal Critical Care Medicine. Silverstein D, Hopper K, eds. St Louis: Saunders, 2009: pp 254–6.
27. Kovacic J. Acid–base disturbances. In: Small Animal Critical Care Medicine. Silverstein D, Hopper K, eds. St Louis: Saunders, 2009: pp 249–53.
28. Russell KE, Hansen BD, Stevens JB. Strong ion difference approach to acid–base imbalances with clinical applications to dogs and cats. Vet Clin North Am Small Anim Pract. 1996;26:1185–201.
29. Stewart P. Strong ions, plus carbon dioxide, plus weak acid, isolated blood plasma and isolated intracellular fluid. In: How to Understand Acid–Base. New York: Elsevier, 1981: pp 110–44.
30. Buckley M, LeBlanc J, Cawley M. Electrolyte disturbances associated with commonly prescribed medications in the intensive care unit. Crit Care Med. 2010;38(6):S253–S263.
31. Buckley M. Electrolyte disturbances associated with medications in the critically ill. Int J Intensive Care 2012;Spring:83–8.

32. DeMorais HA, Bach J, DiBartola S. Metabolic acid–base disorders in the critical care unit. Vet Clin North Am Small Anim Pract. 2008;38(3):559–74.

33. Gunnerson K, Kellum JA. Acid–base and electrolyte analysis in critically ill patients: are we ready for the new millennium? Curr Opin Crit Care 2003;9:468–73.

34. Ke L, Calzavacca P, Bailey M, et al. Systemic and renal haemodynamic effects of fluid bolus therapy: sodium chloride versus sodium octanoate-balanced solution. Crit Care Resus. 2014;16(1):29–33.

35. Raghunathan K, Shaw A, Nathanson B, et al. Association between the choice of IV crystalloid and in-hospital mortality among critically ill adults with sepsis. Crit Care Med. 2014;42(7):1585–91.

36. Yunos N, Bellomo R, Story D, Kellum J. Bench-to-bedside review: chloride in critical illness. Crit Care 2010;14:226–36.

37. Zhou F, Peng Z, Bishop J, etal. Effects of fluid resuscitation with 0.9% saline versus a balanced electrolyte solution on acute kidney injury in a rat model of sepsis. Crit Care Med. 2014;42(4):e270–e278.

38. Haskins SA. Acid-base evaluation. In: Advanced Monitoring and Procedures for Small Animal Emergency and Critical Care. Burkitt C, Davis D, eds. Ames: John Wiley and Sons, 2012: pp 651–64.

39. Stewart PA. Modern quantitative acid–base chemistry. Can J Physiol Pharmacol. 1983;61:1444–61.

40. Badr A, Nightingale P. An alternative approach to acid–base abnormalities in critically ill patients. Contin Educ Anaesth Crit Care Pain 2007;7(4):107–111.

41. Robertson SA. Simple acid–base disorders. Vet Clin North Am Small Anim Pract. 1989;19:289–306.

42. Duranton F, Cohen G, DeSmet R, et al. Normal and pathologic concentrations of uremic toxins. J Am Soc Nephrol. 2012;23:1258–70.

43. Dyck R, Asthana S, Kalra J, et. al. A modification of the urine osmolal gap: an improved method for estimating urine ammonium, Am J Nephrol. 1990;10:359–62.

44. Kamel KS, Ethier JH, Richardson RMA, et. al. Urine electrolytes and osmolality: when and how to use them. Am J Nephrol. 1990;10:89–102.

45. Reddi AS. Fluid, Electrolyte, and Acid–Base Disorders. New York: Springer Science & Business Media, 2014: p 14.

46. Waldrop J. Urinary electrolytes, solutes, and osmolality. Vet Clin North Am Small Anim Pract. 2008;38:503–12.

CHAPTER 8

Oxygenation and ventilation

Christin Reminga and Lesley G. King[†]

University of Pennsylvania, Philadelphia, Pennsylvania

Introduction

Lungs allow the exchange of oxygen (O_2) and carbon dioxide (CO_2) between blood and room air. Respiratory gas transport is essential for cellular metabolism and thus organism sustainability, requiring ventilation, pulmonary gas exchange, and O_2 transport to and from the tissues. Ventilation and oxygenation are distinct but interdependent physiological processes.

Ventilation is the movement of gas into and out of the alveoli. Under the control of brainstem respiratory centers in spontaneously breathing animals, skeletal muscle (diaphragm and intercostal muscles) uses energy to generate the mechanical force responsible for lung expansion. Mechanical expansion of the thoracic cavity creates a negative transpulmonary pressure gradient that causes air to flow into the lungs by conduction. Air from the atmosphere starts at the nares and is conducted through the nasopharynx, larynx, trachea, and into the mainstem bronchi. The bronchi split several times (airway generations), ending in the terminal respiratory units of the lung that are lined with alveoli. Exhalation is a passive process because of thoracic skeletal muscle relaxation and the lung's intrinsic elastic properties [1].

Minute ventilation describes the total volume of air moved into and out of the lungs in one minute, and is determined by the product of the respiratory rate and the tidal volume. Respiratory rate is primarily controlled centrally, while tidal volume depends on the integrity of neural control (including spinal cord and peripheral nerves), respiratory muscles, and the respiratory conduction system. Minute ventilation is primarily controlled by changes in blood CO_2, which alter cerebrospinal fluid (CSF) pH. Changes in CSF pH are then detected by brainstem respiratory centers, which directly alter ventilation in order to maintain CO_2 within a narrow range. Ventilation increases in response to an elevation of arterial CO_2 (hypercapnia), and decreases if there is low CO_2 (hypocapnia). This relationship can change in animals with chronic hypoxemia, when oxygenation can become one of the primary drivers of respiration [2].

While ventilation can be thought of as the delivery system that presents oxygen-rich air to the alveoli, oxygenation is the process of delivering O_2 from the alveoli to the tissues in order to maintain cellular activity. Oxygenation is a complex process that involves the respiratory, cardiovascular, hematological, and cellular transport systems.

In order for O_2 to move from the alveoli to the tissues, the mode of transportation changes from conduction to a more efficient means called diffusion, in which a molecule passively moves along its concentration gradient. O_2 diffuses across the alveolar epithelium,

pulmonary interstitium, and the pulmonary capillary endothelium, where it dissolves in plasma and then binds to hemoglobin (Hgb). The concentration gradient between high atmospheric O_2 and lower venous O_2 allows rapid diffusion in the healthy lung. At the same time, CO_2 readily diffuses from the bloodstream into the alveoli, to be subsequently exhaled.

For adequate pulmonary O_2 diffusion, ventilation and pulmonary capillary perfusion of individual alveolar units need to be in balance. This is described as the ventilation-perfusion (V/Q) ratio. Alterations in V/Q can lead to a decrease in arterial O_2 content (hypoxia) with or without changes in arterial CO_2 [2].

Once dissolved in plasma, O_2 enters erythrocytes to bind to Hgb molecules. Up to four O_2 molecules can bind to one Hgb molecule, with only a small portion of O_2 remaining dissolved in the plasma. Binding of each O_2 molecule results in a conformational change of the Hgb molecule, which facilitates an increased rate of binding of subsequent O_2 molecules. The relationship between the concentration of O_2 dissolved in the plasma and the percent saturation of Hgb with oxygen is therefore nonlinear, characterized by a sigmoid bend (Figure 8.1) [3]. The total amount of O_2 carried in the blood is known as the O_2 content (CaO_2) and is related to the amount of oxygen dissolved in the plasma, the amount of Hgb, and the saturation of Hgb with O_2 (Table 8.1).

Once delivered to the tissues, O_2 bound to Hgb dissociates and diffuses into the cellular mitochondria for energy production. The rate of diffusion is governed mainly by differences in transmembrane partial pressures, but also by gas solubility in the tissue.

CO_2 is the main endproduct of aerobic metabolism and causes respiratory acidosis if it is not promptly removed from the body by alveolar ventilation. It too uses diffusion as the form of transport and is carried to the lungs dissolved in plasma and, to a lesser extent than O_2, attached to Hgb.

Respiratory failure is diagnosed when there is a deficit in arterial O_2 (hypoxemia) or the accumulation of CO_2 (hypercapnia) due to abnormalities within the respiratory system or neurological control of ventilation. It is important to identify a decline in ventilation and oxygenation early in the course of critical illness to prevent the ensuing cascade of detrimental cellular events. Identifying the inciting cause of respiratory failure and anticipating the consequences requires the timely implementation of diagnostic and monitoring procedures.

Diagnostic and monitoring procedures

Patients with oxygenation or ventilation disorders can experience a rapid and life-threatening change at any moment. Hypoxic animals can decompensate rapidly with even minimal restraint. A staged

[†]Deceased.

Monitoring and Intervention for the Critically Ill Small Animal: The Rule of 20, First Edition. Edited by Rebecca Kirby and Andrew Linklater.
© 2017 John Wiley & Sons, Inc. Published 2017 by John Wiley & Sons, Inc.

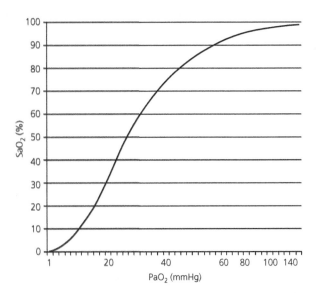

Figure 8.1 Oxyhemoglobin dissociation curve describing the relationship between partial pressure of oxygen (PaO_2, x-axis) and the oxygen saturation (y-axis). Oxygen saturation (SaO_2) is the percentage of arterial hemoglobin that is saturated with oxygen. The nonlinear relationship between the concentration of oxygen and its ability to bind hemoglobin is represented by a sigmoid curve.

strategy for evaluation is essential, addressing the most life-threatening conditions first. Co-morbidities can result in respiratory compromise even though the respiratory physical examination is unremarkable. Therefore oxygenation and ventilation parameters should be evaluated in all hospitalized patients, and ideally continuously monitored in those that are critically ill.

Upon triage, a brief physical examination focusing on the respiratory, cardiovascular, and neurological systems is often all that can be performed in animals with severe respiratory distress. Immediate O_2 supplementation should be provided. An enclosed O_2 cage can provide visualization of the animal while decreasing their stress from hospital transport and handling, especially in cats. Attention is paid to the environmental temperature and CO_2 concentration in any enclosed supplemental O_2 environment. Anxiolytic agents may be indicated if anxiety is compounding the respiratory distress; these should be avoided or used cautiously in patients with respiratory muscle fatigue. Emergent anesthetic induction and endotracheal intubation followed by ventilation with 100% oxygen may be required if the animal is experiencing severe work of breathing.

Often the history and physical examination are the only diagnostic tests possible until the patient has been further stabilized. In-hospital point of care (POC) testing can follow, providing immediate data. Clinicopathological testing and imaging procedures are done to further identify an underlying cause for any respiratory compromise when the patient can tolerate restraint and diagnostics. Throughout the process, careful monitoring and patient support are required to avoid decompensation.

History

The history begins with the signalment (age, sex, breed), with breed predilections for respiratory disease considered (such as brachycephalic syndrome, hypoplastic trachea, and tracheal collapse). Hereditary causes of heart disease could be a cause of pulmonary edema or other respiratory distress. The past medical history could

identify problems such as heart murmur, vomiting, asthma or other findings that could contribute to the onset of breathing abnormalities. The recent history can reveal vaccination status, exposure to other animals or a travel history that may pose a risk for infectious disease. The current problems should be described to include the onset and progression of clinical signs. Exercise intolerance, potential exposure to inhaled toxins (such as smoke, strong perfumes, incense, gases, sprayed chemicals) and a description of any breathing changes, such as coughing, open-mouth breathing or loud breathing, warrant further investigation.

It is important to have a description of the respiratory rate (such as fast, slow, normal) and effort (such as open-mouth, lips drawn back, elbow abducted with neck extended) observed in the patient. A description of any coughing heard can be important. There are three main types of cough that can be described for the dog and cat. Purposeful coughing is the beneficial expelling of foreign material or mucopurulent exudate such as might occur due to foreign body inhalation, infectious tracheobronchitis or pneumonia. This cough is loud and harsh, often occurring in a series until the animal swallows or there is expulsion of sputum or foreign material. Cautionary coughing is a manifestation of a systemic disruption, which can be life-threatening, such as pulmonary edema (congestive heart failure, acute respiratory distress syndrome) and pulmonary hemorrhage (rodenticide, leptospirosis). This type of cough has a soft sound, often occurring in a series. An irritating cough is a nuisance to the patient, as might occur in animals with mild tracheal collapse or chronic bronchitis. This is often a progressive chain of "goose-honking" sounds.

Physical examination

The physical examination is the most important tool to help narrow down the cause of respiratory failure when other diagnostic tools are not possible due to the fragile condition of the patient. Characterizing the respiratory pattern by simple observation can be an incredibly informative initial approach. Common respiratory rates and patterns are described with possible localization within the respiratory tract in Table 8.2. An abnormal breathing pattern develops as an adaptive process to minimize the effect of abnormal forces applied to the respiratory system. Distinct breathing patterns, if observed, may be helpful in determining the underlying pathology and next diagnostic or therapeutic steps.

Patients with mild upper airway disease can have a change in voice, gagging, retching, and coughing. Severe upper airway abnormalities cause noises that are audible without a stethoscope, as well as gasping, retching or vomiting, and orthopnea. Two types of upper airway sounds are recognized. Stertor is a low-pitched or snoring inspiratory sound, due to a lesion located in the nasal passages, soft palate or nasopharynx. Stridor is a coarser, more raspy and higher pitch sound, that is due to a laryngeal or tracheal abnormality. Upper airway sounds may be underappreciated if the patient is enclosed in an O_2 chamber [4]. Upper airway obstruction is associated with an "obstructive" breathing pattern with the loudest sounds on inspiration (such as laryngeal paralysis). Lower airway obstruction primarily affects exhalation [5].

Rapid, shallow breathing suggests a "restrictive" breathing pattern, most compatible with lung parenchymal pathology (such as pulmonary edema, pneumonia, pulmonary fibrosis). Paradoxical respiration is characterized by asynchrony between the movement of the chest and the abdomen, more typical of pleural space disease or of respiratory muscle fatigue [6,7].

Table 8.1 Important arterial and venous oxygenation indices.

Arterial oxygenation indices	Indication	Interpretation
Alveolar-arterial O_2 gradient A-a gradient = $PAO_2 - PaO_2$ Where $PAO_2 = 150 - (PaCO_2/0.8)$	Distinguish hypoxia due to pulmonary parenchymal disease from that induced by hypoventilation; to standardize changes in oxygenation between ABG sampling at different ventilation rates; helps assess integrity of alveolar capillary unit	Normal A-a gradient <20 on room air, higher at higher FiO_2 (normal values not standardized at FiO_2 values >21%). Increased gradient occurs with right to left shunting, pulmonary embolism, ventilation/perfusion mismatch. If lack of oxygenation is proportional to low respiratory effort due to hypoventilation, then the A-a gradient is not increased. A healthy animal that hypoventilates will have hypoxia, but will have a normal A-a gradient. High CO_2 levels from hypoventilation can mask an existing high A-a gradient due to concurrent lung disease
PaO_2/FiO_2 ratio	Used to quantify severity of hypoxemia at varying percentages of inspired O_2; useful when O_2 supplementation cannot be removed during ABG sampling	Normal ratio is >400. A ratio <300 indicates moderate to severe disruption of gas exchange. A ratio <200 is suggestive of ARDS or other severe pulmonary diseases (pneumonia, pulmonary thromboembolism)
Oxygen content $CaO_2 =$ $1.34 \times Hgb \times (SaO_2/100) + [0.0031 \times PaO_2]$	Used to quantify the total O_2 content of blood	Normal = 20 mL/dL. Changes in dissolved O_2 will have much less impact on O_2 content than Hgb disturbances
Tissue O_2 delivery $DO_2 = Q \times CaO_2$ $DO_2 = (HR \times SV) \times 1.34 \times Hgb \times (SaO_2/100) + [0.0031 \times PaO_2]$ where Q = cardiac output (L/min) = HR × SV		Normal = 20–35 mL/kg/min (790 mL/min/m²). As DO_2 decreases, it eventually reaches *critical O_2 delivery* threshold (8–11 mL/kg/min)
Tissue O_2 uptake/consumption $VO_2 = Q \times (CaO_2 - CvO_2)$		Normal = 4–11 mL/kg/min (164 ml/min/m²)
Oxygen extraction ratio (OER) $OER = VO_2/DO_2$		Normal: 20–30% of delivered oxygen is taken up by tissues. Major changes in DO_2 or increases in tissue metabolic demands will increase O_2 extraction. Once DO_2 reaches *critical O2 delivery* threshold, tissue O_2 extraction is limited by insufficient DO_2. DO_2 must be improved to increase O_2 extraction and VO_2
Venous oxygenation indices **Venous O_2 saturation (SvO_2)** O_2 saturation of Hgb as it leaves the right side of the heart; central catheter with tip in pulmonary artery for ABG sample. $ScvO_2$ – central catheter with tip in right atrium for ABG sample.	Important in determining tissue O_2 extraction; provides insight into adequacy of cardiac output during critical illness	SvO_2 and $ScvO_2$ are interpreted in similar manner to monitor changes in O_2 extraction. Normal SvO_2 is 60–80% with $ScvO_2$ >70%. Low SvO_2 indicates increased O_2 extraction. High SvO_2 indicates reduced O_2 extraction (such as might occur in sepsis, carbon monoxide poisoning)

A, alveolar; a, arterial; ABG, arterial blood gas; CaO_2, oxygen content; CO_2, carbon dioxide; CV, central venous; DO_2, oxygen delivery; FiO_2, fraction of inspired oxygen; Hgb, hemoglobin; HR, heart rate; O_2, oxygen; P, partial pressure; Q, cardiac output; S, saturation; SV, stroke volume; v, venous; VO_2, tissue oxygen uptake/consumption.

Body posture can be important in assessing the severity of respiratory distress (Figure 8.2). In cats, open-mouth breathing is commonly a sign of respiratory failure or severe anxiety. In dogs, open-mouth breathing allows direct air flow through the oropharynx rather than the nasopharynx to avoid the increased airway resistance within the nasal turbinates. The neck is extended to straighten the trachea and further decrease airway resistance. Dogs tend to stand or prefer sternal recumbency, and abduct their elbows, all of which optimize thoracic compliance by avoiding compression of the expanding chest. Open-mouth breathing in dogs must be dif-ferentiated from panting secondary to hyperthermia, fear or anxiety. In panting dogs, the tidal volume is small and each breath primarily moves dead space rather than excessively ventilating the alveoli. The minute ventilation and arterial CO_2 remain normal.

During clinical evaluation, a cough should be induced by palpation and compression of the cervical trachea. The resultant cough is categorized as moist or productive, dry or hacking or honking. However, the cough in itself is not pathognomonic for any particular disease process. Differentials for an inducible cough include collapsing trachea, laryngeal and pharyngeal dysfunction, tracheitis,

Table 8.2 Common findings on physical examination reflecting respiratory distress.

Finding	Interpretation	Etiology
Altered facial structure or discharges	Possible impairment of upper airway	Neoplastic, fungal, bacterial or viral disease; in young patient may include congenital abnormalities
Decreased nasal flow	Obstruction of nasal passages or nasopharynx	Neoplastic, fungal, bacterial or viral disease, polyps and foreign object
Pale mucous membranes	Vasoconstriction or anemia	Many
Cyanotic mucous membranes	Decreased oxygen bound to hemoglobin	Altered hemoglobin (toxicity) or hemoglobin desaturation (hypoxemia). Cyanosis may not be seen if anemia is present
Red mucous membranes	Vasodilation or toxicity	Hyperthermia, systemic illness/SIRS, cyanide, CO
Tracheal auscultation	Stertor, stridor, wheezes	See Table 8.3
Thoracic auscultation – wheezes	Lower airway disease	Edema, inflammation, bronchoconstriction, or foreign material/object in lower airways
Thoracic auscultation – increased airway sounds	Nonspecific finding possibly associated with increased respiratory effort	Any airway or lung disease
Thoracic auscultation – crackles (fine or coarse)	Parenchymal or interstitial disease	Fine crackles at end inspiration may indicate fluid accumulation in alveoli and airways, e.g. pneumonia, hemorrhage (contusions), edema, infectious, ARDS, etc. Coarse crackles, often during both inspiration and expiration, may indicate airways snapping open and closing, e.g. idiopathic interstitial fibrosis
Thoracic auscultation – decreased sounds, less commonly pleural friction sounds	Pleural space disease	Pyo-, hemo-, hydro-, chylo-, pneumothorax, masses or lung torsion, diaphragmatic hernia, pleural fibrosis
Thoracic auscultation – gut sounds	Diaphragmatic hernia	Congenital or traumatic diaphragmatic hernia
Cardiac auscultation	Murmurs, gallop sounds (cats), arrhythmias	Cardiac dysfunction – structural, electrical or metabolic disease
Pulse quality	Decreased	Cardiac disease, shock, hemorrhage

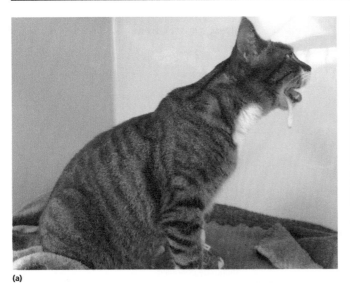
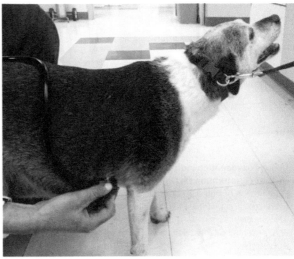

(a)   **(b)**

Figure 8.2 Orthopnea in a dog and a cat. (a) Severe dyspnea in a cat with orthopnea due to congestive heart failure. Note the open-mouth breathing, neck extension, and elbow abduction. Source: courtesy of Dr Dana Clarke. (b) Severe respiratory distress in a dog that presented with congestive heart failure. Note the extended head and neck, open mouth, standing posture, and abducted elbows.

tracheal masses, and bronchitis. A cough may also be elicited in patients with esophageal dilation (megaesophagus), esophagitis, allergic airway disease, asthma, pulmonary hemorrhage, pneumonia, heartworm infection, and pulmonary edema (dogs). Mediastinal masses, pulmonary thromboemboli, tracheobronchial lymphadenopathy, and left atrial enlargement should also be on the differential list. Patients assessed as having a potentially contagious cause of coughing should be in isolation if hospitalized. In dogs, canine infectious respiratory disease complex includes viral and bacterial agents as well as parasites, while in cats contagious diseases targeting the respiratory tract include viruses, *Mycoplasma* species, and lungworms.

A more thorough examination can be performed once life-threatening problems have been stabilized. Common physical examination findings associated with respiratory distress are listed in Table 8.3.

The temperature, pulse rate and intensity, mucous membrane color, and capillary refill time are assessed. The perfusion and hydration status are assessed. The circulatory status and severity of hypoxemia can change the mucous membrane color from pink to

Table 8.3 Physical examination changes observed with respiratory distress.

Respiratory pattern	Description	Suggested localization	Mechanism
Tachypnea	Increased respiratory rate, >12 breaths/minute	Not specific – respiratory or nonrespiratory disease	Build-up of CO_2 causes respiratory acidosis, stimulating the respiratory centers of the brain. Respiratory causes can include any airway or lung disease. Nonrespiratory causes include stress, anxiety, increased activity, drugs, pain
Panting	Open-mouth breathing with short, quick breaths, tongue out (must be distinguished from hyperventilation)	Not specific – respiratory and nonrespiratory problems	Low tidal volume per breath. Peripheral thermal receptors stimulate brain to initiate panting as an effective mechanism of heat exchange in the dog. Many causes: pain, anxiety, fear, exercise, hyperthermia, drugs, respiratory or endocrine disease
Orthopnea, shortness of breath when lying in lateral recumbency	Sternally recumbent or standing with head and neck extended, elbows abducted, open mouth	Not specific – respiratory disease	Improved ventilation perfusion matching in sternal recumbency or standing. Attempting to decrease airway resistance to air flow and optimize thoracic compliance
Stertor	Low-pitched or snoring inspiratory sound	Lesions located in nasal passages, soft palate or nasopharynx	Caused by partial obstruction of airway above the level of the larynx and by vibrations of tissue of the nasopharynx, pharynx or soft palate
Stridor	Coarser, more raspy and higher pitched sound than stertor	Laryngeal or upper tracheal pathology. Inspiratory stridor suggests larynx or cervical trachea; expiratory stridor suggests intrathoracic trachea or mainstem bronchus	Caused by turbulent air flow at or below the larynx
Restrictive	Increased rate, shallow breaths	Primarily lung parenchymal disease, some pleural space diseases	If thoracic or lung compliance is reduced increased respiratory muscle work is required to move a normal tidal volume of air into the lungs. The body compensates by decreasing the tidal volume per breath with an increase in respiratory rate
Small airway obstruction	Prolonged expiration, with abdominal push, wheezes on auscultation. Affected patients tend to have normal inhalation but active exhalation characterized by enhanced abdominal effort	Bronchitis, asthma	Obstruction and collapse of intrathoracic bronchi
Paradoxical respiration (asynchronous or dyssynchronous)	Abdomen and chest move in opposing directions. During inspiration, the thoracic cavity expands while the abdomen sucks inwards	Pleural space disease or any respiratory disease accompanied by respiratory muscle fatigue	Fatigued muscle groups may be overwhelmed by those that are less fatigued; thus, for example, inhalation may be accompanied by diaphragmatic contraction which results in expansion of the abdominal wall, but the caudal part of the thoracic wall may paradoxically collapse inwards at the same time, because of fatigue of the intercostal muscles
Weak chest wall movements	Inadequate contraction of intercostal muscles and diaphragm	Disorders affecting the brainstem, cervical spinal cord, peripheral nerves, myoneural junction, or muscular disorders	Anesthesia/sedation, severe metabolic, toxic, neurological or neuromuscular disease. Severe hypokalemia can also impair ventilation
Agonal breathing	Large gasping motions with an open mouth; patient is usually unaware of surroundings	Severe intracranial disease or impending respiratory or cardiac arrest	Originates from lower brainstem neurons as higher centers become increasingly hypoxic. Agonal respirations can produce clinically important ventilation, oxygenation, and circulation
Apneustic breathing	Deep gasping inspirations with incomplete exhalation	Damage to pons or medulla	Concurrent removal of input from the vagus nerve and pneumotaxic center causes this pattern of breathing. It is an ominous sign, with a generally poor prognosis
Ataxic breathing	Complete irregularity of breathing, with irregular pauses and increasing periods of apnea	Damage to medulla	Damage to the respiratory centers of the brainstem
Kussmaul breathing	Purposeful deep breaths at a normal or slower rate	Associated with extreme metabolic acidosis	Respiratory compensation for metabolic acidosis
Cheyne–Stokes breathing	Cyclic variations between rapid, deep breaths and apnea	Diffuse injury to the cerebral cortex or diencephalon	Instability of respiratory control and results from hyperventilation, prolonged circulation time, and reduced blood gas buffering capacity

(Continued)

Table 8.3 (*Continued*)

Respiratory pattern	Description	Suggested localization	Mechanism
Grunting with respiration	Expiratory grunt	Nonspecific; may be associated with pain, e.g. pulmonary contusions, diaphragmatic hernia, abdominal hemorrhage. Vocalization or whining may be associated with drug-induced dysphoria	Pain on movement of the respiratory muscles
Flail chest	Section of chest moving asynchronously to remainder of chest	Series of adjacent ribs are fractured in at least two places, cranially and caudally	Section of the chest wall becomes unstable and moves inwards during spontaneous inspiration. The physiological impact depends on the size of the flail segment, the intrathoracic pressure generated during spontaneous ventilation, and the associated damage to the lung and chest wall
Cough	Forceful expulsion of air. Can have variable characteristics: Moist Productive Dry Hacking Honking	Variable: may indicate upper or lower airway disease, triggered by mucosal inflammation, external compression or structural distortion or stretch of the airway	Stimulation of airway receptors triggers the afferent neural reflex, with the efferent part causing maximal inhalation, and then initial forced exhalation against a closed glottis. Concurrent bronchial smooth muscle constriction causes a milking action that also moves material towards the oropharynx

pale or white, or even to gray, purple or blue. Pale mucous membranes can occur due to peripheral vasoconstriction or anemia. Anemia decreases the O_2 content of the blood, and can also result in tachypnea. Red mucous membranes occur in animals with peripheral vasodilation or certain toxicities such as cyanide and carbon monoxide exposure. Dark mucous membranes, including those that are gray, purple or blue, indicate severe hypoxemia, termed cyanosis. Cyanosis is the presence of deoxyhemoglobin, and can only be appreciated if sufficient Hgb (>5 mg/dL) is circulating through the capillaries in the mucosa. Cyanosis is not visible in animals with severe anemia, even if they are hypoxic. Cyanosis is a late indication of respiratory dysfunction.

The entire facial structure should be evaluated, including the parts of the palate and dental arcade that can be visualized on an awake oral examination. Nasal discharge can be characterized as serous, mucoid, purulent, sanguineous, or hemorrhagic. Unilateral versus bilateral nasal patency can be assessed by holding a microscope slide in front of each external nares and observing steam upon exhalation. Discharge from the external nares can be due to intranasal or extranasal diseases. As a general rule, younger patients tend to have more infectious or congenital nasal abnormalities whereas older patients are more likely to have neoplastic, fungal or dental-related causes. Immunocompromised patients are prone to secondary bacterial or fungal infections. Hunting dogs are susceptible to inhaled foreign material such as grass or ground debris [8,9].

Auscultation of the cardiorespiratory system (including the larynx, cervical trachea, lungs, and heart while palpating peripheral pulses) can better distinguish the type and location of respiratory disease. Pathology of the conducting airways can manifest as auscultatable stridor, stertor, or wheezes. Depending on the severity of airway obstruction, these sounds can be noticeable without a stethoscope or only evident during auscultation over the trachea. Wheezes are defined as whistling or squeaky sounds, due to obstruction of lower airways, which could be caused by edema, mucus, inflammation, bronchoconstriction or a mass. True wheezes are most prominent during expiration, and are highly suggestive of lower airway disease (such as feline asthma).

Pleural space disease can be suspected if there is a decrease in audible resonance of the lung and heart sounds due to the presence of pleural fluid, air, or tissue. Dull lung sounds can be identified dorsally or ventrally; they can be focal or diffuse, unilateral or bilateral. Ventral dull sounds are more consistent with pleural fluid, whereas air tends to accumulate dorsally. Common pleural diseases include pneumothorax, pleural effusion, masses, and diaphragmatic hernia. These changes on auscultation are often difficult to distinguish in the cat, since lung sounds may be heard throughout their thorax even with pleural space disease. In large dogs, percussion of the chest wall may demonstrate dull sounds with pleural fluid and hyperresonant sounds with pleural air.

Increased bronchovesicular sounds and crackles may be heard in animals with lung parenchymal disease. However, increased or harsh lung sounds may be present in normal animals. Increased bronchovesicular sounds warrant further diagnostics for evidence of lung disease. Crackles are popping, discontinuous sounds that result from the presence of fluid in distal airways and alveoli, or alveolar/bronchial collapse and reexpansion. Crackles can be further characterized as fine end-inspiratory crackles, which confirm parenchymal disease and suggest the presence of fluid such as pulmonary edema, hemorrhage, or inflammatory exudate. This is distinct from loud crackles that can occur during any phase of the respiratory cycle, which indicate stiffening of the lower airways, occurring with bronchitis or pulmonary fibrosis. Often in the cat, the only change on auscultation is that the lung sounds are louder than normal.

An effort is made to auscultate the lungs when the patient is closed-mouth breathing to minimize large airway sounds that can mask the lower airway and lung sounds. All lung fields should be auscultated since focal disease is not uncommon. Cranioventral abnormalities tend to occur due to aspiration pneumonia, whereas perihilar, diffuse or dorsocaudal distribution can be due to cardiogenic pulmonary edema, acute respiratory distress syndrome, hemorrhage, pulmonary thromboembolism, and many other alveolar diseases [5].

Respiratory distress can also be a result of cardiovascular or hematological disorders that can impair oxygen delivery (DO_2). The heart should be auscultated for at least 60 seconds while simultaneously palpating the peripheral pulses. The presence of a murmur, gallop rhythm or arrhythmia warrants further diagnostics for heart failure as a cause of or contributor to labored breathing. Cats are more difficult to diagnose with congestive heart failure on physical examination since they may only have an intermittent murmur or arrhythmia. In cats, an audible gallop rhythm may be the only cardiac abnormality heard. In both dogs and cats, pulse quality may be decreased in the presence of cardiovascular disease, but is often normal in animals with respiratory system disease [10].

The neurological examination is done to evaluate for evidence of cervical or thoracic spinal lesions or brain abnormalities that could affect the control of ventilation. The respiratory centers are located in the brainstem and disease in this area can cause an abnormal depth or rate of breathing (see Table 8.2).

Careful palpation of the abdomen is done to identify any abdominal masses, effusions or gastric distension that could impair ventilation by increasing the intraabdominal pressure and restricting the movement of the diaphragm. In addition, many intraabdominal diseases can be complicated by secondary respiratory distress (such as peritonitis with acute respiratory distress syndrome (ARDS) or acute lung injury (ALI), gastrointestinal (GI) foreign body with aspiration pneumonia or gastric dilation-volvulus with impaired ventilation).

Point of Care testing

The initial POC testing begins with the collection of samples for the packed cell volume (PCV), total protein (TP), blood urea nitrogen (BUN), glucose, electrolytes, venous blood gas, coagulation profile, urinalysis (UA), and cytology of any collected pleural fluid or respiratory tract secretions. When the patient can tolerate the procedure, arterial blood is sampled for an arterial blood gas (ABG). The technique for collecting an arterial sample is outlined in Box 8.1.

Hemoconcentration may indicate dehydration, common with open-mouth breathing, profuse nasal discharge, severe pulmonary edema or pleural effusion. Anemia (low PCV) can be a cause of hypoxemia or a consequence of pleural or pulmonary hemorrhage. Hypoproteinemia (low TP) can be present due to albumin loss and is of concern due to loss of pulmonary capillary colloidal osmotic pressure during fluid therapy (see Chapter 4).

Box 8.1 Procedure for collecting an arterial blood gas.

1. Clip and aseptically clean the site over the artery to be used.
2. Use a preheparinized or lithium heparin coated 1 mL syringe.
3. Use a small (25 gauge) needle.
4. Hold needle at 30–45° angle to the artery over strongest pulse.
5. Palpate artery with nondominant hand.
6. Advance needle slowly toward palpated pulse with dominant hand.
7. Entering the artery, a blood flash is seen in the needle hub.
8. Aspirate sample gently if using standard syringe or allow auto-filling if using arterial blood sampling syringe.
9. Remove needle from artery and apply direct pressure over site, applying tight bandage for 5–10 minutes.
10. Tap any air from the syringe and cap syringe to prevent blood exposure to room air.
11. Transport to laboratory on ice or run sample immediately.

The BUN is evaluated in conjunction with the specific gravity of the urine for the initial assessment of renal function. Uremic pneumonitis and oliguric or anuric renal failure can each affect the fluid balance in the lungs and result in pulmonary edema (see Chapter 13). Prolongation of coagulation times can be associated with lung parenchymal or pleural hemorrhage. A hypercoagulable state can result in pulmonary thromboembolic disease (see Chapter 9).

Venous blood gas analysis

Venous blood gas analysis is performed to assess ventilation and for monitoring acid–base status. Venous samples are collected by direct venipuncture or through a peripherally or centrally placed catheter. Common sites include the saphenous, cephalic, and jugular veins [11]. The sample is collected and handled similar to an arterial sample (see Box 8.1).

If the patient's hemodynamic status is fairly normal, the pH and PCO_2 of venous blood is similar to arterial [12]. In normal animals, the partial pressure of venous CO_2 ($PvCO_2$) is equal to the tissue PCO_2, and is only 3–5 mmHg higher than the partial pressure of arterial CO_2 ($PaCO_2$) [13]. The venous partial pressure of O_2 (PvO_2) should be much lower than and does not correlate with PaO_2. Typically (in normal dogs breathing room air), jugular PvO_2 is 45–65 mmHg and cephalic PvO_2 is 49–67 mmHg [14]. Elevated PvO_2 is related to decreased tissue O_2 extraction, usually due to increased O_2 delivery, decreased O_2 demand, or high flow states [14]. Trends in PvO_2 can be monitored to document the efficacy of hemodynamic resuscitation.

Arterial blood gas analysis

Arterial blood gas analysis provides invaluable and specific data regarding the patient's respiratory status. The PaO_2 and $PaCO_2$ are directly measured. ABG analysis is the gold standard for the diagnosis for respiratory failure, allows quantitation of the severity of disease, and sometimes even allows categorization of the type of respiratory dysfunction. In addition, the ABG provides information regarding the patient's acid–base status [15]. As a general rule, ABG analysis should be performed in dogs exhibiting clinical signs of respiratory failure to assess the severity and cause of signs. However, clinical judgment is required since restraint is needed for sample collection. This test is difficult to perform in cats and is not usually ordered in awake cats.

Arterial blood can be sampled by direct puncture of an artery or using an indwelling arterial catheter. The most common artery used is the dorsal pedal artery (Figure 8.3), but other options include the femoral, auricular, and coccygeal arteries [11]. The sublingual artery can be sampled in anesthetized patients. The method of collection is outlined in Box 8.1. The sample should be run as soon as possible or placed on ice to stop ongoing cell metabolism for transport to a laboratory [16]. Samples should be analyzed within two hours of being obtained. If the PaO_2 is low, it may be difficult to determine whether a sample is arterial or inadvertently obtained venous blood. A known venous sample can be obtained for comparison.

Arterial catheter placement requires a similar technique to puncture the artery. Standard "over-the-needle" peripheral venous catheters can be used, or specialized arterial lines can be placed using the Seldinger technique. Once the catheter is taped in place, it can be capped or attached to a pressure transducer for continuous monitoring of arterial blood pressure (see Chapter 3). Blood samples can be obtained from the catheter using the three-syringe technique, by first withdrawing a "pre-sample" of at least 2 ml of blood mixed with saline, that will be injected back into a venous catheter. Then the actual sample for analysis is withdrawn and the catheter flushed (see Box 10.2). Most modern ABG analyzers require <0.5 ml of blood.

In respiratory patients, ABGs should not be sampled until a steady state has been achieved after ventilator settings have been changed or oxygen supplementation has been started. Typically this requires about 5–10 minutes, but some patients with chronic airway disease may require longer equilibration times.

Guidelines for the interpretation of the respiratory components of the ABG are provided in Table 8.4, with two separate but interconnected values evaluated: PaO_2 and $PaCO_2$. The CO_2 is

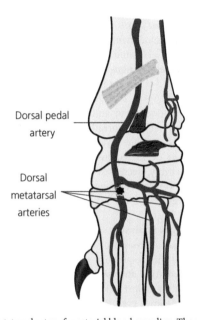

Figure 8.3 Metatarsal artery for arterial blood sampling. The dorsal aspect of the left tarsus is shown with the major regional arterial supply. The most common vessel used for arterial puncture or catheterization is the metatarsal artery, located distal to the dorsal pedal artery between the third and fourth metatarsal bones.

Dorsal pedal artery

Dorsal metatarsal arteries

readily diffusible (about 20 times more diffusible than O_2), therefore the arterial CO_2 ($PaCO_2$) is directly proportional to the minute ventilation. Changes in CO_2 cause predictable alterations in plasma pH; severe changes result in enzymatic and cellular disturbances, potentially leading to life-threatening conditions and even death (see Chapter 7).

Hypercapnia is an elevated $PaCO_2$ and is almost always caused by inadequate ventilation, although on rare occasions it can be caused by severe pulmonary parenchymal disease. Considerations for the cause of ventilatory failure include depressed brainstem function (such as during anesthesia), neuromuscular dysfunction (including electrolyte abnormalities), upper airway obstruction, and respiratory muscle fatigue. The accumulation of CO_2 results in respiratory acidosis. Elevated CO_2 levels are not well tolerated, with $PaCO_2$ values >50 mmHg significant and prompting intervention. $PaCO_2$ values >70 mmHg can quickly lead to life-threatening consequences, such as vasodilation and central nervous system abnormalities (including coma and death) [17]. Immediate intervention requires establishing an airway and providing positive pressure ventilation if the underlying cause cannot be identified and immediately treated [18].

Low $PaCO_2$ values (hypocapnia) occur due to hyperventilation, a rather common physical manifestation of respiratory compromise, anxiety or pain. However, when severe, the hypoxemia caused by pulmonary dysfunction can take over the previously CO_2 driven respiratory control of the brainstem and result in hypocapnia [19].

The PaO_2, representing the O_2 dissolved in plasma, defines the amount of O_2 that can bind to Hgb, therefore the PaO_2 controls the amount of Hgb that is saturated with O_2 (SaO_2). The relationship between the PaO_2 and Hgb-O_2 saturation is represented by a sigmoid curve (see Figure 8.1). As PaO_2 values increase, the SaO_2 rises rapidly and plateaus when the PaO_2 is around 60 mmHg. PaO_2 is the most important determinant of SaO_2, but other variables can cause a shift in the curve. A rise in body temperature, $PaCO_2$, and level of 2,3-DPG in the blood all cause the curve to shift to the right. This reflects a decrease in Hgb O_2 affinity and results in improved release of O_2 to the tissues. A decrease in these variables produces the opposite effect. A $PaO_2 < 80$ mmHg is considered hypoxemic and corresponds with SaO_2 around 93%. Severe hypoxemia is defined as a $PaO_2 < 60$ mmHg. Hypoxic patients require further

Table 8.4 Interpretation of arterial blood gas results.

ABG Value	Interpretation	Effect	Intervention
PaCO₂			
32–43 mmHg (dog)*	Normal	N/A	None
26–36 mmHg (cat)*	Normal		
<32 mmHg (dog)	Hyperventilation	Loss of respiratory drive, respiratory alkalosis, vasoconstriction	Treat underlying disease; alleviate pain, anxiety
<26 mmHg (cat)			
>43 mmHg (dog)	Inadequate ventilation	Respiratory acidosis, vasodilation, coma, death	Identify and treat underlying cause. Intubation and manual or mechanical ventilation if underlying cause cannot be treated
>36 mmHg (cat)			
PaO₂			
80–105 mmHg (dog)*	Must be interpreted based on oxygen supplementation levels	N/A	None
95–115 mmHg (cat)*			
<80 mmHg	Hypoxemia	Poor oxygen delivery to tissues	Oxygen supplementation, or mechanical ventilation
<60 mmHg	Severe hypoxemia		
>100 mmHg	Usually due to oxygen supplementation	Increased likelihood of oxygen toxicity	Discontinue or taper oxygen therapy

* Normal values may vary between laboratory equipment. ABG, arterial blood gas.

investigation of the cause as well as immediate oxygen support and possibly ventilation [2].

Clinicopathological testing

A complete blood count (CBC) and serum biochemical profile should be performed in animals with problems affecting ventilation and oxygenation. An inflammatory leukogram could be compatible with pneumonia, ALI or ARDS as a cause of respiratory failure. The serum creatinine is assessed with the BUN and urinalysis results for evidence of renal disease, with consequences potentially affecting the respiratory tract (see Chapter 13). When pulmonary thromboemboli are suspected, adrenocorticotropic hormone (ACTH) stimulation testing for hyperadrenocorticism, a urine protein:creatinine ratio for glomerular disease, and thromboelastography (TEG) to define the coagulation status can be requested. The Baermann fecal examination is a method used to determine if there are Strongyloides or Aelurostrongylus species of lungworms present.

Several techniques are available to collect samples from the respiratory system to diagnose the underlying etiology. Endotracheal wash, transtracheal wash, bronchoscopic brush, and bronchoalveolar lavage samples can all be collected with fluid or cytology samples sent for laboratory analysis. The cytology of collected fluid is examined for evidence of infectious organisms (fungal infections, bacteria, and parasites) and to classify the disease process (inflammatory, neoplastic). Samples can also be sent for aerobic culture and susceptibility as well as the polymerase chain reaction (PCR) diagnosis of many infectious diseases.

Radiographic, fluoroscopic or ultrasound-guided aspiration of abnormal lung tissue is another way of collecting samples. There is risk of iatrogenic hemorrhage and pneumothorax with this procedure, but the procedure can be well tolerated in many patients. Collected samples may be useful for cytological analysis and culture and susceptibility testing.

A variety of fungal species can infect the pulmonary system in dogs and cats. Fungal antigen and antibody tests are available, requiring relatively noninvasive procedures to collect samples. Reported sensitivity of the urine antigen test for detection of blastomycosis in dogs is as high as 93.5%, and considered more sensitive than serum antibody tests. This urine test can also be used as a tool to monitor clinical remission [20,21]. Other fungal organisms, such as Coccidioides, require serum antibody testing or identification of the organism in collected samples [22].

Diagnostic imaging

Diagnostic imaging is used in the stabilized patient to define the underlying cause of any respiratory failure and, under some circumstances, to demonstrate progression or resolution of the disease over time. Imaging begins with survey thoracic radiographs and can incorporate ultrasound, bronchoscopy, fluoroscopy, and computed tomography (CT) scans.

Thoracic radiographs

Survey thoracic radiographs are done only when the animal can tolerate positioning. Lateral and ventrodorsal positioning is ideal but may not be tolerated by a dyspneic patient. Dorsoventral and standing lateral positioning may be all that can be done in the fragile patient. The integrity of the ribs, spine, and diaphragm are examined for evidence of problems that might impair ventilation. This is followed by an assessment of the lung parenchyma, pleural space, pulmonary vasculature, and mediastinal structures.

The presence of pulmonary interstitial patterns, air bronchograms or intrapulmonary nodules suggests lung parenchymal pathology. A caudodorsal distribution is compatible with etiologies such as neurogenic pulmonary edema or hematogenous pneumonia. A ventral distribution, often isolated to the right middle lung lobe, is suggestive of aspiration pneumonia. Bronchiolar markings indicate an infiltrate around the bronchi, commonly noted with bronchial inflammation or edema (such as with bronchitis or asthma). Hyperinflation of the lungs and flattening of the diaphragm may be seen with feline asthma. Lung atelectasis or torsion will often cause the appearance of a consolidated lung lobe with shifting of the cardiac silhouette. The pleural space is evaluated for the presence of fluid, air, masses or herniated abdominal organs. Pleural space problems can result in inability to follow the pulmonary vasculature out to the thoracic wall.

The pulmonary vasculature is examined, with venous distension potentially due to congestion from heart failure. The loss of radiographic evidence of pulmonary vasculature (lucency) in a lung lobe of a hypoxic animal can suggest a pulmonary thromboembolism. Tortuous pulmonary vasculature can be seen with heartworm disease.

The mediastinum and its structures are also examined, to include the heart shape, size and positioning, the size and patency of the esophagus, the size of the vena cava, tracheal positioning and patency, the location and positioning of the bifurcation of the mainstem bronchi, any discernible lymph nodes or thymus, and any mass lesions. A pneumomediastinum is suspected when the borders of most of the mediastinal structure are highly visible. Severe aerophagia can impede ventilation and is evidenced by an enlarged gas-filled stomach, with air often distending the esophagus, as well.

Fluoroscopy can be done to assess the large airways for stricture or collapse during breathing. It can also be used to guide needle placement for a lung aspirate.

Ultrasound examination

Echocardiography can be done to evaluate the contribution that the heart may make to respiratory failure. Abdominal ultrasound can be used to identify any abnormal size, shape, and position of abdominal organs that might affect oxygenation and ventilation.

Point of care ultrasound examination of patients with respiratory compromise has been gaining popularity due to the wide availability of ultrasound and the noninvasive nature of the examination. The thoracic focused assessment with sonography technique (TFAST) has developed, enabling cage-side ultrasonograpic examination [23]. The TFAST consists of the examination of five sites on the patient.

- Sites 1 and 2 – the chest tube sites (CTS), located between the eighth and ninth ribs (bilaterally) dorsal to the costochrondral junction at the level of the xiphoid (where a chest tube would be placed).
- Sites 3 and 4 – the pericardial sites (PCS), located between the third and fourth intercostal spaces (bilaterally) at the level of the heart.
- Site 5 – the diaphragmatic site (DH), which is located at the ventral midline just caudal to the xiphoid, directed toward the thoracic cavity through the diaphragm.

Findings that can be significant at these locations are summarized in Table 8.5, with additional references provided under Further reading.

Table 8.5 Ultrasound findings in the thoracic cavity using thoracic focused assessment with sonography technique (TFAST) and the Veterinary Bedside Lung Exam (VetBLUE) [24].*

Ultrasound finding	Description	Interpretation
TFAST signs		
Gator sign	Two rib heads ("gator eyes") and associated intercostal space; the brightest line between the rib head represents the pulmonary pleural interface ("bridge of gator nose")	Normal finding
Glide sign	Back and forth motion of the pulmonary pleural interface	Rules out pneumothorax
Ultrasound lung rockets	Previously called comet tails and B-lines, these are points of interface between fluid and air. They are "laser-like" hyperechoic lines that do not "fade" with distance, move back and forth with respirations and originate at the pulmonary pleural interface	Consistent with intraparenchymal fluid (such as edema or contusions), indicates "wet lung"
Step sign	A disruption or step of the normal pulmonary pleural interface	Thoracic wall injury; can also be seen with masses, hematoma, diaphragmatic hernia and pleural effusion
VetBLUE signs		
Dry lung	Glide sign with A lines (bright reverberations of the pulmonary pleural interface)	Normal
Wet lung	Ultrasound lung rockets or B lines, moving back and forth with respirations	Fluid within the lung parenchyma (cardiogenic and noncardiogenic edema, pneumonia, contusions, etc.)
Shred signs	Variable echogenicity with focal hyperechoic regions within poorly echogenic tissue; also referred to as "dirty shadowing"	Significant consolidation of lungs from edema, contusions, pneumonia, torsion, etc.
Tissue sign	Lung tissue is easily visualized, lack of aerated lung, "hepatized lung"	Complete lack of aerated lung; consolidation, torsion
Nodule sign	Well-delineated, focal structure, surrounded by normal or abnormal lung	Mass

* Depth should be set to 4–6cm and frequency to 5–10MHz. VetBLUE, Veterinary bedside lung exam.

The Veterinary Bedside Lung Exam (VetBLUE) is a focused and more detailed ultrasound technique that can be used to evaluate the thoracic cavity in patients with respiratory distress [24]. It requires the examination of four bilateral anatomical sites over the thoracic cavity:

- the caudal lung lobe region between the eighth and ninth intercostal space (bilaterally)
- the perihilar lung lobe region between the sixth and seventh intercostal space (bilaterally)
- the middle lung lobe region, between the fourth and fifth intercostal space (generally over the heart)
- the cranial lung lobe region between the second and third intercostal space (bilaterally).

Findings of the VetBLUE examination are also summarized in Table 8.5 with additional references provided under Further reading.

Bronchoscopy/bronchoalveoar lavage

Bronchoscopy can help define a variety of conditions associated with the larger airways, remove foreign obstructive objects, and assist in the collection of airway samples to help define the underlying etiology. General anesthesia is required and real-time visualization of the airways is possible as the patient ventilates. Samples collected by brushing or lavage of the bronchi can be submitted for cytology, PCR testing, and aerobic culture and susceptibility. Small biopsies of nodules or masses in the airway can be collected for histopathology.

Computed tomography

Computed tomography (CT) has increased the ability to image the pulmonary system and thoracic cavity and also the sensitivity for detecting pulmonary nodules [25]. The CT scan performed with intravenous contrast angiography can demonstrate pulmonary thrombi that are not visible by survey radiography or ultrasonography.

Monitoring procedures

A full physical examination is performed at least twice daily using a systematic approach to appreciate both initial abnormalities and subtle changes. It is important to thoroughly observe, palpate, and auscultate the entire respiratory system, from the nares to the thoracic cavity. However, many physical abnormalities (such as cyanosis) cannot be detected on a physical examination until disease is severe enough to be life threatening. Therefore, any change in the patient's respiratory pattern or auscultation findings should prompt immediate testing of the oxygenation and ventilation.

The Rule of 20 is used to assess the patient at least twice daily. Blood pressure, electrocardiogram (ECG), and physical perfusion parameters provide a minimum for evaluating the cardiovascular status. Fluid, electrolyte, and acid–base balance are of major concern since loss of free water through the respiratory tract occurs with tachypnea, profuse nasal discharge, nasal, endotracheal or tracheal O_2 supplementation, and positive pressure ventilation. Monitoring fluid balance becomes more difficult. Monitoring the pressure or diameter changes in the caudal vena cava as a reflection of central fluid volume can be misleading in light of the effects of pneumothorax or positive pressure ventilation (PPV) on the intrathoracic and vena caval pressures. Body weight and physical perfusion and hydration parameters become even more important. Placing a urinary catheter allows better patient hygiene and an assessment of urinary output. Body weight, albumin levels, and body condition scoring can aid in assessing the nutritional status of the patient (see Chapter 16)

The ABG provides the most direct method of monitoring the PaO_2 and $PaCO_2$ that results from the oxygenation and ventilatory efforts of the animal. Intubated patients with respiratory failure should have an ABG performed within 10–15 minutes of intubation. In mechanically ventilated patients, ABG analysis should be performed approximately every 4–6 hours or any time the patient's respiratory status or ventilator settings change significantly. Less invasive monitoring, such as end-tidal CO_2 (ETCO$_2$) and pulse oximetry (SpO$_2$), should be performed simultaneously with the ABG. If the results of ETCO$_2$ and SpO$_2$ are valid based on the ABG values, these can be substituted and provide continuous real-time data, thereby allowing a decrease in frequency of ABG testing and avoiding unnecessary blood collection.

Pulse oximetry

Pulse oximetry is a noninvasive tool that provides rapid, continuous assessment of oxygenation, allowing detection of minor changes in respiratory status [26]. The pulse oximeter uses both oximetry and plethysmography. Oximetry (measurement of the saturation of Hgb with O_2 (SaO$_2$)) is determined through spectrophotometry. The Beer–Lambert law states that all atoms absorb specific wavelengths of light, which coincides with the concentration of the substance being measured. This principle is used to measure the concentration of oxygenated Hgb in blood, which absorbs red light at a wavelength of about 660 nm, and deoxygenated Hgb, which absorbs infrared light at a wavelength of 940 nm [27]. The pulse oximeter measures light absorption using two light-emitting diodes (660 nm and 940 nm) on one side of the tissue bed and two photodectors on the other. The two photodetectors quantify the transmitted light and calculate the concentration of oxyhemoglobin and deoxyhemoglobin. Oxygenated Hgb is then expressed as a percentage (SpO$_2$). Phlethysmography identifies only arterial pulsatile flow characteristics, distinguishing flow from nonarterial blood. Many pulse oximeters display the pulse rate but also an image of the pulsatile waveform. This can be used for continuous monitoring of heart rate and to confirm the accuracy of the SpO$_2$ reading as well as the strength of the signal (Figure 8.4) [28].

The results from the pulse oximeter have been validated in both canine and feline patients. Normal SpO$_2$ should be greater than 95%, bearing in mind that this may correlate with PaO$_2$ values as low as 70 mmHg (see Figure 8.1). Valid SpO$_2$ values of 91–94% indicate significant hypoxemia that may require intervention. Valid SpO$_2$ values <90% indicate potentially life-threatening hypoxemia

that should be managed by O_2 supplementation or positive pressure ventilation [29,30].

Two main sensors are used in veterinary medicine: transmittance probes, detecting light that passes through the tissue, and reflectance probes, wherein the sensor is placed flat against a tissue. The lingual sensor can be placed on the tongue in sedated or anesthetized patients, or on the outer pinna, lips, prepuce, vulva, toe webbing, or Achilles tendon of awake patients. Wetting and parting or clipping the fur will increase skin contact. When using the lingual sensor, frequent repositioning may be necessary to avoid decreased blood flow due to compression, and tissue dessication can be avoided by placing a wet gauze square between the tongue and the probe. The reflectance probe is a linear probe that is used on the ventral base of the tail (not into the rectum). This type of probe has also been used with success directly over arteries, such as the femoral artery, pedal arteries, on the palmar aspect of the feet, proximal to the carpal or tarsal pad and in the rectum, facing the caudal abdominal aorta. Lubricant does not alter SpO$_2$ readings [31].

Following application of the probe, there is a 10–15 second delay before a reading is obtained because the signal is averaged. Mild to moderately hypoxemic patients may still be on the plateau of the O_2 Hgb dissociation curve where the PaO$_2$ can decrease significantly with little change in the SpO$_2$ reading. In addition, the quality of the signal can significantly alter the accuracy of SpO$_2$ readings, with factors such as motion, skin pigmentation, and anemia affecting the SpO$_2$ result. A list of common causes of inaccurate pulse oximetry readings is given in Table 8.6.

Of note, the concentration of oxygen in arterial blood (CaO$_2$) in anemic animals may be low even if the SpO$_2$ is normal. SpO$_2$ values may be 98–100% in patients receiving O_2 supplementation, regardless of whether the PaO$_2$ is 100 mmHg or 500 mmHg [2]. Therefore, it is necessary to measure PaO$_2$ to assess lung function in these patients. The pulse oximeter does not provide quantitative data regarding ventilation as it provides no measurement of PaCO$_2$ [32].

Continuous pulse oximetry is recommended in sedated or anesthetized patients, including those on ventilators. In awake patients,

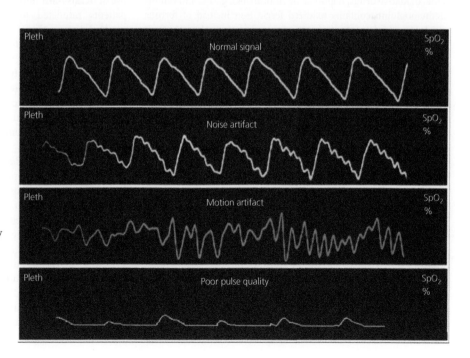

Figure 8.4 The pulsatile oximetry signal (SpO$_2$) is a unitless waveform displayed on certain pulse oximeter devices which directly corresponds with the pulse quality at the probe site. Normal signal showing the sharp waveform. Pulsatile signal with superimposed noise artifact gives a jagged appearance. Motion artifact is represented by an erratic waveform. Pulsatile signal during low perfusion shows a much flatter sine wave.

Table 8.6 Artifacts which alter pulse oximeter readings.

Artifact	Due to
Motion artifact/inability to read pulsatile flow	Shivering, twitching, panting, seizures, ambulation
Inability to read pulsatile flow	Vasoconstriction from medications or shock, hypothermia, shock or peripheral hypoperfusion (thrombus)
Skin pigmentation or disease	Inability of light to pass through
Carboxyhemoglobin	Interpreted as hemoglobin; falsely elevates SpO_2
Methemoglobin	Causes a static SpO_2 reading of around 85% regardless of PaO_2 level
Anemia, when severe (packed cell volume <15)	Erroneously low readings
Ambient (especially infrared heating) lighting	Falsely elevated as signal is picked up by photodetector
Maximum value of SpO_2 (100%)	Regardless of PaO_2

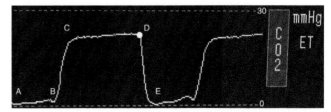

Figure 8.5 A normal capnograph tracing throughout the respiratory cycle. Labels A–B represent a zero baseline because the air passing at the beginning of expiration is from dead space, and therefore does not contain any CO_2. Labels B–C show a sharp increase in CO_2 corresponding with expired gas that is coming from lung units participating in gas exchange mixed with dead space air. Labels C–D is the plateau that corresponds with the latter part of expiration, in which all of the air is coming from ventilated lung units. Labels D–E show a sharp decline, which represents the beginning of inspiration and is devoid of carbon dioxide.

intermittent measurements are indicated on a scheduled timetable or when pertinent clinical signs change. Frequent evaluation of SpO_2 aids in quantification of response to therapy and can provide early detection of deterioration, facilitating intervention.

Other oximeters

While traditional pulse oximeters only measure deoxyhemoglobin and oxyhemoglobin, the co-oximeter also measures methemoglobin and carboxyhemoglobin by using additional wavelengths of light. Smoke inhalation is the most common cause of carboxyhemoglobinemia, which is a stable complex of carbon monoxide (CO) and Hgb. CO has a much higher affinity for Hgb than O_2 (about 200 times), and accumulation of carboxyhemoglobin prevents adequate tissue DO_2.

Exposure to certain intoxicants can cause methemoglobinemia, including acetaminophen, local anesthetics, nitrates, nitrites, nitroglycerin, nitroprusside, certain antibiotics (sulfonamides), benzocaine, oxidative drugs, naphthalene (mothballs), garlic, and onions. Methemoglobin contains oxidized ferric iron instead of ferrous, which has a higher affinity for O_2, thus preventing release of O_2 in tissues. There is normally less than 2% methemoglobin in healthy patients, and it is converted back to Hgb by nicotinamide adenine dinucleotide (NADH)-dependent methemoglobin reductase [33]. Higher concentration of CO or methemoglobin warrants an investigation of cause and specific therapeutic intervention.

A large amount of research has been performed evaluating the benefit of monitoring tissue oxygenation levels (StO_2) with near infrared spectroscopy (NIRS). Oxygen must diffuse down its concentration gradient into the tissues, typically making StO_2 much lower than arterial oxygen levels. Monitoring the StO_2 shows promise for the clinical monitoring of tissue oxygenation in the future [34,35].

Capnography

Capnography uses infrared spectrophotometry to measure the CO_2 level in expired air. By emitting a constant infrared beam from a phototransmitter and detecting absorption on the other side of the sampling compartment, the device continuously quantitates CO_2 during the respiratory cycle. There are two main types of capnographs: sidestream and mainstream. Sidestream devices aspirate air into a side chamber on the instrument for CO_2 measurement, which

can cause a slight delay in the reading and increase dead space, especially in smaller patients. If the aspirated air contains inhalants, it must be returned to the anesthetic machine circuit for safety reasons. Mainstream instruments attach directly onto the endotracheal tube and directly measure CO_2 as exhaled air flows through the device [36].

Because CO_2 is approximately 20 times more rapidly diffusible than O_2, alveolar CO_2 is almost identical to the PCO_2 in the pulmonary capillaries. Alveolar CO_2 is exhaled at the end of each breath ($ETCO_2$), and when measured it can be used as an indirect estimation of PCO_2; there is a small amount of blood shunted (e.g. through bronchiole arterioles and coronary artery) that bypasses the lungs without being oxygenated, accounting for a $ETCO_2$-$PaCO_2$ difference of up to 5 mmHg. The capnograph produces a waveform and numerical display of CO_2 throughout the respiratory cycle (Figure 8.5). The plateau CO_2 level is reported by the instrument as the $ETCO_2$ [37].

End-tidal CO_2 is commonly used as a surrogate for the $PvCO_2$, but variability of the gradient between $ETCO_2$ and PCO_2 makes the use of trends most informative. The capnograph is typically used in patients intubated for an anesthetic event, cardiopulmonary cerebral resuscitation (CPCR), or positive pressure ventilation. The normal $ETCO_2$ range for dogs and cats is 35–45 mmHg. Values greater than 50 mmHg indicate hypercapnia and hypoventilation; those less than 30 mmHg may indicate hyperventilation. A sudden decline in the $ETCO_2$ towards zero may indicate a leak in the ventilator circuit, airway occlusion, severe pulmonary thromboembolism, or cardiopulmonary arrest (CPA). It can help to troubleshoot endotracheal tube placement, as the $ETCO_2$ will be zero if the tube is in the esophagus.

End-tidal CO_2 is influenced by several factors, especially problems that affect the ventilation-perfusion relationship within the lung. Decreased perfusion of alveolar units results in lower concentration of CO_2 in those alveoli. If these alveoli are ventilated, dead space air from the underperfused alveoli mixes with air from perfused alveoli, and the $ETCO_2$ decreases, creating a gradient between PCO_2 and $ETCO_2$. In addition, tachypnea and panting cause decreases in $ETCO_2$ due to mixing of gases within the sampling chamber. Hyperventilation (during anesthesia or CPR) will cause a falsely decreased $ETCO_2$ reading, requiring ventilation to remain fairly constant to obtain a significant reading. Sidestream capnographs aspirate 50–100 mL/min from the circuit, which may require adjustment of minute ventilation, especially in smaller patients.

Capnography is used extensively in ventilated patients because it provides continuous, real-time readings that can be used for ventilator setting adjustment. It can be used to measure dead space using the dead space to tidal volume ratio (VD/VT), which is determined partly from $ETCO_2$ where: $VD/VT = (PaCO_2 - P$ end-tidal $CO_2)/PaCO_2$. This ratio can provide information regarding the presence of V/Q mismatch.

Capnography can also be used to monitor patients with tracheostomy tubes, as well as those that are spontaneously breathing. A sidestream capnograph can be used in combination with a nasal cannula to monitor $ETCO_2$ in the awake, nontachypneic, nonintubated patient [38].

Capnography is an invaluable tool for early detection of apnea and CPA, and is now standard of care for intubated critically ill patients [39]. During a CPA event, the capnograph tracing rapidly becomes zero before the decline of other monitored parameters such as O_2 saturation and electrocardiography. Upon initial intubation during initiation of CPR, the $ETCO_2$ may be elevated due to respiratory failure or zero due to decreased cardiac output. $ETCO_2$ measurement during CPR is directly correlated with efficacy of ventilation and with coronary blood flow [40]. $ETCO_2$ values near zero may indicate esophageal intubation; values greater than 15 during CPR in dogs appear to be predictive of a better outcome [41]. $ETCO_2$ values will rise with an increase in cardiac output and during the return of spontaneous circulation [42].

Disorders of oxygenation and ventilation

Four types of hypoxia have been described:

- hypoxemic hypoxia is caused by a fall in the PaO_2 in the bloodstream and is caused primarily by disorders of respiration
- histotoxic hypoxia occurs when the quantity of oxygen reaching the cells is normal, but the cells cannot use it effectively (such as cyanide poisoning)
- circulatory hypoxia occurs when blood flow to a part of the body is insufficient, making O_2 insufficient
- anemic hypoxia, where the PaO_2 is normal but total oxygen content of the blood is reduced due to the inadequate amount of hemoglobin to carry oxygen to the tissues.

Problems at any location within the respiratory tract or problems involving the neuromuscular control of breathing can cause hypoxemic hypoxia and be a major contributor to patient morbidity and mortality.

The five main causes of hypoxemic hypoxia (Table 8.7) are: hypoventilation, decreased inspired O_2, V/Q mismatch with dead space ventilation (V/Q <1), V/Q mismatch with intrapulmonary shunting (V/Q >1), and diffusion impairment.

Hypoventilation is the delivery of a low volume of inspired air to the alveoli. The $PaCO_2$ is always elevated. Failure of alveolar ventilation also results in a proportional drop in PaO_2. Supplemental O_2 often results in improvement of the PaO_2 to normal because it increases the percentage O_2 within the alveoli. However, O_2 supplementation does not change the volume of O_2 being delivered, which is dependent on the minute ventilation (breaths per minute). Treating hypoventilation (the underlying cause of hypoxemia) may include the reversal of sedation, removal of an upper airway obstruction, or positive pressure ventilation to treat respiratory muscle fatigue or paralysis.

Decreased inspired O_2 is an uncommon cause of hypoxemia at sea level. At altitude, there are fewer O_2 molecules in inhaled air because barometric pressure is lower causing a lower partial pressure of inhaled O_2. At sea level, decreased O_2 in inspired air occurs if there is a problem with the supply of O_2 during anesthesia or while in an enclosed area (such as oxygen cages with insufficient flow, house fires). Patients may compensate by increasing their respiratory rate and can have a low $PaCO_2$ in combination with low PaO_2. As long as there are no irreversible effects of the hypoxemia, this type of hypoxemia can be fully corrected with supplemental O_2.

Ventilation-perfusion mismatch disturbs gas exchange at the capillary-alveolar interface. Normally, ventilation of alveolar units slightly exceeds capillary blood flow, causing the V/Q ratio to be greater than 1.0 [2]. V/Q mismatch causes hypoxemia before it causes hypercapnia, primarily because CO_2 is so much more diffusible than O_2. There are two main reasons for V/Q imbalance: *dead space ventilation* and *intrapulmonary shunting*, both of which are seen in animals with lung disease. Patients with V/Q mismatch compensate for hypoxemia by elevating their respiratory rate. This increases the energy required for breathing, but fails to improve oxygenation. In patients with V/Q mismatch, oxygen supplementation should result in improved PaO_2. V/Q mismatch is the most common reason for poor oxygen delivery to tissues for a variety of etiologies.

Dead space ventilation is defined as areas of the respiratory system that do not participate in gas exchange. Anatomical dead space refers to the conducting airways, where there are no respiratory units and thus no possibility of exposure to capillary blood for gas exchange. A large amount of this dead space occurs in the pharynx, while the oral cavity, trachea, and large bronchi make

Table 8.7 Causes of hypoxemic hypoxia.

Etiology	Examples	Response to oxygen
Decreased inspired concentration of oxygen (FiO_2)	Decreased fresh gas flow, enclosed space, house fire	
Decreased inspired O_2 because of low barometric pressure	High altitude	Return to normal
Hypoventilation	Sedation/anesthesia, airway obstruction, neuromuscular disease, hypoglycemia, hypokalemia	Often improves PaO_2, depending on severity and cause
Ventilation/perfusion (V/Q) mismatch >1	Dead space ventilation: pulmonary thrombus, decreased cardiac output, alveolar overdistension	Usually improves PaO_2
Ventilation/perfusion (V/Q) mismatch <1	Shunting of blood past nonaerated tissue: all forms of alveolar/lower airway disease and anatomical shunts	All but a true anatomical shunt or complete mismatch (V/Q = 0) respond to oxygen
Diffusion impairment	Thickened pulmonary interstitium (fibrosis)	Usually improves PaO_2

up the rest. Physiological dead space refers to areas in which inspired air reaches the respiratory units but is not able to equilibrate with the flowing capillary blood. The combined anatomical and physiological dead space in a healthy patient is about 25–30%. The normal ratio between dead space and tidal volume (VD/VT) is 0.25–0.3 [2].

Three main differentials should be considered in patients suffering from increased physiological dead space ventilation: destruction of the alveolar-capillary interface or impaired capillary blood flow such as occurs with pulmonary thromboembolism, low cardiac output, and overdistension of the alveoli preventing capillary blood flow during positive-pressure ventilation. Increasing the inspired O_2 (FiO$_2$) will usually improve PaO$_2$ by increasing the transmembrane pressure differential and thus the rate of O_2 diffusion. Supplemental O_2 is a noninvasive means to optimize Hgb saturation; however, treating the underlying cause is essential for correction.

In animals with *intrapulmonary shunting*, capillary blood flow exceeds ventilation, causing the V/Q ratio to be <1.0 [2]. Blood flow that is not exposed to ventilated areas is incapable of effectively participating in gas exchange. There are two forms of shunting: true shunt and venous admixture. A true shunt represents complete lack of gas exchange (V/Q = 0). Venous admixture is a decreased V/Q ratio due to incomplete equilibration between the capillary blood and alveolar O_2 (1 < V/Q >0). The amount of intrapulmonary shunting (shunt fraction) that occurs in a healthy patient is about 10% of the cardiac output. Normally, the pulmonary vasculature undergoes local vasoconstriction when a decreased O_2 tension is detected in the alveoli, to prevent unnecessary perfusion to a region that cannot perform gas exchange, thereby reducing the extent of V/Q mismatch. Differentials considered in a patient with a suspected intrapulmonary shunt include all forms of alveolar and lower airway disease, including atelectasis. Shunt is the one cause of hypoxia that fails to improve with supplemental O_2 because of lack of available gas-exchanging units.

Any severe pulmonary pathology that produces thickening of the pulmonary interstitium could result in *diffusion impairment*. The rate of diffusion of a gas depends on the concentration gradient, the surface area, and the thickness or distance the gas molecules must travel. CO_2 is more diffusible than O_2, and thus tends to be unaffected in conditions causing poor diffusion. The primary differential diagnosis is pulmonary fibrosis. O_2 supplementation is a treatment option, improving PaO$_2$ by increasing alveolar O_2 content.

Treatment of hypoxemia

Stabilization of the critical small animal patient with hypoxemia commonly begins with providing anxiolytic/analgesic agents (examples include butorphanol 0.2–0.4 mg/kg IV or IM or acepromazine 0.0025–0.02 mg/kg IV or IM), assuring a patent airway, and providing supplemental oxygen. The SpO$_2$ and PaO$_2$ values can be used to confirm the need for O_2 supplementation and should be provided for critically ill patients with SpO$_2$ < 95% or PaO$_2$ < 80 mmHg. The clinical signs of respiratory distress (such as abnormal breathing pattern, respiratory rate or work of breathing) or poor perfusion will also prompt oxygen support when the patient is not stable enough for testing. Each method of oxygen supplementation has advantages and limitations depending on the patient size, O_2 requirement and tolerance, hypoxemia etiology, clinical skill level, and available monitoring.

There are noninvasive methods of oxygen supplementation that are fast and easy to initiate: flow-by, mask, hood and cage oxygen,

while more invasive nasal cannulas or catheters are used for prolonged oxygen support. Endotracheal intubation and tracheostomy provide a means for controlling the airway and providing therapeutic PPV.

Oxygen supplementation for more than a few hours can cause epithelial desiccation, which leads to inflammation and increased mucus production. Humidification of inspired gas with water vapor is mandatory whenever supplemental O_2 bypasses the nasal turbinates [43]. Humidification is achieved by inserting a canister (Hudson Rci, Temecula, CA) filled with distilled water into the oxygen delivery system. As the O_2 travels out of the diffuser, bubbles are created that rise through the water. Evaporation of water occurs at the contact surface of each bubble, loading the gas passing through with water vapor. Greater quantities of water vapor can be added if the water is heated, the bubbles are smaller or the water is made deeper for longer diffusion times. The humidified O_2 above the water then travels along the tubing to the patient.

Oxygen therapy is not without risk, and hyperoxia and oxygen toxicity must be avoided. As a general rule, a patient should not receive more than 60% FiO$_2$ for more than 12 hours [44]. During mitochondrial aerobic metabolism, highly reactive O_2 species (including hydrogen peroxide, hydroxyl radicals, superoxide radicals) are formed that will disrupt and damage essential cellular lipid membranes, cytoplasmic proteins, and nuclear DNA [45]. Administration of excessive FiO$_2$ for long periods of time results in production of much higher concentrations of these reactive oxygen species [46], causing oxidative injury. Ideally, the lowest possible FiO$_2$ should be used to maintain the patient's O_2 saturation above 93%. However, it may be impossible to avoid use of high FiO$_2$ values in animals with severe respiratory disease.

Chronic hypercapnia in patients with longstanding respiratory disease (such as chronic obstructive lung disease) results in central nervous system adaptations. In these patients, hypoxemia has taken over from hypercarbia as the main trigger for brainstem respiratory centers. Therefore, providing O_2 supplementation to these animals can result in hypoventilation and worsening of their respiratory function [2].

Noninvasive oxygen delivery

Flow-by O_2 is one of the least invasive methods of supplementation, commonly used in the emergency setting while the patient is being evaluated and stabilized. O_2 tubing is placed close to the mouth or nose, with O_2 flow rates of 1–5 L per minute. FiO$_2$ achieved is variable depending on the flow rate, size of the patient, and whether the animal is breathing through the nose or mouth. This technique is not recommended after the initial stabilization of the patient [43].

An O_2 mask acts as a reservoir system. Masks of various sizes have been designed specifically for the dog and cat (Surgivet, Waukesh, WI). The mask size should ideally be slightly larger than the muzzle or head of the patient to prevent rapid equilibration of O_2 with the surrounding air and minimize the accumulation of CO_2, heat, and humidity inside the mask. A flow rate of 2–10 L/minute is recommended to clear the exhaled gas from the reservoir. FiO$_2$ values of 30–90% can be achieved depending on the size of the mask and patient [47]. Frequent monitoring is required to ensure proper mask placement and patient tolerance. This method is best applied in patients with minimal voluntary movement or during initial stabilization to transition to a self-supporting mechanism.

Commercially available oxygen hoods (Oxyhood, Jorgen Kruuse, Denmark) are available or an oxygen hood can be made by taping O_2 tubing to the inside bottom of an Elizabethan collar. The wide

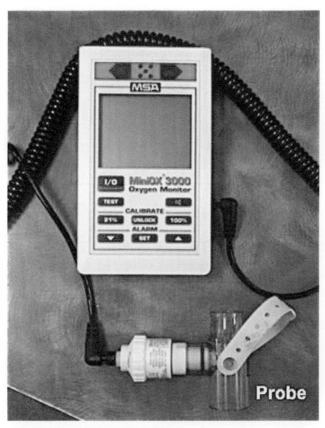

Figure 8.6 Oxygen monitor (MSA, Pittsburg, PA). The probe can be placed inside a cage or a large Elizabethan collar can be used for hood oxygen to determine the inspired fraction of oxygen (FiO_2).

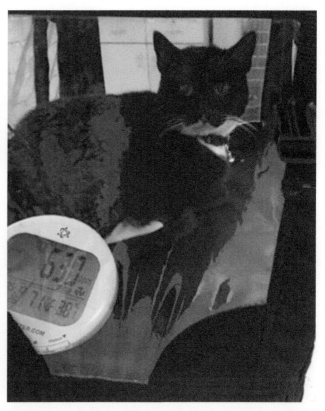

Figure 8.7 Temperature, CO_2, and humidity monitor placed in the small oxygen cage to ensure a safe environment for the patient (CO2Meter.com, Ormond Beach, FL). CO_2 levels = 250–600 parts per million (ppm); up to 1000 is acceptable; >1000 indicates room or cage needs better ventilation [49].

opening of the collar is covered with plastic wrap to create a reservoir system, with a small opening (approximately 5 cm) made at the top of the plastic to allow escape of CO_2 and water vapor. Use of clear material to make the hood allows easy patient monitoring. This system can achieve FiO_2 values of 30–50% or more [48]. Larger patients, and those that are panting, are at risk of hyperthermia when using this technique.

Oxygen cages provide excellent O_2 delivery, controlled humidity, and regulation of chamber temperature. They can be used long term in hypoxic patients, or during the emergency management of stressed patients that cannot handle restraint. FiO_2 levels achieved vary depending on the manufacturer, but values as high as 80–90% should be available for short-term use in a crisis. The main disadvantage is the inability to handle the patient when necessary. Opening the cage immediately results in equilibration to room air. Additionally, temperature regulation may be difficult with larger, panting or brachycephalic dogs, due to the small size of the enclosure. The placement of ice bags inside the cage can help with temperature regulation with regular monitoring of the body temperature recommended. The use of O_2 cages in patients with upper airway obstructions should be avoided because of the inability to hear upper airway sounds when monitoring the patient.

Given the varying ability of cages to control O_2 concentration, oxygen monitors (MSA, Pittsburg, PA) that measure the FiO_2 in the cage are recommended (Figure 8.6). The accumulation of CO_2 is of concern and some cages come with a CO_2 scavenging system built in. When that is not available, CO_2 and temperature monitors

(CO2Meter.com, Ormond Beach, FL) should be placed within O_2 cages to allow intervention if necessary (Figure 8.7).

Invasive oxygen delivery

Nasal or nasopharyngeal O_2 is used for longer supplementation, allowing continuous handling of the patient without fear of O_2 desaturation. FiO_2 values can be as high as 70% with O_2 flow rates up to 150 mL/kg/min [50]. However, rates >100 mL/kg/min have been associated with patient discomfort, with higher flow rates achieved with bilateral nasal lines. Humidification is required to prevent pharyngeal epithelial desiccation. Complications of high O_2 flow rates include nasal mucosal irritation, sneezing, and discomfort manifested by pawing or rubbing the nose. Panting decreases the effective FiO_2. Nasal supplementation should be used cautiously in patients with concurrent head trauma since sneezing can increase intracranial pressure.

Nasal prongs or catheters can be used. Nasal prongs (Cardinal Hill, McGaw Park, IL) provide bilateral nostril flow but are manufactured for human patients and easily slip out of the nares. Application of a strip of tape around the two tubes attached to the prongs and across the dorsal aspect of the muzzle can help to prevent displacement.

Nasal catheter options include 5–10 French red rubber or flexible feeding tubes that can be placed unilaterally or bilaterally when a higher FiO_2 is necessary. The catheter should be premeasured and marked at the level of the medial canthus of the eye. Topical anesthesia, using 2% lidocaine or 0.5% proparacaine ophthalmic solution, is applied by dripping it into the nostril while the nose is held pointed up. The catheter tip is coated with lubricant or lidocaine gel and advanced through the ventral meatus to the level of the mark. It is secured with glue or sutures, one at the lateral aspect of the nostril (alternatively through the nasal planum) and the other on the lateral maxilla or zygomatic arch. The nasal catheter is attached to an adapter and O_2 tubing in order to create a tight seal. An Elizabethan collar is placed to minimize the ability of the patient to remove the tube. Box 20.5 describes nasal oxygen placement.

Nasopharyngeal placement is similar except that the catheter tip is advanced through the ventral meatus into the pharynx. In this case, the catheter is premeasured to the mandibular ramus. Nasotracheal oxygen supplementation is an option as well, but most pets require moderate sedation to maintain the tube in place as coughing may easily dislodge the tube from the trachea.

Endotracheal intubation

Endotracheal (ET) intubation is indicated for patients requiring general anesthesia, developing hypoxia from hypoventilation, respiratory fatigue or apnea and for aggressive or overtly anxious patients that are not tolerating less invasive forms of O_2 supplementation. In addition, animals with upper airway obstruction or those given O_2 but remaining severely hypoxemic ($PaO_2 < 60\,mmHg$) or hypercapnic ($PaCO_2 > 50\,mmHg$) can benefit from an ET intubation and oxygenation.

Prior to ET intubation, all equipment and drugs needed for induction and tube placement, suction, and crisis management should be prepared. There are two main types of ET tubes: the Murphy tube (most common) and the Cole tube. The Murphy tube has a distal side fenestration to allow for continued air flow despite the end being occluded by secretions or anatomical abnormalities. The larger tubes are cuffed, but those less than 3 mm internal diameter are usually uncuffed. Cole tubes are all uncuffed but have a distal shoulder that is placed just rostral to the larynx in order to obtain a tight seal. Both types of tubes are available in a large variety of sizes and different materials, including polyvinyl chloride, rubber, and silicone. Clear tubes are ideal, allowing visualization of secretions within the tube.

Multiple ET tubes in different sizes (the anticipated size, one larger and two sizes smaller) should be readily available prior to induction of anesthesia. The ET tube size selected is based on the normal body weight of the patient and adjusted for anticipated individual variations (such as brachycephalic dogs with hypoplastic tracheas). The recommended ET tube size according to body weight is shown in Table 8.8 for the dog and Table 8.9 for the cat. Cats have a more uniform tracheal diameter.

Intubation of cats tends to be more difficult because their highly sensitive larynx will spasm closed when touched. Avoiding tactile stimulation with the tube and laryngoscope is helpful, along with applying a topical anesthetic such as lidocaine spray.

A source of oxygen and ventilation equipment (either manual or mechanical) is prepared and supplemental oxygen is provided before, during, and after intubation. Rapid-acting injectable anesthetics are necessary to facilitate rapid sequence intubation. It is recommended that an anesthetic agent or combination of agents be chosen that supports the cardiovascular status of the patient. Possible induction agents can include:

- propofol (2–6 mg/kg IV)
- ketamine/benzodiazepine combination (ketamine 1–2 mg/kg and diazepam/midazolam 0.25–0.5 mg/kg)
- alfaxalone (1–3 mg/kg)

Table 8.8 Endotracheal tube size guidelines according to body weight in dogs.

Body weight (kg)	ET tube size (mm)	Body weight (kg)	ET tube size (mm)
2	5.0	**14**	8.5
3.5	5.5	**16**	9
4.5	6	**18**	9.5
6	6.5	**20**	10
8	7	**25**	11
10	7.5	**30**	12
12	8	**>40**	14–16

Table 8.9 Endotracheal tube size guidelines according to body weight in cats.

Body weight (kg)	ET tube size (mm)
1	3.0
2	3.5
3.5	4.0
>4	4.5

- etomidate/benzodiazepine combination (1–3 mg/kg etomidate and 0.25–0.5 mg/kg diazepam or midazolam).

Induction with gas anesthetics is not recommended due to slow speed, stress to the patient, excitatory phase of induction, and exposure to inhalant by personnel.

Preoxygenating the patient with flow-by O_2 for approximately five minutes will help prevent prolonged hypoxemic events. After induction, the patient is positioned in sternal recumbency and an assistant holds the maxilla by placing the finger and thumb behind the canine teeth while pulling the lips dorsally. The mandible can be held open with the other hand by grasping the tongue and pulling it forward and downward (avoid tongue contact with the mandibular canines). Rapid visual assessment of the upper airway increases the chances of successful intubation and can identify upper airway obstruction, abnormal anatomical structures, upper airway secretions, and dynamic functional changes in the pharynx and larynx. It is vital to be prepared for difficult intubations in every critically ill patient, with special emphasis on brachycephalic dogs, small patients, cats, and those with oropharyngeal or orofacial obstructions, trauma or other disease.

A laryngoscope can provide light and open the epiglottis, allowing better visualization and access to the trachea. The chosen lubricated ET tube is advanced orally through the larynx and into the trachea, providing a patent airway. Inflation of a cuff protects the patient from aspiration. O_2 or gaseous anesthetics and PPV can be provided.

With practice, intubating dogs and cats in dorsal recumbency may actually become easier than sternal since it allows the head and neck to be held straight. The laryngoscope can be used as designed for humans (Figure 8.8).

Once the ET tube is advanced through the larynx, the distal end is estimated to lie at or near the thoracic inlet. Tracheal tube placement is confirmed by auscultating both sides of the thoracic cavity for air movement and visualization of thoracic wall excursions during PPV and humidification of the tube during exhalation. $ETCO_2$ is the most accurate indirect method of confirming placement, and values should be >20 mmHg to confirm correct

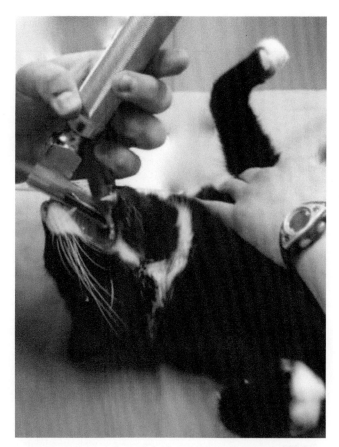

Figure 8.8 Technique of endotracheal intubation with the animal in dorsal recumbency.

Box 8.2 Placement of tracheostomy tubes.

Materials

Sterile drape	Thumb forceps
Towel clamps	Needle holders
#10 or #15 scalpel blade	Metzenbaum scissors
Clippers, scrub	Curved hemostats
Sterile gloves	Umbilical tape
Nonabsorbable suture	Tracheostomy tube
(2–0, 3–0)	

Procedure

1. General anesthesia and endotracheal intubation are provided.
2. Place patient in dorsal recumbency.
3. Clip the ventral neck from thyroid cartilage to thoracic inlet.
4. Scrub area, place drapes, secure with towel clamps.
5. Incise skin with scalpel blade on ventral midline over the 3rd–6th tracheal rings.
6. Bluntly dissect the sternohyoid and sternothyroid muscles on midline down to the fascia overlying the trachea using a hemostat.*
7. Excise the thin fascia over the trachea using Metzenbaum scissors.
8. Incise between the tracheal rings with a scalpel blade. Do not cut more than 50% of the tracheal circumference.*
9. Place two long stay sutures around the tracheal rings immediately cranial and caudal to the incision and leave in place.**
10. Open the tracheal incision using the stay sutures and gently insert the tracheostomy tube.
11. Secure the tracheostomy tube using sterile umbilical tape tied around the back of the neck. Note: Do NOT suture the tube to the skin
12. A gauze bandage is placed to keep the stoma site clean.

* The tracheostomy tube can be inserted at this point if an emergent procedure.
** This step is often performed later when done as an emergency tracheostomy.

placement in the trachea. The ET tube is then secured with a tie anchored around the maxilla in dogs with a long muzzle or behind the ears of cats and brachycephalic dogs.

Endotracheal tube cuffs are inflated to protect the airway and during general anesthesia when PPV or inhalants are being administered. Cuff pressure should be maintained between 25 and 35 cmH$_2$O (18.3–25.7 mmHg). Overinflation of the cuff applies excessive pressure on the tracheal mucosa, causing mucosal ischemia and occasionally tracheal rupture [50,51]. High-volume, low-pressure endotracheal cuffs are recommended for all patients.

Patients predisposed to complications during ET tube placement include cats and brachycephalic dogs, animals with orofacial and dynamic airway abnormalities, and those with suboptimal positioning. Preoxygenating these patients is especially important. Besides multiple ET tube sizes, several red rubber catheters and stiff peripheral intravenous catheters should be available in case tracheal catheterization is required. For patients that are difficult to intubate, it may help to stiffen the softer ET tubes with a guidewire or stylet [52]. However, a stylet should never extend beyond the tip of the ET tube.

Transtracheal intubation

Transtracheal intubation can be a life-saving procedure during an upper airway obstruction. It can also be used for O$_2$ supplementation, to facilitate removal of airway secretions, to provide O$_2$ and gas inhalant to patients undergoing upper airway procedures where ET tube placement is contraindicated, and to decrease anatomical dead space during PPV. There are several approaches to tracheal intubation, including temporary and permanent methods. Temporary procedures include tracheal needle insertion and catheterization or surgical tracheostomy.

Cervical anatomy must be understood to avoid vital cervical structures. The thyroid cartilage is the rostral border of the trachea, and tracheal rings can usually be palpated. Small blood vessels lie along the midline of the trachea, including the thyroid vessels as they branch from the external jugular at the level of the thoracic inlet.

It is ideal to preoxygenate the patient prior to a tracheal procedure [53]. Supplies for an emergency tracheostomy should be readily accessible and are listed in Box 8.2. Tracheal catheter placement is performed as a temporary means to establish partial control over the airway and provide oxygen. The hair is clipped and the skin aseptically prepared over the cranial third of the trachea. A through-the-needle long flexible catheter is percutaneously inserted between the cervical rings on the tracheal midline. Once the needle is in place, the catheter is advanced through the needle into the carina. The needle is then withdrawn from the skin, leaving the catheter in place. Humidified oxygen is provided until upper airway access can be confirmed. Complications include kinking of the catheter at the skin and tracheal entry site, and accidental withdrawal of the catheter so that the tip lies under the skin with subcutaneous insufflation of oxygen. Should this procedure fail to provide sufficient oxygenation and ventilation in an animal with large airway disease, a tracheostomy is performed.

Large airway disorders

Loud stertor or stridor heard without a stethoscope can be an important clinical indication of large airway disease. The large airway includes the nares, nasal passages, pharynx, larynx, trachea, and bronchi. Common large airway disorders encountered in the small animal ICU patient are listed in Table 8.10. Inflammation of the airways will often result in a cough with increased tracheal secretions. Anatomical changes, such as ruptured or collapsing trachea, can impair the ability to provide adequate oxygenation and ventilation. Airway obstruction can be due to a tenacious mucoid or hemorrhagic fluid, foreign body, laryngeal paralysis, collapse (tracheal, pharngeal, laryngeal), mass lesions or compression of the airway. Traumatic intubation can lead to laryngeal edema, hemorrhage, and spasm, as well as increased vagal tone. These patients are at risk for requiring emergent tracheal intubation, requiring that tracheal tubes, ties, gauze, and a laryngoscope be available cage-side to prevent any delays.

The first intervention in patients decompensating from a large airway problem is to provide supplemental oxygen by flow-by or transtracheal routes in preparation for securing an airway by ET intubation as described above. Should the initial attempt at routine ET intubation fail, it should be reattempted with a smaller tube. If there is an obstruction or anatomical abnormality, a long thin catheter or guidewire can sometimes be successfully inserted into the airway, then a small ET tube can be passed over it [54]. In rare circumstances, direct visualization using a fiberoptic light source may aid placement. Blind intubation is also possible using careful palpation to identify known anatomical structures.

Retrograde intubation may be performed using a guidewire or catheter. A needle is placed percutaneously into the tracheal lumen caudal to the larynx and a wire or catheter is advanced retrograde towards the oral cavity. A tube can then be passed using the guidewire or catheter. This can provide at least a narrow lumen for oxygen supplementation and exhalation of CO_2 in preparation for a tracheostomy. Tracheostomy may be required in patients with upper airway obstruction of any etiology (trauma, anaphylaxis, conformational defects).

Tracheostomy

The materials required and method of performing a tracheostomy are listed in Box 8.2. Ideally, tracheostomy should be performed in a controlled situation after a secure airway has been established by endotracheal intubation. Several techniques for tracheostomy have been reported, all of which have similar complication rates and functionality [55,56]. Tracheal tubes are available in several sizes and materials, with and without cuffs and internal cannulas. Size should be chosen such that the tube occupies about two-thirds of the internal diameter of the trachea. Risks of a tracheostomy include obstruction, displacement, hemorrhage, infection, dislodgment, and intolerance by the patient. In addition, drowning, gagging, vomiting, subcutaneous emphysema, pneumothorax, pneumomediastinum, and rare long-term tracheal stricture or stenosis can also occur. Cats tend to form excessive secretions and have a greater risk of acute tube occlusion [57].

Patients with an indwelling tracheostomy tube require continuous monitoring. A dedicated nurse is necessary along with management supplies to immediately address complications such as obstruction with mucus or displacement of the tube [58]. It is unnecessary to inflate the tracheal tube cuff in most spontaneously breathing patients. If the cuff is to be inflated, the minimal degree of distension will help prevent iatrogenic mucosal damage, with the cuff periodically deflated if possible [56].

Table 8.10 Common causes of large and small airway disorders in the small animal ICU patient.

Large airway disorders	Small airway disorders
Nasal passages	**Acute bronchitis**
Obstruction	Infectious, e.g. *Bordetella*
Infection	Inhaled noxious substances
Neoplasia	
Foreign body	**Chronic bronchitis**
Trauma	Parasitic
Inhalation injury	Infectious
	Congenital, e.g. ciliary dyskinesia
Pharynx	Immune mediated
Elongated soft palate	Allergic
Foreign body	Idiopathic
Hemorrhage, hematoma	Bronchiectasis
Erosions, ulceration	
Ingested caustic agents	**Feline bronchial disease**
Polyps	Asthma (allergic, bronchospasm)
Neoplasia	
Granulomas	
Abscess	
Allergic	
Larynx	
Laryngeal paresis or paralysis	
Granulomatous	
Foreign body	
Neoplasia	
Trauma	
Voice abuse (barking)	
Inflammatory laryngitis (cats)	
Trachea	
Infection	
Neoplasia	
Parasitic nodules	
Collapsing trachea	
Hypoplasic trachea	
Aspiration of gastric material	
Trauma	
Rupture	
Foreign body	
Inhaled toxins	
Pressure necrosis (intubation)	
Stricture, stenosis	
Allergic	
Mainstem bronchi	
Infection	
Neoplasia	
Foreign body	
Aspirated material	
Compression from atria	
Inflammation	
Bronchomalacia	

Since cool dry air is now bypassing the upper airway, mucosal desiccation results in inflammation, mucosal swelling, and production of excess mucus. This will accumulate in and around the tracheal tube and incision site, potentially causing a life-threatening obstruction. Nebulization is recommended to decrease tracheal and mucus desiccation. In addition, the tube itself or the inner cannula, when present, should be removed and cleaned every 2–4 hours as needed, based on the presence of audible noises created during breathing. Prior to cannula or tube removal, it is beneficial to preoxygenate the patient and monitor hemodynamics since gagging may induce a vasovagal event [59]. The inner cannula or tube is then removed, rinsed in hydrogen peroxide or chlorhexidine and scrubbed with a sterile brush or pipe cleaner, then thoroughly flushed with sterile saline before being replaced [56,57]. The incision and tube secretions are monitored for signs of infection and the umbilical tape securing the tube should be replaced when soiled.

When removal of the cannula or tube and cleaning does not resolve the airway obstruction, the airway secretions can be moistened by administration of 0.2–0.5 mL/kg of sterile saline directly into the tracheal tube. Continuous nebulization can also be considered in an attempt to further moisten the airways. Airway suction can be performed on an "as-needed" basis, but should be avoided if possible because of stress to the patient, damage to the airway mucosa, and potential for triggering a vagal response. If suctioning is required, the suctioning causes a negative pressure and should be pulsed for 1–2 seconds rather than continuous, with negative pressure applied for no more than approximately 10 seconds at a time [56]. In an unstable patient, a small sterile catheter can be placed down to the carina during suctioning to provide supplemental oxygen during the procedure.

Tracheostomy tubes are a temporary intervention with the decision to remove the tube based on adequate resolution of the underlying airway problem. When the tube is a loose fit in the trachea, occlusion of the end of the tube with a gloved fingertip for 30–60 seconds allows a test of the patient's ability to breathe around the tube. It is almost always safe to extubate a patient that passes this test. However, patients with accumulated mucus or a tight tube can fail the test, but still be ready for extubation. Once the tube has been removed, the patient should be kept quiet, with oxygen provided if needed and observed for several hours. Reintubation may be necessary if airway obstruction recurs. Prior to discharge, the stay sutures can be removed. The stoma heals by second intention over 7–10 days.

Indications for permanent tracheostomy include upper airway obstructions (masses and orofacial trauma), and laryngeal or pharyngeal dysfunction (laryngeal collapse, surgical reconstruction) that cannot be corrected with a definitive surgical procedure [60]. A stoma is formed between the skin and the tracheal lumen. The incised tracheal mucosa is sutured to the dermis adjacent to the stoma. The long-term complication rate in cats is higher than in dogs, because of increased mucus production causing occlusion [59].

Pleural space disorders

Respiratory failure can occur as a result of disease within the pleural space. The presence of fluid, air, mass lesions or herniated organs in the pleural space will cause changes in intrathoracic pressure needed for ventilation and compression of the lungs and pulmonary vasculature. A restrictive breathing pattern can be seen with hypoxia and hypercarbia [61]. Clinical examination findings usually include dull or quiet heart and lung sounds and asynchrony of movement of the chest and abdomen. Common causes of pleural space disorders in the small animal ICU patient are listed in Table 8.11. Stabilization and diagnostic efforts are initially focused on providing supplemental oxygen and removing any pleural fluid or air by needle thoracocentesis. When repeated centesis is required, placement of a thoracostomy tube is indicated.

Thoracocentesis

Thoracocentesis is defined as the removal of fluid or air located in the thoracic cavity using a needle or catheter that is removed at the end of the procedure. When the patient is in respiratory distress,

Table 8.11 Common causes of lung parenchymal and pleural space disorders in the small animal ICU patient.

Lung parenchymal disorders	Pleural space disorders
Neoplasia	**Neoplasia**
Primary	**Heart failure**
Metastatic	**Pyothorax**
	Foreign body
Pneumonia	
Infection (bacterial, viral, fungal, rickettsial)	**Traumatic**
Aspiration	**pneumothorax**
Inhalation	Open
Hematogenous	Closed
	Tension
Allergic pneumonitis	
Interstitial fibrosis	**Spontaneous**
Parasites	**pneumothorax**
Lungworms	**Hemothorax**
Heartworm	Trauma
	Coagulopathy
Pulmonary thromboembolism(s)	Rodenticide toxicity
Cardiogenic pulmonary edema	
Heart failure	**Chylothorax**
Cardiac arrhythmias	**Feline infectious**
	peritonitis
Noncardiogenic pulmonary edema	**Diaphragmatic hernia**
Neurogenic pulmonary edema	Congenital
Electrocution	Traumatic
Snake bite	
Reexpansion edema	**Lung lobe torsion**
Near drowning	
Drowning	
Fresh water	
Salt water	
Smoke inhalation	
Acute respiratory distress syndrome	
Acute lung injury	
Sepsis	
Systemic inflammatory response syndrome diseases	
Lung lobe torsion	
Atelectasis	
Pulmonary contusions	
Pulmonary nodules	
Neoplasia	
Parasitic	
Infectious	
Granulomatous	

therapeutic thoracocentesis will become a priority. The materials required and procedure for thoracocentesis are outlined in Box 8.3. Ultrasound can be used to locate fluid or air pockets and guide needle placement. Diagnostic analysis of any samples can include cell counts and cytological examination (possibly with special staining), biochemical testing and culture and susceptibility testing, as indicated [62].

Risks of thoracocentesis include hemorrhage, development or worsening of pneumothorax by lung laceration, cardiac arrhythmias by inadvertent stimulation of the myocardium, infection, discomfort, distress due to restraint, and a negative aspirate. Reexpansion pulmonary edema is a rare but serious complication that can occur following evacuation of chronic pleural effusion [63–65].

The main contraindications of thoracocentesis are coagulopathy, thrombocytopenia, or a thrombocytopathic disorder. Thoracocentesis should not be performed if there is a pneumomediastinum,

Box 8.3 Performing a thoracocentesis.

Materials

Supplemental oxygen	Sterile gloves
Light sedation	Needle (22–18 G)*
Clippers	Extension set**
Chlorhexidine scrub	Large syringe
Lidocaine	Three-way stopcock
Blood tubes (clot and EDTA)	Culturette

Procedure

1. Connect the three-way stopcock to syringe tip, then the extension tubing to opposite stopcock port.
2. Use ultrasound guidance or perform blind aspiration between the 6th and 9th rib spaces: ventrally for fluid, dorsally for air retrieval.
3. Clip and aseptically prepare a skin area wider than insertion site.
4. Lidocaine can be injected at the insertion site.
5. Insert the needle cranial to the chosen rib to avoid intercostal arteries and nerves.
6. Hold needle perpendicular to the thoracic wall until tip is within the pleural space.
7. Attach extension tubing to needle and apply gentle suction on the syringe until fluid or air enters the tubing.
8. Adjust the needle to lie against the chest wall to avoid trauma to the lung as the pleural space is evacuated.
9. Continue aspiration until all the air or fluid is removed.

---

* A larger bore needle may be needed for exudative fluid.
** A butterfly catheter may be substituted for the needle and extension tubing for cats and small dogs.

Box 8.4 Placing a thoracostomy tube.

Materials

Sterile thoracostomy tube*	Clippers
Continuous suction devices	Chlorhexidine scrub
Connection adapters	Drapes, towel clamps
Suture (nonabsorbable)	Gloves
Bandage material	Syringe (10-65 mL)
Lidocaine	Anesthetic agents
Scalpel	Needle holder
Forceps	Scissors
Carmalt forceps	

Procedure

1. Preoxygenate patient, anesthetic induction, endotracheal intubation, maintenance of anesthesia.
2. Place in lateral recumbency.
3. Clip lateral thoracic wall from 4th intercostal space to the last rib; clip dorsally to the epaxial muscles, ventrally to the sternum.
4. Measure and mark the tube for length from the site of insertion to the 2nd intercostal space.
5. Mark the skin location 2–3 intercostal spaces caudal to thoracic muscle tube insertion site (generally at 9th or 10th intercostal space).
6. Have an assistant pull the skin cranially until the skin insertion site lies directly over the site where the tube will penetrate the thoracic wall.
7. Make an incision slightly larger than the tube diameter in the skin using a scalpel blade.
8. Use a hemostat to bluntly dissect through the underlying fascia and external and internal intercostal muscles.
9. Advance the tube through the pleura into the pleural space by grasping the tube and stylet or by grasping the tube with a curved hemostat near the tip.
10. Advance the tube over the stylet or with hemostats into the thorax, placing it dorsal for air retrieval and ventral for fluid retrieval.
11. Ensure all tube fenestrations are within the thoracic cavity.
12. Remove stylet if present and clamp tube to prevent air entry.
13. Release the skin. The tube is now tunneled through the subcutaneous space to minimize leakage.
14. Secure the tube with a purse-string suture followed by a finger trap suture.
15. Apply a sterile bandage pad and a simple chest bandage or commercial body sleeve.
16. Thoracic radiographs, fluoroscopy or CT is recommended to document correct placement and effective evacuation of the pleural space.

---

* Radiopaque marker required on tube to identify tube by imaging.

diaphragmatic hernia, or a noneffusive pulmonary or pleural mass [66]. Thoracocentesis can be repeated, but each attempt can result in an increased risk of complications. If multiple aspirates are required, an indwelling thoracostomy tube is indicated for continued drainage.

Thoracostomy tube

Thoracostomy tubes are used to aspirate fluid or air intermittently or continuously. Tube placement is indicated when multiple thoracocentesis procedures are necessary, or if a very large volume of fluid or air requires removal (such as tension pneumothorax) [67]. Thoracostomy tubes are also used for the medical management of diseases (such as pyothorax) requiring pleural lavage, for intracavitary chemotherapy or for blood pleurodesis to treat a refractory pneumothorax. Finally, a thoracostomy tube is placed following thoracic surgery to reestablish negative intrathoracic pressure and remove any postoperative effusions. The materials and procedure for thoracostomy tube placement are listed in Box 8.4. A tube is selected that approximates the size of the mainstem bronchus of the patient. An alternative method for placing a thoracostomy tube is to use a catheter and guidewire in a modified Seldinger technique, similar to placing a central venous access line.

Risks of the procedure include hemorrhage, pneumothorax, lung or cardiac puncture, arrhythmias, improper placement, infection, and reexpansion pulmonary edema (after removal of chronic effusions) [68]. The main contraindication is coagulopathy, but in unstable patients the procedure may be required prior to receiving any coagulation test results.

The thoracostomy tube is connected to either a three-way stopcock and syringe for manual aspiration or a continuous suction device that creates a negative pressure of approximately –10 cmH$_2$O (–7.35 mmHg). Intermittent aspiration is typically performed every 4–6 hours, but can be done more frequently if required based on the clinical condition of the patient. Continuous suction is most commonly achieved using a commercial device, such as the Pleurevac® (Teleflex Medical, Research Triangle Park, NC). Medical management of pyothorax should include pleural lavage, performed 4–6 times per day, infusing 10–20 mL/kg of warmed sterile saline, gentle patient agitation, and aspiration of the fluid.

Patients with thoracostomy tubes should be continuously monitored at a 24-hour facility to ensure that the tube does not become dislodged or disconnected. The tube itself should be evaluated using sterile technique at least once daily, and the bandage and dressing should be changed. The most common complication is patient discomfort, so intravenous analgesia or intrapleural analgesia with bupivacaine is an important part of patient management.

The tube is removed once the fluid or air has decreased significantly. Depending on the cause of pneumothorax, air should stop accumulating for a 12–24-hour period prior to tube removal [69]. The presence of the thoracostomy tube causes some pleural inflammation, which results in production of pleural fluid as long as the tube is in place. The tube can be removed once the rate of fluid production is less than 2–5 mL/kg/day [68]. Because tube occlusion or kinking can cause a negative aspiration, thoracic radiographs may be needed to confirm resolution of pleural space disease prior to tube removal.

To remove the tube, the tacking suture is cut and the tube is quickly but carefully pulled out, while holding a sterile gauze square coated with triple antibiotic ointment over the entrance site. Intravenous analgesia can be given prior to removal of the tube. The incision does not require primary closure, but should be covered with a nonadhesive bandage and an overlying adhesive dressing.

Lung parenchymal disorders

Abnormalities within the lung parenchyma are common and often devastating complications in the small animal ICU patient. Abnormal lung function may be the primary complaint or may occur as a complication of the underlying disease (such as aspiration pneumonia, ALI, ARDS, cardiogenic pulmonary edema). Common causes of lung parenchymal disease in the small animal ICU patient are listed in Table 8.11. Aggressive patient support is necessary for the hypoxemic patient while finding the correct diagnosis and initiating the most appropriate therapy for the underlying cause. Most hypoxemic patients with lung parenchymal disease can be treated with supplemental oxygen. However, if this measure fails to improve clinical signs or the patient develops hypoventilation, PPV is the only option for improving oxygenation and ventilation.

Severe hypoxemia can be defined as $PaO_2 < 60$ mmHg ($SaO_2 < 90\%$), while receiving oxygen supplementation. If it is not possible to perform arterial blood gas analysis, pulse oximetry can be used, with a $SpO_2 < 90\%$ despite O_2 support an indication for PPV. The clinician should evaluate the patient as well as the numbers when determining respiratory failure. Some animals with chronic progressive lung disease such as pulmonary fibrosis may be very stable with a PaO_2 of 50 mmHg, and should not be considered candidates for PPV based on the PaO_2 alone. In contrast, a patient with a borderline PaO_2 (PaO_2 65 mmHg) in combination with severe hypocapnia due to excessive hyperventilation is at risk for respiratory fatigue and might benefit from early PPV intervention.

Three main conditions should prompt intervention with PPV [70]: (1) severe hypoxemia despite appropriate therapy and oxygen supplementation, (2) severe hypercapnia, and (3) excessive respiratory effort or impending respiratory muscle fatigue. As a general rule, patients with normal lungs suffering from ventilatory failure (conditions 2 and 3) have a better overall prognosis and require less aggressive PPV therapy [71,72]. Animals with primary lung parenchymal disease require more aggressive PPV therapy and have a higher chance of further decompensation despite intervention. The owner needs to be educated regarding the overall prognosis, quality of life, complication rates, and financial considerations. A 24-hour facility that provides continuous monitoring and supportive care is required. These patients require intense, dedicated nursing care and monitoring (see Chapter 20, Table 20.3).

Severe hypercapnia ($PaCO_2 > 60$ mmHg) requires correction because of the subsequent respiratory acidemia. Cerebral vasodilation is an important systemic side-effect of hypercapnia that can lead to increased intracranial pressure. A marginally elevated $PaCO_2$ may be an indication for PPV in patients with intracranial disease [73].

Mechanical ventilation can be life saving for patients developing respiratory fatigue. A subjective assessment of the work of breathing is the most important diagnostic parameter. Patients may be able to maintain a near normal PaO_2 and $PaCO_2$ at the expense of respiratory muscle fatigue, eventually reaching a point of respiratory failure if PPV is not instituted. As a general rule, if dyspnea is severe and not responding to treatment within a reasonable time period (30 minutes), PPV should be considered.

Mechanical ventilation

Heavy sedation or general anesthesia is usually required for the initiation and maintenance of mechanical ventilation. Inhalants are avoided due to their possible cardiovascular depressant effects and dependence on safe scavenging methods. Selection of intravenous sedatives depends on the type of patient, underlying disease process, and overall stability (see Chapter 22). A multimodal approach is recommended, and typically 2–3 drugs are administered together for induction and provided as a continuous infusion for maintenance of anesthesia during ventilation. Agents such as opioids, benzodiazepines, ketamine, and propofol are commonly used. Table 8.12 provides examples of protocols for the induction and maintenance of anesthesia for PPV. Anesthesia is maintained at the minimum depth required for the patient to tolerate intubation and PPV, requiring frequent monitoring [74,75]. Hypoventilating patients with neurological disease may benefit from tracheostomy tube placement to avoid prolonged anesthesia and allow assessment of neurological progression.

The goals of mechanical ventilation are to optimize pulmonary gas exchange (oxygenation) and to provide adequate ventilation, without inducing additional lung injury. In contrast to the negative airway pressure of spontaneous respiration, during PPV positive pressure is applied to the airway to cause gas flow. Ideal goals of PPV would be to achieve PaO_2 values >80 mmHg and $PaCO_2$ between 35 and 50 mmHg.

Pulmonary oxygenation and ventilation is a dynamic process, requiring frequent adjustments in ventilator settings to meet the needs of the animal. The type of breaths delivered, the option of pressure versus volume to terminate the breath, breath patterns and ventilator settings (such as FiO_2, inspiratory pressure, inspiratory time:expiratory time, tidal volume, and respiratory rate) are variables that can be adjusted to meet the needs of the animal on an ongoing basis. Recommended initial ventilator settings for the dog and cat with normal and diseased lungs are provided in Table 8.13.

The mode of ventilation describes the complex relationship between breath type, control variables, breath patterns, and breath phases. The basis for understanding different modes of ventilation relies on comprehension of the equation of motion, which explains how gas moves by way of mechanical force.

Equation of motion:

$$\text{Muscle pressure} + \text{ventilator pressure} = (\text{resistance} \times \text{flow}) + (\text{tidal volume} / \text{compliance})$$

The total pressure includes the patient-generated force and the pressure exerted by the machine. It depends on the tidal volume,

Table 8.12 Guidelines for induction and maintenance of anesthesia for the small animal ICU patient on mechanical ventilation. With maintenance, usually a combination of medications is necessary.

Drug	Rapid induction or loading dose	Maintenance (constant rate infusion) dose	Notes
Alfaxolone	0.5–3 mg/kg		CRI doses have not been clinically investigated
Atracurium	0.1–0.3 mg/kg	4–9 µg/kg/min	Paralytic, therefore ventilation required, no analgesic or sedative properties, must be combined with anesthesia for humane use; duration 20–30 min
Butorphanol	0.2–0.4 mg/kg	0.1–0.4 mg/kg/h	Minimal analgesia
Dexmedetomidine	0.5–10 ug/kg	0.5–5 µg/kg/h	Vasoconstriction, bradycardia are commonly encountered and may be severe
Diazepam	0.25–1 mg/kg	0.2–0.5 mg/kg/h	May precipitate with many drugs, use dedicated catheter; use with ketamine for rapid induction
Etomidate	1–3 mg/kg	N/A	Use with benzodiazepine for muscle relaxation; may cause adrenocortical suppression
Fentanyl	2–5 µg/kg	0.1–1 ug/kg/min	Minimal cardiovascular depression, can be increased or decreased as needed
Hydromorphone	0.05–0.2 mg/kg	0.01–0.025 mg/kg/h	Minimal cardiovascular depression
Ketamine	1–2 mg/kg	0.1–1 mg/kg/h	Used in combination with benzodiazepine for rapid induction
Lidocaine	2–4 mg/kg (dog) 0.25–0.75 mg/kg (cat)	25–80 µg/kg/min (dog) 10–40 µg/kg/min (cat)	Cautious use in cats due to neurotoxic side-effects
Midazolam	0.1–0.5 mg/kg	0.1–0.5 mg/kg/h	Use with ketamine for rapid induction
Morphine	0.2 mg/kg IM	0.1–1 mg/kg/h (cats max. 0.3 mg/kg/h)	Rapid IV administration may cause histamine release
Propofol	2–6 mg/kg	0.05–0.4 mg/kg/min	Apnea and cardiovascular depression are common

Table 8.13 Recommended initial ventilator settings for normal and diseased lungs.

Parameter	Normal lungs		Diseased lungs
	Cat	Dog	
Fraction of inspired oxygen (FiO$_2$)	100%	100%	100%
Respiratory rate (RR = breaths/min)	8–15	10–20	15–30
Tidal volume (TV = mL/kg)	8–15	8–12	6–10
Peak inspiratory pressure (PIP = cmH$_2$O)	8–10	8–10	<25
Inspiratory time (sec)	0.8–1.0	0.8–1.0	0.5–1.0
Positive end-expiratory pressure (PEEP = cmH$_2$O)	0–4	0–4	4–15
Inspiratory-to-expiratory ratio	1:2	1:2	1:1–1:2
Inspiratory pressure trigger (cmH$_2$O)	−1 – −2	−1 – −5	−1 – −5
Inspiratory flow trigger (L/min)	1–2	1–2	1–2

compliance of the lungs, airway resistance, and flow of gas. Thoracic disease severity influences lung compliance, while the ventilator circuit and patient's airway contribute to airway resistance.

Type of breath

The type of breath is selected. A controlled breath is a mandatory machine-initiated and terminated breath. A spontaneous breath is both initiated and terminated by the patient. An assisted breath is initiated by the patient, but terminated by the machine. A supported breath is used in spontaneously breathing patients, is initiated and terminated by the patient, but pressure support is provided by the ventilator during the breath [76].

Pressure versus volume-limited ventilation

It must then be determined whether the breath is terminated by a set volume or a set pressure. In volume-limited ventilation, the machine is programmed to deliver a set tidal volume, which will result in an airway pressure determined by the amount of disease and the lung mechanics. Once the preset volume is delivered, inspiration is terminated. This type of ventilation requires careful monitoring of the peak airway pressure. If the peak airway pressure becomes elevated, an airway obstruction or decreased lung compliance should be suspected. Ensure the patient is not breathing against the ventilator or coughing. Volume-limited ventilation is not used extensively because of concerns about excessive airway pressures resulting in ventilator-induced lung injury. Tidal volumes of 10–12 mL/kg (ideal weight) are usually selected for patients with normal lungs, while lower tidal volumes are used in patients with lung disease [77–80].

In pressure-limited ventilation, the machine is programmed to provide a breath that terminates at an airway pressure determined by the operator. Ideally, the inflation phase includes a rapid increase in flow rate to achieve the desired pressure at the beginning of inspiration, followed by a tapered decreasing flow to maintain a plateau inflation pressure. The biphasic component to the inspiratory phase may allow increased alveolar recruitment. Since this mode permits adjustments to the peak alveolar pressure, it may decrease the chance of barotrauma/volutrauma and ventilator-induced lung injury. If the airway becomes occluded or lung compliance decreases, hypoventilation or hypoxemia may occur, warranting higher airway pressures to be selected to achieve adequate ventilation. Ideally, peak airway pressure should be maintained less than 25–30 cmH$_2$O to minimize the risk of lung injury.

Breath patterns

Standard ventilators provide two basic breath patterns: assist/control (A/C) and synchronous intermittent mandatory ventilation (SIMV). Adjunctive breathing patterns include pressure support ventilation (PSV) and continuous positive airway pressure (CPAP). Even though an individualized approach is necessary in choosing the mode of ventilation, patients are generally started on A/C mode and later switched to SIMV as part of the early weaning strategy.

The A/C option provides preset ventilator breaths at a minimum rate determined by the operator, with breaths either pressure or volume limited. Mandatory breaths are given by the ventilator at the minimum rate if the patient is apneic. A patient breath can be detected by the ventilator when the patient generates negative inspiratory pressure or air flow. If the patient initiates breaths at the minimum rate, the ventilator times the mandatory breaths to coincide with the spontaneous breaths (Assist). If the patient breathes at a rate higher than the mandatory rate, the ventilator is triggered to provide a full ventilator breath for every patient-initiated breath. Thus, the actual ventilator rate may be higher than the minimum rate set by the operator.

In the A/C mode, the ventilator takes over most of the work of breathing. Each time the ventilator is triggered, it provides a full breath, which can be deleterious in patients with a high respiratory rate because it can cause hyperventilation or breath stacking. As a general rule, the passive expiratory phase of respiration requires about twice as much time as inspiration; thus a typical inspiratory:expiratory ratio (I:E ratio) is 1:2, with an absolute cut-off of 1:1 (as a general rule, expiration should never be shorter than inspiration). When using A/C, it is important to calculate the I:E ratio based on the actual total respiratory rate, rather than the set minimum mandatory rate.

The SIMV mode of ventilation also provides a minimum number of preset mandatory breaths. In addition, the patient can also take spontaneous breaths. SIMV differs from A/C because the spontaneous breaths are not assisted by the ventilator. The machine can integrate mandatory and spontaneous breaths by using a unidirectional valve and two parallel circuits, one for spontaneous breathing and the other for mechanically delivered breaths. During the time cycle, the ventilator waits for the patient to initiate a breath using either a pressure or flow trigger. If the patient does not initiate a breath during this cycle time, the machine will deliver a mandatory breath. When the machine senses a spontaneous breath within that cycle, it will deliver a preset breath known as an assisted breath (synchronous). If the patient continues spontaneously breathing during that time cycle, the machine will not trigger another machine breath until the next time cycle.

Synchronous intermittent mandatory ventilation allows a more physiological breathing pattern, which may aid patient comfort, and it can be useful in tachypneic animals. SIMV has the added advantage of permitting a lower mean airway pressure and more ideal ventilation to perfusion relationship. In addition, it increases the patient's work of breathing to start the weaning process. The operator has the option of adding pressure support to the spontaneous breaths, which helps to overcome the added resistance imposed by the ventilator circuit, which otherwise might cause weaning failure.

Pressure support ventilation (PSV) can be added to spontaneous breaths, thereby increasing the tidal volume and decreasing the patient's work of breathing. Pressure support ventilation allows the patient to initiate and terminate each breath. During a normal breath, air flow rate is highest at the beginning of inspiration, decreasing to zero at peak inspiration. During PSV, when the ventilator detects an inspiratory effort, it provides pressure support until the air flow decreases to a predetermined percent of the peak air flow rate during the breath, usually about 25%. Thus, PSV is sometimes described as a "flow-limited" mode of ventilation. Pressure support can be a useful part of the weaning process as the patient improves. This mode can be added to spontaneous breaths in SIMV or used in patients that are spontaneously breathing without PPV.

Continuous positive airway pressure (CPAP) is best understood as spontaneous breathing with positive end-expiratory pressure (PEEP). In CPAP, all the breaths are initiated and terminated by the patient and there are no positive pressure breaths from the ventilator. However, the baseline pressure between breaths is above zero, which helps prevent deflation and collapse of alveoli and increases

functional residual capacity. PSV can be added to the spontaneous breaths to improve tidal volume if necessary. This mode is used in patients that are initiating breaths on their own but have either pulmonary disease that requires some assistance in preventing alveolar collapse or neuromuscular disease that prevents adequate physiologic PEEP from being maintained.

Ventilator settings

The most important ventilator settings include the tidal volume, respiratory rate, inspiratory pressure, inspiratory time, I:E ratio, trigger sensitivity (pressure or flow triggers), and PEEP.

Peak inspiratory pressure (PIP) is the highest airway pressure during inspiration. The mean inspiratory pressure is the average airway pressure during a respiratory cycle. The inspiratory plateau pressure is usually slightly lower than the peak inspiratory pressure, because of redistribution of air during the plateau inspiratory hold. The difference between the PIP and the inspiratory plateau pressure is greatest when there is airway disease or increased resistance within the ventilator circuit.

Positive end-expiratory pressure is a ventilator setting in which the airway pressure is not allowed to decrease to zero between breaths. Abnormal lung units have decreased or defective surfactant, resulting in collapse. Normal lung units in recumbent patients or during neuromuscular disease can also have atelectasis. Recruitable alveoli are those that collapse completely during expiration and pop open again during inspiration when a PPV breath is received. This repetitive cycle can result in inflammation due to shear stress, and ultimately progression of pulmonary parenchymal disease. PEEP is used to decrease ventilator-induced lung injury and improve oxygenation by increasing functional residual capacity, recruiting already damaged and atelectatic alveoli, and preventing the collapse of unstable but still functional alveoli [81–83]. An individualized approach is required for setting optimal PEEP. PEEP does not usually significantly affect ventilation, but can result in marked improvement of oxygenation, thereby allowing the patient to be managed with a lower FiO_2.

Auto-PEEP occurs when the expiratory time is shorter than the time needed to fully deflate the lungs causing progressive air trapping (hyperinflation), causing adverse respiratory and cardiovascular effects. Intrinsic PEEP can occur due to collapse of the small airways prior to complete exhalation, such as during asthma, chronic bronchitis, and ARDS. Iatrogenic auto-PEEP can also occur when ventilator settings do not allow complete exhalation. Auto-PEEP, either intrinsic or iatrogenic, will increase intrathoracic pressure and result in decreased cardiac preload. It will also cause volutrauma, barotrauma, and leakage of air into the pleural space [81–84].

The respiratory rate is measured in breaths per minute and is usually set between eight and 30 breaths per minute. Higher rates are required for patients with lung disease, particularly if low tidal volumes are being used.

Volume settings include the tidal volume and minute ventilation. The tidal volume (TV) is the amount of gas in a single breath. Patients with ARDS and other forms of severe lung disease that cause decreased compliance are best managed with low tidal volume ventilation [77–80]. The minute ventilation (VE) is the product of tidal volume (liters per minute) and the respiratory rate (breaths per minute). Some ventilators allow the operator to set the inspiratory flow rate, which is usually about 40–60 L/min for both healthy and diseased lungs.

Initiating mechanical ventilation

The patient should be evaluated and most life-threatening complications treated first; if necessary, emergency intubation and manual ventilation may be needed while the therapeutic ventilator is set up.

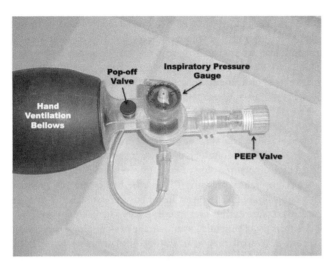

Figure 8.9 Artificial manual breathing unit (AMBU) bag with detachable PEEP valve and detachable inspiratory pressure gauge (Ambu®, Amby Inc, Columbia, MD). Source: courtesy of Angel Rivera.

Ventilator machine internal diagnostic cycles can take several minutes to complete but are necessary to ensure the machine is working properly and all alarms are functional. Hand ventilation with the artificial manual breathing unit (AMBU) bag can provide effective short-term ventilation during resuscitation or to transition the patient to the therapeutic ventilator. AMBU bags are available in varying sizes based on the size of the patient and should have an oxygen source. They can be equipped with an inspiratory pressure gauge and PEEP valve (Figure 8.9); if an AMBU bag is not available, an anesthetic machine (flushed with fresh gas) or an anesthetic ventilator may be used while setting up therapeutic (long-term) ventilation.

Preparation is key when working with a critically ill patient, so having emergency intervention materials can be life-saving if rapid decompensation or machinery failure occurs. This includes emergency CPR drugs, equipment to perform a rapid thoracocentesis, a secondary means of providing supplemental O_2, back-up monitoring devices, multiple ET tube sizes, and other pertinent items for rapid intubation.

Safe initiation of PPV is reliant on swift transition to mechanical breaths. The FiO_2 is usually set at 100% until adequate oxygenation can be confirmed. Humidification of inspired air helps prevent respiratory epithelial desiccation. Warming the inspired air allows it to carry more water vapor, and may help prevent hypothermia.

Once PPV begins, the chest wall movement should be observed during the administration of mechanical breaths, allowing evaluation of patient comfort and quality of chest exertions. Auscultation should be performed frequently. Bilateral breath sounds should be easily heard and if not, a pneumothorax or inadvertent bronchial intubation should be ruled out. Auscultating the upper airway will allow for early detection of ET tube cuff leaks or excessive secretions in the ET or tracheostomy tube.

The settings listed in Table 8.13 provide general guidelines for the initial PPV settings, but each patient will require individual settings according to their unique pulmonary pathology. Initial settings vary depending on the underlying respiratory dysfunction. Hypoventilation usually requires less aggressive settings and minute ventilation is sufficient when the $PaCO_2$ is within the normal range. Most patients start on A/C and then transition to SIMV as the respiratory condition improves, ultimately with use of PSV and possibly CPAP for weaning. Note that all settings should be calculated based on the ideal rather than the actual body weight.

Ventilator settings can be more complicated in the presence of lung disease that causes decreased lung compliance. Lung compliance is defined as the relationship between tidal volume and changes in airway pressure. In diseased lungs with low compliance, a larger change in pressure or higher inspiratory pressures is required to achieve a normal tidal volume. Nevertheless, efforts should be made to avoid positive inspiratory pressure values >25 cmH$_2$O (>18.4 mmHg), because there is increased risk of barotrauma and pneumothorax.

Adjusting and trouble-shooting the ventilator settings

$PaCO_2$ (or $PvCO_2$ if an arterial blood sample is not available) is the first and most important parameter to correct when stabilizing a patient on the ventilator. For most patients, a reasonable goal is to maintain the $PaCO_2$ between 40 and 50 mmHg. Lower values may be necessary in patients with intracranial hypertension. Higher values may be acceptable (termed permissive hypercapnia) in some patients with severe lung disease as long as severe respiratory acidosis does not occur. $PaCO_2$ is linearly related to minute ventilation, and can be manipulated by adjusting either the tidal volume (of assisted breaths or spontaneous breaths) or the respiratory rate. Normal minute ventilation is 150–250 mL/kg/min. Animals with lung disease may require higher than normal minute ventilation, sometimes up to double the normal values. When determining the optimal tidal volume per breath, it is important to observe the chest wall motion of the patient. If the ventilator breath produces insufficient chest wall motion in a patient that has hypercapnia or is difficult to stabilize on the ventilator, it may be necessary to increase the tidal volume in order to make chest excursions look more normal, especially in cats and smaller patients.

Patients with high $PaCO_2$ values experience central respiratory drive due to hypercapnia. Increased central respiratory drive causes the patient to make respiratory efforts (inspiratory or expiratory) that are not related to ventilator breaths, so-called "patient-ventilator" dyssynchrony [85]. It can be difficult to determine whether dyssynchrony is the cause of hypercapnia or a result of it. First, efforts should be made to ensure that the patient is sufficiently anesthetized. If the patient is under deep anesthesia, the next step is to increase the minute ventilation by increasing either the respiratory rate or the tidal volume. If hypercapnia was the cause of the problem, most patients will stop "fighting the ventilator" after a few minutes.

Low tidal volume ventilation in patients with ARDS presents special challenges in regard to hypercapnia. In an effort to avoid ventilator-induced lung injury, each small breath may predominantly ventilate dead space. Thus, it may not be possible to effectively eliminate CO_2, resulting in hypercapnia and respiratory acidosis. In these cases, the clinician must make a compromise between increasing the tidal volume with resultant higher airway pressures and allowing permissive hypercapnia [79–81].

Hypoxemia is the next challenge to address once hypercapnia has been corrected. Initial ventilator settings for almost all patients should include a FiO_2 of 100%. An early goal during PPV is then to decrease the FiO_2 to a value less than 60%, in order to minimize the risk of hyperoxic lung toxicity. Depending on the severity of lung disease, hypoxia (SpO$_2$ < 94%) may be evident at a FiO_2 of 100%, or may become evident as efforts are made to decrease the FiO_2. If hypoxemia occurs as FiO_2 is decreased, the next step is to add PEEP.

Addition of PEEP may allow better oxygenation for a given FiO_2, and helps to prevent ventilator-induced lung injury by preventing cyclical collapse of alveoli [81–83].

If hypoxemia develops in an animal that was previously stable on the ventilator or following a break in the ventilator circuit, consideration can be given to performing a recruitment maneuver, followed by an increase in PEEP. Recruitment maneuvers (RM) consist of a ventilatory strategy that increases the transpulmonary pressure transiently to reopen the recruitable lung units. The three recruitment methods that are most commonly used are sighs (ventilator breath with greater volume than tidal volume), sustained inflation, and extended sigh (stepwise increase in PEEP and decrease in tidal volume over 2 minutes to a CPAP of 30 mmHg for 30 seconds) [86,87]. Maintenance of the patient in sternal recumbency may help to improve oxygenation by optimizing V/Q matching.

If acute hypoxemia occurs during PPV, the first step is to temporarily increase the FiO2 while the underlying problem is being identified. Next, a search is carried out for mechanical or ventilator problems including O_2 source malfunction, circuit breakage or disconnect, ventilator failure, incorrect intubation or dislodged tube. Patient-related factors can include insufficient or excessive depth of anesthesia, progressive lung disease, atelectasis, hyperthermia, mucus obstruction of the endotracheal or tracheostomy tube, or development of pneumothorax or pneumomediastinum.

Once a ventilator alarm is triggered, prompt trouble-shooting of the patient and mechanical ventilator is essential. Alarm ranges are set by the operator and should be reasonable for each individual patient.

The PIP airway pressure alarm range should be set 5–10 mmHg above and below the patient's present PIP. Elevated airway pressures occur because of either a decrease in pulmonary compliance or increase in airway resistance, while an acute drop in airway pressure is usually caused by a leak in the circuit.

The tidal volume alarm should be set 15–20% above and below the current tidal volume of the patient. This alarm is very useful during a pressure-controlled breathing pattern because the tidal volume fluctuates in order to maintain a constant PIP. A low tidal volume alarm will be triggered by a decrease in compliance or increase in airway resistance, or by a circuit disconnect or leak. Minute ventilation alarms should prompt the clinician to similar problems.

Ventilator waveform monitoring is available on most therapeutic ventilators, and may use scalar waveforms (time on the x-axis and pressure, volume or flow on the y-axis) or continuous individual breath waveform loops (pressure-volume loops or flow-volume loops) to identify many problems associated with management of the ventilator patient (leaks, auto-PEEP, various types of dyssynchrony, etc.). Monitoring these waveforms requires thorough understanding of ventilator and patient mechanics.

Monitoring and care for mechanical ventilation

Patients on PPV are completely reliant on a dedicated and experienced 24-hour care team to provide the highest level of continuous monitoring and support. PPV has the potential to cause adverse effects to the cardiovascular, respiratory, neurological, gastrointestinal, and renal systems. Continuous monitoring is essential, including body core temperature, ECG, capnography, oximetry, and arterial blood pressure. In addition, essential frequent monitoring should include thoracic auscultation, breath patterns and efficacy of chest excursions, urine output, anesthetic depth, ET or

tracheostomy tube placement, water trap accumulation, patient positioning, and the detection of pressure sores. Supportive care also includes physical therapy, including passive range of motion, parenteral medication administration, anesthetic adjustments, oral hygiene, tube maintenance and positioning, nutritional supplementation, ocular care, and maintenance of general cleanliness (see Chapter 20 and Table 20.3) [85,86]. Airway management relies on proper tube placement and cuff inflation. Intubation should be as sterile as possible and careful hygiene should be practiced when manipulating the tube or assessing the oral cavity. Humidification is a requirement for long-term mechanical ventilation. Occasional suctioning of the airway becomes a necessity but should not be performed empirically since disconnection of the circuit can cause derecruitment and the potential for ventilator-associated pneumonia.

Positive pressure ventilation differs from spontaneous breathing because negative intrathoracic pressure does not occur during any part of the respiratory cycle. Negative intrathoracic pressure facilitates venous return, and is therefore important for optimal cardiac output. Especially if there is any degree of hypovolemia, PPV can therefore be associated with decreased cardiac output and ultimately decreased tissue perfusion.

Elevated airway pressures may cause overdistension of certain lung units, with distribution of pulmonary blood flow to the unventilated regions, resulting in V/Q mismatch and hypoxia. Ventilator-induced lung injury is associated with high tidal volumes and cyclical recruitment and derecruitment of alveoli [88,89]. Pneumothorax is the most obvious complication of barotrauma/volutrauma, which may cause a rapid decline in the patient's ability to oxygenate and/or ventilate [90]. Identification and early intervention are imperative because continuous administration of mandatory breaths will quickly develop into a life-threatening tension pneumothorax. Treatment involves swift removal of intrathoracic air by thoracocentesis, followed by placement of a thoracostomy tube with continuous negative pressure drainage if the patient is to remain on PPV.

Nosocomial infections are a serious problem in critically ill patients, and ventilator-associated pneumonia continues to be a major complication in both human and veterinary patients. Most cases are thought to be due to either translocation of bacteria into the lungs during ET intubation or aspiration of oropharyngeal contents during PPV [91]. Preventative techniques include strict sterile technique during ET intubation and minimizing ET tube exchanges while on the mechanical ventilator. Decontamination of the oropharynx using an antibacterial oral rinse (such as chlorhexidine solution) and diligent oral hygiene should also be implemented [88]. Routine ET suction maneuvers should be minimized to decrease the chance of dislodging secretions and advancing bacteria into the lower airways. Monitoring the patient for signs of infection is key for early detection, prompt identification, and appropriate treatment. An abnormal temperature (hyperthermia or hypothermia), leukocyte count (leukocytosis, leukocytopenia, presence of left shift, or cytoplasmic toxic change), and purulent respiratory secretions all suggest a systemic infection potentially involving the lungs in the ventilated patient. Thoracic radiographs or CT scans can aid in identifying the presence of pulmonary infiltrates, but have limited sensitivity and specificity since pulmonary infiltrates may be due to pulmonary edema, acute respiratory distress syndrome, atelectasis, hemorrhage, neoplasia, or pneumonia. The diagnosis of ventilator-associated pneumonia includes isolation of the pathogen. Samples are collected from the airway by direct aspiration of secretions or by performing an ET lavage and submitted for culture and susceptibility testing.

Weaning from mechanical ventilation

Discontinuation of mechanical ventilation is a continuous process that begins early during PPV. Efforts to constantly reduce the level of support from the machine to the extent that is tolerated by the patient are ongoing. This is known as "weaning" the patient from the mechanical ventilator. Criteria that must be met prior to considering the patient ready to be weaned include ensuring adequate gas exchange after transition to less aggressive PPV settings, adequate spontaneous ventilation efforts by the patient, and hemodynamic stability [92]. In order for weaning to be possible, the patient usually must be oxygenating effectively on an $FiO_2 < 50\%$ and PEEP values less than $4\,cmH_2O$. Many weaning protocols include transitions from A/C to SIMV with gradual reduction of the number of mandatory breaths and gradual reduction of PSV, followed eventually by transition to CPAP [93,94].

During the final part of the weaning period, which is accompanied by extubation, it is critical that the supportive care personnel monitor the patient continuously because premature or failed trials are not uncommon. Owners should be warned that many patients need repeated periods "on" and "off" the ventilator before weaning is finally successful. Specific parameters to monitor include poor chest exertions, development of hypoxia or hyper/hypocapnia, tachypnea, tachycardia, or discomfort. Arterial blood gas, capnography, and oximetry are necessary to guide the process.

Small airway disorders

Common causes of small airway disorders in the small animal ICU patient are listed in Table 8.10. In dogs, chronic bronchial obstruction can develop due to inflammatory infiltrates (eosinophils, neutrophils, or macrophages), increased mucus production due to goblet cell proliferation, or thickening of the bronchial mucosa due to hyperemia and edema, and early closure of small airways during exhalation, all combining to result in obstructive airway disease.

In cats, the term "asthma" implies a reversible bronchoconstriction related to hypertrophy and hypersensitivity of airway smooth muscle (bronchospasm), hypertrophy of mucous glands, and infiltrates of eosinophils. Asthma in cats is primarily due to type I hypersensitivity reactions. Cats with chronic bronchitis not due to asthma generally have infiltrates of neutrophils or macrophages as well as hypertrophy of mucous glands, hyperplasia of goblet cells, excessive mucus, and ultimately fibrosis secondary to chronic inflammation. Etiologies of bronchitis in cats can include idiopathic disease, bacterial infection, mycoplasmosis, viral and parasitic infections.

Physical examination abnormalities in animals with small airway disease include cough, dyspnea, and wheezes on auscultation. Auscultated wheezes provide very strong evidence of bronchial narrowing. Crackles may be evident occasionally as small airways snap open and closed. In some cats, increased bronchovesicular sounds may be the only abnormality noted on auscultation. If dyspnea occurs, it commonly has a pronounced expiratory component because of early closure of small airways. Open-mouth breathing or panting commonly occurs during periods of stress.

In the emergency setting, lower airway disease can result in airway obstruction and expiratory respiratory distress as a result of bronchoconstriction, mucus accumulation, mucosal thickening due to hyperemia, edema and inflammatory cell infiltrates, and

airway collapse. Feline asthma is defined as the presence of excessive and reversible bronchoconstriction that is triggered by inflammation and causes severe narrowing of the airways and acute dyspnea. Oxygen supplementation, sedation if needed, and specific pharmacological therapies are often necessary to treat dyspnea caused by bronchial disease. Drug treatment for lower airway disease includes antiinflammatories, bronchodilators, and specific treatment for primary causes, for example antibiotic therapy for bacterial infections.

Glucocorticoids should always be the first-line therapy for patients with lower airway disease. Of note, nonsteroidal antiinflammatory drugs are minimally effective in the respiratory tract and are not used to treat airway or lung inflammation. By decreasing airway inflammatory cell infiltrates and mucus production, glucocorticoids result in improved air flow and reduction in coughing. Since inflammation is the cause of bronchial narrowing in dogs with chronic bronchitis and of bronchoconstriction in cats with asthma, glucocorticoids should usually be administered for emergency and long-term treatment of lower airway disease. They are often used in combination with bronchodilators, which can help lower the overall dose of glucocorticoids if long-term systemic side-effects become intolerable [95,96]. In an emergency presentation, antiinflammatory doses of glucocorticoids should be administered parenterally. Inhaled steroids may be used for long-term treatment, but are not appropriate for emergency stabilization because a single dose of an inhaled steroid is ineffective (i.e. steroids are not used as "rescue inhalers"). Twice-daily dosing for at least a week is needed for efficacy.

Bronchodilators are also an important part of acute therapy for animals with bronchial disease, administered either parenterally or by inhalation. These drugs are of particular importance in cats with asthma-induced bronchospasm [97]. Systemic (intramuscular or intravenous) administration of a beta-2 agonist (usually terbutaline) should result in a decrease in respiratory rate and effort within 30–45 minutes. Side-effects can include tachycardia, restlessness, and skeletal muscle tremors. Beta-2 agonist bronchodilators (usually albuterol) may be administered by inhalation.

However, because dogs and cats cannot be trained to maximally inhale when the metered dose inhaler is activated, the drug may not be effectively distributed to the most diseased airways. If the animal is breathing shallowly, it is likely that the majority of the inhaled drug will be distributed to normal airways with lower resistance, while bronchi with more disease and longer time constants (that take longer to open during inhalation) may not open during the breath and therefore not receive the drug. Thus, inhaled drugs are administered to animals using a specialized chamber called a "spacer" and a face mask (Aerokat and Aerodawg, Trudell Medical International, Ontario). By adding a "spacer" into which the drug is discharged, and requiring the animal to take 10 breaths from the chamber, there is a greater chance of drug distribution to the more diseased airways. Additionally, if rebreathing of carbon dioxide occurs within the spacer, this should trigger deeper breaths, which further increase the chance of effective drug distribution to the diseased airways, while avoiding systemic absorption. Dyspneic animals may not tolerate placement of a mask and it may be impossible for them to take 10 breaths from the spacer without exacerbating respiratory distress. Thus, unless systemic use of beta-agonists is contraindicated, for example in a cat with hypertrophic cardiomyopathy, parenteral administration remains the method of choice for emergency situations.

Neuromuscular breathing disorders

Disorders involving the brainstem, cervical spinal cord, intercostal muscles or diaphragm can cause abnormal respiratory rate, rhythm or respiratory muscle activity; neuromuscular diseases (polyradiculoneuritis, tick paralysis or botulism toxicity) or iatrogenic administration of neuromuscular blockers (atracurium, succinylcholine) can also cause hypoventilation. Clinical signs will vary depending upon the severity of the neuromuscular disorder. Severe hypokalemia can be seen in the critically ill patient and can cause respiratory muscle paresis and impair ventilation.

In the most severe situations, cyanosis and respiratory arrest can occur. Clinical signs vary depending on the site of the neuromuscular defect. If the problem is central (i.e. the brainstem), the patient is likely to be comatose, and hypoventilation may be diagnosed because of a low respiratory rate or shallow respiration. In dogs with spinal cord or peripheral neuromuscular disease, nasal flare, open-mouth breathing, cheek-puffing, and anxiety may accompany minimal movement of the chest wall and diaphragm and paralysis of limbs.

Hypoventilation (increased $PaCO_2$) is the most common cause of hypoxemia in these patients. A search is made to identify and treat the underlying cause. Supplementation of O_2 is provided and may suffice in mild situations. However, placement of an ET tube and PPV are often required until the underlying cause can be effectively treated.

References

1. Corne S, Bshouty Z. Basic principles of control of breathing. Respir Care Clin North Am. 2005;11:147.
2. West JB. Respiratory Physiology: The Essentials, 8th edn. Baltimore: Lippincott Williams & Wilkins, 2008.
3. Severinghaus J. Simple, accurate equations for human blood O2 dissociation computation (oxygen-haemoglobin dissociation curve). J Appl Physiol. 1979;26(3):599–602.
4. Amis TC, Kurpershoek C. Pattern of breathing in brachycephalic dogs. Am J Vet Res. 1986;47:2200–4.
5. Harpster NK. Physical examination of the respiratory tract. In: Textbook of Respiratory Disease in Dogs and Cats. King LG, ed. St Louis: Saunders, 2004: pp 67–72.
6. Le Boedek K, Arnaud C, Chetboul V. Relationship between paradoxical breathing and pleural diseases in dyspneic dogs and cats: 389 cases (2011–2009). J Am Vet Med Assoc. 2012;240(9):1095.
7. Tseng LW, Waddell LS. Approach to the patient in respiratory distress. Clin Tech Small Anim Pract. 2000;15(2):53–62.
8. Meler E, Dunn M, Lécuyer M. A retrospective study of canine persistent nasal disease: 80 cases (1998–2003). Can Vet J. 2008;49(1):71–6.
9. Plickert HD, Tichy A, Hirt RA. Characteristics of canine nasal discharge related to intranasal disease: a retrospective study of 105 cases. J Small Anim Pract. 2014;55(3):145–52.
10. Sigrist NE, Adamik KN, Doherr MG, et al. Evaluation of respiratory parameters at presentation as clinical indicators of the respiratory localization in dogs and cats with respiratory distress. J Vet Emerg Crit Care 2011;21(1):13–23.
11. Creedon, Burkitt J, Davis H. Advanced Monitoring and Procedures for Small Animal Emergency and Critical Care. Chichester: Wiley-Blackwell, 2012.
12. Treger R, Pirouz S, Kamangar N, et al. Agreement between central venous and arterial blood gas measurements in the intensive care unit. Clin J Am Soc Nephrol. 2010;5:90.
13. Silverstein D, Hopper K. Small Animal Critical Care Medicine, 2nd edn. St Louis: Saunders Elsevier, 2015.
14. Ilkiw JE, Rose RJ, Martin ICA. A comparison of simultaneously collected arterial, mixed venous, jugular venous and cephalic venous blood samples and the assessment of blood-gas and acid-base status in the dog. J Vet Intern Med. 1991;5:294.
15. Hopper K, Haskins SC. A case-based review of a simplified quantitative approach to acid-base analysis. J Vet Emerg Crit Care 2008;18(5):467.
16. Rezende ML, Haskins SC, Hopper K. The effects of ice water storage on blood gas and acid-base measurements. J Vet Emerg Crit Care 2007;17:67.
17. Masoro EJ, Siegel PD. Acid-base Regulation: Its Physiology, Pathophysiology and the Interpretation of Blood-Gas Analysis, 2nd edn. St Louis: Saunders, 1978.
18. Marik P, Vincent J. Arterial blood gas interpretation. In: Textbook of Critical Care, 6th edn. Vincent JL, ed. Philadelphia: Elsevier Saunders, 2011.
19. DiBartola SP. Introduction to acid-base disorders. In: Fluid, Electrolyte and Acid-base Disorders, 4th edn. DiBartola SP, ed. St Louis: Elsevier Saunders, 2012.
20. Spector D, Legendre AM, Wheat J. Antigen and antibody testing for the diagnosis of blastomycosis in dogs. J Vet Intern Med. 2008;22(4):839–43.
21. Foy DS, Trepanier LA, Kirsch E, Wheat L. Serum and urine Blastomyces antigen concentrations as markers of clinical remission of systemic blastomycosis. J Vet Intern Med. 2014;28(2):305–10.
22. Kirsch EJ, Greene RT, Prahl A. Evaluation of Coccidioides antigen detection in dogs with coccidioidomycosis. Clin Vaccine Immunol. 2012;19(3):343.
23. Boysen SR, Lisciandro GR. The use of ultrasound for dogs and cats in the emergency room: AFAST and TFAST. Vet Clin North Am Small Anim Pract. 2013;43(4):773–97.
24. Lisciandro G. The VetBLUE lung scan. In: Focused Ultrasound Techniques for the Small Animal Practitioner. Ames: Wiley & Sons, 2014: pp 166–88.
25. Alexander K, Joly H, Blond L. Comparison of computed tomography, computed radiography and film-screen radiograph for the detection of canine pulmonary nodules. Vet Radiol Ultrasound. 2012;53(3):258.
26. Fairman NB. Evaluation of pulse oximetry as a continuous monitoring technique in critically ill dogs in the small animal intensive care unit. J Vet Emerg Crit Care 1992;2(2):50–6.
27. Grosenbaugh DA, Alben JO, Muir WW. Absorbance spectra of inter-species hemoglobins in the visible end-near infrared regions. J Vet Emerg Crit Care 1997;7:36–42.
28. Srinivas K, Gopal Reddy L, Srinivas R. Estimation of heart rate variability from peripheral pulse wave using PPG sensor. Proc Int Fed Med Biol Eng. 2007;325–8.
29. Cohn L. Pulmonary parenchymal diseases. In: Textbook of Veterinary Internal Medicine, 7th edn. Ettinger SJ, Feldman EC, eds. St Louis: Elsevier, 2010.
30. Sendak MJ, Harris AP, Donham RT. Accuracy of pulse oximetry during arterial oxyhemoglobin desaturation in dogs. Anesthesiology 1988;68:111–14.
31. Hendricks JC, King LG. Practicality, usefulness, and limits of pulse oximetry in critical small animal patients. J Vet Emerg Crit Care 2003;l3(1):5–12.
32. Toben B. Pitfalls in the measurement and interpretation of hemoglobin, oxyhemoglobin saturation, and oxygen content in point-of-care devices. RT Decision Makers Respir Care 2008;21(1):1–5.
33. Ayres DA. Pulse oximetry and CO-oximetry. In: Advanced Monitoring and Procedures for Small Animal Emergency and Critical Care. Burkitt-Creedon JM, Davis H, eds. Oxford: John Wiley & Sons, 2012: pp 274–85.
34. Engbers S, Boysen SR, Engbers J, Chalhoub S. A comparison of tissue oxygen saturation measurements by 2 different near-infrared spectroscopy monitors in 21 healthy dogs. J Vet Emerg Crit Care 2014;24(5):536–44.
35. Pavlisko ND, Killos M, Henao-Guerrero N, et al. Evaluation of tissue hemoglobin saturation (StO2) using near-infrared spectroscopy during hypoxemia and hyperoxemia in Beagle dogs. Vet Anaseth Analg. 2016;43(1):18–26.
36. Pascucci RC, Schena JA, Thompson JE. Comparison of a sidestream and mainstream capnometer in infants. Crit Care Med. 1989;17:560–2.
37. Raffe M. End tidal capnography. In: Textbook of Respiratory Disease in Dogs and Cats. King LG, ed. St Louis: Saunders, 2004: pp 198–201.
38. Pang D, Heathy J, Caulkett NA, Duke T. Partial pressure of ETCO2 via an intranasal catheter as a substitute for parital pressure of arterial CO2 in dogs. J Vet Emerg Crit Care 2007;17(2):143–8.
39. Trevino RP, Bisera J, Weil MH, et al. End-tidal CO2 as a guide to successful cardiopulmonary resuscitation: a preliminary report. Crit Care Med. 1985;13:910–11.
40. Gudipati CV, Weil MH, Bisera J, et al. Expired carbon dioxide: a noninvasive monitor of cardiopulmonary resuscitation. Circulation 1988;77:234–9.
41. Hofmeister EH, Brainard BM, Egger CM, et al. Prognostic indicators for dogs and cats with cardiopulmonary arrest treated by cardiopulmonary cerebral resuscitation at a university teaching hospital. J Am Vet Med Assoc. 2009; 235:50–7.
42. Sanders AB, Kern KB, Otto CW, et al. End-tidal carbon dioxide monitoring during cardiopulmonary resuscitation. A prognostic indicator for survival. J Am Med Assoc. 1989;262:1347–51.
43. Tseng LW, Drobatz KJ. Oxygen supplementation and humidification. In: Textbook of Respiratory Disease in Dogs and Cats. King LG, ed. St Louis: Saunders, 2004: pp 205–13.
44. Paine JR, Lynn D, Keys A. Observations on effects of prolonged administration of high oxygen concentration to dogs. J Thoracic Surg. 1941;11:151–68.
45. Hitt ME. Oxygen derived free radicals: pathophysiology and implications. Compend Contin Educ Pract Vet. 1988;10(8):939–46.
46. Crapo JD. Morphologic changes in pulmonary oxygen toxicity. Am Rev Physiol. 1986;48:721–31.

47. Loukopoulos P, Reynolds W. Comparative evaluation of oxygen therapy techniques in anaesthetized dogs: face-mask and flow by technique. Aust Vet Pract. 1997;27:34–9.

48. Loukopoulos P, Reynolds W. Comparative evaluation of oxygen therapy techniques in anaesthetized dogs: intranasal catheter and Elizabethan collar canopy. Aust Vet Pract. 1996;26:199–204.

49. Howard MM. Undesirable concentrations of CO_2 in enriched oxygen environments in the clinical setting. J Vet Emerg Crit Care 2014;24(5):491–2.

50. Mann FA, Wagner-Mann C, Allert JA, Smith J. Comparison of intranasal and intratracheal oxygen administration in healthy awake dogs. Am J Vet Res. 1992;53(5):856.

51. Alderson B, Senior AH, Dugdale JM. Tracheal necrosis following tracheal intubation in a dog. J Small Anim Pract. 2006;47(12):754–6.

52. Mitchell SL, McCarthy R, Rudloff E, et al. Tracheal rupture associated with intubation in cats: 20 cases (1996–1998). J Am Vet Med Assoc. 2000;216(10):1592.

53. Mort TC. Preoxygenation in critically ill patients requiring emergency tracheal intubation. Crit Care Med. 2005;33(11):2972–5.

54. McKelvey D, Hollingshead KW. Veterinary Anesthesia and Analgesia, 3rd edn. St Louis: Mosby, 2003: pp 66–74, 166–70.

55. Bryant LR, Mujia D, Greenberg S, et al. Evaluation of tracheal incisions for tracheostomy. Am J Surg. 1978;135(5):675–9.

56. Colley P, Huber M, Henderson R. Tracheostomy techniques and management. Compend Contin Educ Pract Vet. 1999;21(1):44–52.

57. Harvey CE, O'Brien JA. Tracheostomy in the dog and cat: analysis of 89 episodes in 79 animals. J Am Anim Hosp Assoc. 1982:563–6.

58. Fitton, CM, Myer, CM. Practical aspects of pediatric tracheotomy care. J Otolaryngol. 1992;21(6):409–13.

59. Hedlund CS, Tangner CH. Tracheal surgery in the dog – part II. Compend Contin Educ Pract Vet. 1983;5:738–50.

60. Hedlund CS, Tangner CH, Waldron DR, et al. Permanent tracheostomy: perioperative and long-term data from 34 cases. J Am Anim Hosp Assoc. 1988;24:585–91.

61. Dempsey SM, Ewing PJ. A review of the pathophysiology, classification and analysis of canine and feline cavitary effusions. J Am Anim Hosp Assoc. 2011;47:1.

62. American Thoracic Society. Guidelines for thoracocentesis and needle biopsy of the pleura. Am Rev Respir Dis. 1989;140:257.

63. Janocik SE, Roy Ted, Killeen TR. Re-expansion pulmonary edema: a preventable complication. J Ky Med Assoc. 1993;91:143–6.

64. Mahajan VK, Simon M, Huber GL. Reexpansion pulmonary edema. Chest 1979;75:192–4.

65. Worth A, Machon R. Prevention of reexpansion pulmonary edema and ischemia-reperfusion injury in the management of diaphragmatic herniation. Compend Contin Educ Pract Vet. 2006;7:531–8.

66. Hawkins EC, Fossum TW. Medical and surgical management of pleural effusion. In: Kirk's Current Veterinary Therapy, vol. 13. Bonagura JD, ed. Philadelphia: WB Saunders, 2000.

67. Sigrist NE. Thoracostomy tube placement and drainage. In: Small Animal Critical Care Medicine. Silverstein DC, Hopper K, eds. 2nd edn. Philadelphia: Saunders, 2015: pp 134–7.

68. Marques AIDC, Tattersall J, Shaw DJ, et al. Retrospective analysis of the relationship between time of thoracostomy drain removal and discharge time. J Small Anim Pract. 2009;50(4):162.

69. Puerto D, Brockman DJ, Lindquist C, Drobatz K. Surgical and nonsurgical management of and selected risk factors for spontaneous pneumothorax in dogs: 64 cases (1986–1999). J Am Vet Med Assoc. 2002;220(11):1670–4.

70. Hopper K, Haskins SC, Kass PH, et al. Indications, management and outcome of long-term positive-pressure ventilation in dogs and cats (1990–2001). J Am Vet Med Assoc. 2007;230:64.

71. King LG, Hendricks JC. Use of positive pressure ventilation in dogs and cats: 41 cases (1990–1992). J Am Vet Med Assoc. 1994;204:1045.

72. Lee JA, Drobatz KJ, Koch MW, King LG. Indications for and outcome of positive-pressure ventilation in cats: 53 cases (1993–2002). J Am Vet Med Assoc. 2005;226:924.

73. Lumb AB. Nunn's Applied Respiratory Physiology, 7th edn. Oxford: Churchill Livingstone, 2010.

74. Boudreau AE, Bersenas AME, Kerr CL, et al. A comparison of 3 anesthetic protocols for 24 hours of mechanical ventilation in cats. J Vet Emerg Crit Care 2012;22:239.

75. Ethier MR, Mathews KA, Valverde AV, et al. Evaluation of the efficacy and safety for use of two sedation and analgesia protocols to facilitate assisted ventilation of healthy dogs. Am J Vet Res. 2008;69:1351.

76. Haskins SC, King LG. Positive pressure ventilation. In: Textbook of Respiratory Disease in Dogs and Cats. King LG, ed. St Louis: Saunders, 2004: pp 217–29.

77. ARDS Network. Ventilation with lower tidal volumes as compared with traditional tidal volumes for acute lung injury and the acute respiratory distress syndrome. N Engl J Med. 2000;342:1301.

78. Amato MBP, Barbas CSV, Medeiros DM, et al. Effect of a protective ventilation strategy on mortality in the acute respiratory distress syndrome. N Engl J Med. 1998;338:347–54.

79. Brochard L, Roudot-Thoraval F, Roupie E. Tidal volume reduction for prevention of ventilator-induced lung injury in acute respiratory distress syndrome: the multicenter trial group on tidal volume reduction in ARDS. Am J Respir Crit Care Med. 1998;158:1831–8.

80. Brower RG, Shanholtz CB, Fessler HE, et al. Prospective, randomized, controlled clinical trial comparing traditional versus reduced tidal volume ventilation in acute respiratory distress syndrome patients. Crit Care Med. 1999;27:1492–8.

81. Mercat A, Richard JC, Vielle B, et al. Positive end expiratory pressure setting in adults with acute lung injury and acute respiratory distress syndrome: a randomized controlled trial. J Am Med Assoc. 2008;299(6):646–55.

82. Hess DR, Kacmarek RM. Essentials of Mechanical Ventilation, 2nd edn. New York: McGraw-Hill, 2002.

83. Briel M, Meade M, Mercat A, et al. Higher vs lower positive end expiratory pressure in patients with acute lung injury and acute respiratory distress syndrome. J Am Med Assoc. 2010;303:865.

84. Blanch L, Bernabe F, Lucangelo U. Measurement of air trapping, intrinsic positive end-expiratory pressure, and dynamic hyperinflation in mechanically ventilated patients. Respir Care 2005;50(1):110.

85. Hendricks JC. Airway Hygiene. In: Textbook of Respiratory Disease in Dogs and Cats. King LG, ed. St Louis: Saunders, 2004: pp 214–17.

86. Guerin C, Debord S, Leray V, et al. Efficacy and safety of recruitment maneuvers in acute respiratory distress syndrome. Ann Intensive Care 2011;1:9.

87. Lapinsky S, Mehta S. Bench-to-bedside review: recruitment and recruiting maneuvers. Crit Care 2005;9:60–5.

88. Genuit T, Bochicchio G, Napolitano LM, et al. Prophylactic chlorhexidine oral rinse decreases ventilator-associated pneumonia in surgical ICU patients. Surg Infect. 2001;21(1):5–18.

89. Tsuno K, Prato P, Kolobow T. Acute lung injury from mechanical ventilation at moderately high airway pressures. J Appl Physiol. 1990;69:956.

90. Anzueto A, Frutos-Vivar F, Esteban A, et al. Incidence, risk factors and outcome of barotrauma in mechanically ventilated patients. Intensive Care Med. 2004; 30:612.

91. Epstein SE, Mellema MS, Hopper K. Airway microbial culture and susceptibility patterns in dogs and cats with respiratory disease of varying severity. J Vet Emerg Crit Care 2010;20:587.

92. Mellema MS, Haskins SC. Weaning from mechanical ventilation. Clin Tech Small Anim Pract. 2000;15:157.

93. Blackwood B, Alderdice F, Burns K, et al. Use of weaning protocols for reducing duration of mechanical ventilation in critically ill adult patients. Cochrane systematic review and meta-analysis. BMJ. 2011;342:7237.

94. Esteban A, Frutos F, Tobin MJ, et al. A comparison of four methods of weaning patients from mechanical ventilation. N Engl J Med. 1995;332:345.

95. Labiris NR, Dolovich MB. Pulmonary drug delivery. Part II: the role of inhalant delivery devices and drug formulations in therapeutic effectiveness of aerosolized medications. Br J Clin Pharmacol. 2003; 56(6):600–12.

96. Kuehn NF. Chronic bronchitis in dogs. In: Textbook of Respiratory Disease in Dogs and Cats. King LG, ed. St Louis: Saunders, 2004: pp 379–87.

97. Padrid PA, Hornof W, Kurperchoek C, et al. Canine chronic bronchitis: a pathophysiologic evaluation of 18 cases. J Vet Intern Med. 1990;4:172.

Further reading

Lisciandro GR. The thoracic FAST3 (TFAST3) exam. In: Focused Ultrasound Techniques for the Small Animal Practitioner. Ames: Wiley & Sons, 2014: pp 140–65.

CHAPTER 9

Coagulation

Andrew Linklater
Lakeshore Veterinary Specialists, Milwaukee, Wisconsin

Introduction

Coagulation is the ever-present dynamic process of changing liquid blood into a semisolid mass (clot) within the vasculature. The coagulation process is accomplished by interactions of a combination of platelets, activated serine proteases, tissue factor (TF), TF-bearing cells, cell membrane receptors, and natural anticoagulants; the end result is a platelet-fibrin clot. The traditional cascade model of fibrin formation exhibited a sequential activation of the coagulation proteins initiated through extrinsic (outside the bloodstream) and intrinsic (within the bloodstream) pathways (Figure 9.1a).

Research has shown that these two cascading pathways are intricately linked and that platelets and other cellular components of the blood are integral parts of the coagulation process. A cell-based model of coagulation has evolved (Figure 9.1b) which incorporates three overlapping phases of coagulation: initiation, amplification, and propagation. This new model of understanding coagulation emphasizes the role of cells (particularly TF-bearing cells and platelets) along with coagulation factors to accomplish coagulation and has gained prominence. Natural endogenous anticoagulant mechanisms are also present and important in regulating clot formation and fibrinolysis; the anticoagulants are found in blood and on endothelial cells, the endothelial glycocalyx, and platelets.

Evidence indicates that one of the key initiators of coagulation *in vivo* is TF [1]. In normal conditions, cells expressing TF are primarily localized outside the vasculature. Some circulating cells (such as monocytes) and circulating microparticles can express inactive or encrypted TF on their membrane surfaces. Microparticles arise from the plasma membrane of endothelial cells, platelets, and monocytes during normal cell activation, programmed cell death or exposure to shear stress [1].

Alterations in coagulation and anticoagulation can occur in critically ill animals as part of the presenting illness or can develop as a complication of the underlying disease process. When disease causes cells to be activated or injured, a calcium-mediated reaction occurs which brings procoagulant receptors to the cell surface. This process can markedly increase the speed of some coagulation reactions. Cytokines, thrombin, shear stress, and hypoxia can stimulate the formation of additional microparticles from granulocytes and erythrocytes that can stimulate coagulation. The resultant clot formation and eventual fibrinolysis can occur at local sites of injury or at distant sites unrelated to the initial injury in these patients. Thrombosis or a consumptive coagulopathy are potentially life-threatening consequences that can cause organ ischemia or uncontrolled hemorrhage, respectively.

Hemorrhage can also occur as a result of insufficient production of coagulation proteins or alterations in platelet numbers due to peripheral destruction, consumption, or lack of production with bone marrow disease. While less common, hereditary coagulation factor deficiencies or a disruption in the fibrinolytic process may negatively impact the critically ill patient as well.

While all ICU patients deserve to be monitored for a coagulation disorder, a high priority is set for patients that have experienced a potential trigger for systemic coagulation, such as prolonged capillary stasis, severe hypoxia or hypotension, massive tissue damage, and systemic inflammatory response syndrome (SIRS). A list of disease processes known to be associated with coagulopathies is presented in Box 9.1. In addition to the underlying disease process, fluid infusion and a variety of drugs administered as part of the treatment plan can interfere with normal coagulation. It is important to recognize the potential for a coagulation disorder in the ICU patient and to be prepared to intervene.

Monitoring methods

Evaluation of the ICU patient for coagulation disorders begins by reviewing the patient history and assessing the physical examination findings. Early diagnosis of coagulation abnormalities depends in part on identifying changes with regular physical examinations and point of care (POC) testing; monitoring trends of change over time (rather than any single value) on POC testing and correlating those diagnostics with physical exam findings is vital. A definitive diagnosis may require additional clinicopathological testing that is not immediately available. Therapeutic intervention may be necessary while test results are pending. Monitoring the patient's response to treatment is important and contributes to the diagnostic evaluation. The end goal is to avoid an unexpected hemorrhagic or thrombotic crisis.

History
The signalment (age, sex, and breed) is important to assess for potential predilections to coagulopathies. Past medical problems, preventative care, transfusion history, postoperative bleeding, and current medications are all important. The environment is investigated relating to exposure to ticks, toxins, and infectious diseases. Any illness in other animals in the household or related pets may help detect toxic or inherited disorders.

Physical examination
Specific physical examination findings that can reflect an alteration in coagulation status are listed in Table 9.1. Studies in animals have found that hemorrhage identified at more than one site is indicative of a hypocoagulable state [2]. Extremes in body temperature may

---

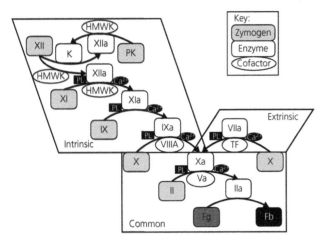

Figure 9.1(a) The cascade model of fibrin formation. This model divides the coagulation system into separate redundant pathways (extrinsic and intrinsic), either of which can result in generation of FXa. The common pathway results in generation of thrombin and subsequent cleavage of fibrinogen to fibrin. Many of the enzyme and enzymatic complexes require calcium (Ca^{2+}) and binding to active membrane surfaces (PL) for full activity. For simplicity, feedback activation of pro-co-factors to co-factors and the many inhibitors of the various enzymes have been omitted. Fb, fibrin: Fg, fibrinogen; HMWK, high molecular weight kininogen; K, kallikrein; PK, prekallikrein; PL, phospholipid membrane. Source: Reproduced with permission from Smith SA. J Vet Emerg Crit Care 2009;19(1):3–10.

alter coagulation; hyperthermia (>106 °F, >41 °C) permanently alters coagulation factors and prolonged hypothermia (<94 °F, <34 °C) prolongs clotting time.

Poor perfusion may be a cause of coagulation abnormalities or occur as a consequence of thrombosis or significant hemorrhage. The findings of a heart murmur, arrhythmia, gallop sounds or muffled heart sounds can be a consequence of volume loss, anemia, pericardial effusion or other cardiac disease. Intrapulmonary thrombosis or hemorrhage can cause tachypnea, labored breathing, altered lung sounds, and hypoxemia. Oropharyngeal hematomas and tracheal mucosal hemorrhage can manifest as stertorous breathing.

Intraabdominal hemorrhage may distend the abdominal cavity and results in a fluid wave on abdominal palpation when blood loss is >40 mL/kg [3]. Red blood found on rectal examination suggests lower gastrointestinal (GI) bleeding while melena is typically due to upper GI bleeding.

The eyes (anterior chamber, retina, and sclera), mouth, and nasal cavity may reveal signs of occult bleeding in the form of hyphema, gingival bleeding or epistaxis, respectively. The integument and mucous membranes (oral and genital) are carefully examined for ecchymosis (Figure 9.2) and petechiae (Figure 9.3). Skin bruising should be outlined with nontoxic permanent marker to monitor progression or resolution.

Clinical signs of a hypercoagulable state, causing central or peripheral thrombosis, will vary depending on the location and degree of obstruction to blood flow. Cats presenting with feline aortic thromboembolism (FATE) will demonstrate paresis or paralysis of one or more limbs. The right forelimb or both hindlimbs are most commonly affected. There will be decreased or absent pulses, often a lowered rectal temperature and discoloration of the paw pads on the affected limb (Figures 9.4 and 9.5) and significant pain.

Problems resulting from thrombosis of blood vessels supplying major internal organs can cause clinical signs compatible with

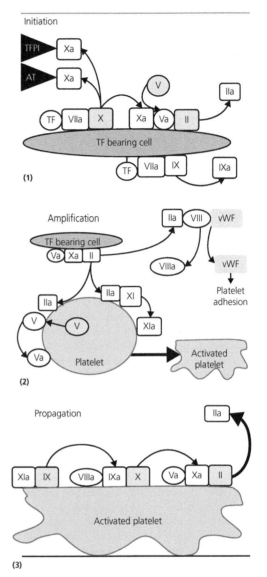

Figure 9.1(b) The cell-based model of fibrin formation. This model incorporates the contribution of various cell surfaces to fibrin formation. In this model, thrombin generation occurs in overlapping phases. (1) Initiation phase. This phase occurs on the TF-bearing cell. It is initiated when injury exposes the TF-bearing cell to the flowing blood. It results in the generation of a small amount of FIXa and thrombin that diffuse away from the surface of the TF-bearing cell to the platelet. (2) Amplification phase. In the second phase, the small amount of thrombin generated on the TF-bearing cell activates platelets, releases vWF and leads to generation of activated forms of FV, FVIII, and FXI. (3) Propagation phase. In the third phase the various enzymes generated in earlier phases assemble on the procoagulant membrane surface of the activated platelet to form intrinsic tenase, resulting in FXa generation on the platelet surface. Prothrombinase complex forms and results in a burst of thrombin generation directly on the platelet. AT, antithrombin; TF, tissue factor; TFPI, tissue factor pathway inhibitor; vWF, von Willebrand factor. Source: Reproduced with permission from Smith SA. J Vet Emerg Crit Care 2009;19(1):3–10.

gastrointestinal dysfunction, acute renal failure, severe abdominal pain, and poor perfusion (shock). Altered mentation, seizures, stupor, coma, and paresis or paralysis are signs compatible with thrombosis or hemorrhage within the central nervous system (see Chapter 12).

Clinicopathological testing

Proper sample collection is mandatory for accurate results (Box 9.2). It is important to remember that *in vitro* coagulation testing may not accurately reflect the exact status of *in vivo* coagulation [4]. Any therapeutic decisions based on coagulation test results must also take into consideration the primary diagnosis, current health status, and anticipated procedures. Clinicopathologcal testing of hemostasis begins at the cage side (point of care testing).

Point of care testing

Point of care testing can provide a rapid impression of the quantity and function of the cells and proteins required for clotting. A list of POC tests to initially assess coagulation is provided in Table 9.2.

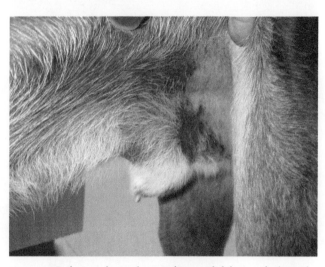

Figure 9.2 Ecchymotic hemorrhage on the ventral abdomen of a dog with a coagulopathy.

Box 9.1 Common processes associated with altered coagulation.

Prolonged capillary stasis
Severe hypotension
Shock
Cardiac disease
Vascular disease
Liver disease
Renal disease (protein-losing nephropathy)
Exposure to anticoagulant toxins/drugs
Severe tissue trauma
Red blood cell lysis
Hypoxia
Severe alterations in body temperature
Hypocalcemia/hypercalcemia
Immune-mediated disease
Systemic inflammatory diseases (SIRS)
Sepsis
Severe gastrointestinal disease
Endocrine disease
Neoplasia
Infectious diseases (tick borne, dirofilariasis, severe bacterial, viral, fungal or parasitic infections)
Medical intervention (IV catheters)

Table 9.1 Physical examination findings associated with coagulation disorders. These physical exam alterations can serve as a trigger to evaluate coagulation, an indication of ongoing hypocoagulation (bleeding) or hypercoagulation (thrombosis).

Triggers to evaluate coagulopathy	Physical evidence of hypocoagulation	Physical evidence of thrombosis (hypercoagulation)
Severe pyrexia (>106 °F, > 41 °C)	Petechiae	Cool skin or limb
Hypothermia (<94 °F, <34 °C)	Ecchymosis	Discoloration (pale or cyanotic) of mucous membranes, foot
Cardiac arrhythmias, murmurs (cat and dog)	Bleeding/bruising	pads or skin
or gallop sounds (cat)	Spontaneous	Labored, rapid breathing
Peripheral edema or vasculitis	At venipuncture site(s)	Cyanosis
Prolonged seizures	Sudden soft tissue swelling	Acute abdominal pain
Organomegaly	Poor perfusion	Absent single pulse
Acute abdominal pain	Altered thoracic auscultation	Sudden change in mentation, consciousness
Evidence of tissue trauma	Labored rapid breathing	Peripheral or central nerve deficits
Severe systemic infection	Synchronous – lung parenchyma	Sudden inability to use limb(s); swelling, painful limbs and
Pale or yellow mucous membranes	Asynchronous – pleural space	over time a firmness to the tissues or vessels
Evidence of infection or systemic	Stertor/stridor – upper airway	Sudden-onset organ dysfunction or failure
inflammation	obstruction or hematoma	Acute-onset seizures
Poor perfusion:	Cyanosis	Acute-onset paresis/paralysis
• Altered heart rate	Muffled or quiet heart sounds	Unexplained anxiety
• Poor pulses	Depressed mentation or change in	Sudden onset of severe pain
• Altered capillary refill time	mentation/consciousness	
• Altered mentation	Seizures or sudden cranial or peripheral	
• Markedly altered blood pressure	nerve changes	
• Pale, injected or cyanotic mucous	Melena or frank blood in stool	
membranes	Marked red/brown pigment of urine	
	Pale or white mucous membranes	
	Abdominal fluid wave	
	Epistaxis	
	Frank blood or digested blood ("coffee	
	grounds") in vomit	
	Retinal hemorrhage or hyphema	
	Gingival bleeding	

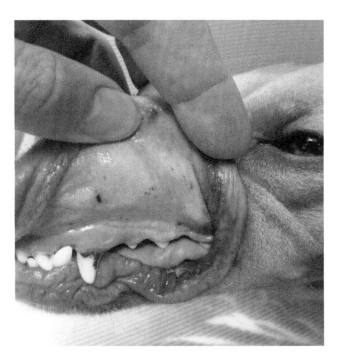

Figure 9.3 Buccal petechiae of a dog with a platelet disorder.

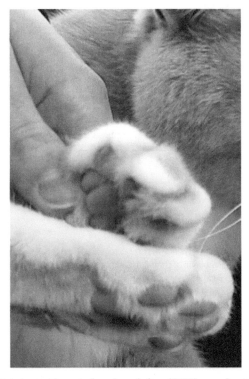

Figure 9.4 A cat with aortic thromboembolism (FATE) secondary to heart disease. Note the pale color of the hindlimb pads (*bottom*) compared to the forelimb pads (*top*).

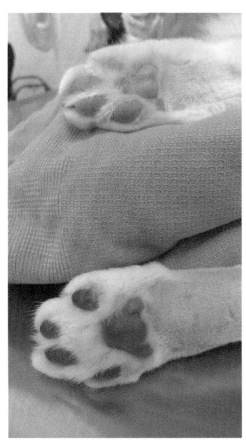

Figure 9.5 A cat with unilateral (right) hindlimb venous thrombosis secondary to neoplasia. Note the cyanotic discoloration to the pads and the swelling of the foot.

Box 9.2 Tips for blood collection for coagulation testing.

Avoid jugular veins if hypocoagulable or head injury
Needle size does not impact common coagulation tests [5]
Perform atraumatic venipuncture
Collect into proper tube
- EDTA for platelet, WBC and RBC evaluation and vWF
- Na citrate for PT, aPTT, vWF and individual factor tests
- Diatomaceous earth with heating block for ACT
- Serum separator or lithium heparin (green top) for common chemistry analysis
Ensure appropriate dilution
- Citrate requires 1:9 dilution (1.8 mL of blood to 0.2 mL of anticoagulant)
Samples with anticoagulant should be gently agitated to ensure even distribution
The tube should be examined visually for clot formation
Bandage should be placed over venipuncture site to limit hematoma formation

---

ACT, activated clotting time; aPTT, activated partial thromboplastin time; PT, prothrombin time; RBC, red blood cell; WBC, white blood cell; vWF, von Willebrand factor.

Minimum database

The minimal database will include packed cell volume (PCV), total protein (TP), blood glucose, blood urea nitrogen (BUN), electrolytes, blood gas (venous or arterial), and blood lactate. A normal or even elevated PCV with a disproportionate decrease in TP may be a reflection of acute hemorrhage in the dog, as the PCV is preserved through splenic contraction. The PCV and TP will both eventually decline after hemorrhage, particularly with fluid resuscitation. Icteric serum warrants concern for hepatic disease or red cell hemolysis, both with potential to cause a

Table 9.2 Point of care coagulation tests and normal values.

Test	Normal*	Collection tube	Notes
Microhematocrit tube		Micro hematocrit tube	Buffy coat should be examined as well as it may indicate alterations in WBC
• PCV	37–55 (D); 25–45 (C)		
• Total proteins (refractometer)	5.8–7.2 (D); 5.7–7.5 (C)		
• Serum color	Clear to light yellow		
Platelet estimate	10–30 per 100× field	Lavender top (EDTA) or capillary tube (EDTA)	Smeared on glass slide, monolayer examined for count; feathered edge examined for platelet clumping
Platelet count	170 000–575 000/ul (D) 200 000–680 000/ul (C)	Lavender top (EDTA)	Within 5 hours room temperature or 24 hours (refrigerated)
BMBT	<4 min (D) <2.5–3 min (C)	N/A	Site should not be disrupted while performing test
PT	13–18 sec (D) 14–22 sec (C)	Blue top (Na citrate)	Run within 1 hour of collection or kept in fridge/shipped with ice
aPTT	10–17 sec (D) 14–18 sec (C)	Blue top (Na citrate)	Run within 1 hour of collection or kept in fridge/shipped with ice
ACT	60–90 sec (D) 45–160 sec (C)	Gray top (diatomaceous earth)	Run immediately and at 37 °C (98 °F) in a heated block or water bath

* Individual laboratory normal values may be different.
ACT, activated clotting time; aPTT, activated partial thromboplastin time; BMBT, buccal mucosal bleeding time; C, cat; D, dog; PCV, packed cell volume; PT, prothrombin time.

Box 9.3 Steps to perform a manual platelet count.

1. Collect sample in an atraumatic fashion
2. The sample may be stored in an EDTA tube (lavender top)
3. A drop of blood is placed on a microscope slide
4. A second slide is used to create a "bullet"-shaped smear, producing a monolayer and feathered edge
5. The monolayer is examined under 100X magnification
6. Platelet numbers are counted in 10 high-power (100X) fields and averaged
7. Multiply this number by 15 000 and this is the estimated number of platelets/µL
8. 10–30 platelets/hpf is considered normal, which is equivalent to 150 000–450 000/µL

Table 9.3 Differential diagnoses for causes of platelet disorders.

Thrombocytopenia	Thrombocytopathy	Thrombocytosis
Destruction Primary Immune mediated Systemic lupus **Secondary** Drugs Vaccination Neoplasia FeLV/FIV	**Drug related** Aspirin Clopidogrel Antibiotics Cardiac drugs Hydroxyethyl starch Barbiturates Heparin Massive transfusion	**Systemic illness** Neoplasia GI disease Endocrine disease **Immunological** Rebound from IMHA, ITP therapy, blood loss or trauma
Consumption/ sequestration Hemorrhage Disseminated intravascular coagulation Splenic torsion Sepsis Hepatic disease Hypothermia Severe uremia	**Systemic illness** Uremia Anemia Acidemia Severe hepatic disease Hypothermia Myeloproliferative disease Ehrlichiosis and other tick-borne disease Snake envenomation	**Drugs** Steroids Chemotherapy (e.g. vincristine)
Decreased production Post vaccination Radiation Tick-borne infection Bone marrow aplasia	**Other** Vasculitis Hyperadrenocorticism Hypocalcemia Von Willebrand's Congenital disorder	**Other** Fractures Post splenectomy

FeLV, feline leukemia virus; FIV, feline immundeficiency virus; GI, gastrointestinal; IMHA, immune-mediated hemolytic anemia; ITP, immune-mediated thrombocytopenia.

coagulopathy. Blood in the gastrointestinal tract can elevate the BUN when there is normal renal function. A low BUN can direct diagnostics for liver dysfunction. Calcium is an important component of the coagulation process and hypocalcemia is a potential cause of prolonged clotting times and bleeding. The detrimental effects of acidosis on coagulation include depleted fibrinogen levels and platelet counts, prolonged clotting times, and increased bleeding times. Monitoring lactate levels can provide a measure of restoration of oxygenation to tissue beds affected by significant hemorrhage or thrombosis.

Blood smear

A thin, even blood smear with a monolayer is part of the minimum database to evaluate red blood cell (RBC) and platelet morphology and to estimate the platelet count. The presence of spherocytes, schistocytes or dacrocytes suggests RBC destruction. Reticulocytes, polychromasia and nucleated RBCs (nRBCs) are compatible with regeneration; nRBCs are also seen with heatstroke and other critical illness.

A manual platelet estimate should be performed (Box 9.3). The feathered edge of the blood smear is examined for platelet clumping and platelet morphology. Large platelets suggest young platelets while small platelets may be seen with immune-mediated thrombocytopenia (ITP) [6]. A declining trend in platelet numbers may provide the earliest indication of a coagulation disorder involving both the primary (platelets) and secondary (serine proteases) hemostatic mechanisms.

A moderate reduction in platelet count (50 000–150 000/uL) can occur associated with a variety of underlying diseases (Table 9.3) and commonly reflects increased platelet consumption, dilution or sequestration. Following a trend in the platelet count over time can help detect ongoing consumptive processes such as disseminated intravascular coagulation (DIC). Patients are typically at risk for spontaneous hemorrhage when platelet numbers are less than 30 000–50 000/uL.

Buccal mucosal bleeding time

Buccal mucosal bleeding time (BMBT) is a method of evaluating *in vivo* primary hemostasis. The test uses a cartridge to create a standard size incision on the buccal mucosal surface to determine the time required for cessation of capillary bleeding. It should not be run if the platelet count is low. The steps to perform BMBT are noted in Box 9.4.

Prolonged BMBT (see Table 9.2) found with normal platelet count suggests von Willebrand's disease or other abnormal platelet function. Factors such as operator error and extreme abnormalities in hematocrit can alter the bleeding time. The BMBT can also be used to monitor patients receiving antiplatelet drugs (such as aspirin or clopidogrel) to assess the effect of the drug on platelet function [7]. Unfortunately, BMBT is a poor predictor of surgical bleeding [8].

POC coagulation tests (PT, aPTT, ACT)

Determination of the prothrombin time (PT), activated partial thromboplastin time (aPTT), and activated clotting time (ACT) can be done through POC testing. Normal values for these tests are listed in Table 9.2.

The PT reflects both the function and quantity of the coagulation factors in the extrinsic (factor VII) and common (factors I, II, V, and X) coagulation pathways (see Figure 9.1a). Potential causes of prolongation of PT are listed in Table 9.4. A substantial decrease

---

Box 9.4 Steps to perform a buccal mucosal bleeding time.

1. Turn the patient's lip up, and secure with gauze around the maxilla
2. Place the lancet device securely against the lip, rostral to the gauze and deploy
3. Start timing immediately (and end when bleeding ceases)
4. Blot away blood that drains from incision with filter paper, taking care not to touch or disrupt the incision site/clot in any way
5. Monitor the site for continued bleeding

(≥70%) of one or more of these clotting factors is needed for the PT to be prolonged. Prothrombin time is often the first coagulation test altered when there is a consumptive coagulopathy, inadequate production of coagulation proteins or rodenticide toxicity. This is because factor VII has the shortest half-life, and formation of TF receptor complex, which activates factor VII, is stimulated by circulating cytokines (inflammatory proteins) commonly found in critically ill animals. The PT is used to monitor the effectiveness of anticoagulant drugs such as coumadin, with the therapeutic goal of prolonging the PT 1.5–2.5 times beyond the pretreatment value. A shortened time for the PT result is not significant and more likely represents a collection or lab error; it does not represent a hypercoagulable state.

The aPTT reflects the function and quantity of coagulation factors in the intrinsic (factors VIII, IX, XI, XII) and common (factors I, II, V, X) coagulation pathways (see Figure 9.1a). Similar to PT, the aPTT becomes prolonged when there is a functional or quantitative decrease of ≥70% of one or more of these coagulation factors. A list of possible causes of prolonged aPTT is provided in Table 9.4. It is important to note that prolonged aPTT in dogs that have sustained trauma has been correlated with nonsurvival [9]. Patients receiving heparin therapy can be monitored using aPTT, with the goal of increasing the aPTT by 1.5–2 times the pretreatment value. A shortened aPTT is not significant and more likely to represent a collection or lab error; it does not represent a hypercoagulable state. PT and aPTT testing do require specialized equipment, but are widely available and affordable, making other clotting parameters less utilized [10].

The activated clotting time (ACT) tests the coagulation factors of the intrinsic and common pathways. While similar to the aPTT, it is less sensitive; a functional or quantitative decrease in coagulation factors of >90% is required to prolong the ACT. The ACT, however, can be tested with minimal equipment, making it an option for clinics that do not have PT and aPTT testing available. The ACT test only requires appropriate tubes with diatomaceous earth and a heating block or water bath kept at 98 °F (37 °C). An i-STAT® cartridge (Abbott, Princeton, NJ) that runs a kaolin-based ACT test is also available.

The results of coagulation testing should always be interpreted with the clinical picture of the patient (signs of blood loss, PCV/TP, etc,). If an intervention is deemed necessary (transfusions, vitamin K, etc.), it is appropriate to recheck these values to ensure the therapeutic benefit has been achieved.

Table 9.4 Assessment of PT and aPTT in small animal ICU patients.

PT	aPTT	Differential	Additional testing
Normal	Normal	No coagulopathy or early stages or mild disease or lab error	Investigate other sources of disease, CBC (platelets count/function), BMBT
Prolonged	Normal	"Early" vitamin K deficiency (toxic or therapeutic anticoagulants), severe liver failure, DIC, FVII or other factor deficiency (rare)	Blood levels of anticoagulants, FVII testing, liver tests, CBC
Normal	Prolonged	FVIII deficiency (hemophilia A), FIX deficiency (hemophilia B), FXII deficiency (primarily seen in cats and not associated with bleeding), von Willebrand's disease, other (rare) factor deficiencies	Liver tests, individual factor testing, CBC, von Willebrand's quantification
Prolonged	Prolonged	Severe liver disease, "late" anticoagulant toxicity, DIC, common pathway deficiency (FI, II, V, X), severe malabsorptive disease (bowel disease, cholestatic disease), heparin therapy, acute traumatic coagulopathy/trauma-induced coagulopathy, severe sepsis or other SIRS disease	Liver function tests, CBC, individual factor testing, anticoagulant rodenticide blood tests, TEG, FDP, D-dimers, fibrinogen

aPTT, activated partial thromboplastin time; BMBT, buccal mucosal bleeding time; CBC, complete blood count; DIC, disseminated intravascular coagulation; FDP, fibrin degradation product; PT, prothrombin time; SIRS, systemic inflammatory response syndrome; TEG, thermoelastography.

Blood profiles, imaging, and other supportive diagnostics

The complete blood count (CBC), serum biochemistry, and urinalysis provide important information for detecting metabolic or physical problems that can cause or be caused by a coagulation disorder. A high white blood cell count with a left shift can be compatible with inflammation or infection and warrants further patient evaluation for a SIRS disease. Red blood cell hemolysis sets the stage for intravascular coagulation. Significant elevations in RBC count or serum proteins can have a negative effect on capillary rheology, contributing to capillary status and intravascular coagulation. Blood testing for *Dirofilaria*, hyperthyroidism, hyperadrenocorticism, and tick-borne disease may be necessary in select patients.

Radiographs or ultrasound of the chest, and possibly echocardiography, may be necessary to evaluate for neoplasia, abscesses, fluid in the pericardial or pleural space, heart size and function, pulmonary parenchymal fluid or hemorrhage, size and prominence of pulmonary vasculature and any evidence of heartworm disease. Radiographs and ultrasound of the abdomen can identify abdominal fluid, masses, organ enlargement or displacement, infiltrative disease, and gastrointestinal changes. Animals with a compatible history can be quickly evaluated for free abdominal and thoracic fluid with the focused assessment with sonography techniques [11]. The presence of free fluid warrants centesis for fluid evaluation.

Advanced imaging techniques (Table 9.5) are required for detection of intravascular clots. Echocardiography can be used to demonstrate echogenic thrombi in the heart and large vessels. Ultrasound can demonstrate echogenic thrombi in abdominal and peripheral vasculature (Figure 9.6). Intravenous contrast angiography may be used with computed tomography (CT) or fluoroscopy to indirectly visualize thrombi. Contrast administration can be contraindicated in patients with renal injury. Ventilation/perfusion scans (scintigraphy) use radioisotopes to aid in the diagnosis of large pulmonary thromboemboli.

Information from these tests is used to further direct diagnostic and monitoring procedures. Patients with concern for pulmonary thrombosis should have their ability to oxygenate monitored via pulse oximetry, co-oximetry or arterial blood gas. Indirect evidence of reperfusion injury (history, hyperkalemia, hyperphosphatemia) can warrant monitoring for cardiac arrhythmias or renal failure.

Cats with evidence of thrombosis warrant echocardiographic evaluation of the heart, systemic blood pressure measurement, thoracic radiographs, and thyroid function testing. Advanced coagulation testing may be necessary to better define the presence of a coagulopathy, determine the inciting cause, and direct therapy that is specific for the patient.

Advanced clinicopathological testing

While POC evaluation of a patient with a coagulopathy remains necessary in the emergency setting, additional diagnostics may be necessary in the critically ill for further assessment, definitive diagnosis, and even specific intervention. Many of the tests discussed are not available at many emergency hospitals, require specialized or expensive equipment or do not have established points of intervention.

Advanced techniques for assessing platelet function and factors, coagulation protein quantity and function, clot formation, clot dissolution, and natural anticoagulant components are gaining momentum and accessibility in veterinary medicine. Normal values and how to interpret abnormalities revealed through advanced coagulation testing are provided in Table 9.5.

Monitoring platelet function and related factors
Platelet function

Platelets are identified as having three functions with respect to coagulation: control of thrombin generation, support of fibrin formation, and regulation of fibrin clot retraction. Platelet function analyzers evaluate the ability of the platelet to aggregate and form a platelet plug. There is less operator variability with these tests compared to BMBT.

The PFA-100® (Siemens, Malvern, PA) (see Table 9.5) monitors blood flow through an aperture, which stimulates platelet function, as it is coated with epinephrine or collagen. The "closure time" is the length of time for cessation of blood flow through the aperture due to platelet plug formation. The VerifyNow® (Accriva Diagnostics, San Diego, CA) measures light transmittance through a fibrinogen-coated bead bed that initiates platelet aggregation. This instrument is more commonly used to assess the therapeutic response to platelet inhibitory drugs rather than for diagnosis of a clinical thrombocytopathy.

Platelet flow cytometry and ELISAs (i.e. platelet antibody test; see Table 9.5) are available to detect platelet-bound IgG. These tests aid in the diagnosis of idiopathic thrombocytopenia purpura and immune thrombocytopenia [12]. The results do not differentiate primary from secondary immune-mediated disease. Other specific platelet function tests include light aggregometry and current impedance and flow cytometry. However, the significance of the results from these test procedures in small animals is unknown at this time.

Von Willebrand factor

Von Willebrand factor (vWF) is a protein required for platelet adhesion. Deficiency is commonly hereditary but can be acquired as a result of disease or medications. vWF is measured in comparison to a species normal and is reported as a percentage of normal (see Table 9.5). Platelet function testing is abnormal in von Willebrand's disease, while the platelet count, PT, and aPTT are typically normal. This is most commonly diagnosed in young animals that experience excessive bleeding during routine surgical procedures.

Bone marrow evaluation

Bone marrow aspiration or biopsy is used to evaluate the cause of thrombocytopenia. Recent evidence suggests that bone marrow evaluation for thrombocytopenia without concurrent pancytopenia (low white blood cell and RBC counts) may not provide significant diagnostic information [13]. Bone marrow aspirate is generally considered to be safe in patients with only thrombocytopenia. Concurrent submission of a complete blood count for pathologist review and/or bone marrow biopsy may be warranted.

Monitoring clot formation and fibrinolysis
Fibrinogen

Fibrinogen (factor I) is cleaved by thrombin to produce the fibrin strands that form the stable blood clot. Low fibrinogen levels have been shown to provide an indication of risk for spontaneous hemorrhage (when <5%) or surgical bleeding (when <20%) [14,15]. However, the significance of fibrinogen levels can be difficult to interpret. As fibrinogen is also an acute-phase protein, levels can be elevated in response to inflammation; in addition, normal removal of circulating fibrinogen by the liver may be impaired by liver disease.

Table 9.5 Advanced clinicopathological testing and imaging to define coagulation status.

Test	Normal value*	Interpretation/indication	Limitations/notes*
Fibrinogen (I)	2–400 mg/dL (D) 50–300 mg/dL (C)	Low levels: consumption; DIC, thrombosis; lack of production: liver disease, malnutrition, congenital disorders, use of plasma expanders, snake envenomation Elevated: systemic inflammation, liver dysfunction, tissue necrosis, ongoing coagulopathy	Na citrate tube or EDTA depending on methodology, refrigerate or freeze Heparin, phenobarbital and fibrinolytic agents may decrease values
FDPs	<10 μg/mL (serum; D and C)	Increased: DIC, SIRS, liver and renal disease, protein-losing disease, hemorrhage, trauma, gammopathies, burns, parvovirus, hyperadrenocorticism, pulmonary or other thromboembolic disease, regardless of cause	Na citrate or FDP tubes depending on laboratory method Fibrinolytic agents will increase values
D-dimer	<25 μg/mL (D and C)	Same as FDPs and heart disease	Collection method depends on lab, fibrinolytic agents will increase values
Antithrombin	65–145% (D) 75–120% (C)	Decreased: consumption: DIC, thromboembolism; poor production: liver disease, heparin therapy or increased loss with protein-losing enteropathy and nephropathy	Na citrate tube
INR	Target 2.0–3.0 baseline 2.5–3.5 for heart valve replacement	Monitoring patient on warfarin or coumarin	Several labs may run this test which is then compared to an in-house normal to give a ratio
PIVKA	16–24 sec (D) 16–25 sec (C)	Anticoagulant rodenticide toxicity, severe liver, GI, pancreatic or biliary disease leading to fat malabsorption, disease that results in decreased vit K absorption; inherited factor deficiencies, DIC, neoplasia	Markedly prolonged with anticoagulant toxicosis
vWD	70–180% of control	Primary hemostatic disorder with normal platelet numbers and/or abnormal BMBT	Values <50% indicate vWF deficiency, <25% poses a risk of bleeding, <1% is diagnostic for severe (type III) vWF deficiency
TEG	Normals are laboratory dependent	See Figure 9.7	Helpful with hyper- and hypocoagulable states; points of intervention are not established
PFA-100	<98 sec (ADP) <300 sec (epinephrine)	Results are listed as closure time. Prolonged times indicate primary platelet dysfunction. Should only be run when platelet numbers are normal as thrombocytopenia will prolong results	Citrate tubes, must be run within 4 h of collection
Anti-Xa activity	0.1–0.2 U/mL	These are suggested target goals for monitoring patients on UH or LMWH	There are no well-established target goals
Bone marrow aspirate	Laboratory dependent	Of most diagnostic value when pancytopenia is present	Should be interpreted concurrently with a CBC and pathologist review
Anticoagulant levels	Anything above 0	Anticoagulant rodenticide toxicity suspected	Must be sent to reference laboratory; point of care detection is not useful
Protein C (APC)	75–135% (D) 65–120% (C)	Liver disease, DIC, sepsis, portosystemic shunts, vit K deficiency (rodenticide, coumarin therapy, cholestasis)	Na citrate. Protein C plays a role in coagulation (inactivates FV and FVIII) as well as inflammation
Individual clotting factors	Expressed as a percentage of normal with a range	Patients with suspected hemophilia or prolonged PT or aPTT	VIII, IX deficiencies are most common in dogs; VIII, IX and XII deficiencies in cats (XII deficiency rarely causes clinical hemorrhage)
Anti-Xa	Suggested values: 0.35–0.7 U/mL (D)	Monitoring patients receiving heparin therapy	Studies determining target ranges for therapeutic monitoring are lacking
Platelet antibody	Negative	ITP, other autoimmune disorders	Flow cytometry is most commonly used, ELISA and IFA are alternative methods; does not differentiate primary from secondary disease
Angiography	Normal anatomy and flow	Cardiovascular disease and congential abnormalities (e.g. cardiac shunts, portovascular anomalies, valvular disease and stenosis, thromboembolic disease – venous or arterial)	Advanced procedure that should be performed and interpreted by someone with skill in the diagnostic arena. Selective and nonselective methods are possible
Nuclear medicine (scintigraphy)	Uniform distribution of radioactive isotope in lungs	Suspected pulmonary thrombosis or right to left cardiac shunts	Must be performed in a facility with appropriate equipment

Table 9.5 (*Continued*)

Test	Normal value*	Interpretation/indication	Limitations/notes*
Ultrasound	Normal anatomy and blood flow	Identification of underlying disease that may contribute to embolic complications (e.g. neoplasia or liver disease) or identification of hemorrhage (hypoechoic to mixed echogenic fluid); identification of echogenic thrombi	FAST and TFAST scans can easily be performed by most clinicians to identify cavitary effusions/hemorrhage; experience is often required to identify echogenic thrombi
Echocardiography	Normal anatomy and blood flow	Identification of underlying cardiac disease	Echocardiograms are often performed by individuals with experience in this field

* Reference values and collection methods will vary depending on species, methodology, and laboratory used.

aPTT, activated partial thromboplastin time; BMBT, buccal mucosal bleeding time; C, cat; CBC, complete blood count; D, dog; DIC, disseminated intravascular coagulation; ELISA, enzyme-linked immunosorbent assay; FAST, focused assessment with sonography for trauma; FDP, fibrin degradation products; GI, gastrointestinal; IFA, immunofluorescence assay; INR, international normalized ratio; ITP, immune-mediated thrombocytopenia; LMWH, low molecular weight heparin; PIVKA, protein induced in vitamin K absence/antagonism; PT, prothrombin time; SIRS, systemic inflammatory response syndrome; TEG, thromboelastography; TFAST, thoracic FAST; UH, unfractionated heparin; vWD, von Willebrand.

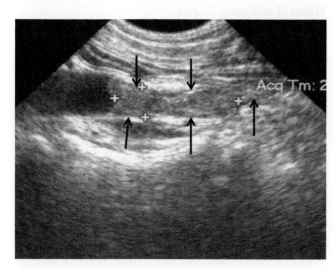

Figure 9.6 Ultrasound image showing an echogenic thrombus in a large vessel, outlined by measurement points.

Individual clotting factors

Individual coagulation protein factor assays can be quantitated from blood samples. Identification of specific factor deficiencies is necessary for the diagnosis of hemophilia A (factor VIII deficiency) or hemophilia B (factor IX deficiency), as well as Hageman factor (factor XII) deficiency in cats. Other individual clotting factor deficiencies (I, II, VII, X, XI, XII) occur but are much less common.

Viscoelastic coagulation assessment

Thromboelastography (TEG) and thromboelastometry (TEM) (also called rotational thromboelastography – ROTEM) are viscoelastic assays that determine the efficiency and speed of blood coagulation. They provide an evaluation of whole clot formation, platelet function, clot strength, kinetics of fibrin formation and cross-linking and fibrinolysis; they are amongst the few tests that can be used to identify a hypercoagulable state. The results are displayed as a tracing that shows the development of the clot. Coagulation variables that are measured include reaction time (R), clotting time (K), speed of fibrin accumulation and cross-linking (α angle), clot strength (maximum amplitude, MA), and fibrinolysis (LY60), as seen in Figure 9.7.

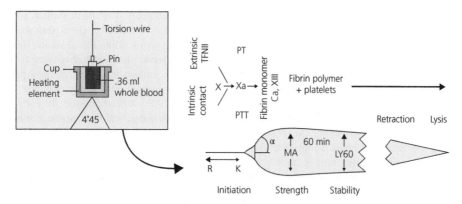

Figure 9.7 Thromboelastogram. The thromboelastography tracing (thromboelastogram) provides a visual representation of hemostasis. The reaction time (R) represents the time of latency from test initiation until beginning of fibrin formation, measured as an increase in amplitude of 2 mm. The clotting time (K) is the time to clot formation, measured from the end of R until an amplitude of 20 mm is reached. The angle (α) represents the rapidity of fibrin accumulation and cross-linking. Maximum amplitude (MA) represents clot stregth. LY60 reflects fibrinolysis, determined by the percentage decrease in amplitude 60 minutes following MA. *Source*: Reproduced with permission from Hackner SG, White CR. Bleeding and hemostasis. In: Tobais JM, Johnston SA, eds. Veterinary Small Animal Surgery, vol. 1. St Louis: Elsevier Saunders, 2012: pp 100.

One of the advantages of these viscoelastic assays is the ability to identify a hypercoagulable state, which traditionally has been quite difficult. A group of veterinary specialists have attempted to identify known information and knowledge gaps that are present in TEG evaluations of veterinary patients [16–21]. Each site that runs these tests is encouraged to develop its own normal values [17,20]. As with many coagulation assays, specific and consistent collection and storage of blood samples are recommended; samples that are not run in a timely fashion may falsely demonstrate hypercoagulability [18].

Thromboelastography has been used to identify hypercoagulable states and predict thromboembolic events in human surgical patients [22]. TEG and ROTEM are also potential tools for diagnosing DIC in human sepsis [23]. Sequential measurements have been necessary to understand the TEG/ROTEM coagulation patterns seen during sepsis as well as during other underlying diseases. Fibrinogen levels and platelet counts are reported to have a major influence on TEG variables [24].

The TEG results of decreased α angle and decreased MA with a prolonged aPTT in dogs with severe trauma have shown significance in predicting the need for blood transfusion and an increase in mortality [9]. A positive correlation has been made between TEG results that indicate reduced clotting ability and bleeding tendencies in dogs. The importance of these findings and the use of the TEG results during various stages of disease and therapeutic intervention in small animals are under investigation.

Fibrin degradation products

Fibrin degradation products (FDPs), also called fibrin split products, are the fragments of protein produced when fibrin is broken apart by plasmin during fibrinolysis. The FDPs produced have a short half-life and are cleared by the liver. An elevation in FDPs suggests that active coagulation and fibrinolysis are occurring systemically. However, other disease states can have elevated FDPs, such as severe liver disease, renal disease, monoclonal gammopathy, and burns. Elevated FDPs have been reported in dogs with pulmonary thromboembolism (sensitivity 80%, specificity 30%). In this study, an absence of thrombosis was found when FDP levels were below 103 µg/mL (sensitivity 100%) [25].

D-dimers

D-dimers are specific FDPs that occur after fibrinolysis of cross-linked (by factor XIII) fibrin and contain two "D domains" of the original fibrin molecule. D-dimers are only elevated when the coagulation and fibrinolytic systems have been activated. Because D-dimers are more specific than FDPs for active fibrinolysis and have a short half-life, the measurement of D-dimers has gained favor for detecting thrombosis or DIC. However, D-dimers can be elevated with many disease processes (see Table 9.5) so are not specific for DIC [26–29]. D-dimers and antithrombin levels have been examined in cats with cardiac disease; further investigation may help us define if any of these factors are indicative of impending thromboembolic events [30].

Anticoagulant therapy monitors
International normalized ratio (INR)
The INR is essentially a PT test that is "standardized" across laboratories as a means of accounting for inequality in the clotting agent used in coagulation testing. The formula for INR is:

$$INR = \left(PT_{test} / PT_{normal}\right)^{ISI}$$

The ISI is the international sensitivity index of the tissue factor used, which varies between 1.0 and 2.0. The INR is used primarily to assess the effectiveness of warfarin or coumadin therapy. Target INR values in dogs for anticoagulant therapy are 2.0–3.0 times baseline [31].

Anti-factor Xa
Anti-factor Xa is also called the heparin assay and is used to monitor patients receiving heparin therapy. It is a functional assay that facilitates the measurement of AT-catalyzed inhibition of factor Xa by unfractionated heparin (UH) and the direct inhibition of factor Xa by low molecular weight heparin (LMWH). The results are expressed in units of anticoagulant per mL. Studies in dogs have reported that anti-Xa activity of 0.35–0.7 U/mL as a goal for effective heparin therapy, but investigation of this target range and outcome is necessary [32,33].

Natural anticoagulants
Antithrombin
Antithrombin (AT), also termed AT III, is an endogenous anticoagulant which inhibits coagulation factors IX, X, XI, XII, and II (thrombin). Plasma AT activity is first tested and reported as a percentage of normal activity. Low levels of AT activity predispose the animal to thrombosis or embolization. An AT deficiency can be due to increased consumption (e.g. DIC, thromboembolic disease), poor production (e.g. liver disease) or loss (e.g. protein-losing nephropathy). The anticoagulant properties of heparin are due to heparin binding to AT which significantly increases the rate of AT-thrombin binding. Therefore, patients that are AT deficient will be resistant to heparin therapy [34].

Activated protein C
Activated protein C (APC) is a vitamin K-dependent anticoagulation factor that inhibits the activity of factor Va and factor VIIIa. It is activated on the surface of endothelial cells and requires protein S as a co-factor. In addition to the anticoagulant functions, APC has cytoprotective effects such as modulation of inflammation, antiapoptotic effects, and endothelial barrier protection; these cytoprotective effects were postulated to provide an observed therapeutic benefit in human septic patients. Human recombinant APC (drotrecogin alpha) was approved for use in humans with sepsis, when initial studies demonstrated improved survival; however further studies have found differing results. The use of recombinant APC in human sepsis remains controversial, and the product is no longer available.

Decreased APC concentration in the plasma of traumatized dogs has been associated with an increased need for blood product administration [9]. In addition, dogs with thrombosis have been found to have decreased levels of APC [35]. A study of dogs with snakebite found no correlation between survivors and nonsurvivors and their serum APC concentration [36]. Further evaluation is required to determine the diagnostic and therapeutic use of APC in veterinary patients.

Test for anticoagulant rodenticides
Identification of rodenticides in blood, tissue, vomitus or bait with mass spectroscopy or gas chromatography may be helpful to confirm the diagnosis of anticoagulant toxicity; this may help guide the duration of required vitamin K1 therapy. These tests, however, take several days and cannot guide emergency therapy. Recently, a study

evaluated a POC test for anticoagulant rodenticide intoxication in dogs and found it was not reliable [37].

The Protein Induced Vitamin K Antagonism (or Absence; PIVKA) test is actually a modification of the PT test. Coagulation factors II, VII, IX, and X are produced in the liver as nonfunctional coagulation protein precursors. The final carboxylation step requires a vitamin K1-dependent carboxylase. Since anticoagulant rodenticides are vitamin K antagonists, there is an elevation in nonfunctional precursors in the serum. A study of the PIVKA test in dogs found that a PIVKA time of >150 seconds has a 91% sensitivity and 99% specificity for making a positive diagnosis of anticoagulant rodenticide toxicity [38]. However, both false-negative and false-positive results have occurred with PIVKA. The PIVKA test offers little or no advantage over the more widely available and rapid PT test for the diagnosis of rodenticide toxicity under most circumstances [38].

Disorders of coagulation

Initial stabilization

Due to the wide variation and severity of emergency presentation due to coagulopathies, urgent stabilization to treat symptoms of respiratory distress, shock, pain, etc. is often necessary prior to POC diagnostics, let alone definitive diagnosis of the underlying problem. The initial stabilization of patients with overt clinical signs of a coagulopathy could require aggressive intervention such as hemostasis, respiratory support, circulatory support, and careful patient handling. Drugs that are used to treat specific coagulation disorders and their indications are listed in Table 9.6.

Any source of hemorrhage must be quickly identified and hemostasis provided. A compression bandage or digital pressure is placed on the site of superficial bleeding. Tracheal hemorrhage or

Table 9.6 Medications commonly administered for coagulopathies.

Medication	Indication	Dose
Aspirin	Thromboembolic disease, IMHA	0.5 mg/kg PO q 24 h
Clopidogrel	Thromboembolic disease, IMHA	18.25 mg PO q 24 h (cat) 1–3 mg/kg PO q 24 h (dog)
Warfarin	Refractory thromboemoblic disease; thrombosis	0.22 mg/kg PO q 12 h then adjusted based on PT (target PT 1.25–1.3 times normal)
Unfractionated heparin	Thromboembolic disease	50–300 U/kg SC q 6–8 h
Dalteparin (LMWH)	Thromboembolic disease	150 U/kg SC q 8 h
Enoxaparin (LMWH)	Thromboembolic disease	0.8 (dog), 1.5 (cat) mg/kg SC q 6–12 h
Vincristine	Thrombocytopenia	0.5 mg/m² IV through new IV catheter as delivery outside the vein causes tissue sloughing
Leflunomide	Immune-mediated thrombocytopenia	4–6 mg/kg PO q 24 h (dog)
Prednisone (or alternative steroid)	Immune-mediated thrombocytopenia	2–4 mg/kg/day
Doxycycline	Tick-borne disease	5–10 mg/kg PO or IV q 12 h
Antivenom	Snakebite envenomation	1–10 vials as directed and indicated based on coagulopathy, pain, and clinical judgment
DDAVP (desmopressin)	Von Willebrand's disease, platelet inhibitory drugs, FVIII deficiency	Intranasal product 1–4 µg/kg SC to control bleeding or preoperatively; parenteral product should be given slow and lower doses, 0.3–1 µg/kg SC or IV
Activated protein C	Sepsis	No clinical dose has been published
Antithrombin	Disseminated intravascular coagulation	Not investigated clinically, may be administered with plasma and more effective with concurrent heparin administration
hrVIIa	Bleeding from coagulopathies, sepsis, DIC	90 µg/kg bolus q 2 h until hemostasis
Epsilon-aminocaproic acid	Hyperfibrinolysis, Greyhounds	50–100 mg/kg IV loading then 15 mg/kg/h CRI q 8 h or 15–40 mg/kg IV followed by 500–1000 mg PO q 8 h
Ca-gluconate	Hypocalcemia	50–150 mg/kg (0.5–1.5 mL/kg of 10% solution) slow IV, monitor ECG, stop infusion with bradyarrhythmia
Rivaroxaban (Xa inhibitor)	Thromboprophylaxis	0.5–1 mg/kg PO q 12–24 h
Vitamin K1	Liver disease, anticoagulant drugs or toxicity	2.5–5 mg/kg SC or PO q 12–24 h
Cyclosporine	Immune-mediated thrombocytopenia	5–10 mg/kg PO q 12 h
Azathioprine	Immune-mediated thrombocytopenia	2 mg/kg PO × 2 weeks then q 48 h
Mycophenolate	Immune-mediated thrombocytopenia	10–20 mg/kg PO q 12 h
S-adenosylmethionine	Liver failure/disease	20 mg/kg PO q 24 h (dog)
Silymarin	Liver failure/disease	20–50 mg/kg/day (dog)
Vitamin E	Liver failure/disease	200–600 U/day (dog)
Protamine sulfate	Heparin toxicity	1 mg for every 100 U heparin slow IV
Tranexamic acid	Hyperfibrinolysis	10–15 mg/kg SC or IM, slow IV q 6–8 h
Human IV immunoglobulin	Immune thrombocytopenia	0.5–1 g/kg IV over 6–12 h once
Yunnan baiyao	Neutraceutical but may be helpful with prolonged bleeding	Dog: <15 kg 1 capsule PO q 12 h, 15–30 kg 2 capsules PO q 12 h, >30 kg 2 capsules PO q 8 h Cats: ½ capsule PO q 12 h

DIC, disseminated intravascular coagulation; ECG, electrocardiogram; IMHA, immune-mediated hemolytic anemia; LMWH, low molecular weight heparin; PT, prothrombin time; SC, subcutaneously.

pharyngeal hematomas may obstruct the airways and necessitate orotracheal intubation or tracheostomy for stabilization. Abdominal counterpressure [3] may be required to blunt ongoing abdominal hemorrhage until definitive treatment can be initiated. Patients with pleural or pericardial hemorrhage often benefit from (ultrasound-guided) centesis to evacuate blood. Blood evacuated by cavitary centesis should be collected aseptically and preserved for potential analysis and autologous blood transfusion [39,40].

Pulmonary thromboembolism and pleural or lung parenchyma hemorrhage can lead to life-threatening impairment of oxygenation and ventilation. Patients with mild signs benefit from oxygen support, while more severe respiratory distress may require tracheal intubation and mechanical ventilation until the problem has resolved (see Chapter 8).

Capillary stasis plays a role in the initiation and perpetuation of all forms of coagulation disorders that occur as a complication of disease. The administration of IV crystalloids appropriate for the underlying condition will contribute to the maintenance of vascular flow and hydration of the ICU patient. If a hypercoagulable condition is anticipated, such as DIC or thromboembolism, the addition of hydroxyethyl starch to the fluid protocol can help retain fluid in the vasculature and provide mild anticoagulation effects [41]. Low normal resuscitation endpoints are targeted for fluid infusion (also called permissive hypotension) in patients with a history of trauma or hemorrhage to avoid dislodging a life-saving or fragile clot (see Chapter 2). Patients with a suspected SIRS disease can benefit from high normal resuscitation endpoints. Acidosis and hypothermia contribute to the prolonged clotting times and must be identified and corrected (see Chapters 7 and 17).

Critical patients experiencing significant or ongoing hemorrhage may require the infusion of blood components to supplement RBCs, coagulation proteins, albumin, and antithrombin. A guide for the selection of blood products and the dose is provided in Table 9.7. Acute and delayed transfusion reactions are possible and require close patient monitoring for fever, hypotension, vomiting, labored breathing, facial swelling or urticaria. It is ideal to

Table 9.7 Blood product administration for patients with coagulopathies.

Product	Indication	Dose
Stored whole blood	As frozen plasma with concurrent need for RBCs	Target Hgb of 7–9 mg/dL
Fresh whole blood	As fresh frozen plasma with concurrent need for RBCs	Target Hgb of 7–9 mg/dL
Fresh frozen plasma	Rodenticide ingestion, hemophilia A and B, DIC, liver failure, von Willebrand's disease	6–12 mL/kg minimum or until bleeding stops
Frozen plasma	Rodenticide ingestion, hemophilia B	6–12 mL/kg minimum or until bleeding stops
Cryoprecipitate	Hemophilia A or von Willebrand's disease	1 U/10 kg
Platelet-rich plasma	Thrombocytopenia	To a platelet level of 5–10 000/μL or 50 000/μL if invasive procedure planned (checked 1 h after transfusion)
Platelet concentrate	Thrombocytopenia	As above

DIC, disseminated intravascular coagulation; RBC, red blood cell.

determine the blood type and to cross-match the donor blood to the patient blood prior to transfusion to minimize adverse reactions. Dogs that are DEA 1.1 positive are considered to be universal recipients and DEA 1.1 negative dogs, universal donors.

General nursing care

Careful handling of the patient and limited phlebotomy are essential. Cage rest with padded bedding can minimize patient trauma during hospitalization. Venipuncture for laboratory sampling is done infrequently by using a small gauge needle and a peripheral limb vessel. Compression bandages are placed where indicated. The patient is carefully examined several times daily for evidence of bleeding from the mucosal surfaces or into the skin. Locations and quantity of bleeding are documented in the medical record. Skin bruises are outlined with a marker to document the progression or regression of the hemorrhage.

Coagulation disorders

Coagulation disorders can result in bleeding, thrombosis or a combination of both. DIC, acute traumatic coagulopathy (ATC), rodenticide toxicity, and thromboembolic disorders are the most frequently diagnosed coagulation disorders in ICU patients. Microscopic damage (not grossly detected) will occur before clinical signs become apparent. Since any type of coagulopathy can have devastating consequences, early recognition is optimal for a successful outcome.

Disseminated intravascular coagulation

Disseminated intravascular coagulation (DIC) is a syndrome that develops through multiple stages as a consequence of any systemic disease that has inflammation or capillary stasis as a key component. In DIC, platelets are activated by circulating inflammatory mediators, contact with subendothelial collagen and exposure to the disrupted cell membranes of endothelial cells, RBCs, and platelets. At the same time, there is activation of the coagulation proteins as a result of their exposure to circulating inflammatory mediators, TF, and activated platelets. Initially, a hypercoagulable state develops with microthrombi produced. The fibrinolytic system is activated and FDPs and D-dimers are produced. When the platelet and clotting factor utilization (or consumption) becomes greater than their production, a consumptive hypocoagulopathy dominates with evidence of spontaneous or induced (through surgery or phlebotomy) bleeding.

No single laboratory test will make the definitive diagnosis of DIC. A clinical diagnosis is made when a patient has a predisposing illness, significant capillary stasis, a declining trend in platelet numbers, prolonged POC clotting times (PT, aPTT, ACT), and elevated FDPs or D-dimers. Schistocytes may be evident on a blood smear reflecting RBC trauma from intravascular fibrin deposition. Antithrombin levels are often declining. The TF-activated TEG tracing in dogs with suspected DIC was found to vary from normal to hypercoagulable to hypocoagulable status. It was suggested that the normal TEG tracings reported in these dogs with DIC could have reflected the transition point between hyper- and hypocoagulability rather than "normal" coagulation; in this same study, patients with a hypocoagulable tracing had higher fatality rates [42].

The cornerstone of treating critical animals with DIC is elimination of capillary stasis and effective treatment of the underlying condition. Figure 9.8 provides an algorithm to assist in decision making in patients suspected of having DIC.

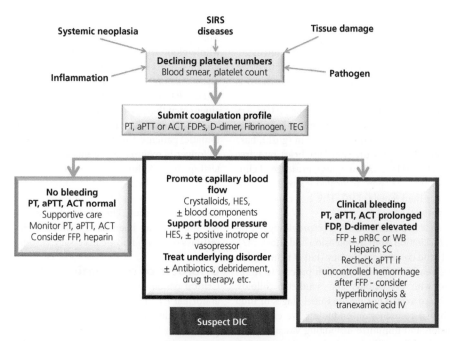

Figure 9.8 Algorithm for approaching small animal ICU patients with suspected disseminated intravascular coagulation. Disease processes listed in purple are some of the most prevalent in the veterinary ICU that may initiate DIC. Declining platelet numbers should alert the clinician to a possible consumptive coagulopathy. POC coagulation profiles to include blood smear, PT, aPTT, ± ACT are analyzed and FDP, D-dimer, and TEG submitted when available. Treatment should begin with promoting capillary blood flow and supporting blood pressure. The administration of HES with crystalloids can provide some mild anticoagulant support in the early stages of this hypercoagulable problem. SIRS patients or cardiac patients might require positive inotropic support of blood pressure if depressed cardiac function is contributing to hypotension. Vasopressor therapy is used only after aggressive fluid infusion in nonresponsive shock and assessment of the Rule of 20 has ruled out other causes of hypotension. Whole blood or pRBCs and FFP may be required during initial stabilization. Treatment of the underlying disorder is essential and examples are given. However, FFP with heparin can be of benefit if surgery or other invasive procedure is planned or the disease status is declining. Evidence of clinical bleeding and prolongation of PT, aPTT with elevations in FDPs or D-dimer warrants more aggressive management. Fresh frozen plasma is given and subcutaneous heparin therapy initiated. If uncontrolled hemorrhage is occurring after adequate FFP infusion, hyperfibrinolysis is considered. The administration of tranexamic acid IV is considered. ACT, activated clotting time; aPTT, activated partial thromboplastin time; FDPs, fibrin degradation products; FFP, fresh frozen plasma; HES, hydroxyethyl starch; IV, intravenous; pRBC, packed red blood cells; PT, prothrombin time; SC, subcutaneous; TEG, thromboelastography; WB, whole blood.

Intravenous fluid therapy with a combination of crystalloids and hydroxyethyl starch (colloid) will promote blood flow through capillaries and provide a mild anticoagulant effect with the colloid (see Chapter 2). This may be adequate to treat DIC in patients without clinical evidence of bleeding or thrombosis.

Patients with clinical bleeding attributed to DIC might benefit from whole blood or plasma administered to replace RBCs, coagulation proteins, albumin, and AT lost through hemorrhage. Patients found to have hypercoagulation from DIC may be at risk from thrombosis. Heparin therapy (see Table 9.8) and fresh frozen plasma (see Table 9.7) to replace consumed coagulation factors and AT are options for treatment of ongoing DIC. Specific therapeutics such as human recombinant APC, human recombinant factor VII, antithrombin, and tissue factor pathway inhibitor are under investigation and may provide options for treating DIC in the future. Thromboprophylaxis with heparin or antiplatelet drugs could be considered early in the treatment of patients predisposed to developing DIC, but studies to determine efficacy are lacking.

Acute trauma coagulopathy

Acute traumatic coagulopathy (ATC) (also called trauma-induced coagulopathy and acute coagulopathy of trauma) is a severe coagulopathy described in human and veterinary trauma patients. A combination of key factors is the driving force in the initiation and propagation of ATC: tissue damage, inflammation, hypoperfusion, hemodilution, hypothermia, and acidosis. There are three hypotheses that account for how ATC develops: ATC is a form of DIC with a profibrinolytic state, ATC has an enhanced thrombomodulin-thrombin protein C pathway, or ATC results from catecholamine-induced endothelial damage from a substantial sympathoadrenal response [43]. A central role is played by hypotension, acidosis, and hypothermia, resulting in a vicious cycle that can lead to uncontrolled hemorrhage and mortality [44].

Severe trauma-induced tissue damage initiates a complex series of events that result in inflammation, DIC, and hyperfibrinolysis. Hypothermia contributes to the coagulopathy by causing platelet dysfunction, reduced coagulation factor activity, and induction of fibrinolysis. Acidosis impairs most if not all of the coagulation process. Platelets change their structure and shape at low blood pH. Also, acidosis increases degradation of fibrinogen. Dilutional coagulopathy becomes part of the pathogenesis due to aggressive crystalloid and synthetic colloid resuscitation. Hydroxyethyl starches can cause a dose-dependent coagulopathy.

Human trauma centers make the diagnosis and guide therapy of ATC based on TEG. Human studies have shown that the relative risk of multiple organ dysfunction and death is substantially higher in severely injured patients with acute coagulopathy than in those without [45]. Until TEG results become readily available to veterinary trauma centers, clinical signs and POC coagulation test results will have to provide a high index of suspicion for ATC. A combination of declining platelet numbers, increased PT and aPTT and declining PCV and hemoglobin in a trauma patient with tissue damage, shock, hypothermia, acidosis, and acute hemorrhage is highly suggestive of ATC.

The Trauma Associated Severe Hemorrhage scoring system was developed to predict the need for massive transfusion in humans utilizing the following parameters: blood hemoglobin (g/dL), base excess (mmol/L), systolic blood pressure (mmHg), heart rate, free intraabdominal fluid (detected by FAST imaging), presence of clinically unstable pelvic fractures or open/dislocated femoral fracture, and gender (male greater than female) [46]. This has not yet been adapted to veterinary patients.

The therapeutic struggle in patients with ATC is providing hemostasis and adequate resuscitation from hypotension and shock [47]. Fresh whole blood or blood component therapy (target hemoglobin of 7–9 g/dL) is required early in the resuscitation process to minimize further dilution with crystalloids and synthetic colloids. Hypothermia should be corrected during the initial stages of fluid resuscitation. Low normal resuscitation endpoints are chosen to promote organ perfusion and minimize dislodging vascular clots. The blood pH is monitored for acidosis with the goal of pH >7.2. Sodium bicarbonate is given if the acidosis is nonresponsive to fluid resuscitation. Blood lactate is monitored as a reflection of tissue perfusion and source of acidosis. Blood calcium is monitored and supplemented if the equivalent of one half or more of the total blood volume (90 mL/kg dog; 65 mL/kg cat) has been given.

Without established TEG values as a guideline, veterinary patients meeting the above criteria for ATC and experiencing uncontrollable hemorrhage after aggressive transfusion therapy may benefit from antifibrinolytic therapy (tranexamic acid and epsilon-aminocaproic acid). Kelmer et al. evaluated 68 dogs with bleeding disorders treated with blood products and tranexamic acid (Hexakapron®, Teva Pharmaceutical, Israel) (mean dosage of 8.6 ± 2.2 mg/kg q 6–8 h) [48]. The dogs given tranexamic acid received fewer blood transfusions and a lower blood component dose with only two dogs experiencing vomiting as an adverse effect.

Vitamin K antagonist rodenticide toxicity

Vitamin K antagonist rodenticides (i.e. bromodiolone, diphacinone, brodifacoum, diphenadione, warfarin, and others) interfere with the carboxylation of factors II, VII, IX, and X in the hepatic vitamin K cycle. The initial suspicion of toxicity is based on a history of exposure, observed ingestion of product or rodent, appearance of product in vomit or feces, or a sudden onset of clinical signs associated with bleeding, which vary depending on location of hemorrhage. Ninety two percent of patients with acute ingestion (<6 hours) may be successfully treated with only gastrointestinal decontamination [49]. If the animal is asymptomatic, emesis is induced with apomorphine (0.03 mg/kg IV) and/or activated charcoal (1–4 g/kg) is administered orally.

Animals presenting with or developing severe hemorrhage will require stabilization. Bleeding around the pharyngeal area can obstruct the airway and require endotracheal or transtracheal intubation. Intrapulmonary hemorrhage may cause hypoxemia and necessitate oxygen supplementation or mechanical ventilation. Thoracocentesis might be necessary to improve oxygenation and ventilation. Any blood from the pleural or abdominal cavity is collected aseptically for autotransfusion should it be needed (this blood is only useful for volume replacement and RBCs as it will not correct the coagulopathy). Actively bleeding animals will benefit from plasma transfusion to provide coagulation proteins and/or whole-blood transfusion to provide RBCs if needed (see Table 9.7). Frozen plasma is adequate for rodenticide intoxication if only coagulation factors are needed.

The PT is measured at presentation and 2–6 hours after emergency therapy (vitamin K1 and plasma) for bleeding patients or 48–72 hours after initial treatment for acute ingestion (asymptomatic) patients. Vitamin K1 (2.5–5 mg/kg PO) therapy for 30 days or longer is required for animals that have prolonged PT at either testing time. Animals that are actively bleeding may require the initial dosage of vitamin K1 by injection. The PT should be normal within 24–48 hours of administration or the vitamin K1 dose should be increased. The PT is rechecked 48–72 hours after vitamin K1 therapy has been discontinued [49] as prolonged therapy (60 days or more) may be necessary in some patients.

Disorders of coagulation factors

Critical patients with adequate platelet numbers and function but abnormal PT or aPTT typically have a problem related to clotting factor production or function. A list of differential diagnoses is provided in Table 9.4.

Severe liver dysfunction can cause a deficiency in factors I, II, V, VII, IX, X, and XI, all of which are made in the liver. Decreased production of vitamin K-dependent clotting factors (II, VII, IX, and X) in the liver can be due to problems with vitamin K intake, absorption or action. The biliary system assists in the absorption of fat-soluble vitamin K, such that severe hepatic, GI or obstructive biliary disease may potentially contribute to hypocoagulation.

Some degree of a dilutional coagulopathy is anticipated after aggressive IV fluid resuscitation that does not involve the administration of plasma products. Medications such as anticoagulants, vitamin K antagonists, and hydroxyethyl starch can interfere with clotting factor function. Iatrogenic coagulopathies may occur with dialysis or continuous renal replacement therapy that often uses either heparinization or citrate therapy.

Inherited coagulopathies are rare and diagnosed more commonly in young animals (<1 year old) that bleed after sustaining minor trauma or surgery. Hemophilia A (factor VIII deficiency) and hemophilia B (factor IX deficiency) are among the most common causes of prolongation of aPTT without elevation of PT. Hageman factor (XII) deficiency has been reported in cats demonstrating prolonged aPTT and no clinical evidence of hemorrhage. A review of the history and quantification of specific coagulation factors are required to make the diagnosis of a specific factor deficiency.

Along with supportive care, coagulation factor disorders are generally treated with transfusions and vitamin K1. A list of transfusion components and doses is provided in Table 9.7. The specific choice of blood product depends on the need for red cells and which coagulation factors are required. Stored or frozen plasma is adequate for anticoagulant rodenticide toxicity or iatrogenic warfarin intoxication. Fresh frozen plasma is necessary for most other coagulopathies requiring coagulation proteins (DIC, hemophilia, liver failure). Desmopressin may provide additional support for animals with hemophilia A. Medications that support liver function can be an adjunct to therapy and are listed in Table 9.6.

Thromboembolic disorders

Thrombosis is the formation of a blood clot within a blood vessel obstructing the blood flow. Thrombi results from platelet adherence and aggregation occurring simultaneously with fibrin

Table 9.8 Known etiological factors for thromboembolic events.

Category	Disease
Endocrine	Hypercortisolism
	Diabetes mellitus
Immune mediated	IMHA
	Protein-losing eneteropathies
Renal	Protein-losing nephropathies
Inflammatory/infectious	Parvovirus
	Pancreatitis
	Sepsis
	Dirofilaria immitis
Neoplasia	Acute leukemia
	Solid tumors
Cardiac	Infective endocarditis
	Dirofilaria immitis
	Primary cardiac disease (cats)
Altered coagulation	Greyhounds (anecdotal)
Liver disease	Microangiopathies and other diseases

IMHA, immune-mediated hemolytic anemia.

strand formation associated with the exposure of blood to TF or subendothelial collagen. Tissue factor can be released at the site of tissue damage or can be circulating in the bloodstream on cells or TF-bearing microparticles [50].

Virchow's triad identifies three major contributors to thrombus formation: (1) injury to vascular endothelium, (2) alterations in normal blood flow, and (3) a hypercoagulable state; these can arise from a variety of disease states. The resulting vascular obstruction causes hypoxic injury to the cells, tissues, and organs distal to the clot. Venous thrombi usually develop in low flow states and consist predominantly of erythrocytes and fibrin (red thrombi). Arterial thrombi develop in areas of high shear stress and consist predominantly of platelets with relatively little fibrin or red cells (white thrombi).

The consequences of arterial thromboembolisms are frequently acute and often catastrophic. FATE is one of the most common examples. The most common site for arterial thromboembolism in the dog and cat is the caudal aorta, although other large arteries are possible. Venous thromboses (with or without embolism) are more common in the pulmonary arteries and large vessels such as the vena cava. These red clots are seen secondary to hypercoagulable states, associated with problems such as heartworm, DIC, sepsis, hyperadrenocorticism, nephrotic syndrome (protein-losing nephropathy), immune-mediated hemolytic anemia (IMHA), and neoplasia. A list of diseases that have a known association with thrombus formation is provided in Table 9.8.

The diagnosis of a thromboembolic disorder initially depends on a high index of suspicion. A review of the history might help to identify any of the underlying disease processes. Physical examination findings that include a sudden onset of labored breathing, a change in mentation, seizures or other neurological signs, acute pain, loss of heat and pulse in a limb, or rapid patient deterioration warrant consideration of a thromboembolic disorder. Ruling out other causes of patient decline is paramount.

Clinicopathological testing and imaging can further support the diagnosis. TEG is one of the few coagulation tests to reliably detect a hypercoagulable state. A normal chest radiograph in a hypoxemic animal is highly suggestive of a pulmonary thromboembolism. Advanced imaging such as ultrasound, echocardiography, contrast angiography, contrast CT scan or ventilation/perfusion scans can be used to reveal the presence and location of a thrombus or embolism.

Therapy for thromboembolic disorders will direct efforts towards four ultimate goals: (1) treat the inciting disease, (2) support the function of organs affected by clot formation, (3) minimize the growth of existing thrombi, and (4) prevent additional thrombus formation. Anticoagulant drug therapy is initiated to minimize growth of existing clots and prevent the formation of new clots. Thromboprophylaxis can be indicated in patients diagnosed with a disease known to cause thrombus formation. Unfortunately, the negative consequences of thrombolytic therapy reported in the dog and cat limit this as a good therapeutic option.

Controlled trials comparing the different anticoagulant drugs in thromboembolic diseases in animals are lacking [51]. Drug choices classically include one or more of the following types of agents: platelet inhibitors (aspirin, clopidogrel), heparin (unfractionated, low molecular weight), and vitamin K antagonists (warfarin). New classes of drugs (e.g. antiXa inhibitors such as rivaroxaban) may prove useful as more information on their effectiveness and safety becomes available. A list of the available drugs and recommended initial doses can be found in Table 9.6. Monitoring the effectiveness of therapy is essential.

The two most common oral antiplatelet drugs used in small animals are aspirin and clopidogrel, with little documentation of superiority of one drug over the other [52]. Aspirin inhibits cyclo-oxygenase which decreases thromboxane A2 production and permanently inhibits the ability of treated platelets to aggregate. Clopidogrel specifically inhibits the binding of ADP to the platelet P2Y12 receptor, decreasing platelet aggregation. The benefit of monitoring antiplatelet therapy with platelet function tests is unknown. The clinical safety and efficacy of the platelet-inhibiting drugs abciximab and eptifibatide in small animals are not known, and these are not recommended.

The goal of heparin therapy is to halt the progression of the thromboembolic process and provide time for natural clot lysis. A choice must be made between unfractionated heparin and low molecular weight heparin. A goal for therapy with either form of heparin is to increase aPTT to 1.5–2.5 times the baseline value or INR to 2–3. Protamine sulfate will reverse the anticoagulant effects of both types of heparin and is used to treat heparin overdose or toxicity.

Unfractionated heparin can prevent new clot formation and the expansion of existing clots. Unfractionated heparin activity is variable based on bioavailability and can have unpredictable effects. Therefore, monitoring the effect of this form of heparin on clotting times (aPTT or INR) is essential. Recent evidence indicates that dosing unfractionated heparin guided by anti-factor Xa monitoring reduced fatalities in dogs with IMHA [53]. The unfractionated heparin-induced thrombocytopenia reported in people has not been documented in veterinary species.

Low molecular weight heparin (e.g. enoxaparin, dalteparin) is described as having improved bioavailability, causing fewer bleeding tendencies and requiring less frequent dosing than unfractionated heparin in people. These differences have not been clearly demonstrated in veterinary species. Using anti-Xa activity to monitor dosing, it was determined that dogs require at least twice-daily doses of low molecular weight heparin to achieve the therapeutic benefits [54,55]. Cost of these medications is often a limiting factor.

Warfarin therapy is an option for patients that require long-term management of thromboembolic disease or have been refractory to other anticoagulant drugs. Warfarin therapy induces an initial hypercoagulable state as it also inhibits the natural anticoagulants protein C and protein S. Heparin administration is therefore required during the first 2–3 days of warfarin therapy. Due to the narrow therapeutic index of warfarin, regular monitoring of INR is required; a target goal of 2.0–3.0 of baseline is appropriate. A higher therapeutic goal may be required when animals undergo heart valve replacement [56].

The use of thrombolytic agents (streptokinase, tissue plasminogen activator, urokinase) to lyze established clots has provided inconsistent results, an increased risk of bleeding, and has shown no proven benefit to outcome [57]. The few reports of surgical procedures for removal of thrombi in veterinary patients have described poor outcomes. Catheter-guided procedures (endovascular management) of thromboses to administer thrombolytic drugs at the site of the clot or physical clot removal are options that require investigation in veterinary medicine.

Direct factor Xa inhibitors (xabans) are a new class of anticoagulant drugs that can provide an alternative to warfarin and heparin. The efficacy, benefits, and side-effects of xabans in veterinary medicine have yet to be defined.

Feline aortic thromboembolism

Feline aortic thromboembolism (FATE) occurs as a consequence of turbulent blood flow in the heart and affects approximately 30% of cats with heart disease [58]. A dilated left atrium is one of the greatest risk factors for thrombosis. Neoplasia and thyroid disease have also been associated with FATE.

Blood stasis, hypercoagulability, and endothelial damage occurring in cats with heart disease set the stage for thrombus formation. Spontaneous contrast ("smoke") or low auricular blood flow may be observed in the left atrium on echocardiography as a precursor to clot formation. Clots found in the left atrium can remain static, continue to grow and interfere with outflow into the left ventricle, or break apart and travel to a distal part of the body. Close to 90% of cats with a thromboembolism have a clot that lodges in the terminal aorta. Other potential sites for embolization are brachial, visceral, and cerebral arteries. Ultrasound and Doppler evaluation of accessible vessels can be used to demonstrate vascular blood flow and identify a thrombus when present.

The thromboembolism not only occludes the artery where it lodges but also impairs collateral circulation. It is theorized that the thromboembolus releases serotonin and thromboxane A2 which causes vasoconstriction of the collateral vessels. However, treatment with serotonin and thromboxane antagonists has no apparent benefit [59]. The potential for ischemic tissues makes it important to evaluate renal function as well as serum potassium, sodium, phosphorus, and lactate levels during the crisis stage.

Therapeutic management of FATE will first focus on treating the pain (see Chapter 19); pure mu agonists such as methadone, hydromorphone or fentanyl are recommended. Concurrent congestive heart failure may occur with the sudden increase in cardiac afterload, making stabilization of the consequences of cardiac disease essential; therapy may include oxygen, furosemide, vasodilators, and medications to treat the specific cardiac disorder (see Chapter 11). Blood pressure support may be required with judicious IV fluid administration and possibly positive inotropes (see Chapter 3). Reperfusion injury or renal thrombosis may lead to life-threatening hyperkalemia; IV regular insulin (0.5 U/kg) followed by IV dextrose (0.5 g/kg) is administered to decrease serum potassium levels when indicated.

No specific therapy has proven more effective than supportive therapy alone for the established thrombus. Heparin is often recommended but evidence of effectiveness is lacking; thrombolytic drugs (streptokinase, urokinase, and tPA) have been used but none has shown therapeutic benefit over more conservative care and they can result in serious side-effects in cats. Rheolytic (catheter-guided) thrombectomy with fluoroscopy has been described in a small number of cats as well. Survival to discharge is similar for conservative management and those receiving thrombolytic therapy or endovascular management. Further research is needed before recommendations for thrombolytic agents or catheter-directed clot removal can be made [60,61].

Supportive therapy with unfractionated heparin (300 U/kg SQ q 8 h) is routinely recommended. The proposed goal is a prolongation of aPTT by 1.5–2.5 times baseline. Adjunctive therapy for FATE in cats could include massage and heat therapy of limbs with obstructed blood flow. Pain management must be continuous and visceral organs such as the kidneys and GI tract supported if blood flow has been affected. The effects of hyperbaric oxygen and hemoglobin-based oxygen carrier solutions in cats with FATE warrant investigation in the future.

Recommendations for prophylactic treatment to avoid thromboembolism in cats are under investigation. Cats with FATE have been shown to have a worse prognosis when aspirin or clopidogrel was not part of their maintenance therapy [62]. Preliminary evidence favors the use of clopidogrel (18.75 mg/cat q 24 h) over aspirin (81 mg/cat q 72 h) for improved survival time and improved time before clot recurrence [63]. Warfarin has been used at a starting oral dose of 0.06–0.09 mg/kg/day, with heparin necessary the first 2–3 days of warfarin therapy, and dose adjusted based on coagulation monitoring. Close monitoring of coagulation parameters is essential and concern for risk of bleeding often limits use of this drug. Starting doses for low molecular weight and unfractionated heparin are given in Table 9.6.

Immune-mediated hemolytic anemia

The majority of dogs with IMHA have been found to be in a hypercoagulable state, and the role of thromboembolism in IMHA is multifactorial and complex [64]. The presence of both venous and arterial thrombosis suggests dysregulation of both coagulation and platelets. While pulmonary thromboembolisms are very common, other venous sites for thrombosis have been reported to include cranial vena cava, portal vein, cephalic vein, splenic vein, and hepatic vein. Arterial sites documented include pulmonary, myocardial, splenic, renal, iliac, pituitary, and mesenteric arteries.

Dogs with IMHA express excessive platelet activation and activation of coagulation as evidenced by decreased AT, thrombocytopenia, prolonged aPTT and PT, and elevated D-dimers. Activated platelets, damaged RBCs, and microparticles found in IMHA are procoagulant. Studies in humans and laboratory animals suggest that activated endothelium plays a central role in thrombosis associated with hemolytic disease. Free hemoglobin results in the scavenging of nitric oxide, which contributes to increased TF expression and platelet aggregation. It is possible that inflammatory cytokines, activated monocytes, and free hemoglobin induce endothelial cell TF expression, as well. In addition, TF-expressing microparticles derived from monocytes bind to endothelium and contribute to thrombosis. The exposure of TF activates factor VII and initiates coagulation. Reticulocytes or antibody-induced spherocyte formation seen in IMHA result in excessive RBC binding to endothelial cells.

Treatment of IMHA in dogs typically involves the administration of one or more immunosuppressive agents such as glucocorticosteroids, azathioprine, cyclosporine, and cyclophosphamide. Human IV immunoglobulin G has been given to dogs to inhibit pathological antibodies and modulate complement activation, but it has not uniformly demonstrated success. However, the immunosuppressive agents used to treat IMHA and other supportive measures could contribute to thrombosis. Human IV immunoglobulin G has been found to be prothrombotic in dogs. Glucocorticosteroids increase circulating levels of some coagulation factors and decrease fibrinolysis, but it is unknown if they contribute to thrombosis in dogs with IMHA. The IV catheter is a supportive measure that has been associated with thrombosis [51].

Thromboprophylaxis in dogs with IMHA appears to be warranted with drugs that target coagulation. Unfractionated heparin affects many of the pathways that seem to contribute to the prothrombotic state in IMHA. Unfortunately, the dosage required is highly variable and individualized monitoring of the therapeutic effect is recommended (aPTT and anti-factor Xa activity). Survival was significantly higher in a study in dogs given individually adjusted doses of unfractionated heparin compared to a constant dose of 150 U/kg q 6 h [32]. Further studies are needed for definite recommendations. At this time, however, the initial dosage of heparin is 150 U/kg q 6–8 h, adjusted to reach the target of prolonging aPTT to 1.5–2.5 baseline control and an anti-factor Xa activity of 0.35–0.7 U/mL. Low molecular weight heparin has been suggested as an alternative, but its efficacy for reducing the risk of thrombosis and a target range for anti-factor Xa monitoring is unknown and requires further study at this time.

Treatment with prednisone, ultra low-dose aspirin (0.5 mg/kg), and azathioprine had improved long- and short-term survival in an outcome study in dogs with IMHA [65]; however, demonstrable *in vivo* effects of aspirin at this dose have not been seen in healthy dogs. Clopidogrel provided similar short-term survival rates as the 0.5 mg/kg/day aspirin dose or when the two antiplatelet drugs were combined [52]. Heparin combined with low-dose aspirin may prove to be beneficial, but controlled trials comparing differing anticoagulation drugs are warranted [33].

Pulmonary thromboembolism

Pulmonary thromboembolism (PTE) occurs when venous thrombi produced in large, deep veins travel through the right side of the heart and lodge in the pulmonary arterial bed. Underlying diseases associated with PTE include hyperadrenocorticism, SIRS diseases, IMHA, diabetes mellitus, heartworm, neoplasia, protein-losing nephropathy or enteropathy, cardiomyopathy, vasculitis, and polycythemia. The caudal lung lobes are more likely to be involved because they receive most of the right ventricular output.

Pulmonary consequences of PTE include hypoxemia, bronchoconstriction, ventilation-perfusion (V/Q) mismatch, hyperventilation, atelectasis, pulmonary edema, and pleural effusion. There is an increase in right ventricular afterload and ventricular oxygen demand. Cardiac ischemia, arrhythmias, or right ventricular failure could occur with severe elevations in pulmonary arterial pressure (pulmonary hypertension). Decreased cardiac output secondary to obstruction of pulmonary blood flow and decreased pulmonary venous return can cause hypotension and poor systemic perfusion.

Definitive diagnosis of PTE is difficult. The first indication can be sudden onset of tachypnea, labored breathing, and hypoxemia in an animal with a compatible underlying disease process. An arterial blood gas will show hypoxemia and possibly low or normal carbon dioxide due to hyperventilation. Echocardiography can show flattening of the interventricular septum or dilation of the pulmonary trunk, right atrium or right ventricle. A normal echocardiogram does not rule out PTE. Chest radiographs may be normal or show evidence of pleural effusion, alveolar infiltrates, areas of oligemia, hyperlucent lung regions, cardiomegaly or enlarged main pulmonary artery. Advanced imaging, such as spiral CT or V/Q scans with radioisotopes, are necessary for diagnosis of pulmonary thrombi.

Patient management is first centered on providing an airway if necessary, ensuring adequate breathing, and promoting circulation. Hypoxemia seen in these patients may or may not be responsive to oxygen supplementation. However, patients with severe PTE may require endotracheal intubation and mechanical ventilation until the crisis has passed (see Chapter 8). Even though the current PTE may dissolve without treatment within hours, a prothrombotic condition exists warranting thromboprophylaxis. The potential devastating consequences of PTE have promoted the recommendation for intravenous administration of heparin. A loading IV dose of 80–100 U/kg is given followed by 18 U/kg/h in dogs and a loading dose of 100 U/kg IV followed by 10–30 U/kg/h in cats. The aPTT is checked prior to heparin infusion and 6 hours post IV loading dose. The goal is aPTT 1.5–2 times baseline. Antiplatelet therapy is also initiated with low-dose aspirin or clopidogrel. A safe and effective protocol for thrombolytic therapy has not been documented for small animals and it is not recommended at this time.

Disorders of natural anticoagulants

An abnormal quantity or function of natural anticoagulants can cause hypercoagulation. Proteins S and C are vitamin K-dependent anticoagulants made in the liver which inhibit the function of factors Va and VIIa. These factors are decreased in the early stages of warfarin therapy and cause a prothrombotic state. Antithrombin (AT) is also made in the liver. Any disease that causes albumin loss (such as SIRS, protein-losing nephropathy or enteropathy) is likely to cause loss of AT molecules as well. Consumption of AT can occur in DIC and ATC, making heparin therapy ineffective until AT is replaced. Diseases associated with thrombotic events are listed in Table 9.8. Fresh frozen plasma can be administered to supplement natural anticoagulant concentrations (see Table 9.7 for dose).

Platelet disorders
Thrombocytopenia

Thrombocytopenia can result from decreased platelet production, increased platelet sequestration, increased platelet consumption, and increased platelet destruction (Table 9.3 gives a list of differential diagnoses). Immune destruction of platelets often results in the most significant drop in platelet numbers. Clinical bleeding is likely with platelet numbers <30 000 platelets/µL.

The initial diagnosis of thrombocytopenia is based on a low platelet count. Historical information includes past medical problems, recent vaccination, exposure to ticks or an endemic area, FeLV, FIV and heartworm status, and drug exposure. Physical examination findings suggestive of a platelet disorder include petechiae, bleeding from the gums, and melena. Splenomegaly suggests an underlying disease process associated with the thrombocytopenia.

Diagnostics that are routinely recommended include CBC and blood smear to look for macrothrombocytes, indicating bone marrow response, platelet clumping, PCV/TP to evaluate for bleeding, serum biochemistry, imaging, evaluation for tick-borne disease. A bone marrow sample is collected when pancytopenia is present. The diagnosis of immune-mediated thrombocytopenia (ITP) is based on the findings of moderate-to-severe thrombocytopenia and lack of other coagulation abnormalities, platelet sequestration or underlying disease. Demonstration of antiplatelet antibodies will support the immune-mediated diagnosis but is often not performed.

Mild-to-moderate thrombocytopenia (50 000–200 000/μL) rarely requires specific intervention, but requires investigation and treatment of the underlying pathology. Bleeding associated with severe thrombocytopenia (<30 000–50 000/μL) can be temporarily blunted by infusion of platelet concentrate, platelet-rich plasma or fresh whole blood (see Table 9.7). These blood components deliver a low number of platelets with a limited lifespan, but may be adequate while definitive therapy is provided.

Medication options used to treat specific platelet disorders are provided in Table 9.6. Vincristine can release platelets from megakaryocytes in the bone marrow and increase circulating platelet numbers; it is not clear if these platelets are functional. Prednisolone therapy directed at suppressing the immune destruction of platelets is initiated when ITP is the working diagnosis. Azathioprine, cyclosporine, mycophenylate, luflonemide or other medications can be added as indicated if there is a poor response to prednisolone. Human IVIG administered early for canine ITP patients has been shown to improve platelet number recovery time and decrease hospitalization time [66–68]. It must be remembered that ICU patients receiving immunosuppressive therapy are at risk of (hospital-acquired) infections and may have side-effects from administered drugs. Splenectomy is an intervention for ITP but is reserved for patients with chronic or recurrent disease [69]. Doxycycline is often indicated to treat infectious causes of thrombocytopenia pending serology of suspected arthropod vector diseases.

Thrombocytopathy, von Willebrand's disease, and thrombocytosis

Thrombocytopathy should be suspected when platelet numbers are normal, BMBT is prolonged, and coagulation times are normal.

Congenital defects and vWD are less common, but can be present in young animals experiencing excessive bleeding with their first mild trauma or elective surgical procedure (spay or neuter). There is a breed predilection for vWD, which includes Doberman Pinschers, German Shepherds, Golden Retrievers, Miniature Schnauzers, Pembroke Welsh Corgis, Shetland Sheepdogs, Basset Hounds, Scottish Terriers, Standard Poodles, and Manchester Terriers.

In a patient known or suspected to have vWD, desmopressin acetate (DDAVP; see Table 9.6) may be administered and is reported to shorten clotting times associated with vWD; fresh frozen plasma or cryoprecipitate may alleviate clinical signs of bleeding as well. Desmopression may also alleviate clinical sings of bleeding secondary to aspirin administration [70] (i.e. prior to emergency therapy). Significant ongoing hemorrhage from any cause of thrombocytopathy will include transfusion with fresh whole blood, cryoprecipitate or fresh or fresh frozen plasma transfusion to provide vWF.

Thrombocytosis is an uncommon diagnosis in veterinary medicine and investigation of underlying disease is necessary. Therapy to specifically treat thrombocytosis is usually not required unless there is evidence of thrombosis.

Disorders of fibrinolysis

Fibrinolysis must occur for normal blood flow to be reestablished after clot formation. The fibrin mesh of a clot is cleaved in multiple locations by the enzyme plasmin during fibrinolysis. Endothelial cells begin to secrete tissue plasminogen activators (tPA) that convert plasminogen to plasmin to start dissolving the thrombus. Clot lysis results in circulating FDPs, which are subsequently cleared by circulating proteases or processed by the kidney and liver. The fibrinolytic system is closely linked to the inflammatory response (complement system) with FDPs potentially contributing to increased vascular permeability.

Dogs appear to have accelerated fibrinolysis compared to humans. Studies in Greyhounds with posttraumatic and postoperative bleeding have identified hyperfibrinolysis as a probable cause. The venom of pit vipers (and other species) contains fibrinogenases that rapidly dissolve clots after envenomation. Trauma patients with substantial tissue damage can have overwhelming activation of TF with concurrent hyperfibrinolysis. In addition, the lysis of RBCs can enhance tPA-mediated fibrinolysis.

Bleeding associated with hyperfibrinolysis can range from mild bruising at an incision site to life-threatening hemorrhage. Diagnosis of fibrinolytic disorders is supported by elevated FDPs and D-dimers, prolonged thrombin clotting time, RBC changes (see Chapter 10) and TEG tracings reflecting hyperfibrinolysis.

Excessive fibrinolysis resulting in a coagulopathy requires very specific therapy. Derivatives of the amino acid lysine, epsilon-aminocaproic acid and tranexamic acid inhibit fibrinolysis (doses are given in Table 9.6). Recommendations to administer epsilon-aminocaproic acid to Greyhounds prior to surgical intervention have been made [71,72]. The therapeutic value after surgery, trauma or envenomation is unknown.

Victims of snake envenomation, particularly pit vipers, benefit primarily from the administration of antivenin. Species-specific or polyvalent antivenin binds to and limits the effects of excessive enzymatic degradation and spreading of the venom. The use of antifibrinolytics for snakebite victims is thought to offer minimal or no benefit [73].

Plasma transfusions to provide clotting factors are of limited value for arresting hemorrhage in animals affected by excessive fibrinolysis, but may be helpful to restore volume or if a concurrent consumptive coagulopathy is present. Red blood cell transfusions may be indicated for excessive blood loss or hemolysis.

References

1. Smith SA. The cell-based model of coagulation. J Vet Emerg Crit Care 2009;19(1):3–10.
2. Hackner SG. Bleeding disorders. In: Small Animal Critical Care Medicine. Silverstein DC, Hopper K, eds. St Louis: Elsevier Saunders, 2014: pp 507–14.
3. Herold L, Devey J, Kirby R, Rudloff E. Clinical evaluation and management of hemoperitoneum in dogs. J Vet Emerg Crit Care 2008;18(1):40–53.
4. Taggart R, Austin B, Hans E, Hogan D. In vitro evaluation of the effect of hypothermia on coagulation in dogs via thromboelastography. J Vet Emerg Crit Care 2012; 22(2):219–24.
5. Greenwell CM, Epstein SE, Brain PH. Influence of needle gauge used for venipuncture on automated platelet count and coagulation profile in dogs. Aust Vet J. 2014; 92(3):71–4.
6. Brooks MB, Catalfamo JL. Immune-mediated thrombocytopenia, von Willebrand disease and platelet disorders. In: Textbook of Veterinary Internal Medicine, 7th edn, vol. 1. Ettinger SJ, Feldman EC, eds. St Louis: Elsevier Saunders, 2010: pp 772–83.
7. Brooks MB. Canine IMHA and feline ATE: how can we improve outcomes? In: Hemostasis and Hypercoagulability in the Critically Ill. Proceedings of the American

College of Veterinary Emergency and Critical Care Multidisciplinary Review, February 17, 2007, Orlando, FL.

8. Brooks M. Evaluation of the bleeding patient: point of care tests. Clin Brief 2006:83–6.

9. Holowaychuk MK, Hanel RM, Darren Wood R, Rogers L, O'Keefe K, Monteigh G. Prospective multicenter evaluation of coagulation abnormalities in dogs following severe acute trauma. J Vet Emerg Crit Care 2014;24(1):93–104.

10. Harrell K. Activated vlotting time. In: Blackwell's Five Minute Veterinary Consult: Laboratory Tests and Diagnostic Procedures, Canine and Feline. Vaden SL, Knoll JS, Franks WK, Tilley LP, eds. Ames: Wiley-Blackwell, 2009: pp 24–5.

11. Boysen SR, Lisciandro GR. The use of ultrasound for dogs and cats in the emergency room: AFAST and TFAST. Vet Clin North Am Small Anim Pract. 2015:43(4):773–97.

12. Brooks MB, Catalfamo JL. Current diagnostic trends in coagulation disorders among dogs and cats. Vet Clin North Am Small Anim Pract. 2013;43(6):1349–72.

13. Miller MD, Lunn KF. Diagnostic use of cytologic examination of bone marrow from dogs with thrombocytopenia: 58 cases (1994–2004). J Am Vet Med Assoc. 2007;231(10):1540–4.

14. Brooks MB. Coagulation factors. In: Blackwell's Five Minute Veterinary Consult: Laboratory Tests and Diagnostic Procedures, Canine and Feline. Vaden SL, Knoll JS, Franks WK, Tilley LP, eds. Ames: Wiley-Blackwell, 2009: pp 176–8.

15. Corn S. Fibrinogen. In: Blackwell's Five Minute Veterinary Consult: Laboratory Tests and Diagnostic Procedures, Canine and Feline. Vaden SL, Knoll JS, Franks WK, Tilley LP, eds. Ames: Wiley-Blackwell, 2009: pp 303–5.

16. Goggs R, Brainard B, de Laforcade AM, et al. Partnership on Rotations ViscoElastic Test Standardization (PROVETS): evidence-based guidelines on rotational visco-elastic assays in veterinary medicine. J Vet Emerg Crit Care 2014;24(1):1–22.

17. McMichael M, Goggs R, Smith S, et al. Systematic evaluation of evidence on veterinary viscoelastic testing. Part 1: System comparability. J Vet Emerg Crit Care 2014;24(1):23–9.

18. Flatland B, Koenigshof AM, Rozanski EA, et al. Systematic evaluation of evidence on veterinary viscoelastic testing. Part 2: Sample acquisition and handling. J Vet Emerg Crit Care 2014;24(1):30–6.

19. De Laforcade A, Goggs R, Wiinberg B. Systematic evaluation of evidence on veterinary viscoelastic testing. Part 3: Assay activation and test protocol. J Vet Emerg Crit Care 2014;24(1):37–46.

20. Hanel RM, Chan DL, Conner B, et al. Systemic evaluation of evidence on veterinary viscoelastic testing. Part 4: definitions and data reporting. J Vet Emerg Crit Care 2014;24(1):47–56.

21. Brainard BM, Goggs R, Mendez-Angulo JL, et al. Systematic evaluation of evidence on veterinary viscoelastic testing. Part 5: Nonstandard assays. J Vet Emerg Crit Care 2014;24(1):57–62.

22. Kashuk JL, Moore EE, Sabel A, et al. Rapid thromboelastography (r-TEG) identifies hypercoagulability and predicts thromboembolic events in surgical patients. Surgery 2009;146(4):764–72.

23. Muller M, Meijers J, Vroom M, Juffermans N. Utility of thromboelastography and/or thromboelastometry in adults with sepsis: a systematic review. Crit Care 2014;18(1):R30.

24. Bolliger D, Seeberger MD, Tanaka KA. Principles and practice of thromboelastography in clinical coagulation management and transfusion practice. Transfus Med Rev. 2012;26(1):1–13.

25. Epstein SE, Hopper K, Mellema MS, Johnson LR. Diagnostic utility of D-dimer concentrations in dogs with pulmonary embolism. J Vet Intern Med. 2013;27(6):1646–9.

26. Stokol T. D-dimer. In: Blackwell's Five Minute Veterinary Consult: Laboratory Tests and Diagnostic Procedures, Canine and Feline. Vaden SL, Knoll JS, Franks WK, Tilley LP, eds. Ames: Wiley-Blackwell, 2009: pp 217–19.

27. Nelson OL, Andreasen C. The utility of plasma D-dimer to identify thromboembolic disease in dogs. J Vet Intern Med. 2003;17:830–4.

28. Griffin A, Callan MB, Shofer FS, Giger U. Evaluation of a canine D-dimer point-of-care test kit for use in samples obtained from dogs with disseminated intravascular coagulation, thromboembolic disease, and hemorrhage. Am J Vet Res. 2003;64:1562–9.

29. Monreal L. D-dimer as a new test for the diagnosis of DIC and thromboemobolic disease, Editorial. J Vet Intern Med. 2003;17:757–9.

30. Stokol T, Brooks M, Rush JE, et al. Hypercoagulability in cats with cardiomyopathy. J Vet Intern Med. 2008;22(3):546–52.

31. Brooks MB. Prothrombin time. In: Blackwell's Five Minute Veterinary Consult: Laboratory Tests and Diagnostic Procedures, Canine and Feline. Vaden SL, Knoll JS, Franks WK, Tilley LP, eds. Ames: Wiley-Blackwell, 2009: pp 504–5.

32. Helmond SE, Polzin DJ, Armstrong PJ, Finke M, Smith SA. Treatment of immune-mediated hemolytic anemia with individually adjusted heparin dosing in dogs. J Vet Intern Med. 2010;24(3):597–605.

33. Kidd L, Mackman N. Prothrombotic mechanisms and anticoagulant therapy in dogs with immune-mediated hemolytic anemia. J Vet Emerg Crit Care 2013;23(1):3–13.

34. Davis DG. Antithrombin III (ATIII). In: Clinical Veterinary Advisor, Dogs and Cats, 2nd edn. Cote E, ed. St Louis: Elsevier Mosby, 2011.

35. Bauer N, Mortiz A. Characterisation of changes in the haemostasis system in dogs with thrombosis. J Small Anim Pract. 2013;54(3):129–36.

36. Hadar G, Kelmer E, Segev G, et al. Protein C activity in dogs envenomed by Vipera palaestinae. Toxicon 2014;87(Sep):38–44.

37. Istvan SA, Marks SL, Murphy LA, Dorman DC. Evaluation of a point-of-care anticoagulant rodenticide test for dogs. J Vet Emerg Crit Care 2014;24(2):168–73.

38. Mount ME, Kim BU, Kass PH. Use of a test for proteins induced by vitamin K absence or antagonism in diagnosis of anticoaglant poisoning in dogs: 325 cases (1987–1997). J Am Vet Med Assoc. 2003;222(2):194–8.

39. Higgs V, Rudloff E, Kirby R, Linklater A. Autologous blood transfusion in 24 dogs with thoracic and/or abdominal hemorrhage. J Vet Emerg Crit Care 2015;25(6):731–8.

40. Linklater A. Treatment of acute hemoabdomen in a dog. Clin Brief 2013;11(1):13–15.

41. Glover PA, Rudloff E, Kirby R. Hydroxyethyl starch: a review of pharmacokinetics, pharmacodynamic, current products, and potential clinical risks, benefits and use. J Vet Emerg Crit Care 2014;24(6):642–61.

42. Wiinberg B, Jensen AL, Johansson PI, et al. Thromboelastographic evaluation of hemostatic function in dogs with disseminated intravascular coagulation. J Vet Intern Med. 2008;22(2):357–65.

43. Palmer L, Martin L. Traumatic coagulopathy Part 1: Pathophysiology and diagnosis. J Vet Emerg Crit Care 2014;24(1):63–74.

44. Palmer L, Martin L. Traumatic coagulopathy Part 2: Resuscitative strategies. J Vet Emerg Crit Care 2014;24(1):75–92.

45. Maegele M, Spinella PC, Schochi H. The acute coagulopathy of trauma: mechanisms and tools for risk stratification. Shock 2012;38(5):450–8.

46. Yucel N, Lefering R, Meaegle M. Trauma Associated Severe Hemorrhage (TASH) Score: probability of mass transfusion as surrogate for life threatening hemorrhage after multiple trauma. J Trauma 2006;60(6):1228–36.

47. Abelson AL, O'Tolle TE, Johnston A, Respess M, de Laforcade AM. Hypoperfusion and acute traumatic coagulopathy in severely traumatized canine patients. J Vet Emerg Crit Care 2013;23(4):395–401.

48. Kelmer E, Marer K, Bruchim Y, et al. Retrospective evaluation of the safety and efficacy of tranexamic acid (Hexakapron) for the treatment of bleeding disorders in dogs. Israel J Vet Med. 2013;68(2):94–100.

49. Pattinger GE, Otto CM, Syring RS. Incidence of prolonged prothrombin time in dogs following gastrointestinal decontamination for acute anticoagulant rodenticide ingestion. J Vet Emerg Crit Care 2008;18(3):285–91.

50. Furie B. Pathogenesis of thrombosis. Hematol Am Soc Hematol Educ Progr. 2009;255–8.

51. Kidd L, Mackman N. Prothrombotic mechanisms and anticoagulant therapy in dogs with immune-mediated hemolytic anemia. J Vet Emerg Crit Care 2013;23(1):3–13.

52. Mellett AM, Nakamura RK, Bianco D. A prospective study of clopidogrel therapy in dogs with primary immune-mediated hemolytic anemia. J Vet Intern Med. 2011;25(1):71–5.

53. Helmond SE, Polzin DJ, Armstrong PJ, Finke M, Smith SA. Treatment of immune-mediated hemolytic anemia with individually adjusted heparin dosing in dogs. J Vet Intern Med. 2010;24(3):597–605.

54. Lunsford KV, Mackin AJ, Langston VC, Brooks M. Pharmacokinetics of subcutaneous low molecular weight heparin (enoxaparin) in dogs. J Am Anim Hosp Assoc. 2009;45(6):261–7.

55. Scott KC, Hansen BD, DeFrancesco TC. Coagulation effects of low molecular weight heparin compared with heparin in dogs considered to be at risk for clinically significant venous thrombosis. J Vet Emerg Crit Care 2009;19(1):74–80.

56. Orton EC, Hackett TB, Mama K, Boon JA. Technique and outcome of mitral valve replacement in dogs. J Am Vet Med Assoc. 2005;226(9):1508–11.

57. Brooks MB. Canine IMHA and feline ATE: how can we improve outcomes? In: Hemostasis and Hypercoagulability in the Critically Ill. Proceedings of the American College of Veterinary Emergency and Critical Care Multidisciplinary Review, February 17, 2007, Orlando, FL.

58. Rush JE, Freeman LM, Fenollosa NK, et al. Population and survival characteristics of cats with hypertrophic cardiomyopathy: 260 cases (1990–1999). J Am Vet Med Assoc 2002;220(2):202–7.

59. Kittleson MD. Thromboembolic disease. In: Small Animal Cardiovascular Medicine. Kittleson MD, Kienle RD, eds. St Louis: Mosby, 1998: pp 540–7.

60. Beal M. Proceedings of the Central Veterinary Conference, November 1, 2010, San Diego, CA

61. Marshall HC, Koors T. How to handle feline aortic thromboembolism. Available at: http://veterinarymedicine.dvm360.com/how-handle-feline-aortic-thromboembolism

62. Borgeat K, Wright J, Garrod O, etal. Arterial thromboembolism in 250 cats in general practice: 2004–2012. J Vet Intern Med. 2014;28(1):102–8.

63. Hogan D, Fox P, Jacob K, et al. Analysis of the Feline Arterial Thromboembolism: Clopidogrel vs Aspirin Trial (FAT CAT). Proceedings of the ACVIM Forum, June 4–7, 2013, Seattle, WA.

64. Johnson V, Dow S. Management of immune mediated hemolytic anemia in dogs. In: Kirk's Current Veterinary Therapy XV. Bonagura JD, Twedt DC, eds. St. Louis: Elsevier Saunders, 2014: pp 275–9.

65. Weinkle TK, Center SA, Randolph, JF, Warner KL, Barr SC, Erb HN. Evaluation of prognostic factors, survival rates, and treatment protocols for immune-mediated hemolytic anemia in dogs: 151 cases (1993–2002). J Am Vet Med Assoc. 2005;226(11):1869–80.

66. Balog K, Huang AA, Sum S, et al. A prospective randomized clinical trial of vincristine versus human intravenous immunoglobulin for acute adjunctive management of presumptive primary immune-mediated thrombocytopenia in dogs. J Vet Intern Med. 2013;27(3):536–41.

67. Bianco D, Armstrong PJ, Washabau RJ. A prospective, randomized, double-blinded, placebo-controlled study of human intravenous immunoglobulin for the acute management of presumptive primary immune-mediated thrombocytopenia in dogs. J Vet Intern Med. 2009;23(5):1071–8.

68. Bianco D, Armstrong PJ, Washabau RJ. Treatment of severe immune-mediated thrombocytopenia with human IV immunoglobulin in 5 dogs. J Vet Intern Med. 2007;21(4):694–9.

69. Jans HE, Armstrong PJ, Price GS. Therapy of immune mediated thrombocytopenia. A retrospective study of 15 dogs. J Vet Intern Med. 1990;4(1):4–7.

70. Di Mauro FM, Holowaychuk MK. Intravenous administration of desmopressin acetate to reverse acetylsalicylic acid-induced coagulopathy in three dogs. J Vet Emerg Crit Care 2013;23(4):455–8.

71. Marin LM, Iazbik MC, Zaldivar-Lopez S, Guillaumin J, McLoughlin MA, Couto CG. Epsilon aminocaproic acid for the prevention of delayed postoperative bleeding in retired racing greyhounds undergoing gonadectomy. Vet Surg. 2012;41(5):594–603.

72. Marin LM, Iazbik MC, Zaldivar-Lopez S, et al. Retrospective evaluation of the effectiveness of epsilon aminocaproic acid of the prevention of postamputation bleeding in retired racing Greyhounds with appendicular bone tumors: 46 case (2003–2008). J Vet Emerg Crit Care 2012;22(3):332–40.

73. Rojnuckarian P, Intragumtornchai T, Sattapiboon R, et al. The effects of green pit viper (Trimeresurus albolabris and Trimeresurus macrops) venom on the fibrinolytic systems in humans. Toxicon 1999;37(5):743–55.

Further reading

Brooks MB. Von Willebrand factor. In: Blackwell's Five Minute Veterinary Consult: Laboratory Tests and Diagnostic Procedures, Canine and Feline. Vaden SL, Knoll JS, Franks WK, Tilley LP, eds. Ames: Wiley-Blackwell, 2009: pp 716–17.

Mintzer DM, Billet SH, Chmielewski L. Drug-induced hematological syndromes. Adv Hematol. 2009; Article ID 495863. Drugs and mechanisms of action for impact on coagulation and other hematological syndromes: Table 1.

Smith SA. The cell-based model of coagulation. J Vet Emerg Crit Care 2009;19(1):3–10. A review of cell-based coagulation.

CHAPTER 10

Red blood cells and hemoglobin

Andrew Linklater[1] and Veronica Higgs[2]

[1] Lakeshore Veterinary Specialists, Milwaukee, Wisconsin
[2] Metropolitan Veterinary Specialists and Emergency Services, Louisville, Kentucky

Introduction

Alterations in the red blood cell (RBC or erythrocyte) and hemoglobin (Hgb) content of the blood are common in the critically ill small animal patient. Changes in these blood parameters can occur as part of the primary disease or, potentially, as a complication of diagnostic testing or treatment. The effects can cause life-threatening problems due to impaired perfusion and poor tissue oxygenation, warranting diligent monitoring with timely intervention for a successful patient outcome.

Erythrocytes or RBCs consist mainly of Hgb, a complex metalloprotein. The iron (Fe) atoms of the four heme groups (tetramers) of the Hgb molecule temporarily bind to oxygen molecules. Inhaled oxygen easily diffuses from the alveoli through the cell membrane of the erythrocyte as the cell traverses the pulmonary capillaries. The majority of oxygen found in arterial blood is bound to Hgb, with a much lesser amount dissolved in the plasma (Box 10.1). This makes the RBCs and Hgb molecules critical to the delivery of oxygen (DO_2) to the tissues. In addition to oxygen transport, the Hgb molecule will transport a portion of the carbon dioxide from the tissues to the lungs for exhalation.

The RBC is made in the bone marrow by a process called erythropoiesis, and is under the control of the hormone erythropoietin (EPO). Juxtaglomerular cells in the kidney produce EPO in response to decreased oxygen delivery (as in anemia and hypoxia) and increased levels of androgens. The mechanism of oxygen concentration detection is through hypoxia inducible factor 1 which is a transcription activator that is oxygen sensitive. The RBC development process is controlled and influenced by a number of different factors, including EPO, cytokines (interleukin (IL)-3 and IL-4), and granulocyte-macrophage colony stimulating factor. In addition to EPO, RBC production requires adequate supplies of substrates, mainly iron, vitamin B12, and folate.

During the initial phase of erythrocyte production, the multipotential myeloid stem cell differentiates into the erythroid stem cell. From here, the first erythrocyte precursor, the proerythroblast (also called rubriblast), is formed, which has a nucleus and is under the influence of EPO. This cell becomes the basophilic erythroblast, which gains its color from the ongoing production of basophilic staining Hgb in the cytoplasm. This cell transforms into the last RBC precursor capable of mitosis, the smaller polychromatic erythroblast (or prorubricyte). The next stage, called the normoblast (or rubricyte), finds the cell smaller with a small dense nucleus and not capable of mitosis. The reticulocyte (metarubricyte) follows, which has extruded the nucleus and has a slight basophilic staining and webbing of the cytoplasm. These cells can carry oxygen and can normally be found in small numbers in the bloodstream. The final product of erythropoiesis is the erythrocyte or RBC, which is released from the bone marrow into the circulating bloodstream.

The shape of the mature RBC is a biconcave disk, depressed and flattened in the center. This distinctive shape optimizes the flow properties of blood in the large vessels. The membrane of the RBC plays many roles that aid in regulating their surface deformability, flexibility, adhesion to other cells, and immune recognition. These functions are highly dependent on its three-layer composition: the carbohydrate-rich glycocalyx on the exterior; the lipid bilayer containing transmembrane proteins; and the membrane skeleton, a structural network of proteins located on the inner surface of the lipid bilayer.

The mature RBC diameter is approximately 7 microns in the dog, with a life span of 110–120 days. In the cat, the RBC diameter is 5.8 microns with a life span of 65–76 days. The normal RBC count in the dog is 4.8–9.3 million/microliter with a packed cell volume (PCV) of 35–55%. In the cat, the normal RBC count is 5.91–9.93 million/microliter with a PCV of 29–45%. Healthy dogs will have <1.5% reticulocytes and healthy cats <1% reticulocytes. Old RBCs are removed from circulation by the spleen and liver.

The spleen acts as a filter for the blood, recognizing and removing old, malformed, or damaged RBCs. The RBCs must pass through a maze of narrow passages, with healthy blood cells simply passing through and continuing back into the circulation. Most old or damaged RBCs are removed from the bloodstream by phagocytosis. The iron is stored as either ferritin or bilirubin, and eventually returns to the bone marrow where Hgb is made.

The spleen will also act as a storage unit for blood. The canine and feline spleen both have a large storage capacity, estimated as 10–20% of the circulating RBC mass. Within the spleen there are three pools described in which the RBCs circulate. The majority (~90%) of the circulating blood enters the rapid pool and traverses through the organ in about 30 seconds. Approximately 9% of the red blood cells enters the intermediate pool and circulates through within eight minutes. The remaining 1% traverses through the slow pool, which can take nearly an hour to complete its circulation through the spleen.

Under conditions of stress, hypoxemia, heavy exercise, and excessive blood loss, up to 98% of the splenic blood volume is shifted to the rapid pool through splenic contraction to significantly increase the circulating blood volume. The interaction of splenic innervation and adrenal medullary hormones appears to be responsible for splenic contraction in the cat and dog [1,2].

Monitoring and Intervention for the Critically Ill Small Animal: The Rule of 20, First Edition. Edited by Rebecca Kirby and Andrew Linklater.
© 2017 John Wiley & Sons, Inc. Published 2017 by John Wiley & Sons, Inc.

Box 10.1 Formula for arterial content of oxygen. Normal value is 19-21 ml/dl.

$CaO_2 = (1.34 \times Hgb \times SaO_2) + (0.003 \times PaO_2)$

CaO_2 = arterial content of oxygen
Hgb = concentration of hemoglobin in the blood (g/dL)
SaO_2 = percent saturation of Hgb with oxygen
1.34 = mL of oxygen bound per mg of Hgb when saturated
PaO_2 = arterial partial pressure of oxygen

Disorders of Hgb or RBC content in the circulating blood can be categorized as *anemia*, when there is a low RBC count and Hgb content, *erythrocytosis*, when there is an elevated RBC count and Hgb content, or *dyshemoglobinemia*, when there are abnormalities in the hemoglobin molecule. Many of the abnormalities associated with RBCs and Hgb content can be identified through the history, physical examination, and other diagnostic testing tools. Monitoring the critical small animal ICU patient for signs associated with altered RBC and Hgb content is essential.

Diagnostic and monitoring methods

The majority of diagnostic data used for detecting the presence of anemia or erythroctosis can be obtained through the history, physical examination, and cage-side point of care (POC) testing. The rapid return of POC diagnostic information can be used to select and guide any emergent therapy that may be required. Additional clinicopathological laboratory testing and imaging may be necessary to make a definitive diagnosis of the underlying disease process.

History

The history begins with the signalment (breed, age, sex). Any possible breed-related problems are considered, such as sighthounds with higher PCVs,; pyruvate kinase deficiency in Basenjis, Beagles, and Cairn Terriers; stomatocytosis in Alaskan Malamutes; hemolytic anemia in American Cocker Spaniels; and phosphofructose kinase deficiency in English Springer Spaniels. Past medical history should highlight vaccination status, indoor or outdoor activity (exposure to infectious disease), retroviral status in cats, and possible exposure to toxins. A list of common drugs and toxins that can cause anemia in the dog and cat is provided in Table 10.1. Chronic administration of diuretics could cause dehydration and erythrocytosis. Drugs such as nonsteroidal antiinflammatory drugs (NSAIDs) or glucocorticosteroids could cause gastrointestinal (GI) ulceration and anemia from blood loss. The excessive supplementation of zinc or the administration of acetaminophen could be a cause for anemia. Recent halothane anesthesia can cause sequestration of RBCs in the spleen and other body areas in the dog [3].

The travel history can warrant suspicion of exposure to infectious agents (such as babesiosis) that can cause anemia. A recent history of intestinal parasites might indicate a hookworm or whipworm infestation as a cause of blood loss anemia. The altitude where the patient lives is important since the lower oxygen of higher altitudes results in a higher PCV in normal dogs and cats. Semimoist cat food contains propylene glycol that can cause oxidant injury and Heinz bodies in the RBC of the cat. Although these cats are not usually anemic, RBC life span is reduced.

The consequences of anemia or erythrocytosis are often quite apparent to owners, with lethargy, inappetance, increased

Table 10.1 Common drugs and toxins associated with anemia in the dog and cat. The category of the mechanism of anemia is in bold. NSAIDs = nonsteroidal anti-inflammatory drugs, DIC = disseminated intravascular coagulation, EPO = erythropoietin.

Drugs	Toxins
Oxidative	**Oxidative**
Acetaminophen (paracetamol)	Crude oil
Benzocaine	Naphthalene
Propofol	Copper
	Zinc
Blood loss	Propylene glycol
Dapsone	
NSAIDS	**Blood loss**
Anticoagulants	Dicoumarol
Aspirin, clopidogrel or other antiplatelet	Anticoagulant rodenticides
drugs or antithrombotic drugs	Snakebite (DIC)
Glucocorticosteroids	
	Hemolysis
Immune-mediated hemolysis	Onions
Cephalosporins	Garlic
Penicillins	
Sulfonamides	**Decreased marrow production**
	Lead
Hemolysis	Propylene glycol
Fenbendazole	
Heparin	
Decreased marrow production	
Amphotericin	
Chloramphenicol	
Cephalosporins	
Fenbendazole	
Griseofulvin	
Phenobarbital	
Phenothiazine	
Recombinant human EPO	
Sulfonamides	

DIC, disseminated intravascular coagulation; EPO, erythropoietin; NSAID, nonsteroidal antiinflammatory drug.

respiratory rate, weakness, collapse, yellow discoloration to skin or blood in the urine or feces as features in the presenting complaint. Behavioral changes, neurological abnormalities noted at home or changes in energy level can be a complaint associated with either anemia or erythrocytosis.

The observation of frank red blood in the vomitus or stool, black, tarry stool or "coffee ground" flecks in the vomitus suggests GI bleeding as a source of RBC and Hgb loss. Abnormal urine color could be indicative of hemoglobinuria or bilirubinuria secondary to RBC lysis.

Physical examination

Physical examination begins with the temperature, pulse rate and intensity, respiratory rate and effort, mucous membrane color, and capillary refill time (CRT). Table 10.2 lists common abnormal physical examination findings associated with anemia and erythrocytosis.

Basic physical examination parameters can vary dramatically depending on the rate of RBC or Hgb changes. Physical signs of anemia and dyshemoglobinemia are associated with poor oxygen delivery to the tissues and can include tachycardia, increased respiratory rate, altered mentation, severe lethargy, weakness, weak pulses, pale or white mucous membranes, and prolonged or absent CRT. Patients with dyshemoglobinemias may have muddy or brown

Table 10.2 Common physical examination findings occurring with abnormal erythrocyte and hemoglobin concentrations.

Anemia	Erythrocytosis
Weakness	**Absolute erythrocytosis**
Pale mucous membranes (pallor)	Red, injected or gray mucous membranes
Rapid or slow capillary refill time	Rapid (<1 sec) capillary refill time
Tachycardia	Tachycardia
Altered pulses: bounding or weak	Bounding pulses
Decreased mentation	Heart murmur
Lethargy	Tachypnea
Tachypnea	Injected/tortuous retinal vessels
Increased or decreased lung sounds	Epistaxis
Heart murmur	Hyphema
Yellow mucous membranes (jaundice)	Gastrointestinal bleeding
Pale or yellow skin color	Absent pulses, cold limbs (thrombosis)
Pigmenturia	Focal neurological deficits
Melena or frank blood on rectal exam	Central neurological changes: seizures, tremors, ataxia, blindness, behavior changes
Epistaxis	
Decreased size of ocular blood vessels	**Relative erythrocytosis**
Pendulous abdomen or fluid wave	Clinical signs of dehydration
	Clinical signs of hypovolemia
	Hyperthermia (heatstroke)
	Burns
	Differential cyanosis (congenital)
	Third body fluid spacing

Box 10.2 Three-syringe technique for collecting blood from a central venous catheter.

1. Swab the catheter hub with alcohol.
2. Remove 2–4 mL of blood (volume based on length of catheter) into syringe #1.
3. Collect only the amount of blood needed to perform the blood test into syringe #2.
4. Replace the blood collected in syringe #1 back into the catheter.
5. Flush the line with heparinized saline with syringe #3.

skin or mucous membranes when there is methemoglobinemia or brick red mucous membranes with carboxyhemoglobinemia. The blue tongue and membrane coloration of cyanosis is evident when there is 5 g/dL of deoxygenated Hgb. The brown coloration of methemoglobin requires only 1.5 g/dL of deoxygenated Hgb.

Cardiac murmurs may be noted on auscultation of an animal with anemia or erythrocytosis due to the changes in blood rheology and turbulence of the cardiac blood flow. Icterus noted in the skin and mucous membranes, along with pigmenturia, may be seen in patients with RBC hemolysis. The oral cavity, mucous membranes, integument, and rectal examination can provide physical evidence of bleeding. While blood loss through petechiae, ecchymoses or bruising is impossible to quantify, substantial quantities of RBCs can be lost within these affected tissues. Areas of bruising or ecchymoses in the skin should be outlined with a waterproof nontoxic marker to monitor for changes in size over time. Any skin or subcutaneous abnormal swellings or masses could be related to hemorrhage and should be outlined with a marker and monitored for progression. A thorough exam for external parasites can reveal a heavy infestation of fleas or ticks that can cause a severe anemia.

The abdomen is palpated and balotted for fluid waves. A positive ballotment of the abdomen suggests that there is a large volume of fluid within the cavity. The abdomen and limbs can be measured and the circumference tracked for evidence of expansion that could be due to internal bleeding.

Point of care testing

The site of collection of blood samples must be considered and commonly includes small veins or capillary beds (such as clipped nails or ear veins) for microhematocrit tubes and peripheral (such as cephalic or saphenous veins) or central veins (such as the jugular vein or through a central catheter) for larger volumes of blood. Using a central catheter for blood collection can avoid repeated entry into a vein by a needle. The three-syringe technique (Box 10.2) is used for blood collection from a catheter to minimize blood loss and to avoid iatrogenic dilution of blood samples due to the catheter flushing solution.

The POC testing should include the packed cell volume (PCV), total protein (TP), blood glucose, blood urea nitrogen (BUN), electrolytes, acid–base status, coagulation profile, blood smear, blood lactate, fecal exam for parasites, and urinalysis. Normal values for PCV/TP, Hgb, and other complete blood count (CBC) values are noted in Table 10.3 [4].

When indicated, saline agglutination testing is done to identify autoagglutination as a cause of RBC intravascular hemolysis. Cross-match testing kits (Rapidvet®-H, DMS Laboratories Inc., Flemington, NJ) are available for POC testing prior to the administration of a blood transfusion. Canine and feline blood typing (Rapidvet®-H, Dms Laboratories Inc., Flemington, NJ) agglutination test cards are also available as POC testing.

The PCV and spun hematocrit (Hct) are interchangeable names for the simple and inexpensive method of assessing the percentage of centrifuged anticoagulated whole blood in a microhematocrit tube, that is, RBCs. The PCV result can normally vary by up to 5% between measurements. The true hematocrit is technically a value calculated by automated hematology analyzers, using the formula: MCV × RBC count/10, where MCV is the mean corpuscular volume. Spectrophotometry has also been used to determine the hematocrit value.

The PCV and Hct will each provide data for identifying anemia or erythrocytosis. Trends of change should be monitored by consistently using the same method (PCV or calculated Hct) throughout hospitalization.

The TP and state of hydration of the patient are important when evaluating the significance of changes in the PCV or Hct. Common alterations observed in the PCV and TP with anemia and erythrocytosis and possible etiologies are listed in Table 10.4. Transient erythrocytosis can occur when a dog is anxious or excitable due to splenic contraction. This transient increase in RBCs is particularly noticeable in large breed dogs and usually subsides within one hour [5]. Splenic contraction may occur in response to hemorrhage to maintain a normal PCV. However, there is no reserve for protein, causing a relative decrease in TP compared to the PCV. Both the PCV and TP will continue to drop after hemorrhage due to fluid resuscitation and redistribution of body fluids.

It is also important to observe the size of the buffy coat (white blood cells and platelets) and serum color (straw colored = normal, red = hemoglobin or less likely, myoglobin, white = lipemia, yellow = icterus) of the spun microhematocrit tube. Icteric or hemolyzed serum may indicate RBC destruction.

Table 10.3 Normal laboratory values for the dog and cat [4].*

Parameter (units)	Definition	Dog normal	Cat normal
PCV(%)	Packed cell volume; volume of blood cells in a sample after it has been centrifuged in a hematocrit tube	35–57%	30–45%
TP (mg/dL)	Total protein; plasma protein	6.0–7.5	6.0–7.5
Hgb (g/dL)	Hemoglobin	11.9–18.9	9.8–15.4
RBC (×10⁶/μL)	Red blood cell count	4.8–9.3	5.9–9.4
Hct (%)	Hematocrit; % of RBCs in blood; calculated from MCV × RBC count/10	35–57%	30–45%
MCV (fL)	Mean corpuscular volume; measure of the average volume of a RBC	66–77	39–55
MCHC (g/dL)	Mean corpuscular hemoglobin concentration; measure of the concentration of hemoglobin in a given volume of packed RBCs	32.0–36.3	30–36
MCH (pg)	Mean corpuscular hemoglobin; measure of the average mass of hemoglobin in a RBC	21.0–26.2	13–17

* Values will vary between laboratory analyzers.

Table 10.4 Possible mechanisms of anemia and polycythemia related to changed in the PCV and TP.

Changes in PCV and TP	Possible etiology
↑ PCV ↑ TP	Dehydration Polycythemia w/dehydration Polycythemia w/hyperproteinemia
↑ PCV **N** TP	Polycythemia Splenic contraction (stress)
↑ PCV ↓ TP	Blood loss (early) w/splenic contraction Dehydration w/hypoproteinemia
N PCV ↓ TP	Acute hemorrhage w/splenic contraction Hypoproteinemia
↓ PCV ↑ TP	Anemia w/dehydration Anemia w/hyperproteinemia
↓ PCV **N** TP	Chronic anemia
↓ PCV ↓ TP	Acute blood loss Anemia w/hypoproteinemia Intravascular fluid overload

N, normal; PCV, packed cell volume; TP, total protein; w/= with.

An elevation in BUN can be a reflection of renal disease, which can impact EPO production and the occurrence of anemia. BUN may also be elevated with dehydration (prerenal azotemia), so PCV or Hct may be falsely elevated. In addition, the presence of free Hgb can cause renal failure. However, blood within the GI tract can also cause an increase in BUN. A low BUN warrants further investigation for liver dysfunction, which is a potential cause of anemia.

Hyperglycemia can cause severe dehydration that can increase the PCV and TP results. Hyperkalemia can be seen with the destruction of RBCs in the Akita. Hypophosphatemia can cause lysis of the RBC cell membrane. The presence of thrombocytopenia or a coagulopathy can cause blood loss anemia. Erythrocytosis can be associated with a hypercoagulable state (see Chapter 9).

The carbonic anhydrase within the RBC plays a vital role in the rapid response to respiratory acidosis. The acid–base balance appears to be corrected by reduction of the RBC carbonic anhydrase activity in the case of alkalosis, and by an increase in RBC carbonic anhydrase activity in the case of acidosis [6].

Elevations in blood lactate provide an assessment of anaerobic metabolism in the tissues. Elevated lactate levels at presentation (4.8 mmol/L vs 2.9 mmol/L) have been associated with nonsurvival in dogs with immune-mediated hemolytic anemia [7]. However,

a change in lactate over time is of more predictive value than a single admission lactate.

Evaluation of the urine specific gravity provides insight into the concentrating abilities of the kidney, with isosthenuria suggestive of renal disease. Hematuria can be microscopic or gross and a source of chronic blood loss. However, hematuria rarely causes blood loss significant enough to be the primary cause of anemia. Hemoglobinuria (free Hgb) causes red coloration of the urine identical to hematuria. However, when the urine is centrifuged, the supernatant will be clear with hematuria and remain red with hemoglobinuria. Bilirubinuria provides a greenish brown coloration to the urine and can be a consequence of extravascular hemolysis or other causes of icterus. The microscopic examination of a fecal preparation is performed to detect hookworms or whipworms that can be an important source of blood loss.

Blood smear

A blood smear allows an initial assessment of the RBC morphology. A search is made for the bone marrow response and any underlying cause of anemia. A list of the common microscopic changes in the erythrocyte and brief interpretation of the finding is provided in Table 10.5. Blood collected for detecting *Mycoplasma* in the cat is best sampled from a peripheral vein and smeared immediately on a glass slide to maximize the potential identification of these organisms. When searching for *Babesia*, blood is collected from a peripheral capillary, such as the ear pinna, and smeared and stained immediately. A search of the RBC membrane surfaces and interior is made for the presence of bacteria or parasites that might be the cause of the RBC disorder.

The color of erythrocytes is due to the heme group of hemoglobin. When combined with oxygen, the resulting oxyhemoglobin is scarlet, and when oxygen has been released the resulting deoxyhemoglobin is of a dark red burgundy color.

Low numbers (<10%) of single, small Heinz bodies may be seen on erythrocytes in healthy cats. These "endogenous" Heinz bodies may be seen in increased numbers (up to 50%) in cats on semi-moist food that contains propylene glycol that causes oxidant injury. Healthy cats also can have a few Howell–Jolly bodies in erythrocytes in peripheral blood. In large blood vessels, RBCs sometimes occur as a stack, flat side next to flat side. This is known as rouleaux formation, and it occurs more often if the levels of certain serum proteins are elevated, such as during inflammation.

Table 10.5 Microscopic erythrocyte changes and associated etiologies for anemia.

Finding	Description	Significance/etiologies
Spherocytosis	Lack of central pallor (dogs)	Primary or secondary immune-mediated hemolytic anemia, recent blood transfusion, blood parasites, zinc toxicity, snake envenomation
Microcytosis	Small red blood cells	Iron deficiency (or chronic blood loss), portovascular anomalies, congenital or acquired, hyponatremia, normal in some breeds
Macrocytosis	Large red blood cells, may have concurrent polychromasia	Regenerative anemia, FeLV, myelodysplasia, hypernatremia
Hypochromasia	Pale color to cells	Chronic anemia
Polychromasia	Variation in cell color staining (pale, to normal to purple)	Regenerative anemia
Anisocytosis	Variation in cells size	Regenerative anemia
Keratocytes and shistocytes	Keratocytes are helmet shaped, shistocytes are fragments of RBCs (i.e. half moon)	DIC, congestive heart failure, glomerulonephritis, myelofibrosis, hemangiosarcoma, doxorubicin toxicosis, burns
Acanthocytes	Irregularly spiculated cells	DIC, portovascular anomaly, chronic liver disease, lymphosarcoma, glomerulonephritis
Echinocytes	Even spacing between blunt to sharp projections from RBC membranes	Artifact, lymphosarcoma, glomerulonephritis
Heinz bodies	Single, light-colored rounded protrusions of the RBC membrane	Onion, vitamin K, acetaminophen, methylene blue, propylene glycol, lymphosarcoma
Basophilic stippling	Small, dark blue inclusions	Lead poisoning
Nucleated RBCs	Dark purple nucleus in a normal-sized RBC	Regenerative anemia, splenic disease, corticosteroids
Parasites that may be visualized	*Babesia*: large tear drop or ring shaped, often in pairs *Cytauxzoon*: small, irregular intracellular rings *Hemobartonella canis*: chain of small cocci or rods across the surface of RBCs. *Mycoplasma felis*: nonrefractile cocci, rods or ring structures on periphery of RBCs	*Babesia, Cytauxzoon, Mycoplasma, Hemobartonella* infection

DIC, disseminated intravascular coagulation; FeLV, feline leukemia virus; RBC, red blood cell.

Saline agglutination

A saline agglutination test is an easy and inexpensive way to screen for autoagglutination and should be a part of the POC evaluation of anemia. The steps for performing a saline agglutination test are outlined in Box 10.3. Agglutination of the RBCs must be differentiated from rouleaux formation. This evaluation can also be used to assess response to therapy when the saline agglutination is positive.

Clinicopathological laboratory testing

A CBC, with review by pathologist, and serum biochemical profile are submitted to characterize changes in the RBCs, identify an underlying cause, and assess for consequences of disorders of RBCs and Hgb. Additional testing can include bone marrow aspirate and core biopsy, serum titers for infectious diseases, and Coombs testing for immune-mediated anemia.

The white blood cell (WBC), RBC, and platelet counts are assessed to determine whether the disorder affects other cell lines. The total WBC count must be corrected for the presence of circulating nucleated RBCs (rubricytes) when they are present.

Hemoglobin is measured by a spectrophotometer in a suspension of lyzed RBCs. Substances, such as lipemia, that increase the optical density of the solution can cause spuriously high readings. The numerical value for Hgb should be approximately one-third of the PCV value [8].

The MCV and mean corpuscular Hgb concentration (MCHC) are measured with the CBC and normal values are provided in Table 10.3. The MCV is a measure of the average volume of a RBC. In patients with anemia, it is the MCV measurement that allows

classification as a microcytic anemia (low MCV; chronic disease, blood loss, iron deficiency), normocytic anemia (MCV within normal range) or macrocytic anemia (high MCV; B12 and folic acid deficiencies). Normocytic anemia is typically seen in acute conditions (blood loss, hemolysis) when the bone marrow has not yet responded with a change in cell volume. The MCHC is a measure of the concentration of Hgb in a given volume of packed RBCs. MCHC is diminished or hypochromic in microcytic anemias, and normochromic in macrocytic anemias.

When anemia is present, the RBC morphology is examined for evidence of a bone marrow response (regeneration). It may take 3–5 days for a normal regenerative response from the bone marrow to be recognized. The presence of polychromasia, reticulocytosis, anisocytosis, macrocytosis, and hypochromasia can support regeneration. The reticulocyte count can be used to determine the degree of regeneration (Box 10.4). Special staining with new methylene blue is required to identify the reticulocytes (Figure 10.1). The absolute reticulocyte count is a percentage of RBCs that are reticulocytes. However, as Hgb drops and anemia is persistent, several things happen: (1) reticulocytes are mixed with a lower percentage of circulating mature erythrocytes, (2) immature reticulocytes are released earlier (called shift reticulocytes), and (3) reticulocytes persist longer in circulation; these result in a falsely high impression of reticulocytes with an absolute count. Corrected reticulocyte percentage and absolute reticulocyte counts correct for (1); reticulocyte production index (in dogs) corrects for (1), (2), and (3) [9]. The significant reticulocyte values and formulas for these corrections are provided in Box 10.4. While nucleated red blood cells may

Box 10.3 Saline agglutination test.

1. Draw blood into an EDTA tube.
2. Place one drop of blood and three drops of saline on a glass slide.
3. Rock the slide back and forth for 1–2 minutes.
4. Look for gross macroagglutination (clumping of the red blood cells).
5. Examine the slide under a low-power microscope for evidence of microagglutination.

Agglutination appears as red blood cells clumped together in a random fashion (often described as "clusters of grapes") compared to rouleaux formation which is grouped in an organized fashion (often described as "stacks of coins," which may branch).

A positive agglutination test is indicative of antibodies against RBC membranes and can be used as part of the diagnosis for immune-mediated hemolytic anemia.

The following pictures demonstrate (a) gross agglutination on a slide, (b) microscopic agglutination under 40 × power, no stain, and (c) rouleaux formation under 100 × power, modified Wright-Giemsa or "Diff-quick" stain. Source: (b) and (c) courtesy of Mandy Nonnenmacher.

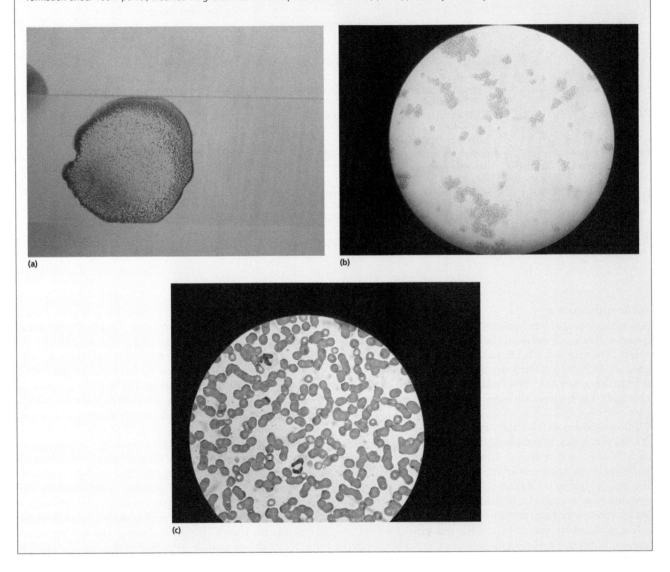

(a)

(b)

(c)

be noted with regeneration, their presence is not a reliable indicator of a regenerative response. The cat has two kinds of reticulocytes: *aggregate* reticulocytes and *punctate* reticulocytes. Punctate reticulocytes can remain in circulation for up to three weeks. It is the aggregate reticulocytes that must be counted when evaluating anemia for a current regenerative response. Aggregate reticulocytes can be identified by their linear aggregates of ribosomes, rather than individual (punctate) structures as seen in punctate reticulocytes (see Figure 10.1).

The serum biochemical profile is evaluated for evidence of hepatic or renal disorders, hypoalbuminemia (or hypoproteinemia), hypophosphatemia (as a cause of hemolysis), and hyperbilirubinemia. The finding of renal disease can implicate impaired production of EPO as a source of RBC problems, or implicated free Hgb, when present, as a cause. Chronic disease of any etiology can have anemia as a consequence. Hypothyroid patients can also develop an anemia. PCR or serum testing for RBC parasites may also be useful in select patients or geographic regions.

Box 10.4 Reticulocyte indices [9,10].

1. Observed reticulocyte percentage (%)
   Count performed with new methylene blue stain and expressed as a percentage of total erythrocytes
   Normal (dogs): <1%
   Normal aggregate type (cats): <0.4%
   Normal punctate type (cats): <10%
2. Corrected reticulocyte count = observed reticulocyte % × (patient hematocrit/normal hematocrit)
   (Normal hemotocrit = 45 in the dog and 37 in the cat)
3. Absolute reticulocyte count
   Reticulocyte % × RBC count

Degree of response	Reticulocyte count/µL (dog)	Reticulocyte count/µL (cat)
Nonregenerative	<60 000–80 000	<15 000–42 000
Slight	80 000–150 000	42 000–70 000
Moderate	150 000–300 000	70 000–100 000
Marked	>500 000	>200 000

4. Reticulocyte production index (RPI) (dogs only)
   RPI = observed reticulocyte % × [observed Hct %/normal Hct % (45 in dogs)] × [1/blood maturation time]
   Maturation times:
   Hgb of 15 (Hct = 45%): maturation time = 1.0 day
   Hgb of 12 (Hct = 35%): maturation time = 1.5 days
   Hgb of 8 (Hct = 25%): maturation time = 2.0 days
   Hgb of 5 (Hct = 15%): maturation time = 2.5 days
   RPI is the increase in erythrocyte production; an RPI of >2 (or two times the normal erythrocyte production) is considered a regenerative response.

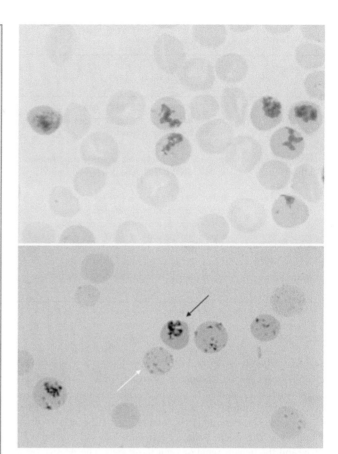

Figure 10.1 An image of canine (*top*) and feline (*bottom*) reticulocytes stained with new methylene blue. Feline aggregate (*black arrow*) and punctate (*white arrow*) reticulocytes are shown. Source: Courtesy of Dr Karen Young, University of Wisconsin-Madison.

Further coagulation testing may be indicated to identify an occult source of hemorrhage. A positive D-dimer or fibrin split product test and low or falling plasma fibrinogen concentration are highly suggestive of disseminated intravascular coagulation [11]. Individual factor testing for congenital or acquired hemophilia and von Willebrand's disease screening may be indicated as well (see Chapter 9).

Serum levels of erythropoietin may be indicated if an absolute erythrocytosis or an unexplained nonregenerative anemia is found. Toxicology screening can diagnose heavy metal, rodenticide, acetaminophen or other toxicities causing anemia. Co-oximetry may be necessary to further evaluate dyshemoglobinemias.

Iron is a necessary metal required not only for the synthesis of hemoglobin but also for many cellular enzymes and co-enzymes. Iron is transported in serum bound to the protein transferrin. Normally, only about one-third of the available binding sites on transferrin are occupied by iron. The total iron binding capacity is found in serum; therefore, it includes the amount of iron already bound to the transferrin (serum iron) plus the amount of iron required to saturate the unoccupied binding sites of transferrin. However, because the liver produces transferrin, alterations in function (such as cirrhosis, hepatitis, or liver failure) must be considered when performing this test.

The determination of serum iron total iron binding capacity (TIBC) and percent transferrin saturation is useful in the differential diagnosis of anemias and other iron disorders. Iron deficiency anemia will have a low serum iron, a high TIBC, and a low percentage of transferrin saturation. Anemia of chronic disease will have a low serum iron, a low TIBC, and a normal percentage of transferrin saturation. In chronic disease, the body produces less transferrin.

The Coombs test and other anti-RBC antigen-antibody assays (such as flow cytometry) should be considered if there is a high degree of suspicion for an immune-mediated hemolytic anemia. Several diagnostic criteria can be used to make the diagnosis of an immune-mediated hemolytic anemia and are listed in Table 10.6.

Examination of the bone marrow is provided by aspiration and core biopsy to evaluate erythropoiesis. Obtaining bone marrow samples requires heavy sedation or anesthesia, with samples collected with an Illinois bone marrow needle or Jamshidi bone biopsy instrument. Common sites of collection include the humerus, tibia, femur, and wing of the ilium. Bone marrow aspirates and biopsy samples should be submitted along with a peripheral blood sample for CBC.

Diagnostic imaging

Survey radiographs of the chest and abdomen are often the first imaging technique performed. Metallic (gastric) foreign objects are easily identified, with zinc, copper or lead known to cause anemia. Abdominal fluid is anticipated with loss of serosal detail, abdominal distension, splenic or hepatic masses or loss of detail in the retroperitoneal space.

Abdominal ultrasound may help determine if there is free fluid in a body cavity (peritoneal, pleural, pericardial, or retroperitoneal)

Table 10.6 Diagnostic criteria for immune-mediated hemolytic anemia. Not every parameter will be present in every patient.

Diagnostic criteria	Methodology
Anemia	PCV/TP hematocrit or CBC with hemoglobin
Evidence of anti-RBC antibodies	Gross or microscopic agglutination (see Box 10.3),* Coombs test,* flow cytometry
Evidence of RBC destruction	Spherocytosis,* hemolyzed serum, icterus (elevated total bilirubin), bilirubinuria or hemoglobinuria
Lack of other (primary) disease	Routine screening tests including thoracic and abdominal radiographs and/or abdominal ultrasound, screening for tick-borne disease or other infectious, inflammatory or neoplastic disease
Response to therapy	Appropriate therapy and monitoring; may not be immediately evident
Evidence of regeneration	Polychromasia, anisocytosis, macrocytosis, hypochromasia, reticulocyte count, bone marrow analysis

* For definitive diagnosis, one or more of the following hallmarks needs to be present [11].

and may identify as a source of hemorrhage. Brief ultrasound examinations can be invaluable when searching for potentially life-threatening cavitary hemorrhage. The abdominal focused assessment technique for trauma (AFAST) examines for free fluid in four areas of the abdomen: the diaphragmatic-hepatic or subxiphoid view, the spleno-renal or left flank view, the cysto-colic view, and the hepato-renal or right flank view. The AFAST technique can be used for trauma, as a triage tool, and to track the progress of the patient over time [12]. The thoracic focused assessment with sonography technique (TFAST) can be used to determine if there is pleural effusion or evidence of pulmonary hemorrhage or pericardial hemorrhage (see Chapters 8, 15 and Further reading).

If blood is identified from either body cavity, a sterile centesis sample is obtained and the PCV or Hct and TP compared to the peripheral blood. Should significant volumes of blood be removed, the collected blood is saved in a sterile blood collection bag and available for autotransfusion if necessary.

Video endoscopy (such as rhinoscopy, GI endoscopy, cystoscopy) may identify mucosal bleeding from ulcerative disease. Advanced imaging techniques such as computed tomography or magnetic resonance imaging may be helpful in select cases. Echocardiographic examination of patients with cardiac murmurs may be essential to help rule out underlying cardiac disease (see Chapter 11).

Bedside monitoring techniques

Monitoring begins with the peripheral perfusion parameters (pulse rate and intensity, mucous membrane color, CRT) to assess the systemic effects of blood volume and the circulatory system. Blood pressure evaluation is important, with hypertension possible with renal disease and hypotension if severe anemia and hypovolemia (see Chapter 3). Body temperature and general physical and mental status are important to monitor during a blood transfusion, looking for signs of facial swelling, urticaria, vomiting, diarrhea, hyperpnea or shock. Observations should be made every five minutes for the first 20 minutes, every 15 minutes for the first hour and then hourly during initial assessment and resuscitation.

Monitoring the PCV and TP is important for determining the trend of change in the amount of RBCs available for tissue oxygenation. The frequency is dependent upon the severity and progression of the illness. Many critically ill patients require multiple blood samples and the volume withdrawn should be kept to a minimum to prevent iatrogenic blood loss anemia. A variety of techniques are available to minimize blood loss: use of microhematocrit tubes, blood smear evaluation, three-syringe collection techniques, and ear prick blood draws (Table 20.2). Patients receiving extracorporeal therapy such as dialysis are also at high risk of iatrogenic blood loss.

If hemorrhage is a concern, monitoring the size or diameter of the area at risk can often detect continued blood loss before changes in perfusion become obvious. An assessment of the volume of blood loss should be made and the progression or resolution monitored. Diarrhea and vomit that resembles frank hemorrhage can be collected onto disposable pads and weighed. Fluids that can be collected from nasogastric tube suctioning can also be quantified. Fluid recovered from centesis and from various catheters (such as thoracostomy tube, urinary catheter, wound drains, peritoneal catheter), should be quantified and the PCV recorded. If the PCV of the fluid matches or is within 5 points of peripheral blood, it can be assumed that hemorrhage has occurred and concern for active, ongoing hemorrhage is warranted.

When estimating surgical blood loss, blood-soaked sponges, suctioned blood, bloody diarrhea/vomit, blood remaining on surgical equipment and drapes, and an estimate of removed blood clot volumes should all be included. A completely soaked 4×4 gauze can hold an average of 10 mL of blood [13,14]. Canisters that collect blood from a suction apparatus should be marked with the blood volume.

Pulse oximetry measures the oxygen saturation of Hgb, not the quantity of Hgb. In patients with dyshemoglobinemia, pulse oximetry can give a falsely elevated reading, promoting a sense of false confidence. Co-oximetry, which can measure carboxyhemoglobin and methemoglobin concentrations, is more useful (see Chapter 8).

Disorders caused by red blood cells

Increasing demands for oxygen delivery (DO_2) occur when there is an increased rate of oxygen consumption (VO_2). In the small animal ICU patient, an increase in VO_2 can be a consequence of surgery, trauma, burns, inflammation, sepsis, pyrexia, shivering, seizures, agitation/anxiety/pain, adrenergic drugs, or even weaning from ventilation. The Hgb contained within the RBC is the main transporter of oxygen for distribution to the tissues. A deficit (anemia) or an excess (erythrocytosis) of RBCs will eventually affect blood flow and viscosity, resulting in insufficient DO_2 to meet the demands of the cell. When left untreated, the resultant tissue hypoxia causes organ dysfunction and cell death.

Identifying anemia or erythrocytosis is not the most difficult challenge; however, rapid recognition of potentially life-threatening consequences of anemia or erythrocytosis is the initial focus. Resuscitation may be required prior to a definitive diagnosis of the underlying RBC disorder.

Anemia

Anemia is defined as a reduction in the oxygen-carrying capacity of blood due to a decrease in Hgb concentration and RBC mass. Values used to diagnose anemia are PCV <37%, and Hgb <12 g/dL in the dog and PCV ≤27% and Hgb ≤9 g/dL in the cat. An algorithm

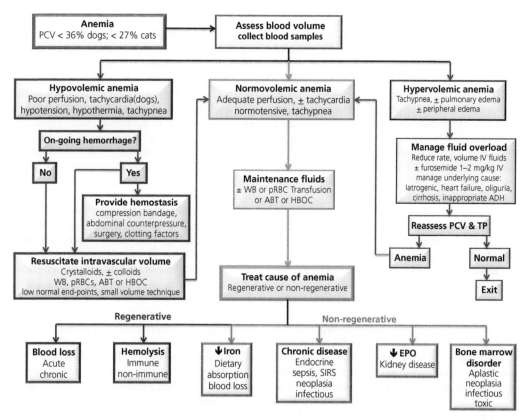

Figure 10.2 A decision-making algorithm for the diagnosis and treatment of the small animal ICU patient with anemia. ABT, autologous blood transfusion; HBOC, hemoglobin-based oxygen carrier; PCV, packed cell volume; pRBC, packed red blood cells; SIRS, systemic inflammatory response syndrome; TP, total protein; WB, whole blood.

to guide the initial decision-making processes when managing the small animal ICU patient with anemia is provided in Figure 10.2.

The presence of anemia will trigger important compensatory responses. To increase oxygen delivery to the tissues, the body will try to: (1) increase RBC or Hgb mass, (2) increase blood flow, and (3) increase oxygen unloading from Hgb in the capillaries [15]. These adaptations are possible due to mechanisms that increase cardiac output, redistribute blood flow, decrease the affinity of Hgb for oxygen, and increase oxygen extraction.

The shift to the right of the oxyhemoglobin dissociation curve in anemia is primarily the result of increased production of 2,3-diphosphoglycerate (2,3-DPG) in the RBCs. This enables more oxygen to be released to the tissues at a given partial pressure of oxygen, offsetting the effect of the reduced oxygen-carrying capacity of the blood. The dog has relatively high levels of red cell 2,3-DPG with relatively high oxygen affinity. Increased 2,3-DPG levels can be seen within four hours after significant hypoxia in the dog [16]. The cat, however, has low oxygen affinity hemoglobin that interacts weakly with 2,3-DPG, and low concentrations of red cell 2,3-DPG [17].

The most important determinant of the cardiovascular response to anemia is the blood volume status of the patient (left ventricular preload). Acute blood loss often results in anemia and hypovolemia and is termed hypovolemic anemia (see Figure 10.2). Clinical signs of hypovolemia may be noted when as little as 15% of blood volume is removed from healthy donor dogs [18]. With hypovolemic anemia, tissue hypoxia can occur from volume-induced decreased cardiac output (circulatory hypoxia) as well as decreased

oxygen-carrying capacity (anemic hypoxia). The sympathetic nervous system redistributes the available cardiac output to vital organs by increasing arterial tone. The body will also initially increase RBC and Hgb mass through splenic contraction. The renin-angiotensin-aldosterone system is stimulated to retain water and sodium in an effort to increase blood volume. The loss of >15% of blood volume can result in increased heart rate (dogs) and decreased arterial blood pressure. Blood is rapidly shunted from the splanchnic, skeletal, and cutaneous organs towards the brain and the heart (see Chapter 2).

An increase in cardiac output will also occur as a compensatory response to anemia when there is a normal blood volume, termed normovolemic anemia. An inverse relationship between the cardiac output and Hgb level exists as the Hgb declines below 12 g/dL [19]. Anemia causes a decrease in blood viscosity that reduces the resistance to blood flow. The net effect is an increase in blood flow to and from the heart (increased preload and decreased afterload). Increases in heart rate and myocardial contractility play only a minor role as long as normovolemia is maintained. Patients with normovolemic anemia may not have a change in blood pressure with the increase in cardiac output until anemia is severe. When severe, the heart rate will increase as well.

At the systemic level, normovolemic anemia triggers a redistribution of blood flow to areas of high demand and with higher oxygen extraction ratios (heart, brain). At the microcirculatory level, three mechanisms may increase the amount of oxygen supplied to the tissues at the capillary networks: recruitment of previously closed capillaries, increased capillary flow, and increased oxygen extraction from existing capillaries [20]. There is decreased vascular resistance, which will increase blood flow, attributed to reduced inactivation of nitric oxide and an increased production of nitric oxide synthase [21].

As hemodilution increases, blood viscosity decreases, resulting in an increased rate of flow and a decrease in time spent in capillaries [22]. Blood viscosity is highest in postcapillary venules where flow is slowest. At this site, a disproportionate decrease in blood viscosity occurs as anemia worsens and, as a consequence, venous return is augmented for a given venous pressure [23,24]. When these mechanisms have increased to their maximum levels, further tissue hypoxia can result in signs of altered mentation, arrhythmias, and poor cardiac performance.

The aggressive addition of fluids that do not contain RBCs or the inability to excrete water can cause a significant drop in the RBC count, PCV and Hgb concentration and intravascular volume overload. This is termed hypervolemic anemia. While there is a decrease in blood viscosity, there is also an additional demand on the cardiovascular system to handle the additional preload and vascular volume. An increase in glomerular filtration rate will enhance the excretion of excess water and electrolytes. Iatrogenic causes associated with fluid administration are first suspected in hypervolemic anemia in the ICU patient. However, underlying diseases such as liver cirrhosis, heart failure, acute oliguric renal failure, and increased antidiuretic hormone (such as head injury) can also cause hypervolemia and hemodilution. This form of anemia should be transient, with the restoration to a normal fluid balance the main mechanism of compensation. A recheck of the PCV and Hgb concentration is required when the fluid balance is corrected to evaluate for the persistence of anemia.

Treatment of hypovolemic anemia

Patients with hypovolemic anemia will require resuscitation of their cardiovascular system prior to or simultaneously with definitive treatment for the underlying cause of anemia. Emergent treatment is primarily directed at ensuring hemostasis, restoring RBC and Hgb concentrations, and safely reestablishing an adequate circulating blood volume. Providing supplemental oxygen during resuscitation can increase oxygen transport by ensuring that the blood Hgb is fully saturated and by raising the quantity of oxygen carried in solution in the plasma [25]. However, dissolved oxygen provides very little of resting tissue oxygen requirements and replacement of RBCs and Hgb is necessary.

The baseline physical perfusion parameters (heart rate, pulse intensity, mucous membrane color, CRT) and blood pressure are assessed and 1–2 intravenous catheters placed for fluid resuscitation. Anemic animals in the decompensatory stage of shock or with ongoing, poorly controlled hemorrhage will require transfusion with whole blood (WB) or packed red blood cells (pRBCs) as part of the initial fluid resuscitation plan (see Blood transfusion below). A combination of isotonic balanced crystalloids and whole blood or crystalloids, synthetic colloid (such as hydroxyethyl starch) and pRBCs are infused to low-normal resuscitation endpoints using small-volume titration techniques (see Chapter 2).

Fortunately, dogs do not have clinically significant preformed naturally occurring antibodies against the RBC antigens most often implicated in immediate hemolytic transfusion reactions (dog erythrocyte antigen (DEA) 1.1), making the first RBC transfusion a low risk for incompatibility but a high risk for sensitization. In cats, most fatal transfusion reactions are caused by incompatibilities in type B cats receiving type A RBCs. However, there may be more

blood types in cats (such as Mik) that are not fully characterized. When blood is urgently needed, the risk of uncross-matched RBCs must be weighed against the risk of delaying the transfusion. In the urgent setting, for dogs, DEA 1.1-negative blood should be given if available. In both species, subsequent transfusions should be cross-matched. A blood type is always recommended in cats [26].

If blood products are not available, and the patient has hemothorax or hemoabdomen, the blood retrieved from these cavities can be administered as an autologous blood transfusion (ABT). If hemoglobin-based oxygen carrier (HBOC) solutions are available, the HBOC can be infused instead of the WB, pRBCs or ABT. The physical perfusion parameters and blood pressure are closely monitored throughout the resuscitation period.

The patient history and physical examination are quickly assessed for indications of the possible source, severity, and longevity of hemorrhage. Providing hemostasis (when possible) becomes an immediate priority. A compression bandage may dampen the superficial flow of blood until definitive treatment can be provided. Ultimately, utilizing pressure to arrest hemorrhage depends on normal hemostatic mechanisms. Clamping with the tip of a hemostat for 3–5 minutes may be sufficient for small vessels. Large vessels will require ligation or electrocautery after local or general anesthesia.

There are a variety of external and internal hemostatic agents available to assist in arresting hemorrhage. These hemostatic agents work through a variety of mechanisms: causing obstruction to blood flow, providing a framework for clotting to occur, absorbing water to increase effectiveness of natural clotting or stimulating the coagulation cascade; some of these are summarized in Table 10.7. Most of these products are intended for human use, and many are absorbable and do not need to be removed, but should be used with care in surgical wounds as they may inhibit healing [27].

Ongoing abdominal hemorrhage can be slowed or stopped by temporarily applying abdominal counterpressure, allowing a more detailed assessment and possible intervention once stabilized. It is important that the rear limbs are included in this bandage (Figure 10.3). The procedure for placing abdominal and hindlimb counterpressure is outlined in Box 10.5.

Significant blood loss can occur from coagulopathies such as anticoagulant rodenticide toxicosis, liver failure, disseminated intravascular coagulation, trauma-induced coagulopathies and congenital or acquired factor deficiencies. Stabilization may require treatment with vitamin K1, plasma products, antivenom, desmopressin or other medications, depending on the cause, to promote coagulation (see Chapter 9).

In cases of active internal hemorrhage, surgical intervention may be required to ligate vessels or tamponade diffusely bleeding organs in order to stabilize the animal. Box 10.6 outlines the steps required for an emergency laparotomy for hemorrhage control. Blood removed from any body cavity should be collected aseptically, quantified, and stored in blood collection bags for possible ABT.

Blood transfusion

A variety of Hgb-containing blood products may be administered, depending on the underlying cause of anemia. A list of blood products, indications for use, and initial dose is provided in Table 10.8. There is no specific PCV or Hgb value at which a patient requires a transfusion. Recent human studies have determined that the administration of transfusions can be an independent predictor of mortality. Patients who received the more conservative strategy (Hgb ~7 g/dL) of transfusions had improved outcomes [31–33]. Animals with chronic anemia have time for compensatory changes

Table 10.7 Examples of hemostatic agents by category [28,29].

Category/ mechanism	Examples	Manufacturer	Notes
Caustic agents.			
Coagulating proteins, tissue necrosis, eschar formation			
	Aluminum Cl, ferric sulfate, silver nitrate, Zn Cl	Many manufacturers including Vet One (GF Health Products, Atlanta, GA), Kwik-Stop (ARC Laboratories, Atlanta, GA)	Silver nitrate will cause pigmentation, Zn Cl is rarely used; often applied with an applicator stick or powder; external use only
Noncaustic Agents.			
Primarily create a physical mesh facilitating platelet aggregation and amplification and propagation of coagulation			
	Gelatins; provide a matrix for clot formation, activated thrombin	Gelfoam (Pfizer, Memphis, TN), Vetspon (Ethicon, Somerville, NJ)	Requires blood in field, not a sealing agent
	Microporous polysaccharide hemispheres (MPH) from potato starch; hydrophilic and concentrate blood	Hemablock (Abbott, Abbott Park, IL)	Increase in volume of the spheres
	Oxidized regenerated (methyl) cellulose (plant cellulose) – physical barrier for clotting, provides a matrix for clotting	Surgicell (Ethicon)	Acidic and therefore bactericidal
	Microfiber collagen (bovine collagen) – aggregation and degranulation of platelets	Instat (Ethicon), Helistat (Integra, Plainsboro, NJ)	Wound should be dried and product applied with pressure using gauze
	Physiological hemostatics (fibrin, thrombin, platelet gels, antifibrinolytics)	Aminocaproic acid (Hospira, Lake Forest, IL), others	Topical use may not be effective; little reported data
	Fibrin glue – activates conversion of fibrinogen to fibrin	Tisseel/Tissucol (Baxter, Deerfield, IL), Hemaseel (Haemacure, Sarasota, FL), Evisel (Ethicon)	Dry field preferred, spray delivery
	Glutaraldehyde adhesives – cross-linking cell to cell proteins	Bioglue (Cryolife, Kennesaw, GA)	Dry field preferred
	Waxes; malleable and form physical block as well as clotting surface	Bone wax (Aesculap, Center Valley, PA)	Difficult to apply to flat surface, may delay healing
Hemostatic dressings.			
Used as wound dressings to prevent bleeding			
	Alginate dressing – seaweed protein, absorbs fluids through ion exchange reaction, releases calcium	Sorbosan (UDL Laboratories, Rockford, IL)	Not effective in high-pressure bleeding nor for intracavitary use
	Mineral zeolite – kaolin-impregnated polyester gauze, kaolin immediately activates XII, XI; absorbs water	Quickclot (Z-Medica, Wallingford, CT)	Foreign body reaction; early products were exothermic
	Chitin (chitosan) dressing, from crab exoskeletons, adheres to and seal wounds	Celox gauze and powder (Medtrade, Crewe, UK)	May also be antimicrobial

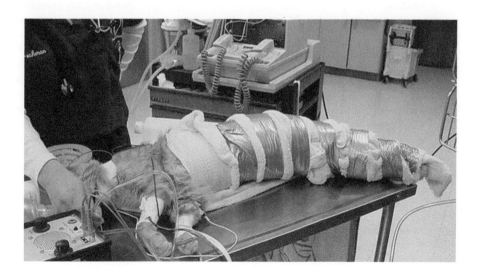

Figure 10.3 Abdominal and hindlimb counterpressure.

Box 10.5 Application of external abdominal and hindlimb counterpressure [30].*

1. Provide sedation, analgesia and support of cardiovascular status.
2. Place urinary catheter if time allows.
3. Place patient in lateral recumbency.
4. Place rolled hand towel between the hindlegs for padding.
5. Place a rolled towel along ventral midline from xiphoid to pubis.
6. Wrap towels or roll cotton tightly around the circumference of the feet in a spiral pattern, ascending to the limbs, over the pelvis and around the abdomen to the xiphoid.
7. Assess degree of tamponade – should be snug but allow hand to slide between abdomen and bandage. Adequate ventilation efforts should be observed.
8. Place duct tape or stretch bandage in a spiral pattern from toes to xiphoid to secure position of bandage.
9. Monitor physical perfusion parameters, ventilation efforts, urine output, blood pressure, and PCV and TP for evidence of ongoing hemorrhage.
10. Allow bandage to remain in place until patient stabilized for >4 hours or until aseptic preparation needed for surgical intervention begins.
11. Release the tape first, strip by strip, in the direction from xiphoid to toes and monitor for decompensation for at least five minutes per section.
12. Loosen the towels or roll cotton slowly in the direction of xiphoid to toes, but leave in place in case counterpressure needs to be reapplied. Monitor for decompensation (should take at least 5–10 minutes).
13. Remove the towels or roll cotton slowly from xiphoid to toes, and monitor for decompensation (should take 5–10 minutes).

---

* Patients with hindlimb or pelvic fractures may not be able to tolerate this procedure without general anesthesia or epidural analgesia.

Box 10.6 Steps for emergency surgery for abdominal hemorrhage.

1. Have personnel, equipment, and medications (doses calculated) ready at time of induction (see also Tables 22.3 and 22.4).
2. Clip and aseptically prepare patient prior to anesthetic induction.
3. Use multimodal analgesia and anesthesia that supports blood pressure (see Chapter 22).
4. Make 10–15 cm incision on midline below xiphoid to allow digital compression of anterior aspect of aorta for immediate hemostasis (compression for 10 minutes maximum).
5. Collect free peritoneal blood aseptically in sterile suction container for autologous blood transfusion if necessary.
6. Extend midline incision caudally to pubis.
7. Pack abdomen with sterile towels to provide hemostasis by tamponade.
8. Explore each quadrant and ligate bleeding vessels as indicated.
9. Control bleeding from massive crush injuries by placing large surgical towels or laparotomy pads to pack off organs, limit hemorrhage and contamination and apply internal abdominal pressure (called damage control technique).
10. Close the abdomen with towels in place, applying internal tamponade to oozing organs.
11. Reexplore in 12–36 hours for definitive therapy.

to occur, and may be able to tolerate a PCV as low as 15% without need for a transfusion.

Indications for transfusion of WB or pRBCs include hypovolemic anemia from blood loss, extreme lethargy or weakness, imminent anesthesia and impending invasive or physically stressful procedures. A study of dogs suffering blunt force trauma found that an admission base excess cut-off of –6.6 was 88% sensitive and 73% specific for transfusion requirement (P <0.001), and a cut-off of –7.3 was 81% sensitive and 80% specific for survival (P <0.001), with no difference in admission PCV between survivors and non-survivors [35].

There is some evidence to support the use of leukoreduction filters at the time of blood collection from dogs. The resultant decrease in leukocytes and platelets prevents the release of cytokines (IL-1, IL-6, tumor necrosis factor) and other compounds that may cause systemic consequences in the recipient [36]. The blood is passed through a leukoreduction filter with the negatively charged leukocytes adhering to the filter material by Van der Waal and electrostatic forces [37]. This adhesion is an active process with the advantage of allowing larger pore size for higher flow rate through the filter.

Blood is administered to the patient through a blood administration set with an in-line microfilter (pore size ranging from 170 to 260 μm) (210 μm filters by Pfizer, previously Hospira, New York, NY) or the detachable 18 micron blood filter (Hemo-Nate® Filters, Utah Medical Products Inc., Midvale, UT). The blood should be at least room temperature when it enters the patient.

There is evidence that canine RBCs had a decreased survival time when administered by volumetric and syringe pumps compared to gravity drip methods [38]. Most patients will receive between 10 and 22 mL/kg. A suggested formula to calculate the amount of WB required is:

$$\text{Volume(mL)} = \left[85\left(\text{dog}\right) \text{ or } 60\left(\text{cat}\right) \times \text{BW}\left(\text{kg}\right) \right]$$
$$\times \left[\left(\text{desired PCV} - \text{actual PCV}\right) / \text{donor PCV} \right]$$

For pRBC or plasma, the average infusion volume is 6–12 mL/kg. The rate of administration will depend upon the urgency of the need. In general, a rate of 0.25–1.0 mL/kg/h is ideal for the first 20 minutes, closely observing for transfusion reactions, by checking respiratory rate and effort, heart rate and temperature at a minimum. The slow administration of blood products (over 4–6 hours) to monitor for reactions and prevent fluid overload is ideal, but not always possible. Only crystalloids that do not contain calcium should be administered simultaneously through the blood infusion catheter.

Storage lesion is a catch-all term that describes the physiological changes that occur in RBCs while kept in cold storage. Adverse changes to RBCs include hemolysis (which can lead to free hemoglobin), altered energy metabolism, rheological and deformability changes to the RBC, microparticle accumulation, ammonia accumulation, and release of proinflammatory cytokines [36].

Canine and feline blood types

It is ideal to determine the blood type and perform a cross-match prior to administration of RBCs to minimize the likelihood of adverse transfusion reactions. There are three major blood groups in cats: A, B, and AB. Group A is the most common, but Group B is common in certain pedigree breeds (breeds vary by country). Group AB appears to be rare in all breeds. Blood group B cats all have naturally occurring high levels of anti-A antibodies as part of their immune system. If a type B cat receives type A blood,

Table 10.8 Choice of product, indications, and dose for small animal transfusions [30,34].

Product	Indication	Dose
Fresh whole blood (FWB)	Acute hemorrhage, anemia with hypoproteinemia, coagulopathy	2 mL/kg to raise PCV 1% (often 10–20 mL/kg) until stable
Stored whole blood	Same as FWB; NOT factor V or VIII deficiency	Same as FWB
Autologous blood	Volume resuscitation or RBC administration	Entire salvaged volume can be infused, avoid volume overload
Frozen plasma	Hypoproteinemia, coagulation factor deficiency (NOT V, VIII), augment COP	Coagulopathy: 6-20 mL/kg PRN to stop hemorrhage Hypoalbuminemia: 45 mL/kg to raise albumin 1 g/dL
Fresh frozen plasma	Coagulopathy without anemia, augment COP	Same as frozen plasma
Packed red blood cells	Anemia, without coagulopathy	1 mL/kg to raise PCV 1% or until PCV supports oxygen delivery
Platelet concentrate	Thrombocytopenia with life-threatening hemorrhage	1 Unit/10 kg PRN to arrest bleeding or until platelet count $\geq$30–50 000 platelets/μL
Platelet-rich plasma	Thrombocytopenia with life-threatening hemorrhage	1 Unit/3 kg
Cryoprecipitate	Von Willebrand's disease, hemophilia A, hypofibrinogen	1 Unit/10 kg
Hemoglobin-based oxygen carriers	Anemia when allogenic blood is not available, may help with concurrent hypotension	Dog 1–5 mL/kg, titrated to effect Cat 0.5–1 mL/kg, titrated to effect CRI 0.8 mL/kg/h

COP, colloid oncotic pressure; PCV, packed cell volume; PRN, pro re nata (as needed).

life-threatening and often fatal immune reactions will occur. Some Group A cats have naturally occurring anti-B antibodies. Therefore, only type-specific blood should be administered to cats.

A feline blood group antigen alloantibody distinct from the AB blood groups was recently reported and named Mik. Anti-Mik alloantibodies are naturally occurring in Mik-negative cats and capable of causing an acute hemolytic transfusion reaction [39].

Compatible cross-matched and type-specific pRBCs used together to confirm compatibility provided a higher posttransfusion PCV in cats compared to type-specific noncross-matched blood [40]. If blood typing is not available, a compatible cross-match is mandatory prior to blood administration in the cat.

The dog has seven internationally recognized blood groups. DEA 1.1 is known to be extremely antigenic and is the DEA antigen routinely determined in both patients and donors. In dogs, DEA 1.1-negative donor blood can be administered to any blood type recipient dog as a first-time transfusion. However, DEA 1.1-negative dogs exposed to DEA 1.1-positive RBCs will likely become sensitized and produce anti-DEA 1.1 antibody.

Another canine antigen referred to as the Dal antigen has been described and found to have no correlation to known DEA antigens [41]. Further studies will be needed to determine the frequency of its occurrence as well as the clinical significance of the anti-Dal antibody.

Transfusion complications
A recent retrospective analysis of dogs receiving blood transfusions reported an overall incidence of transfusion reaction of 28% [42]. The most common type of reaction reported in veterinary medicine is a febrile nonhemolytic transfusion reaction. The cause is attributed to the presence of WBCs in the administered product, resulting in increased cytokines in the banked blood. Collection of blood through a leukoreduction filter is reported to reduce the incidence of these transfusion reactions [43].

Immune-mediated reactions include hemolytic transfusion reactions, acute hypersensitivity reactions, leukocyte and platelet sensitivity reactions, and delayed immune-mediated reactions. Acute hypersensitivity reactions are type I hypersensitivity reactions mediated through IgE and usually occur within 45 minutes of the start of the transfusion. Leukocyte and platelet sensitivity reactions result from the binding of recipient antibodies to donor WBCs or platelets. These types of reactions are often referred to as febrile, nonhemolytic transfusion reactions.

Hemolytic transfusion reactions are antigen-antibody-mediated type II hypersensitivity reactions (predominantly IgG mediated in the dog, IgM mediated in the cat). This leads to acute hemolysis secondary to donor–recipient incompatibility. Delayed transfusion reactions can occur 2–21 days post transfusion. The hallmarks of delayed reactions are a shortened survival of transfused RBCs and a falling PCV. This type of reaction includes immune-mediated hemolysis and posttransfusion purpura characterized by acute thrombocytopenia.

Signs of tachycardia, fever, or urticaria can be early indications of a transfusion reaction, with immediate discontinuation of the transfusion recommended. Diphenhydramine (1–2 mg/kg IM) can be given to blunt the reaction to histamine release. If the vital signs return to normal, the transfusion may be restarted in 10–30 minutes at half of the previous rate. For severe anaphylactic reactions, resuscitation with intravenous fluids ($\pm$ epinephrine, 0.01 mg/kg IV) may be required and the transfusion permanently discontinued.

Transfusion-related acute lung injury (TRALI) is a clinical syndrome characterized by severe tachypnea and dyspnea, with concurrent hypoxemia that occurs within six hours of transfusion. Characteristic radiographic findings include bilateral infiltrates on thoracic radiographs. The pulmonary fluid produced in TRALI has a high protein and/or cellular content, so administration of furosemide alone may be ineffective. The incidence of TRALI in humans is much higher than has been reported in veterinary medicine and is the most common cause of transfusion-related deaths, with a fatality rate reported at 1–10% [44]. The etiology or TRALI is likely multifactorial, and associated with activated endothelium, sequestered neutrophils and reaction of donor leukocyte antibodies with leukocyte antigen on recipient neutrophils. The incidence of TRALI was 3.7% in one study of 54 dogs who had received a transfusion [45].

Finally, transfusion-related immunomodulation (TRIM) describes the transient depression of the immune system after transfusion. An increased incidence of postoperative infection following transfusion in critically ill human patients has been noted but a causal relationship between the two has yet to be determined. TRIM is a complication seen in human medicine that has not been identified in veterinary patients [44].

Nonimmune-mediated hemolysis refers to destruction of donor RBCs before transfusion, occurring secondary to inappropriate collection, storage or administration. Transfusion-associated sepsis may be secondary to contaminated blood products. Circulatory overload may occur when large volumes are administered. The possibility of hypocalcemia from citrate toxicity secondary to large volumes of blood product administration requires monitoring ionized calcium when administering more than 10–15 mL/kg.

Massive transfusion is defined as administration of more than one whole-blood volume in 24 hours, or more than half the blood volume in a short period of time (3–4 hours). Massive transfusion predisposes patients to a variety of potential disturbances, including electrolyte (K, Ca, Mg) abnormalities (46–49), citrate toxicity (hypocalcemia), coagulopathies including thrombocytopenia (46,50), hypothermia (46), metabolic acidosis (49,51), potentially delayed wound healing, and increased infection rates (49,52,53). Air emboli can occur during transfusion administration if lines are not fluid filled. When old blood products are administered or patients with severe hepatic dysfunction are administered stored blood products, hepatic encephalopathy may occur from elevations in blood ammonia.

Infectious disease transmission is a rare complication of blood administration. Patients that are immunosuppressed or may have had a splenectomy are at increased risk. Screening donors for infectious disease on a regular basis is part of routine pretransfusion testing, and ACVIM consensus guidelines should be followed [54].

Thrombus formation can occur in stored or autologous blood; all blood should be administered through a filter to prevent such a complication.

Alternatives to stored blood

When banked blood products are not available, other forms of Hgb transfusion may be needed in life-threatening situations. Autologous blood transfusion, HBOC, and xenotransfusion are options to consider.

Autologous blood can be easily collected from the pleural or abdominal cavities and administered as an ABT. Blood can be collected by syringe and needle centesis or suctioned into a sterile collection canister. Suction pressures should be kept below 100 mmHg and blood–air interfaces should be minimized. Cell salvage machines (Cell Saver®, Haemonetics, Braintree, MA) are available that could potentially improve the viability and quality of the ABT administered but these are expensive and not commonly available [36].

Autologous blood is much more commonly collected through pleural or abdominocentesis or with manual or mechanical suction during an open surgical procedure. During collection, blood–air interface and foaming should be minimized and suction pressures kept below 100 mmHg; the blood may be collected into a canister or blood bag and administered IV or IO through a filter. The addition of anticoagulants is not necessary unless the blood is fresh from ongoing hemorrhage at the time of collection.

Advantages of ABT include immediate availability and compatibility, normothermic blood products, no transmission of new infectious agents, higher levels of RBC 2,3-DPG than stored blood, and decreased overall cost [55]. Administration of ABT to patients with gross GI contamination of the collected blood or neoplasia as the source of hemorrhage is still considered valuable when the alternative is exsanguination and death. Studies in humans undergoing surgery for cancer have demonstrated no worse outcome in patients with ABT compared to banked blood [56,57]. If the ABT is

contaminated, culture, susceptibility, and antibiotic therapy are warranted. Blood that has been in a peritoneal cavity for prolonged periods may contain inflammatory mediators that could contribute to systemic inflammation, warranting careful monitoring for systemic inflammatory response syndrome (SIRS). ABT has been reported in patients with vascular injury (from trauma, gastric dilation-volvulus (GDV) and after ovariohysterectomy), neoplasia, and anticoagulant rodenticide intoxication [58].

A xenotransfusion is the transfusion of blood from one species to a different species. In veterinary medicine, this specifically refers to canine blood administered to a feline patient, with some evidence to support its use [59]. Xenotransfusion may be considered a potential option if donor-appropriate type-specific (allogenic or autologous) feline blood is not available and the patient is suffering a life-threatening anemia or hemorrhage. A review of xenotranfsuion discussed that cats do not appear to have naturally occurring antibodies against canine RBC antigens. Minimal severe adverse reactions were reported in the cats receiving a single transfusion of canine whole blood [59]. The transfused cells had a short life span (<4 days). Repeated xenotransfusion is not recommended since the onset and magnitude of adverse effects are unknown at this time, and severe adverse reactions have been reported.

Commercial stroma-free HBOC solutions, such as Oxyglobin®, provide an alternative to blood transfusion. Although Oxyglobin is currently unavailable, there is potential for future availability and it warrants discussion. The Oxyglobin solution contains bovine Hgb that has been polymerized. It is a colloid with ≥50% of the molecules 65 000–150 000 daltons in size. One gram of the Hgb in the solution could bind 1.3 mL of oxygen, with the oxygen unloading at 40 mmHg capillary pressure. The red color of Oxyglobin changes the color of the plasma and could interfere with some serum biochemical analysis. Bilirubinuria was a frequent finding after administration.

The Hgb is polymerized to reduce the vasoconstrictive effects of free Hgb. However, mild vasopressor activity (through nitric oxide (NO) scavenging) still occurred, potentially an advantage when resuscitating from hypovolemic anemia. Careful monitoring was required for evidence of systemic or pulmonary hypertension. Oxyglobin has been administered as a rapid IV infusion with crystalloids to restore IV volume and blood pressure in dogs (1–5 mL/kg increments, titrated to effect). A more conservative approach has been used in cats (0.5–1.0 mL/kg increments, titrated to effect), followed by a continuous infusion (0.8 mL/kg/h) if needed for Hgb, colloidal, and vasopressor support.

Treatment of hypervolemic anemia

Critically ill and injured patients can undergo massive fluid resuscitation throughout their course of stabilization, which may lead to an iatrogenic hypervolemia. The volume status of the patient cannot be predicted based solely on the volume of fluids administered. Underlying diseases such as heart failure, oliguric renal failure, liver cirrhosis, and increased antidiuretic hormone can cause the retention of water and hypervolemia.

An excess of intravascular fluids that do not contain RBCs will have a dilutional effect on the RBC numbers and Hgb concentration. Anemia initially diagnosed based on the PCV, Hct, RBC count and Hgb concentration could be a "dilutional anemia" rather than a true decrease in RBC numbers.

Hypervolemia can have many detrimental effects on the patient. A change in capillary dynamics can result in peripheral edema, third body fluid spacing, and pulmonary edema. A study in dogs found that hypervolemia combined with anemia was associated with an increase in cardiac output, with the anemia being the primary factor [60].

It is important to reestablish a normal intravascular fluid volume. Reducing the amount of fluids administered is the first step. The administration of a diuretic (furosemide 1–2 mg/kg IV) may be necessary to promote the loss of sodium and water; patients with renal failure may require dialysis. Treatment of any underlying condition that causes hypervolemia is mandatory. Once the patient is normovolemic, the PCV, RBC count, and Hgb concentration are reassessed to determine if a true anemia is present, and if so, the patient is treated as normovolemic anemia.

Treatment of normovolemic anemia

The initial goal of treating hypovolemic anemia and hypervolemic anemia is to reestablish a normal fluid balance (see Figure 10.2). The critical small animal patient with normovolemic anemia is more likely to have cardiovascular stability, unless the anemia is quite severe (PCV <15%) or there is underlying cardiovascular disease. When blood transfusion is required strictly to restore the RBCs and Hgb, the slow infusion of pRBCs is ideal to minimize the intravascular volume infused and minimize volume overload.

Once the blood volume and anemia have stabilized, the diagnosis of the underlying cause of the anemia will direct the treatment plan. An assessment of the reticulocyte count (see Box 10.4) will categorize the anemia as either regenerative or nonregenerative. However, it must be remembered that 3–5 days are required for the appearance of a reticulocyte response in the dog and cat. The MCV is used to characterize the RBCs as microcytic, normocytic or macrocytic and the MCH and MCHC as either normochromic or hypochromic.

The most common mechanisms of anemia are blood loss, RBC destruction, poor production or a combination of these mechanisms. A list of common causes in each category and the typical RBC characteristics and regenerative response associated with each mechanism is provided in Table 10.9. Abnormal erythropoiesis may occur in critically ill patients or patients with chronic diseases. Anemia resulting from chronic inflammatory disease is believed to occur from elevations of IL-6, which results in a reduced Fe carrier protein, limiting the body's access to iron. Chronic renal disease can result in anemia from lack of erythropoietin production. Erythropoietin can be supplemented with erythropoietin administration (Epogen®, Amgen, Thousand Oaks, CA) at a dose of 100 U/kg subcutaneously three times per week to achieve a hematocrit of 37–45 in dogs (cats 30–40). The frequency is then decreased to 1–2 times per week. The patient is closely monitored for signs of hypertension throughout treatment. Patients may develop antibodies against erythropoietin, minimizing its long-term efficacy.

The ingestion of toxins necessitates decontamination of the GI tract. Removal of any metallic foreign objects by endoscopy or surgery is necessary and supportive care is then provided.

Immune-mediated hemolytic anemia (IMHA) is most often treated with immunosuppressive doses of glucocorticosteroids, anticoagulant medications [61], and other immunosuppressive medications, as indicated. Criteria to make the diagnosis of IMHA are discussed in Table 10.6. A list of medications that have been recommended for the treatment of IMHA, with reported doses and mechanisms of action, is provided in Table 10.10. The ideal combination of medications is not known. Treatment with prednisone in combination with low-dose aspirin or clopidogrel and a secondary immunosuppressive agent such as azathioprine

Table 10.9 Common causes and characterization of anemia in the critical small animal ICU patient.*

Category	Regeneration*	Indices	PCV/TP
Blood loss			
Acute blood loss			
Iatrogenic, trauma surgery, drugs, neoplasia, GI, urinary coagulopathies	Yes	Normocytic Normochromic	N PCV/↓TP or ↓ PCV/↓TP
Chronic blood loss			
Drugs, severe parasitism, neoplasia, coagulopathies	Yes	Microcytic hypochromic	N PCV/↓TP or ↓ PCV/↓TP
RBC destruction			
Immune mediated			
Hemolytic anemia, toxin, drug, infectious	Yes	Normocytic or Macrocytic, hypochromic	↓PCV/N TP icteric or red serum
Nonimmune			
Inherited, infectious, chemical, drug, hypophosphatemia, mechanical, cancer, splenic or hepatic disease, heavy metals	Yes	Normochromic	↓ PCV/N TP icteric or red serum
Decreased production			
Chemicals, toxins, renal failure, aplastic anemia, infectious, immune mediated, neoplasia, radiation, inherited, cobalamin malabsorption, B12 deficiency, folate deficiency, idiopathic, chronic disease, retrovirus, hypothyroidism	No	Normocytic Normochromic	↓ PCV/N TP
Iron deficiency	No	Microcytic hypochromic	↓PCV/N TP

* After sufficient time for regeneration.

or cyclosporine has been recommended [62]. There is some evidence to support the use of clopidogrel in conjunction with ultra low-dose aspirin [63].

Doxycycline or other antimicrobials may be necessary for patients suspected of having RBC parasites or tick-borne diseases while test results are pending. Anthelmintic medications are administered in patients with the potential for RBC loss due to a heavy intestinal parasite burden. Patients suffering from hypophosphatemia (most commonly occurring secondary to refeeding syndrome or treatment of diabetic ketoacidosis) may requires phosphorus supplementation (see Chapter 6).

Erythrocytosis

Erythrocytosis is a relative or absolute increase in the number of circulating RBCs, resulting in a PCV increased above reference ranges (>55% dogs, >45% cats). Although some use the term *polycythemia* interchangeably with erythrocytosis, the two are not

Table 10.10 Medications, mechanism of action, and suggested doses for treating dogs and cats with immune-mediated hemolytic anemia.

Medication	Mechanism of action	Dose (dog)
Prednisone	Glucocorticoid receptor agonist	1–2 mg/kg PO q 12 h or 50 mg/m^2
Dexamethasone	Glucocorticoid agonist	0.2–0.6 mg/kg IV q 24 h
Azathioprine	Purine metabolism antagonist	2 mg/kg PO q 24 h initially
Cyclosporine	Binds cyclophilin to inhibit calcineurin and ultimately inhibit transcription of IL-2	2.2 mg/kg PO q 24 h
Mycophenolate	Reversible inhibitor of IMPDH which inhibits guanosine synthesis	12–16 mg/kg PO q 24 h
Leflunomide	Not fully determined; suggested to be related to interference with cell cycle progression	2 mg/kg PO q 12 h
Human intravenous immunoglobulins	Competitively block gamma Fc receptors, preventing phagocytosis and other mechanisms	0.5–1.5 g/kg IV once
Aspirin	Inhibits synthesis and release of prostaglandins	0.5 mg/kg PO q 24 h
Clopidogrel	Prevents binding of ADP to its platelet receptor, impairing GPIIb/IIIa	2–3 mg/kg PO q 24 h
Heparin – unfractionated	Increases the activity of antithrombin to inhibit thrombosis	1–300 U/kg SC q 6–8 h. Dose should be adjusted based on coagulation monitoring
Heparin – low molecular weight – dalteparin	Increases the activity of antithrombin to inhibit thrombosis	150–U/kg q 8 h (monitor coagulation times)
Heparin – low molecular weight – enoxaparin	As above	0.8 (dog), 1.5 (cat) mg/kg SC q 6–12 h (monitor coagulation times)
Doxycycline	Inhibitor of bacterial protein synthesis	5 mg/kg PO q 12 h

ADP, adenosine diphosphate; IMPDH, inosine 5'-monophosphate dehydrogenase.

synonymous. Polycythemia in precise terms refers to an increased number of any hematopoietic cell in blood, be it RBCs, platelets or leukocytes. An increase in RBC number in the circulation (whether relative to changes in body water or an absolute increase in RBC mass) is more precisely called erythrocythemia. Sighthounds and Dachshunds have a naturally occurring mild erythrocytosis (PCV up to 65%) when compared to standard canine reference ranges without underlying pathology.

There are three major mechanisms responsible for an elevation in PCV and Hgb concentration: (1) loss of intravascular water (hypovolemic erythrocythemia), (2) hypoxia stimulating erythrocyte production, and (3) an abnormal production of RBCs by the bone marrow with normal blood oxygen concentrations. The latter two mechanisms have normal or increased blood volume associated with the increase in PCV. Figure 10.4 provides an algorithm to guide the decision-making process when evaluating and treating a small animal ICU patient with erythrocythemia.

While erythrocytosis will increase the oxygen content of blood, this potential benefit to oxygen delivery is offset by a decrease in cardiac output. This fall in cardiac output has been attributed to an increase in systemic vascular resistance caused by the rise in viscosity of the erythrocythemic blood. However, heart rate fails to increase with erythrocytosis as might be expected if the heart were confronted by an afterload burden [64].

The cardiovascular effects of erythrocythemia and hypoxia were studied in normovolemic dogs [65]. Erythrocythemia (PCV >60%) and hypoxemia (PaO$_2$ ~41 mmHg) were induced separately, and then in combination. The combined hypoxia and erythrocythemia increased pulmonary vascular resistance by ~30%, an effect significantly greater than that of hypoxia or erythrocythemia alone. In contrast, systemic vascular resistance increased with erythrocythemia by ~90% whereas hypoxia had no effect on systemic vascular resistance. Erythrocythemia decreased cardiac output by ~50% whereas hypoxia had no significant effect alone or in combination with erythrocythemia. Combined hypoxia and erythrocythemia

decreased oxygen transport by ~50%, an effect greater than that of hypoxia or erythrocythemia alone.

Hypovolemic erythrocythemia

In the critical care setting, intravascular and interstitial fluid losses occur from problems such as lack of intake and loss through diarrhea, vomiting, urine, mechanical ventilation or extravasation into third body fluid spaces. The loss of plasma water results in a proportional rise in the RBC volume in the hematocrit tube. This reason for an increase in the PCV is termed a "relative erythrocytosis." However, there is not an increase in the number of RBCs, just an increase in the proportion of RBCs compared to plasma. The hypovolemia is driving the cardiovascular response in this situation, with tachycardia (dogs) and clinical signs of poor peripheral perfusion. In the acute hemorrhagic diarrhea syndrome of dogs, previously termed hemorrhagic gastroenteritis, hypovolemia occurs and splenic contraction was found to contribute to the relative erythrocythemia [66].

Intravascular fluid resuscitation is the treatment of choice for relative erythrocythemia. Crystalloids, with or without colloids, such as hydroxyethyl starch, are infused to reach high normal resuscitation endpoints using large-volume infusion techniques in the dog and small-volume titration techniques in the cat (see Chapter 2). The physical perfusion parameters and blood pressure are closely monitored throughout resuscitation. The PCV and TP are reassessed when resuscitation is complete. When erythrocythemia persists, a search for underlying causes of absolute erythrocytosis associated with normovolemia is initiated.

Normovolemic/hypervolemic erythrocytosis

A true increase in the number of RBCs in the bloodstream is termed an "absolute erythrocytosis." This increase in the number of cells in the blood most typically is associated with normovolemia, or even hypervolemia. The increase in blood viscosity and decrease in blood flow predispose these animals to arterial and venous thrombosis.

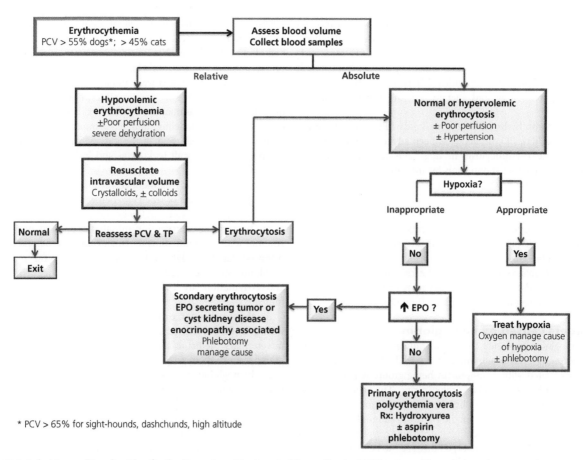

Figure 10.4 A decision-making algorithm for the diagnosis and treatment of the small animal ICU patient with erythrocytosis.

The most common presenting signs are neurological and include seizures, tremors, behavioral changes, and ataxia. The cardiovascular signs will vary depending upon the degree of erythrocytosis, the intravascular volume status, the presence or absence of hypoxemia, and the underlying disease.

An investigation is initiated to determine if the patient is hypoxic. An arterial blood gas ($PaO_2 < 80$ mmHg) or pulse oximetry ($SpO_2 < 90$–95%) is required. When hypoxia is present, the erythrocytosis is labeled as "appropriate." The decrease in the oxygen level influences EPO production in the kidneys and liver by initiating EPO gene transcriptional activation. The number of EPO-generating cells activated is directly related to the degree of hypoxia. With increasing hypoxia, more EPO is released, increasing the plasma level. This stimulates mitosis and differentiation of RBC progenitor cells in the reticuloendothelial tissues. The goal is to improve the oxygen-carrying capacity of the blood by increasing the number of circulating RBCs.

The treatment of appropriate absolute erythrocytosis begins with oxygen supplementation and a search for the cause of chronic hypoxemia. Pulmonary, cardiac, and neurological problems can each cause chronic hypoxemia. The most common cause of this form of erythrocytosis in the dog and cat is congenital heart defects, such as reversed patent ductus arteriosus, ventricular septal defects with right-to-left shunting, and tetralogy of Fallot. Phlebotomy may be required to reduce the RBC mass and correct hypervolemia during the diagnostic and therapeutic phases of patient care. Crystalloid ($\pm$ colloid) fluids are administered during or after phlebotomy to maintain normovolemia if necessary (see below).

When hypoxemia is not present, the absolute erythrocytosis is labeled "inappropriate." A quantitation of the amount of EPO in the blood can aid in determining the underlying cause. A low or normal serum EPO suggests primary erythrocytosis (also called polycythemia vera) [67,68]. This is an acquired myeloproliferative disease and has been reported in cats and dogs.

Elevated EPO levels are indicative of secondary erythrocytosis. EPO-secreting tumors of the kidneys or other organs, or nonneoplastic renal disorders (such as amyloidosis or renal inflammation) resulting in renal hypoxia with EPO production, may cause inappropriate secondary erythrocytosis. Endocrinopathy-associated erythrocytosis results from hormones other than EPO (such as cortisol, androgen, thyroxine, growth hormone) that stimulate erythropoiesis. The mild erythrocytosis in dogs with adrenocortical hyperactivity or in cats with hyperthyroidism or acromegaly is insufficient to cause clinical signs [69].

Treatment begins with supportive care. Patients with a PCV >70% from primary or secondary absolute erythrocytosis or with significant clinical signs can benefit from phlebotomy. An initial volume between 5 and 20 mL/kg of blood is removed. The target hematocrit from phlebotomy is <55% in dogs and <50% in cats [67]. Studies in people, however, indicate that a lower Hct (target <45%) may decrease the incidence of thrombus formation [70]. Care is taken to maintain circulating blood volume by replacing the volume of blood removed with crystalloids ($\pm$ colloids) or the plasma from the phlebotomized blood. When using crystalloids alone for volume replacement, the dose is generally calculated as three times the amount of whole blood removed (such as 750 mL of crystalloid for

250 mL of blood removed). When the patient is going to receive their own plasma, the blood must be collected into a blood collection bag with appropriate anticoagulant. The RBCs are separated from the plasma by centrifugation, and the plasma administered through a blood administration filter. Efforts are made to identify an underlying etiology and therapy for the specific cause is initiated.

Treatment with hydroxyurea (30 mg/kg/day, PO, for 7–10 days, then 15 mg/kg/day, PO, titrated) has been advocated for inappropriate absolute erythrocytosis in dogs and cats. Hydroxyurea induces bone marrow suppression by inhibiting DNA synthesis. Careful monitoring of the CBC is required with anemia, leukopenia, and thrombocytopenia as potential complications. Gastrointestinal upset may be noted. Drug–drug interactions should be investigated prior to administration of hydroxyurea.

Antithrombotic therapy with either platelet inhibitors or vitamin K antagonists has been administered in human patients with polycythemia vera to decrease the risk of thrombosis [71]. Information on the use of these drugs in veterinary patients with inappropriate absolute erythrocytosis is limited at this time.

Disorders caused by hemoglobin

The hemoglobin molecule consists of four globular protein subunits (tetramer). Each subunit is composed of a protein chain tightly associated with a nonprotein heme group. A heme group consists of an Fe ion held in a porphyrin ring. The Fe ion is bound in the center and may be in either the Fe^{2+} or Fe^{3+} state. This is the site of oxygen binding; however, the Fe^{3+} form cannot bind oxygen, so Fe must exist in the 2+ oxidation state to bind oxygen. In binding, oxygen temporarily and reversibly oxidizes Fe^{2+} to Fe^{3+} while oxygen temporarily turns into superoxide.

Besides the oxygen ligand, other ligands can act as competitive inhibitors (such as carbon monoxide) and allosteric ligands such as carbon dioxide and NO. Nitric oxide is bound to specific thiol groups in the globin protein, which dissociates into free nitric oxide and thiol again, as the Hgb releases oxygen from its heme site. This NO transport to peripheral tissues is hypothesized to assist oxygen transport in tissues by releasing vasodilatory nitric oxide to tissues in which oxygen levels are low [72].

Some nonerythroid cells contain Hgb. In the brain, these include some of the dopaminergic neurons, astrocytes in the cerebral cortex and hippocampus, and all mature oligodendrocytes [73]. It has been suggested that brain Hgb in these cells may enable the storage of oxygen to provide a homeostatic mechanism in anoxic conditions. Outside the brain, Hgb has nonoxygen-carrying functions as an antioxidant and a regulator of Fe metabolism in macrophages, alveolar cells, and mesangial cells in the kidney.

The Hgb molecule and heme subunit are important for cell survival. However, extracellular Hgb from hemolysis has been found to trigger specific problems that are associated with adverse clinical outcomes in patients. Acute and chronic vascular disease, inflammation, thrombosis, and renal impairment can be complications from free Hgb and its byproducts (heme Fe^{2+}; hemin -Fe^{3+}). After hemolysis, Hgb exists in a dynamic equilibrium of tetramer and dimer in the plasma. The dimers are of a relatively small molecular size and will translocate across endothelial barriers, entering the subendothelial and perivascular spaces and the lymph fluid. Among the molecular characteristics of the presence of the dimers and heme, oxidative and nitric oxide reactions, hemin release, and molecular signaling effects of hemin appear to be the most critical [74].

Systemic and, to some extent, pulmonary hypertension are the most apparent effect of free Hgb from intravascular hemolysis [74]. The mechanisms driving acute elevations in blood pressure are Hgb translocation into subendothelial spaces, local NO depletion within the vessel wall, and subsequent vasoconstriction. Vascular complications of chronic or intermittent Hgb exposure are likely to involve inflammation, localized oxidative reactions, thrombosis, vascular remodeling, and renal impairment [75]. In renal tubular epithelial cells and in the kidney, heme potently induces chemokines that recruit leukocytes and increase vascular permeability [76].

There is no specific treatment at this time to directly counteract the deleterious effects of free Hgb, heme, and hemin after hemolysis. Identifying the cause of the hemolysis is critical, with appropriate therapeutic intervention initiated as soon as possible (see Anemia above). Fluid diuresis can promote renal excretion of intravascular free Hgb and its subunits. Careful monitoring of blood pressure, renal parameters to include urine output and coagulation are essential, with intervention provided as indicated.

An abnormality of the oxygen-carrying ability of the Hgb located within the RBC is termed a dyshemoglobinemia. While uncommon in veterinary medicine, identification of the problem and specific therapy can be required.

Methemoglobinemia occurs when the Fe^{2+} of normal hemoglobin is changed to Fe^{3+}, impairing the ability of the Hgb molecule to pick up oxygen and to release bound oxygen. Methemoglobin causes a brown discoloration of the blood and mucous membranes in addition to signs of anemia. It is most commonly caused by exposure to toxic agents including acetaminophen, ibuprofen, local anesthetic agents, and exposure to skunk musk.

Treatment of methemoglobinemia includes oxygen therapy minimizing stress, administration of acetylcysteine (for acetaminophen toxicity, 140 mg/kg as 5% solution PO or IV, followed by 3–5 additional treatments of 70 mg/kg q 4h) to limit oxidative damage, fluid therapy, and transfusions when necessary. The administration of methylene blue (1% – 1 mg/kg IV) can offset a crisis by transforming Fe^{3+} back to Fe^{2+}. The response is rapid, but the dose may need to be repeated. Careful monitoring for Heinz body anemia in both the dog and cat is essential after methylene blue administration and can necessitate transfusion. Treatment for the specific toxin is necessary.

Carboxyhemoglobinemia (CO-Hgb) is a result of carbon monoxide (CO) poisoning and occurs most commonly in small animals after exposure to smoke from house fires and exhaust from faulty heating systems or a running vehicle. Patients with CO poisoning may have red mucous membranes. CO binds to the same site on Hgb as oxygen, but the affinity of CO for Hgb is 240 times higher than oxygen. This decreases oxygen binding and transport on Hgb and also decreases offloading of oxygen in the tissues. CO also affects cellular mitochondria, inhibiting normal generation of adenosine triphosphate through inhibition of cytochrome c oxidase (similar to cyanide poisoning). Supplemental oxygen is the primary treatment, with hyperbaric oxygen an option when available. Specific therapy for CO-Hgb is rarely indicated, but management of upper airway inflammation, lower airway fluid accumulation and noncardiogenic pulmonary edema may be required from the inhalation of the toxic gases. Pulse oximetry will report CO-Hgb as O2-HgB and is not reliable. The use of co-oximetry is necessary to definitively diagnose and quantitate the CO-Hgb.

References

1. Greenway CV, Stark RD. Vascular response of the spleen to rapid haemorrhage in the anaesthetized cat. J Physiol. 1969;204(1):169–79.

2. Ramlo JH, Brown JR. Mechanism of splenic contraction produced by severe hypercapnia. Am J Physiol.1959;197:1079–82.

3. Merin RG, Hoffman WL, Kraus AL. The role of the canine spleen in cardiovascular homeostasis during halothane anesthesia. Circ Shock 1977;4(3):241–6.

4. Mahaffey EA. Quality control, test validity, and reference values. In: Veterinary Laboratory Medicine Clinical Pathology, 4th edn. Ames: Iowa State University Press, 2003.

5. Rebar AH. Erythrocytes. In: A Guide to Hematology in Dogs and Cats. Rebar AH, MacWilliams P, Feldman B, et al., eds. Jackson: Teton New Media, 2001: pp 29–68.

6. Taki K, Takamura M, Sotani H, Wakusawa R. Management of the acid–base balance by the red blood cell carbonic anhydrase (RCA). I. Correlation of the RCA activity and acid–base balance in the in vitro and in vivo experiments. Tohoku J Exp Med. 1983;139(4):339–48.

7. Holahan ML, Brown AL, Drobatz KJ. The association of blood lacate concentration with outcome in dogs with idiopathic immune-mediated hemolytic anemia: 173 cases (2003–2006). J Vet Emerg Crit Care 2011;20(4):413–20.

8. Cotter S. Evaluation of erythrocytes. In: A Guide to Hematology in Dogs and Cats. Rebar AH, MacWilliams P, Feldman B, et al., eds. Jackson: Teton New Media, 2001: pp 16–17.

9. Duncan RJ, Prasse KW, Mahaffey EA. Veterinary Laboratory Medicine: Clinical Pathology, 3rd edn. Ames: Iowa State University Press, 1994: p 17.

10. Cowgill ES, Neel JA, Grindem CB. Clinical application of reticulocyte counts in dogs and cats. Vet Clin North Am Small Anim Pract. 2003;33:1223–44.

11. Giger U. Regenerative anemias caused by blood loss or hemolysis. In: Textbook of Veterinary Internal Medicine, 6th edn. Ettinger SJ, Feldman EC, eds. St Louis: Elsevier Saunders, 2005: pp 1886–907.

12. Lisciandro G. The abdominal FAST3 (AFAST3) exam. In: Focused Ultrasound Techniques for the Small Animal Practitioner. Ames: Wiley & Sons, 2014: pp 14–17.

13. Kolb KS, Day T, McCall WG. Accuracy of blood loss termination by health care professionals. Clin Forum Nurse Anesth. 1999;10:170–3.

14. Larsson C, Saltvedt S, Wiklund I, et al. Estimation of blood loss after cesarean section and vaginal delivery has low validity with a tendency to exaggeration. Acta Obstet Gynecol. 2006;85:1448–52.

15. McLellan SA, Walsh TS. Oxygen delivery and haemoglobin. Contin Educ Anesth Crit Care Pain 2004;4(4):123–6.

16. Litwin SB, Rosenthal A, Skogen W, Laver M. Long-term studies of hemoglobin-oxygen affinity in hypoxemic dogs with a right-to-left cardiac shunt. J Surg Res. 1980;28(2):118–23.

17. Bunn HF. Differences in the interaction of 2,3-diphosphoglycerate with certain mammalian hemoglobins. Science 1971;172(3987):1049–50.

18. Ferreira RR, Gopegui RR, de Matos AJ. Volume-dependent hemodynamic effects of blood collection in canine donors – evalution of 13% and 15% of total blood volume depletion. Ann Acad Bras Cienc. 2015;87(1):381–8.

19. Cane RD. Hemoglobin: how much is enough? Crit Care Med. 1990;18:1046–7.

20. Hebert PC, Hu LQ, Biro GP. Review of physiologic mechanisms in response to anemia. Can Med Assoc J. 1997;156(11 suppl).

21. Ni Z, Morcos S, Valiri ND. Up-regulation of renal and vascular nitric oxide synthase in iron-deficiency anemia. Kidney Int. 1997;52(1):195–201.

22. Mirhashemi S, Ertefai S, Messmer K, et al. Model analysis of the enhancement of tissue oxygenation by hemodilution due to increased microvascular flow velocity. Microvasc Res. 1987;34(3):290–301.

23. Hebert PC, Hu LQ, Biro GP. Review of physiologic mechanisms in response to anemia. Can Med Assoc J. 1997;156(11):suppl.

24. Hebert PC, van der Linden P, Biro G, Hu LQ. Physiologic aspects of anemia. Crit Care Clin. 2004;20(2):187–212.

25. Batement NT, Leach RM. Acute oxygen therapy. BMJ. 1998;317(7161):798–801.

26. Tocci LJ, Ewing PJ. Increasing patient safety in veterinary transfusion medicine: an overview of pretransfusion testing. J Vet Emerg Crit Care 2009;19(1):66–73.

27. Anderson DM. Surgical hemostasis. In: Veterinary Surgery Small Animal, vol. 1. Tobais KM, Johnston S, eds. St Louis: Elsevier, 2012: pp 214–20.

28. Flick, JB, Kaur, RR, Siegel D. Achieveing hemostatsis in dermatology Part II: Topical hemostatic agents. Indian Dermatol Online J. 2013;4(3):172–6.

29. Galanakis I, Vasdev N, Soomro N. A review of current hemostatic agents and tissue sealants used in laparoscopic partial nephrectomy. Rev Irol. 2011;13(3):131–8.

30. Herold LV, Devey JJ, Kirby R, Rudloff E. Clinical evaluation and management of hemoperitoneum in dogs. J Vet Emerg Crit Care 2008;18(1):40–53.

31. Herbert PC, Wells G, Blajchman M, et al. A multicenter, randomized, controlled clinical trial of transfusion requirements in critical care. N Engl J Med. 1999;340:409–17.

32. Corwin HL, Gettinger A, Pearl R, et al. The CRIT Study: anemia and blood transfusion in the critical ill – current clinical practice in the United States. Crit Care Med. 2004;32(1):39–52.

33. Vincent JL, Baron JF, Reinhart K, et al. Anemia and blood transfusion in critically ill patients. J Am Med Assoc. 2002;288(12):1499–507.

34. Giger U. Transfusion medicine. In: Small Animal Critical Care Medicine. Silverstein D, Hopper K, eds. St Louis: Elsevier Saunders, 2009: pp 281–6.

35. Stillion JR, Fletcher DJ. Admission base excess as a predictor of transfusion requirement and mortality in dogs with blunt trauma: 52 cases (2007–2009). J Vet Emerg Crit Care 2012; 22(5):588–94.

36. Kisielewicz C, Self IA. Canine and feline blood transfusions: controversies and recent advances in administration practices. Vet Anaesth Analg. 2014;41(3): 233–42.

37. Dzik S. Leukodepletion blood filters: filter design and mechanisms of leukocyte removal. Transfus Med Rev. 1993;7:65–77.

38. McDevitt Tuaux CG, Baltzer WI. Influence of transfusion technique on survival of autologous red blood cells in the dog. J Vet Emerg Crit Care 2011;21(3):209–16.

39. Weinstein NM, Blais MC, Harris K, et al. A newly recognized blood group in domestic shorthair cats: the mik red cell antigen. J Vet Intern Med. 2007;21:287–92.

40. Weiltman JG, Fletcher DJ, Rogers C. Influence of cross-match on posttransfusion paced cell volume in feline paced red blood cell transfusion. J Vet Emerg Crit Care 2014;24(4):429–36.

41. Blais MC, Berman L, Oakley DA, et al. Canine Dal blood type: a red cell antigen lacking in some Dalmatians. J Vet Intern Med. 2007;21:281–6.

42. Holowaychuk MK, Leader JL, Monteigo G. Risk factors for transfusion-associated complications and nonsurvival in dogs receiving packed red blood cell transfusions: 211 cases (2008–2011). J Am Vet Med Assoc. 2014;244(4):431–7.

43. Blajchman MA. Landmark studies that have changed the practice of transfusion medicine. Tranfusion 2005;45(9):1523–30.

44. Prittie JE. Controversies related to red blood cell transfusion in critically ill patients. J Vet Emerg Crit Care 2010;20(2):167–76.

45. Thomovsky EJ, Bach J. Incidence of acute lung injury in dogs receiving transfusions. J Am Vet Med Assoc. 2014;244(2):170–4.

46. Jutkowitz LA, Rozanski EA, Moreau J, et al. Massive transfusion in dogs: 15 cases (1997–2002). J Am Vet Med Assoc. 2002;220(11):1664–9.

47. Meikle A, Milne B. Management of prolonged QT interval during a massive transfusion: calcium, magnesium, or both? Can J Anesth. 2000;47(8):792–5.

48. Ho KM, Leonard A. Risk factors and outcomes associated with hypomagnesemia in massive transfusion. Transfusion 2011;51(2):270–6.

49. Wilson RF, Mammen E, Walt AJ. Eight years of experience with massive transfusion. J Trauma 1971;11(4):275–85.

50. Reiss RF. Hemostatic defects in massive transfusion: rapid diagnosis and management. Am J Crit Care 2000;9(3):158–65.

51. Cosgriff N, Moore EE, Sauaia, et al. Predicting life-threatening coagulopathy in the massively transfused trauma patient: hypothermia and acidosis revisited. J Trauma 1997;42(5):857–61.

52. Argarwal N, Murphy JG, Cayten CG, et al. Blood transfusion increases the risk of infection after trauma. Arch Surg. 1993;128(2):171–6.

53. Ford CD, van Moorleghem G, Menlove RF. Blood transfusion and postoperative wound infections. Surgery 1993;113(6):603–7.

54. Wardrop KJ, Reine N, Birkenheuer A, et al. Canine and feline blood donor screening for infectious disease. J Vet Intern Med 2005;19:135–42.

55. Purvis D. Autotransfusion in the emergency patient. Trans Med. 1995;25(6): 1291–304.

56. Ubee S, Kumar M, Athmanathan N, et al. Intraoperative red blood cell salvage and autologous transfusion during open radical retropubic prostatectomy: a cost-benefit analysis. Ann R Coll Surg Engl. 2011;93(2):157–61.

57. Brewster DC, Ambrosino JJ, Darling R, et al. Intraoperative autotransfusion in major vascular surgery. Am J Surg. 1979;137(4):507–13.

58. Higgs VA, Rudloff R, Kirby R, Linklater AK. Autologous blood transfusions in dogs with thoracic or abdominal hemorrhage: 25 cases (2007–2012). J Vet Emerg Crit Care 2015;25(6):731–8.

59. Bovens C, Gruffydd-Jones T. Xenotransfusion with canine blood in the feline species: review of the literature. J Feline Med Surg. 2103;15(2):62–7.

60. Fowler NO, Bloom WL, Ward J. Hemodynamic effects of hypervolemia with and without anemia. Circ Res. 1958;(6):163–7.

61. Sharpe KS, Center SA, Randolph J, et al. Influence of treatment with ultralow-dose aspirin on platelet aggregation as measured by whole blood impedance aggregometry and platelet P-selectin expression in clinically normal dogs. Am J Vet Radiol. 2010;71(11):1294–304.

62. Weinkle TK, Center SA, Randolph JF, et al. Evaluation of prognostic factors, survival rates and treatment protocols for immune mediated hemolytic anemia in dogs: 151 cases (1993–2002). J Am Vet Med Assoc. 2005;226(11):1869–80.

63. Mellet AM, Nakamura RK, Bianco D. Prospective study of clopidogrel therapy in dogs with primary immune mediated hemolytic anemia. J Vet Intern Med. 2001;25(1):71–4.

64. Lindenfeld J,.Weil J, Travis V, Horwitz L. Regulation of oxygen delivery during induced polycythemia in exercising dogs. Am J Physiol Heart Circ Physiol. 2005;289(5):H1821–5.

65. McGrath RL, Weil JV. Adverse effects of normovolemic polycythemia and hypoxia on hemodynamics in the dog. Circ Res. 1979;43(5):793–8.

66. Unterer S, Busch K, Leipig M, et al. Endoscopically visualized lesions, histologic findings and bacterial invasion in the gastrointestinal mucosa of dogs with acute hemorrhagic diarrhea syndrome. J Vet Intern Med. 2014;28:52–8.

67. Hasler AH. Polycythemia. In: Textbook of Veterinary Internal Medicine, 6th edn. Ettinger SJ, Feldman E, eds. St Louis: Elsevier Saunders, 2005: pp 215–18.

68. Shell L. Polycythemia. Canine Associated Database. 2006. www.vin.com.

69. Randolph JF. Overview of erythrocytosis and polycythemia. In: The Merck Veterinary Manual, 10th edn. Whitehouse Station: Merck & Co., 2010: pp 40–2.

70. Marchioli R, Finazzi G, Specchia G, et al. Cardiovascular events and intensity of treatment in polycythemia vera. N Engl J Med. 2013;368:22–3.

71. Hernandez-Boluda JA, Arellano-Rodrigo E, Cervantes F, et al. Oral anticoagulation to prevent thrombosis recurrence in polycythemia vera and essentail thrombocythemia. Ann Hematol. 2015;95(6):911–18.

72. Jensen FB. The dual roles of red blood cells in tissue oxygen delivery: oxygen carriers and regulators of local blood flow. J Exp Biol. 2009;212(21):3387–93.

73. Biagioli M, Pinto M, Cesselli D, et al. Unexpected expression of alpha- and beta-globin in mesencephalic dopaminergic neurons and glial cells. Proc Natl Acad Sci USA 2009;106(36):15454–9.

74. Schaer DJ, Buehler PW, Alayash A, et al. Hemolysis ad free hemoglobin revisited: exploring hemoglobin and hemin scavengers as a novel call of therapeutic proteins. Blood 2013;121(8):1276–84.

75. Buchler PW, Back JH, Lisk C, et al. Free hemoglobin induction of pulmonary vascular disease: evidence for an inflammatory mechanism. Am J Physiol Lung Cell Mol Physiol. 2012;303(4):L312–L326.

76. Wagener FA, Eggert A, Boerman OC, et al. Heme is a potent inducer of inflammation in mice and is counteracted by heme oxygenase. Blood 2001;98(6):1802–11.

Further reading

Anderson DM. Surgical hemostasis. In: Veterinary Surgery Small Animal, vol. 1. Tobais KM, Johnston S, eds. St Louis: Elsevier, 2012: pp 214–20.

Lisciandro G. The abdominal FAST3 (AFAST3) exam. In: Focused Ultrasound Techniques for the Small Animal Practitioner. Ames: Wiley & Sons, 2014: pp 17–43.

Yagi K and Holowaychuk M, eds. Manual of Veterinary Transfusion Medicine and Blood Banking. Ames: Wiley Blackwell, 2016.

CHAPTER 11

Heart rate, rhythm, and contractility

Dennis E. Burkett

Hope Veterinary Specialists, Malvern, Pennsylvania

Introduction and physiology of heart rate, rhythm, and contractility

The primary function of the cardiovascular system is to provide oxygen and substrate to the tissues for energy production. The heart is the pump that controls the flow of blood and must continuously adjust to meet the demands of the body for oxygenated blood. This cardiac pump has a right and left side, each composed of an atrium resting above a heavily muscled ventricle (Figure 11.1). The left ventricular wall is normally significantly thicker than the right. Cup-shaped valve leaflets (tricuspid on the right, mitral on the left) separate the atria from the ventricles. A thick muscular septum separates the right from the left ventricle. The right atrium receives blood from the systemic circulation and delivers it to the right ventricle. From here, the blood is pumped through the pulmonary artery into the pulmonary circulation for oxygenation and passive diffusion of carbon dioxide. The left atrium receives the oxygenated blood from the pulmonary veins and delivers it to the left ventricle. From here it is pumped into the systemic circulation through the aorta.

This pumping action of the heart occurs in a cyclical fashion through myocardial contraction and relaxation. This is described as the cardiac cycle and is illustrated in Figure 11.2. The myocardial cells undergo electrical depolarization, triggering calcium movement within the cell, illustrated in Figure 11.3. The period of ventricular contraction is termed *systole* and the period of relaxation is called *diastole*. Systole and diastole are further divided into phases of cardiac activity. Although the atria also have periods of systole and diastole, the cardiac cycle focuses on ventricular contraction and relaxation [1,2].

The cardiac output (CO) is the driving force for systemic blood flow and is defined as the volume of blood pumped by the heart per unit time. It is a product of the stroke volume × heart rate and can be expressed as liters per minute. Multiple variables can impact each of the components of CO (Figure 11.4) and can contribute to patient compensatory or decompensatory cardiovascular events.

The overall performance of the heart rests with the stroke volume. This is a delicate interplay between the contractility (inotropic state) of the heart, the afterload (forces opposing the pumping action of the heart), and the preload (forces acting to fill the heart during its quiescent phase). Cardiac performance is also influenced by heart rate, ventriculoatrial coupling, ventricular synchrony, and pericardial properties. The cardiac performance can be further modified by neural control, drugs, hormones, and metabolic products [1].

Preload is the first determinant of contraction (systolic wall motion). It is the force that determines the amount of stretch placed on the contractile elements in the myocardial cell (myocardial sarcomere) at the end of diastole [3]. This increase in diastolic force stretches the sarcomeres and increases the volume in the ventricle at the end of diastole (end-diastolic volume, EDV). Starling's law of the heart states that increased sarcomere stretch results in a more forceful contraction, and decreased stretch results in a less forceful contraction [1,4–6]. This gives the heart the ability to regulate stroke volume on a beat-to-beat basis and allows the body to acutely increase cardiac output by increasing venous return to the heart [7].

Afterload is the second determinant of wall motion. It opposes muscle shortening and impedes contraction. The forces producing contraction and the forces opposing contraction should be equal and opposite. The pressure that a ventricle generates during systole is usually the same as the systolic systemic arterial blood pressure and is determined by aortic resistance to flow (impedence) [8], stroke volume, and velocity of flow into the aorta. The radius of the systemic arterioles is the primary determinant of resistance and impedance. Afterload is increased when (1) intraventricular pressure is increased (such as arteriolar constriction or aortic stenosis), (2) chamber volume (radius) is increased, or (3) ventricular wall thickness is decreased during systole.

The third determinant of stroke volume and systolic wall motion (contraction) is myocardial contractility. Contraction and myocardial contractility are different. Contractility is myocardial performance (force, velocity, and extent of contraction) independent of preload and afterload [4]. Contractility is an inherent myocardial cellular property which, when combined with preload and afterload, influences the force and velocity with which the fundamental contractile unit within the myocardial cell (sarcomere) contracts. Consequently, these factors will change the amount of wall motion or contraction. The primary determinants of contractility include, but are not limited to, (1) increased amount and rate of calcium release by the sarcoplasmic reticulum, (2) increased sensitivity to the released calcium, (3) phosphorylation of proteins within the cell, and (4) cellular adenosine triphosphate (ATP) production [1].

Heart rate (HR) is the number of contractions of the heart per unit time (beats per minute, bpm) and is the remaining component of the CO equation. The normal resting heart rates for the dog and cat are listed in Table 11.1. Tachycardia is a fast heart rate at rest and bradycardia is a slow heart rate at rest. The heart rate can vary according to the physical needs of the patient, to include the need to absorb oxygen and excrete carbon dioxide. Activities that can provoke HR changes include physical exercise, sleep, anxiety, stress,

Monitoring and Intervention for the Critically Ill Small Animal: The Rule of 20, First Edition. Edited by Rebecca Kirby and Andrew Linklater.
© 2017 John Wiley & Sons, Inc. Published 2017 by John Wiley & Sons, Inc.

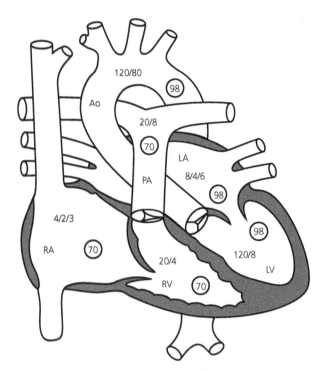

120/80
98
Ao
20/8
70
LA
PA
8/4/6
98
98
4/2/3
RA
70
20/4
120/8
98
LV
RV
70

Figure 11.1 Normal anatomy, pressures (systolic/diastolic/mean), and oxygen saturations (in circles) in the chambers of the heart, systemic circulation, and pulmonary circulation. Source: Kittleson MD, Kienle RD, eds. Normal clinical cardiovascular physiology. In: Small Animal Cardiovascular Medicine. St Louis: Mosby. 1998. Used with permission of Elsevier [1]. Ao, aorta; LA, left atrium; LV, left ventricle; PA, pulmonary artery; RA, right atrium; RV, right ventricle.

pain, illness, and drugs. An arrhythmia occurs when the heart is not beating in a regular pattern.

Each beat of the heart is set in motion by an electrical signal from within the heart muscle. In a normal, healthy heart, each beat begins with a signal from the sinoatrial (SA) node (pacemaker) located in the right atrium. There are important physiological differences between nodal cells and ventricular cells. The specific differences in ion channels and mechanisms of polarization give rise to the unique spontaneous depolarizations necessary for the pacemaker activity of the SA node. This signal stimulates the atria to contract, and then travels to the atrioventricular (AV) node, located in the interatrial septum. After a delay, the stimulus diverges and is conducted through the left and right bundles of His to the respective Purkinje fibers within each side of the heart, then to the endocardium at the apex of the heart, and finally to the ventricular epicardium (Figure 11.5). The left ventricle contracts an instant before the right ventricle. As the signal passes, the walls of the ventricles relax and await the next signal. This process continues over and over as the atria refill with blood and more electrical signals come from the SA node.

On the microscopic level, the wave of depolarization propagates to adjacent myocardial cells by way of gap junctions located on the intercalated disks. Electrical impulses propagate freely between cells in every direction. This allows the myocardium to function as a single contractile unit. This property allows rapid, synchronous depolarization of the myocardium.

In order to maximize efficiency of contraction and CO, the conduction system of the heart must have the following characteristics: substantial atrial to ventricular delay to allow ventricular filling,

coordinated contraction of ventricular cells to provide adequate systolic pressure, and ventricular contraction beginning at the apex of the heart to facilitate upward ejection of blood into the great arteries. After contracting, the heart muscles must relax to fill the chambers again. This relaxation is possible due to rapid repolarization of cardiac muscle caused by a temporary inactivation of certain ion channels.

The heart rate is rhythmically generated by the SA node, but is also influenced by central factors mediated through sympathetic and parasympathetic nerves [9]. The medulla oblongata stimulates activity through sympathetic stimulation of the cardioaccelerator nerves, and decreases heart activity through parasympathetic stimulation through the vagus nerve. During rest, both centers provide slight stimulation to the heart, contributing to autonomic tone. Normally, vagal stimulation predominates.

The ventricles are more richly innervated by sympathetic fibers than parasympathetic fibers. Sympathetic stimulation causes the release of norepinephrine at the neuromuscular junction of the cardiac nerves. This shortens the repolarization period, speeding the rate of depolarization and contraction. Norepinephrine binds to beta-1 receptors and opens chemical- or ligand-gated sodium and calcium ion channels, allowing an influx of positively charged ions [10].

The vagus nerve sends branches to both the SA and AV nodes, and to portions of both the atria and ventricles. Parasympathetic stimulation releases acetylcholine at the neuromuscular junction, which slows HR by opening chemical- or ligand-gated potassium ion channels to slow spontaneous depolarization. Repolarization is also extended, increasing the time before the next spontaneous depolarization occurs.

The cardiovascular centers receive input from a series of visceral receptors, including proprioreceptors, baroreceptors, and chemoreceptors. Baroreceptors are located in the aortic arch and carotid body and sense tension or stretch in the blood vessels. Decreased intravascular circulating fluid volume is sensed by these receptors, and normal inherent vagal input is decreased. This allows the sympathetic tone to become more prevalent and results in an increased heart rate. The increased heart rate functions to compensate for decreased myocardial contraction from a reduced preload and to maintain cardiac output and blood pressure. With increased pressure and stretch, the rate of baroreceptor firing increases, and the cardiac centers decrease sympathetic stimulation and increase parasympathetic stimulation, slowing the HR.

The atrial reflex (or Bainbridge reflex) is stimulated when increased venous return stretches the walls of the atria and stimulates specialized baroreceptors. These atrial baroreceptors increase their rate of firing and stimulate the cardiac center to increase sympathetic stimulation and inhibit parasympathetic stimulation, resulting in an increased HR. The opposite is true when there is a decreased rate of atrial baroreceptor firing.

Increased metabolic byproducts associated with increased metabolic activity, such as declining oxygen levels and increased carbon dioxide, hydrogen ions and lactic acid, are detected by chemoreceptors innervated by the glossopharyngeal and vagus nerves. These chemoreceptors provide feedback to the cardiovascular centers about the need for increased or decreased blood flow, based on the relative levels of these substances.

Critical illness can place significant metabolic demands on the heart. Problems encountered in the small animal patient, such as hypovolemia, hypotension, hypoxia, and systemic inflammation, can initiate compensatory cardiovascular responses that require

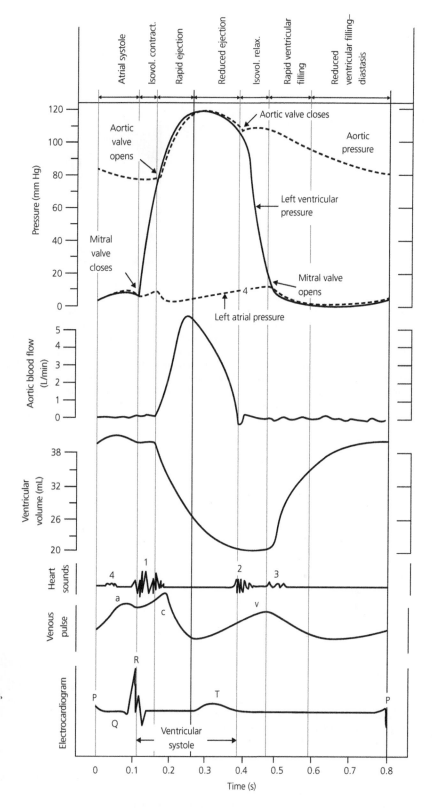

Figure 11.2 Schematic drawings of left heart pressures, aortic flow, left ventricular volume, heart sounds, venous pressure, and electrocardiogram on the same time scale. Events within the cardiac cycle are labeled. Source: Kittleson MD, Kienle RD, eds. Normal clinical cardiovascular physiology. In: Small Animal Cardiovascular Medicine. St Louis: Mosby. 1998. Used with permission of Elsevier [1].

an immediate and sustained increase in cardiac output. The heart must be capable of adjusting the heart rate and increasing the myocardical contractile forces to meet the needs for oxygen delivery to the tissues; however, prolonged or excessive tachycardia can result in myocardial hypoxia and ischemia. It is important to identify potential causes of abnormalities in cardiac rate, rhythm or contractility early in the course of treatment and determine the effects that these changes can have on the tissues.

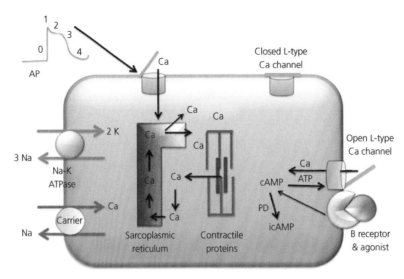

Figure 11.3 A schematic diagram of the movements of calcium during excitation-contraction coupling in cardiac tissue. Excitation-contraction coupling is the process whereby an action potential triggers a myocyte to contract. When a myocyte is depolarized by an action potential, calcium ions enter the cell during phase 2 of the action potential through calcium channels located on the cell membrane. This triggers a subsequent release of calcium stored in the sarcoplasmic reticulum (SR) through calcium release channels. Calcium released by the SR increases the intracellular calcium concentration with the free calcium binding to the troponin of the regulatory complex attached to the thin filaments. A conformational change results in movement ("ratcheting") between the myosin and the actin, shortening the sarcomere length. Ratcheting cycles occur as long as the cytosolic calcium remains elevated. At the end of phase 2, calcium entry into the cell slows and calcium is sequestered by the SR via an ATP-dependent calcium pump, thus lowering the cytosolic calcium concentration and removing calcium from the troponin. To a smaller extent, cytosolic calcium is transported out of the cell by the sodium-calcium exchange pump. The reduced intracellular calcium induces a conformational change in the troponin complex, leading to inhibition of the actin binding site. Beta-adrenergic stimulation, which occurs when sympathetic nerves are activated, increases cAMP which in turn activates protein kinase to increase calcium entry into the cell through L-type calcium channels. ATP, adenosine triphosphate; icAMP, inactive cyclic adenosine monophosphate; PD, phosphodiesterase.

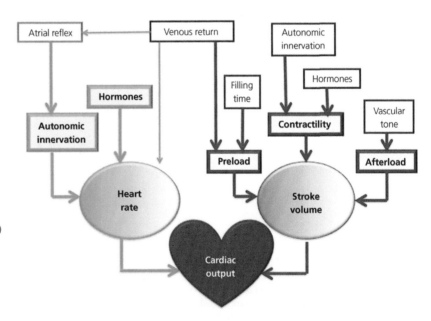

Figure 11.4 Factors influencing cardiac output. Cardiac output is the product of heart rate multiplied by stroke volume. Stroke volume (*in blue*) is the result of the preload, myocardial contractility, and afterload. Vascular tone, venous return, and autonomic innervation are some of the factors that will influence these components. The heart rate (*in green*) is regulated by autonomic innervation, circulating hormones, and venous return.

Table 11.1 Normal resting heart rates for dogs and cats.

Species	Normal (bpm) resting	Tachycardia (bpm) resting	Bradycardia (bpm) resting
Dog – small breeds	60–160	>180	<90
Dog – medium size	60–160	>160	<60
Dog – large breed	60–160	>160	<60
Cat	150–220	>220	<120

bpm, beats per minute.

Initial diagnostic and monitoring procedures

Any tissue that requires oxygen can be affected by poor cardiac performance. Unfortunately, no easy procedure is available to directly measure cardiac output in the small animal patient. Instead, historical and physical examination findings, point of care (POC) and clinicopathological laboratory testing, diagnostic imaging and monitoring procedures must be used to gather information that reflects potential causes and effects of cardiac disorders. Patients that have labored breathing or poor perfusion will require

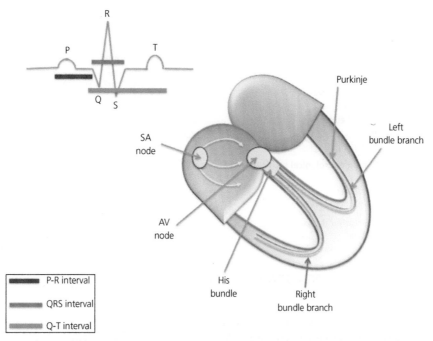

Figure 11.5 Schematic of the cardiac electrical conduction system and the corresponding ECG waveforms. The P wave is the result of atrial depolarization which starts in the sinoatrial (SA) node. These signals from the pacemaker cells of the SA node are transmitted to the right and left atria. The impulse is sent to the atrioventricular (AV) node where it is slowed and passed through the His bundle, then through the right and left bundle branches and finally to the Purkinje fibers for myocardial contraction through excitation coupling. The letters Q, R, and S are used to describe the QRS complex and represent ventricular depolarization. The T wave represents repolarization of the ventricles. The criteria for identifying the QRS waves are: Q: the first negative deflection after the P-wave. If the first deflection is not negative, the Q is absent; R: the first positive deflection; S: the negative deflection after the R-wave. Intervals are then measured and demonstrated by the colored bars above. The PR interval represents the AV conduction time, measured from where the P-wave begins to the beginning of the QRS; the QRS interval is measured from the end of the PR interval to the end of the S wave; the QT interval is measured from the beginning of the QRS complex to the end of the T-wave; indicates time of ventricular activity to include depolarization and repolarization.

Table 11.2 Breed predilections to cardiac disease.

Disease	Breed/signalment/disease predilection
Dilated cardiomyopathy	Doberman Pinscher, Boxer, Great Dane, Labrador Retreiver, American Cocker Spaniel, large hounds, St Bernard, Old English Sheepdog, cats fed a taurine-deficient diet
Myxomatous mitral valve disease	Cavalier King Charles Spaniel; small breeds
Hypertrophic cardiomyopathy	Uncommon in dogs, common in cats; seen in cats with hyperthyroidism
Restrictive and unclassified cardiomyopathy	Cats

therapeutic intervention (such as oxygen supplementation) to support tissue oxygenation throughout the diagnostic period.

History

The history begins with the species and signalment (age, sex, breed). Dogs are more commonly diagnosed with mitral regurgitation and dilated cardiomyopathy as a cause of heart disease, and cats are more likely to have hypertrophic changes causing cardiac disease. Heart disease is diagnosed more commonly in older dogs and cats, with male dogs reported to have an increased incidence of

heart disease compared to females. Certain breeds of dogs and cats can have a genetic predisposition to heart disease (Table 11.2).

The vaccination and heartworm status should be known and any past diagnosis of a heart murmur, gallop or cardiac arrhythmia reported. Past medical problems can identify disorders such as hyperthyroidism, hypothyroidism, heartworm disease, periodontal disease, malnutrition, diabetes mellitus, cancer or immune-mediated disorders that can have an effect on cardiac function. A review of prescribed and over-the-counter medications and of any exposure to potential toxins might identify a possible cardio-toxic agent. Table 11.3 provides a list of common toxins that can affect cardiac performance in the dog and cat.

Identifying when the pet was last completely normal helps to determine whether any cardiovascular changes are acute or chronic. A history of trauma, sudden collapse or syncope warrants immediate concern for acute cardiac disorders. Reported clinical signs of coughing, respiratory difficulty, lameness, and exercise intolerance are common presenting complaints with heart, airway, thrombotic or pulmonary disease and suggest a more chronic problem. In the cat, the clinical signs of heart disease can be quite varied and as subtle as anorexia and depression.

Physical examination

The physical examination begins with the vital signs (temperature, heart rate, pulse intensity, respiratory rate and effort, mucous membrane color, and capillary refill time (CRT)). Hypothermia can be a consequence of poor perfusion due to insufficient CO and is a common finding in cats. A fever can be an early consequence of

Table 11.3 Cardioactive toxins.

Zootoxins	Plant toxins
Bufo toads (cardioactive glycoside)	Foxglove
	Milkweed
Puffer fish (tetrodotoxin)	Kalanchoe
Anemones and jelly fish (Cnidarians, Na and K channel blockers)	Lilly of the valley
	Oleander
	Star of Bethlehem
Snake envenomation (uncommon)	Yew
	Nicotine
Methylxanthines	**Human neurological medications**
Chocolate	Antipsychotics
Terbutaline/Aminophylline	Antidepressants
	ADHD medications
Common cardiac, asthma or antiarrhythmic medications	**Illicit/other drugs**
See Table 11.13	Cocaine
Beta-agonists (albuterol)	Amphetamines
	Alcohol

Table 11.4 Abnormal heart sounds with point of maximal intensity and their clinical significance.

Abnormal heart sound	Significance
Murmur, PMI over the PA valve	May indicate pulmonic stenosis
Murmur, PMI over the Ao valve	May indicate aortic stenosis
Murmur, PMI over the RAV valve	May indicate tricuspid valve insufficiency
Murmur, PMI over the LAV valve	May indicate mitral valve insufficiency
Gallop	May indicate cardiomyopathy
Muffled sounds	May indicate pleural or pericardial fluid or mass
Sounds not synchronous with pulses	May indicate arrhythmia

Ao, aorta; PA, pulmonary artery; LAV, left atrioventricular valve; PMI, point of maximum intensity; RAV, right atrioventricular valve.

Table 11.5 How to grade heart murmurs.

Grade	Characteristics
I	Minimally auscultable with a stethoscope
II	Soft, but easily heard with a stethoscope
III	Intermediate or moderate loudness with a stethoscope
IV	Loud murmur with sound that radiates to other areas of the chest (PMI may be difficult to determine), no thrill (vibration) palpated
V	Very loud with stethoscope barely touching chest, a palpable thrill (vibration) is present
VI	Very loud with stethoscope, is audible with or without stethoscope, palpable thrill (vibration of chest wall) is present

PMI, point of maximum intensity.

valvular endocarditis or systemic inflammatory response syndrome (SIRS) disease with the associated cardiac changes. The presence of sustained tachycardia or bradycardia warrants concern for shock, arrhythmias or poor cardiac performance. The coronary arteries fill during the diastolic phase of the cardiac cycle, and any sustained increase in heart rate could be detrimental. Evaluation of the physical peripheral perfusion parameters (heart rate, pulse quality, mucous membrane color, CRT) can very quickly identify if cardiac output is affecting systemic tissue perfusion. The heart beat and pulse should be synchronous, with irregularities suggestive of an arrhythmia. Distension of the jugular veins can be a result of right heart failure, volume overload, pericardial tamponade or obstruction of the superior vena cava.

The breathing pattern is assessed for evidence of lung parenchymal disease, pleural effusion or small airway disease (see Chapter 8). Auscultation of the thorax should begin at the periphery of the thoracic cavity, listening for the softer sounding lung parenchyma and small airways and then moving to more centrally located and louder sounding large airways and heart. Pleural effusion or pulmonary edema can each be a life-threatening consequence of heart failure. Muffled heart sounds can suggest pericardial fluid or pleural fluid or air accumulation.

The heart is auscultated from both sides of the thoracic cavity, with auscultation requiring at least 1–2 minutes of focused listening to rule out the presence of a murmur or gallop heart sound. Closure of the mitral and tricuspid valves (also called AV valves) is associated with the first heart sound and closure of the aortic and pulmonic (semilunar) valves is associated with the second heart sound. When blood inappropriately leaks through an abnormal closed heart valve, it causes turbulence, creating an auscultable murmur. A third heart sound (gallop sound) is often heard in a patient with cardiac disease at or near the peak of rapid ventricular filling.

When a murmur is identified, the point of maximum intensity is determined in an effort to isolate the valve most likely diseased (Table 11.4). A murmur can be due to anatomical defects (pathological murmurs) or physiological problems such as anemia, hyperthyroidism, hypertension, fever, and excitement (physiological murmurs).

The timing of the murmur to systole or diastole is recorded. Diastolic murmurs suggest stenosis of the AV valves or regurgitation of the semilunar valves. Causes of systolic murmurs can include

stenosis of the semilunar valves, regurgitation of the AV valves, atrial or ventricular septal defects, hypertrophic obstructive cardiomyopathy or physiological flow murmurs. Continuous, combined systolic and diastolic murmurs can be heard with patent ductus arteriosus, coarctation of the aorta, or acute severe aortic regurgitation. The intensity of the murmur is graded, which aids in assessing for changes over time (Table 11.5). Cardiac auscultation must be repeated after intravascular volume resuscitation. Hypovolemia can significantly reduce the volume of regurgitant blood, thereby minimizing or obliterating the sound of the murmur. Restoring the intravascular volume should restore the murmur if valvular regurgitation is present.

Abnormal heart sounds (murmur, gallop) in the cat are frequently intermittent rather than present with each heart beat. This necessitates a focused cardiac auscultation for at least two full minutes to determine whether or not the abnormality is present in the cat. Most feline murmurs have a very focal point of maximum intensity that is generally located just left of the sternum. The neck of the cat should be carefully palpated for evidence of enlarged thyroid glands (thyroid slip), common in hyperthyroid cats (a cause of cardiac disease).

The peripheral limbs of the patient are carefully examined for evidence of interstitial edema resulting from cardiogenic changes in the intravascular hydrostatic pressure. The abdomen is carefully palpated to determine if there is hepatomegaly or abdominal effusion, each a potential consequence of right heart failure.

Point of care testing

A minimum database is provided through POC testing and should include the packed cell volume (PCV), total protein (TP), blood glucose, blood urea nitrogen (BUN) electrolyte panel, blood lactate, blood gas, coagulation profile, blood smear, and urinalysis. As the PCV or hematocrit decreases, blood viscosity decreases and can cause a functional heart murmur. An elevated PCV can be a consequence of chronic hypoxia resulting from cardiac disease (see Chapter 10). Hypoglycemia can affect vascular tone (preload) and myocardial contractility, with insufficient energy substrate available. An elevated BUN and isosthenuria on urinalysis might direct further investigation for kidney disease, a potential consequence of insufficient CO. Electrolyte disorders affecting sodium, potassium, magnesium, calcium or chloride and severe acidemia or alkalemia can each impact cardiac rate, rhythm, myocardial contractility, and vascular tone.

Elevated lactate may indicate that there has been poor oxygen delivery to tissues, and resolution of this may be an important parameter to monitor in patients with cardiogenic shock. Evidence of microfilaria may be seen on a blood smear. Heartworm (*Dirofilariasis immitis*) serology is most commonly performed as a snap test (4DX, Idexx, Westbrook, ME or Accuplex, Antech, Irvine, CA). Current dirofilariasis tests detect antigens only on female heartworms, providing a false-negative result when there are solely male worms present.

Clinicopathological laboratory testing

A complete blood count (CBC) and serum biochemical profile with thyroid panel will provide data pertaining to possible causes and effect of abnormalities in cardiac rate, rhythm or myocardial contractility. The CBC can better define anemia or erythrocytosis when present. An elevation in serum creatinine and BUN directs further investigation for kidney disease and possible renal hypertension which can affect preload and afterload. Elevated liver enzymes can occur with heartworm infestation or hepatic congestion from right heart disease. Hyperthyroidism and hypothyroidism can each affect cardiac performance. Feline patients with chronic thyrotoxicosis may have "masked" renal injury (due to increased renal blood flow), requiring close monitoring of renal parameters during treatment. Additional testing is often required and could include serology for inciting pathogens (cause of SIRS-related cardiac changes) and fluid analysis with culture and susceptibility.

Many of the drugs that are administered for cardiac disease (such as digoxin, furosemide, angiotensin converting enzyme (ACE) inhibitors) require baseline bloodwork and urinalysis at the start of therapy to help avoid side-effects and to tailor drug therapy for the individual patient over time.

Several cardiac biomarkers (such as cardiac troponin I, NT-pro-BNP) are used in human medicine to determine if cardiac injury is immediately present. The significance of these biomarkers in the diagnosis and treatment of heart disease in the dog and cat has not been completely elucidated. Their usefulness might be in differentiating cardiac from noncardiac disease or determining if significant cardiac disease is present prior to the onset of heart failure [11–17]. In addition, these biomarkers might be used to monitor changes in the heart over time [16,18]. Cardiac troponin I and NT-pro-BNP have also been investigated as prognostic indicators in dogs with dilated cardiomyopathy [19] and dogs with myxomatous mitral valve disease [20]. However, these test results should

not be used as a sole diagnostic or prognostic indicator. While elevation in the test results might indicate myocardial injury, the results do not differentiate the etiologies of myocardial injury [15,21,22]. However, two studies have demonstrated that elevated NT-pro-BNP can be supportive of a cardiac cause of respiratory distress in cats [23,24].

Diagnostic imaging

Imaging of the cardiovascular system is an essential component of cardiac evaluation. Imaging most commonly involves thoracic radiographs and echocardiography, including color flow Doppler, and electrocardiography (ECG). Occasionally ultrasound imaging will be used to assess the size and patency of vessels for determining blood flow.

Survey thoracic radiographs are reviewed for evidence of cardiac disease. Radiographic findings that are suggestive of cardiac disease are listed in Table 11.6. The thoracic radiographs can be used to determine the vertebral heart score, performed to document the presence or absence of cardiomegaly. The procedure for assessing this heart score is outlined in Box 11.1.

Ultrasound imaging of the heart and great vessels (termed echocardiography) has changed the way in which cardiac anatomy is clinically evaluated and is complementary to radiographic imaging. The rapid rate of image acquisition allows evaluation of cardiac motion over time, making it possible to evaluate cardiac function noninvasively. Doppler echocardiography (spectral and color flow Doppler) adds the ability to evaluate blood flow direction and velocity and patterns of blood flow within the heart and great vessels. Transesophageal echocardiography is increasingly used in human intensive care medicine but has not yet become widely available in veterinary medicine.

Because echocardiography can demonstrate cardiac anatomy, cardiac function, and blood flow patterns, it has supplanted cardiac

Table 11.6 Survey radiograph findings suggestive of cardiac disease in the dog and cat.

Disease	Radiographic findings
Dilated cardiomyopathy	Enlarged heart (VHS >10.7 in a dog), ± evidence of CHF, enlarged LA
Hypertrophic cardiomyopathy	May be normal, when severe, cardiomegaly and LA enlargement; valentine-shaped heart and evidence of CHF
Mitral valve disease	Enlarged heart (VHS >10.7 in a dog), ± evidence of CHF, enlarged LA
HWD (*Dirofilaria immitis*)	Right ventricular and atrial enlargement, dilated and tortuous pulmonary arteries, interstitial changes to lungs
Pericardial effusion	Globoid appearance to heart
Pulmonary hypertension	May be normal; right heart enlargement
Pulmonary thromboembolism	May be normal, right side of heart may be enlarged, attenuation (small size) of pulmonary arterial vessels
Congestive heart failure, CHF (dog)	Left atrial enlargement, cardiomegaly, perihilar interstitital to alveolar pulmonary pattern
Congestive heart failure, CHF (cat)	Cardiomegaly may or may not be present, pleural effusion may or may not be present, pulmonary edema may present as variable, diffuse or patchy interstitial to alveolar pattern

CHF, congestive heart failure; LA, left atrium; VHS, vertebral heart score;

catheterization as the preferred method for critically evaluating the heart in clinical veterinary medicine. Although echocardiography is a powerful diagnostic aid, it should not be used in isolation. Rather, it must be considered as one component of a complete cardiovascular examination [1].

Box 11.1 Method for calculating the vertebral heart score (VHS) from survey radiographs in dogs and cats.

1. Perform measurements on a lateral thoracic radiograph.
2. Measure the long axis from the carina (branching of the mainstem bronchus) to the apex of the heart.
3. Measure the short axis of the cardiac silhouette at a 90° angle to the long axis, at the widest part of the cardiac silhouette.
4. Compare the short and long axis lengths to vertebral lengths starting at the cranial aspect of vertebral body of the fourth thoracic vertebra.
5. Add the length of each of these together to determine the VHS.
6. Normal values: dog <10.7 for most breeds; cats <8.0. Pictured below is a dog with a VHS of 9.

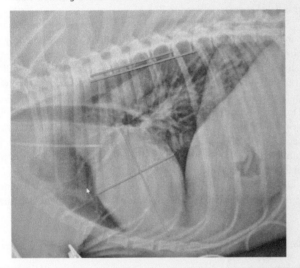

Echocardiography

The two-dimensional examination usually begins on the right side of the thorax and proceeds to the left caudal and ultimately left cranial views. Long axis and short axis view planes can be consistently obtained in most dogs and cats (Figures 11.6, 11.7, and 11.8). The examination can demonstrate the chamber sizes of the heart, wall thickness and movement, valvular movement and lesions, fractional shortening, pericardial changes, and pleural space abnormalities. Normal values for the dog are dependent on the body weight, with normograms provided in the software by the manufacturer of most veterinary ultrasound equipment. Normal values for the cat are listed in Box 11.2. Detailed information regarding how to perform a two-dimensional and M-mode echocardiogram and Doppler flow studies can be found in the references.

Preload, afterload, and contractility determine systolic wall motion and are assessed by the amount of wall contraction seen on an echocardiogram. This is measured by calculating the fractional shortening (FS%). When examining how these factors change in cardiovascular disease, the change in the EDV of the ventricle, the end-systolic volume (ESV) of the ventricle, the wall thickness, and the ability of the ventricle to eject blood into the aorta are determined [1]. The formula for calculating the FS% is presented in Box 11.3, with the result used as an indication of ventricular performance. These variables have been illustrated on the M-mode echocardiogram tracing shown in Figures 11.9 and 11.10. Normal canine long axis echocardiographic images can be found in Figure 11.11 and short axis images in Figure 11.12. Two-dimensional echocardiographic images in the normal cat are illustrated in Figure 11.13.

Myocardial contractility is difficult to define and measure in the clinical setting. No measures of contractility that are entirely independent of preload and afterload are routinely available to the clinician in practice. The FS% can be used as an indicator of myocardial contractility.

Electrocardiogram

The ECG is performed with the patient in right lateral recumbency as a matter of convention, and leads should always be placed on the appropriate limb with a proper conductive agent (electrode gel).

Right parasternal location
Long-axis four-chamber view

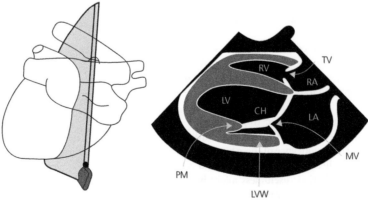

Figure 11.6 Long axis echocardiography views. With the beam plane oriented nearly perpendicular to the long axis of the body, parallel to the long axis of the heart, and with the transducer index mark pointing toward the heart base (dorsal), two views are usually obtained. The first is a four-chamber view with the cardiac apex (ventricles) displayed to the left and the base (atria) to the right. The second, obtained by slight clockwise rotation (when viewed from the bottom of the transducer) of the transducer from the four-chamber view into a slightly more craniodorsal-to-caudoventral orientation, shows the left ventricular outflow tract, aortic valve, aortic root, and proximal ascending aorta. Source: Kittleson MD, Kienle RD, eds. Normal clinical cardiovascular physiology. In: Small Animal Cardiovascular Medicine. St Louis: Mosby. 1998. Used with permission of Elsevier [1].

Long-axis left ventricular outflow viwe

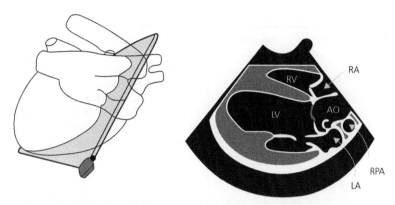

Figure 11.7 Schematic representations of the long axis echocardiography views obtained from the right parasternal window. The black circle at the top of the sector indicates the index mark. Source: Keinle RD, Thomas WP. Echocardiography. In: Veterinary Diagnostic Ultrasound. Nyland T, Mattoon J, eds. Philadelphia: WB Saunders, 1995. Used with permission of Elsevier. AO, aorta; LA, left atrium; LC, left coronary cusp of the aortic valve; LV, left ventricle; RPA, right pulmonary artery; RV, right ventricle.

Right parasternal location

Short-axis views

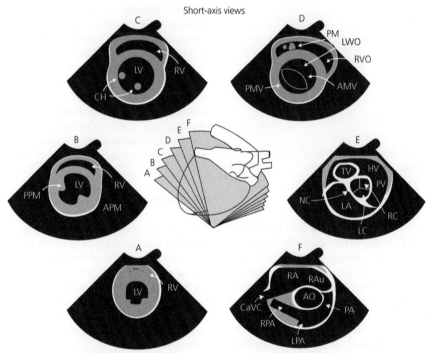

Figure 11.8 Short axis echocardiography views. By rotating the transducer approximately 90° clockwise from the four-chamber view so that the beam plane is oriented close to the long axis of the body and perpendicular to the long axis of the heart and the transducer index mark is pointing cranially (or cranioventrally), a series of short axis views are obtained. Proper short axis orientation is identified by the circular symmetry of the left ventricle or aortic root. Short axis planes are commonly obtained at the level of the left ventricular apex, papillary muscles, chordae tendineae, mitral valve, and aortic valve by angling the beam from the apex (ventral) to the base (dorsal). In most animals, further dorsal angulation and slight rotation allow imaging of the proximal ascending aorta, right atrium, and pulmonary artery branches. The images should be displayed with the cranial part of the image to the right and the right heart encircling the left ventricle and aorta clockwise (the right ventricular outflow tract and pulmonary valve to the right). Source: Kittleson MD, Kienle RD, eds. Normal clinical cardiovascular physiology. In: Small Animal Cardiovascular Medicine. St Louis: Mosby. 1998. Used with permission of Elsevier [1]. AMV, anterior mitral valve leaflet; AO, aorta; APM, anterior papillary muscle; AV, aortic valve; CaVC, caudal vena cava; CH, chorda tendineae; LA, left atrium; LC, left coronary cusp of the aortic valve; LPA, left pulmonary artery; LV, left ventricle; LVO, left ventricular outflow tract; MV, mitral valve; NC, noncoronary cusp of the aortic valve; PA, pulmonary artery; PM, papillary muscle; PMV, posterior mitral valve leaflet; PPM, posterior papillary muscle; PV, pulmonary valve; RA, right atrium; RC, right coronary cusp of the aortic valve; RPA, right pulmonary artery; RV, right ventricle; RVO, right ventricular outflow tract; TV, tricuspid valve; VS, interventricular septum.

Box 11.2 Normal values for feline echocardiogram.

Parameter	Value (mm)	Parameter	Value (mm)
IVSTd	3–6	RVIDd	3–7
LVIDd	10–21	RVWd	<3
LVPWd	3–6	Ao systole	6–12
IVSTs	4–9	LAd	7–15
LVIDs	4–11	LA:Ao	0.8–1.4
LVPWs	4–10	FS	>40%
EPSS	0–3	EF	>70%

Ao, aorta; d, diastole; EF, ejection fraction; EPSS, E point to septal separation; FS, fractional shortening; IVST, interventricular septal thickness; LA, left atrium; LVID, left ventricular internal diameter; LVPW, left ventricular posterior wall; mm, millimeters; RVID, right ventricular internal diameter; RVW, right ventricular wall; s, systole

Box 11.3 Calculation for the fractional shortening and ejection fraction determined by echocardiogram.

Fractional shortening

$$FS(\%) = \left[(LVDd - LVDs) / LVDd\right] \times 100$$

Normal FS (%) = 35–55% (dog), 39–61% (cat), with compensated typical mitral regurgitation, >45%.

Ejection fraction

$$EF(\%) = SV / EDV$$

where: SV = EDV-ESV
EDV, end-diastolic volume; ESV, end-systolic volume; LVD, left ventricular diameter; SV, stroke volume.

The lead II ECG strip is the most commonly recorded rhythm strip for the ICU patient. The ECG measures time on the horizontal axis and amplitude or millivolts on the vertical axis. These should be standardized prior to recording the tracing. Electrocardiographic paper usually has "hatch" marks along the top or the bottom of the paper, which occur either every 50 mm (standard) or 75 mm to aid in identifying a specific length (time frame) [1].

Assessment of the ECG begins with determining the heart rate. Counting the heart rate on a portion of the ECG recorded at 25 mm/ sec is easier and uses less paper. To determine the number of complexes in six seconds, identify a segment of the ECG that is 150 mm in length. The number of complexes within this span are counted and multiplied by 10 to give the number of complexes in one minute. The longer the time over which the heart rate is counted, the more accurate the count will be.

The location of the positive and negative recording leads will determine the characteristics of the waveforms. The limb leads record the ECG in the coronal (dorsal-ventral) plane, and can be used to determine the electrical axis. The limb leads are called leads I, II, III, AVR, AVL, and AVF.

Determining the rate at which an ectopic focus is firing or the rate at which an escape rhythm is depolarizing at any point is often useful when determining treatment options. Arrhythmias commonly produce irregularities in the heart rate (varying intervals between complexes). Consequently, the heart rate can vary from beat to beat. Normally the sinus node acts as the pacemaker of the heart, and normal myocardium cannot depolarize spontaneously. However, damaged myocardium can depolarize spontaneously. It can do this for periods and then stop. If a region of ventricular myocardium was damaged and started to depolarize spontaneously and it did so at a rate faster than the sinus node, it would take over the cardiac rhythm. The faster a ventricular ectopic focus such as this fires, the more malignant the arrhythmia is likely to be. To determine how fast it is firing, the distance between the last sinus complex and the first ventricular premature complex is measured. If one second is present between these complexes, there is one complex each second, and the rate at which the ventricular site is firing is 60 beats/min. If 0.5 seconds are between them, that would mean that two complexes are present every second (1/0.5), so the rate would be 120 beats/min. The formula for determining this "instantaneous" heart rate is: rate = 60 (sec/min) ÷ R-R interval (sec/beat), where R-R is the distance between two QRS complexes measured in seconds [1].

The ECG is most commonly used to determine heart rhythm. Several electrocardiographic complex height and interval measurements are evaluated. Lead II is always used to measure heights and intervals. Whenever possible, calipers are used to make ECG measurements. Normal values for intervals between complexes, durations of P-QRS-T complexes, and heights of these complexes are listed in Table 11.7. Whenever measuring intervals, heights, and durations, do not include the width of the line in the measurement. Line width can often be 1 mm which, if included in a measurement, can produce significant error [2]. Box 11.4 discusses an easy five-step approach for the evaluation of the ECG. While the mean electrical axis can be determined from the electrocardiogram, advances in echocardiography have made the clinical use of this parameter of less importance.

Monitoring procedures

The physical peripheral perfusion parameters (heart rate, pulse intensity, mucous membrane color, CRT) provide the basics for monitoring the effects of cardiac performance on perfusion in the critical small animal patient. The fluid balance and blood pressure are monitored as important factors that affect the CO. Equipment-based monitoring of indices associated with cardiac performance can include ECG, blood pressure, central venous pressure, echocardiographic parameters, and, rarely, thermodilution catheter techniques.

Arterial blood pressure is the product of CO multiplied by systemic vascular resistance. Both indirect and direct methods of arterial blood pressure measurement are detailed in Chapter 3. The heart rate is always assessed with the blood pressure. Common causes of hypotension can include insufficient preload (ventricular filling), inadequate myocardial contractility or decreased systemic vascular resistance (vasodilation). The blood pressure can be within the normal range due to compensatory tachycardia stimulated by hypovolemia that is detected by the baroreceptors. Very rapid heart rates, regardless of the cause, can be detrimental to the heart muscle and will eventually contribute to diminished cardiac output and worsening hypotension. Hypertension can be a result of cardiac disorders or contribute to cardiac dysfunction (see Chapter 3). Monitoring the trends of change in blood

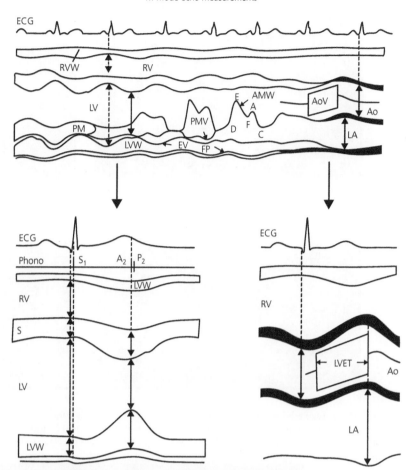

Figure 11.9 Variables of M-mode echocardiography. Recommended methods for echocardiographic measurements from the M-mode echocardiogram. The standard M-mode sweep from the level of the left ventricular papillary muscles to the level of the aorta and left atrium, showing the locations and timing of chamber dimension and wall thickness measurements. Source: Keinle RD, Thomas WP. Echocardiography. In: Veterinary Diagnostic Ultrasound. Nyland T, Mattoon J, eds. Philadelphia: WB Saunders, 1995. Used with permission of Elsevier. For abbreviations see Figures 11.6 and 11.7.

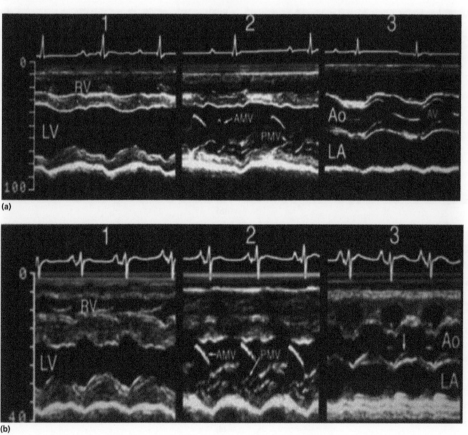

Figure 11.10 M-mode echocardiographic images from a normal dog and cat. (a) Normal canine M-mode echocardiograms recorded at the level of the (1) left ventricle, (2) mitral valve, and (3) aorta and left atrium. (b) Normal feline M-mode echocardiogram recorded at the same levels as in (a) (arrow indicates the aortic valve). Source: Keinle RD, Thomas WP. Echocardiography. In: Veterinary Diagnostic Ultrasound. Nyland T, Mattoon J, eds. Philadelphia: WB Saunders, 1995. Used with permission of Elsevier. For abbreviations see Figures 11.6 and 11.7.

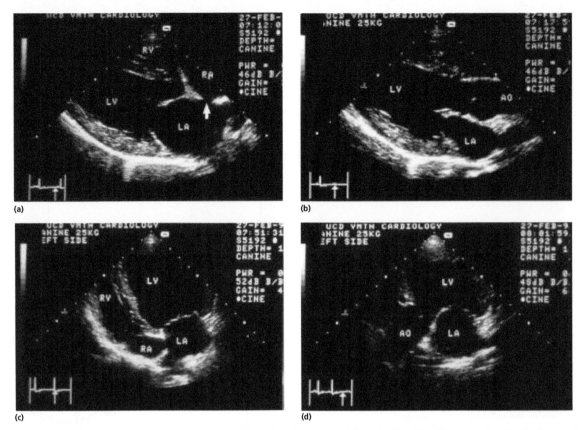

Figure 11.11 Long axis echocardiographic images from a normal dog. (a) Right parasternal four-chamber view. The arrow identifies the fossa ovalis, which may falsely appear to be a septal defect. (b) Right parasternal long axis view. (c) Left caudal (apical) parasternal four-chamber view. (d) Left caudal (apical) parasternal long axis view (five-chamber view) [25]. For abbreviations see Figures 11.6 and 11.7.

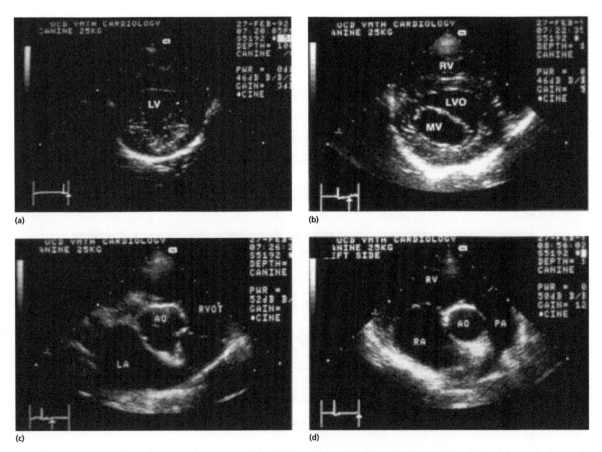

Figure 11.12 Short axis echocardiographic images from a normal dog. (a) Right parasternal short axis view at the level of the left ventricular papillary muscles. (b) Right parasternal short axis view at the level of the mitral valve. (c) Right parasternal short axis view at the level of the aortic valve. (d) Left cranial parasternal short axis view at the level of the aortic valve [25]. For abbreviations see Figures 11.6 and 11.7.

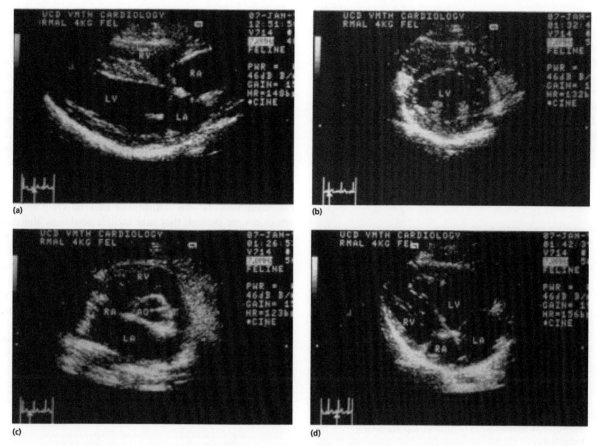

Figure 11.13 Two-dimensional echocardiographic images from a normal cat. (a) Right parasternal four-chamber view. (b) Right parasternal short axis view at the level of the left ventricular papillary muscles. (c) Right parasternal short axis view at the level of the aortic valve. (d) Left caudal (apical) parasternal four-chamber view [25]. For abbreviations see Figures 11.6 and 11.7.

Table 11.7 Normal values for heart rate, intervals between complexes, durations of P-QRS-T complexes, and heights of complexes. At paper speed of 25 mm/sec, each small box = 0.04 sec. At paper speed of 50 mm/sec, each small box = 0.02 sec. s = seconds, mV = milivolts, bpm = beats per minute.

	P (s)	PQ/PR (s)	QRS (s)	QT (s)	HR (bpm)	P (lead II) mV	R (lead II), mV
Dog	0.04	0.06–0.13	0.05–0.06	0.15–0.28	60–160	0.4	2.5–3.0
Cat	0.04	0.05–0.09	Up to 0.04	0.12–0.20	140–240	0.2	0.9

bpm, beats per minute, mV, millivolts; s, seconds.

pressure, in conjunction with the assessment of the physical perfusion parameters, is important for evaluating the impact of therapy and any improvement or decline in the status of the patient.

Continuous ECG monitoring is important in any patient with severe systemic disease, trauma, anesthesia or a potential for cardiac dysfunction. The heart rate and rhythm are assessed on an ongoing basis, allowing rapid intervention should declining trends of change occur. Decisions pertaining to drug therapy for any identified dysrhythmia or arrhythmia are based on the ECG findings, blood pressure, and physical parameters of the patient [26].

Cardiac output monitoring by placement of a pulmonary artery catheter is not widely utilized in clinical veterinary medicine. Few guidelines are available for placement of catheters in the dog and cat and complications associated with invasive monitoring can be high. No consensus currently exists regarding the interpretation of data obtained from the pulmonary artery catheter in the dog and cat.

Additional information regarding pulmonary artery catheter placement and the data obtained can be found in the further reading and references.

Methods such as pulse contour analysis, transesophageal echocardiography, and thoracic bioimpedance are considered less invasive, but have still not been widely adapted for monitoring cardiac output in the dog and cat. Pulse contour analysis is invasive, requiring placement of a central venous catheter and peripheral arterial catheter.

Disorders of cardiac performance

Cardiac performance is influenced by many factors, including heart rate, rhythm, myocardial contractility, valvular function, alterations in preload and afterload, and pericardial properties (Table 11.8, Figure 11.14). It may be further modified by neural control, drugs, hormones, and metabolic products [1]. Clinical signs can vary, ranging from syncope and seizures to respiratory distress, abdominal effusion, and even cardiac arrest.

Circulatory shock can be a consequence of any cause of poor cardiac performance. Yet, abnormalities of heart rate and rhythm are treated quite differently from abnormalities of myocardial contractility. Therefore, careful evaluation of the physical signs manifested by the patient and the diagnostic data collected is required to develop a therapeutic plan that is specific for the patient and for their cardiac disorder.

Box 11.4 Five steps for interpreting the electrocardiogram (ECG).

1. Identify the leads, paper speed, amplitude, and species.
   At 25 mm/sec: big square = 0.2 sec; small square = 0.04 sec
2. Identify the waveforms: PQRST
   P – depolarization of atria
   Q – first negative deflection after P-wave
   R – positive deflection after P-wave
   S – negative deflection after R-wave
   T – repolarization of the ventricles
3. Determine HR: fast? slow? normal?
4. Identify the predominant underlying rhythm.
   Is the QRS wide or narrow?
      Most wide and bizarre QRS are ventricular in origin
      Most narrow QRS are supraventricular in origin
   Are the R-R intervals regular, irregular or irregularly irregular?
      Regular: sinus rhythm, AV block, sinus bradycardia, ventricular tachycardia, sinus tachycardia, supraventricular tachycardia
      Irregular: sinus arrhythmia, bursts of ventricular or sinus tachycardia, intermittent (2°) AV block
      Irregularly irregular: atrial fibrillation, sick sinus syndrome, premature ventricular or atrial beats
   Are there P-waves? Associated with the QRS?
      Always associated: sinus or atrial rhythm, atrial premature complexes
      Sometimes associated: 2° AV block, premature ventricular or junctional complexes
      Never associated: 3° AV block, ventricular tachycardia
5. Identify other abnormalities: premature beats, paroxysmal (bursts) of tachycardia, AV blocks, alterations in QRS complexes, wandering pacemaker.
   Larger amplitude R-wave – left ventricular hypertrophy
   Tall T – consider hyperkalemia as cause
   Tall, tented P-wave – right atrial enlargement
   "M"-shaped P-wave – left atrial enlargement
   Large S-wave – right ventricular hypertrophy
   S-T segment depression – consider hypoxia, pericarditis

Disorders of cardiac rate and rhythm

A cardiac arrhythmia is a condition where the heart rate is too fast, too slow or irregular. The arrhythmia is a consequence of an abnormality within the cardiac conduction system (see Figure 11.5). The major mechanisms causing conduction disturbances include excessive stimulation or inhibition of the SA node, automaticity, reentry phenomenon, and fibrillation.

The cause of heart arrhythmias in the critical small animal patient can include one or more of the following: organic heart disease, myocardial trauma, hypoxia or inflammation, severe systemic disease with circulating chemical mediators (sepsis), catastrophic alterations in body temperature, severe hypotension or hypertension, electrolyte abnormalities, hypoxemia, and hypercarbia. Many patients with arrhythmias have no symptoms. When symptoms are present, they may include weakness, shortness of breath, exercise intolerance, hypotension, and syncope. While many arrhythmias are not serious (such as sinus arrhythmia, premature atrial contractions), some can predispose to complications such as hypotension, pulmonary edema, thromboembolism, and cardiac arrest. It is important to identify any contributing cause (such as hypoxemia, hyperkalemia, vasovagal reflex) and manage those during the course of treatment.

Arrhythmias are diagnosed by evaluating the ECG. While lead II is the primary rhythm strip examined, leads I and III can provide additional data regarding the mean electrical axis of the heart. The ECG waveforms and intervals to measure are illustrated in Figure 11.5.

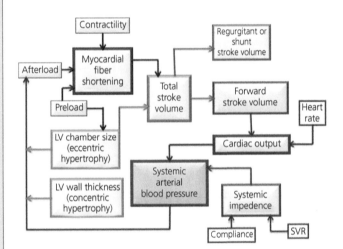

Figure 11.14 Factors involved in systolic function of the heart, factors that determine cardiac output, and factors involved in determining systemic arterial blood pressure and their interrelationships [1]. LV, left ventricle; SVR, systemic vascular resistance.

Table 11.8 Etiologies of poor cardiac output by category.

Decreased heart rate	Decreased Preload	Increased Afterload	Decreased contractility	Structural abnormalities
Arrhythmias Shock Electrolyte abnormalities Severe acidemia or alkalemia Cardiac arrest	Hypovolemia Hemorrhage Obstructions to preload (gastric dilation-volvulus, adrenal or other neoplasia, pericardial effusion) Severe tachycardia Hypertrophic cardiomyopathy	Pulmonary hypertension, systemic hypertension, valvular stenosis	Dilated cardiomyopathy End-stage valvular disease	Valvular disease Congenital heart disease

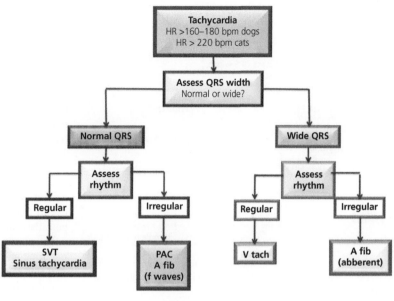

Figure 11.15 A decision-making algorithm to aid in determining the ECG diagnosis when there is a tachycardia. A Fib, atrial fibrillation; HR, heart rate; PAC, premature atrial contraction; SVT, supraventricular tachycardia; V Tach, ventricular tachycardia.

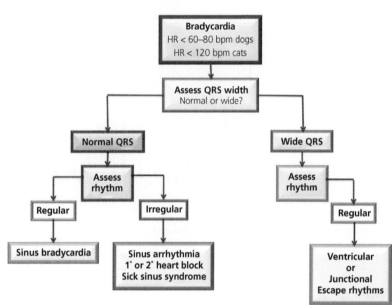

Figure 11.16 A decision-making algorithm to aid in determining the ECG diagnosis when there is bradycardia. HR, heart rate.

The five-step approach to assessing the ECG is provided in Box 11.4. The heart rate is identified as fast (tachycardia), slow (bradycardia) or normal. Algorithms to guide the identification of common arrhythmias in the dog and cat are provided for tachycardia in Figure 11.15, bradycardia in Figure 11.16, and normal heart rates in Figure 11.17. Extra beats can occur with normal or fast heart rates and include premature atrial contractions and premature ventricular contractions.

The more common arrhythmias seen in the small animal ICU patient are listed according to heart rate in Tables 11.9, 11.10, and 11.11, with the ECG criteria for diagnosis and treatment options. Some arrhythmias may require specific therapy and others may simply warrant close patient monitoring while the underlying cause is investigated and treated. The decision for pharmacological intervention should be based on factors such as impaired perfusion due to the arrhythmia, the rate and that the inciting cause can be corrected, the presence of a prefibrillatory arrhythmia (such as R on T phenomena, ventricular flutter, torsade de pointes) and any immediate plans for anesthesia or surgery for the patient.

Tachyarrhythmias that are causing poor perfusion, rapidly progressing, pathologically rapid (impairing ventricular filling) or prefibrillatory warrant pharmacological intervention. Tachyarrhythmias commonly diagnosed in the small animal critical patient are listed in Table 11.9, with the criteria for ECG diagnosis and therapeutic options. Antiarrhythmic agents are divided into classes and are listed in Table 11.12 with their mechanism of action, examples of drugs, and indications for use. Drug doses and possible side-effects for the antiarrhythmic agents can be found in Table 11.13. Refractory atrial fibrillation can predispose to thromboembolic events and has been successfully treated with biphasic transthoracic cardioversion and transesophageal cardioversion in the dog [27].

Clinically significant bradyarrhythmias result in signs of poor perfusion, weakness or depressed mentation and can require pharmacological intervention. Drug options for treatment include atropine, glycopyrrolate, sympathomimetics (such as dopamine, dobutamine, isoproterenol), terbutaline or aminophylline. Doses for these drugs are listed in Table 11.13.

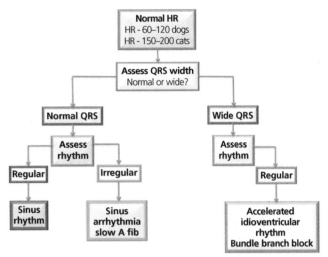

Figure 11.17 A decision-making algorithm to aid in determining the ECG diagnosis when there is a normal heart rate. A Fib, atrial fibrillation; HR, heart rate.

Indications for cardiac pacemaker placement include failure of bradycardia to respond to drug therapy and primary organic cardiac conduction disorders causing poor cardiac output. Bradyarrhythmias that can require pacemaker therapy include third degree AV block, second degree AV block, atrial standstill, sick sinus syndrome, and others.

Temporary cardiac pacing can be achieved with transvenous pacing, transesophageal pacing, transthoracic pacing, epicardial pacing, and thump pacing as a temporary maneuver. Of these, transvenous and transthoracic pacing are used more commonly in veterinary medicine. Transvenous pacing (Medtronic, Minneapolis, MN) is safe and reliable but requires the appropriate equipment and training for placement. Transthoracic pacing is easy to apply to patients. Many defibrillators have the ability to provide this pacing, but require general anesthesia due to pain associated with the procedure; skin burns are another potential complication (LifePak®, Physio-Control, Redmond, WA).

Permanent pacemaker placement is a surgical procedure requiring an experienced cardiac surgeon. Complications associated with permanent transvenous pacemaker implantation include lead dislodgment, infection, hematoma formation, skeletal muscle

Table 11.9 Common ECG tachycardia rhythms in the dog and cat with common characteristics and possible treatment options.

Sinus tachycardia - normal P-QRS-T complexes

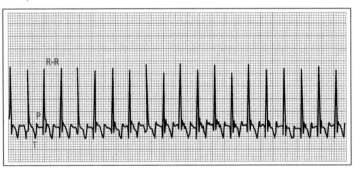

Treat pain, anxiety, hypotension, hypovolemia or other underlying problems

Atrial fibrillation – narrow QRS, irregularly irregular rhythm, f waves

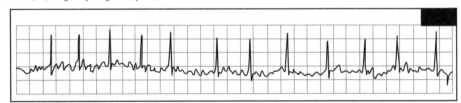

Treat ventricular response rate to optimize perfusion. Often requires diltiazem or digoxin. Ablation or cardioconversion have been utilized if unresponsive to drug therapy.

Ventricular tachycardia – wide QRS, not associated with P-wave

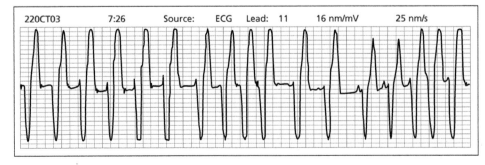

Treat if poor perfusion, hypotension, R on T phenomenon, torsade de pointes, multiform waves. Lidocaine IV following by CRI typical first choice antiarrhythmic drug.

Table 11.9 (*Continued*)

Ventricular premature contractions – individual wide, bizarre QRS not associated with P-wave

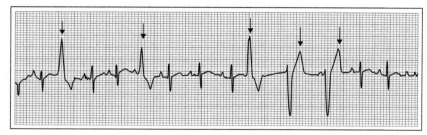

Treat underlying conditions. Lidocaine is given if poor perfusion and hypotension persist.

Run of ventricular tachycardia – wide bizarre QRS, rapid, in a series intermittent with normal beats

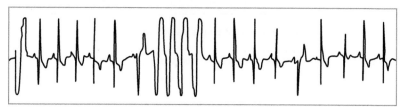

Treatment same as for ventricular tachycardia.

Accelerated idioventricular rhythm – wide QRS, rate 80–150

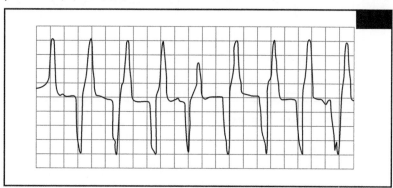

Treat underlying problems. Lidocaine IV and CRI if associated with persistent hypotension.

Ventricular flutter to fibrillation – no recognizable P-QRS-T, chaotic, rhythm of arrest

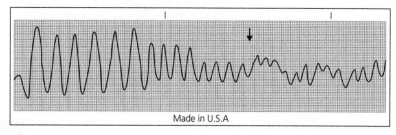

Treat by immediately initiating CPR, defibrillate as soon as possible.

Other tachyarrhythmias
Pulseless ventricular tachycardia – appears similar to ventricular tachycardia, rhythm of arrest.
Treat by immediately initiating CPR.
Torsades de pointes – wide QRS, similar to ventricular tachycardia with oscillation of the peaks of R and T-waves. Treat first with magnesium sulfate, followed by lidocaine or other antiarrhythmic if nonresponsive.
Paroxysmal supraventricular tachycardia – narrow QRS, P-wave morphology may vary depending upon origin of beats. Treat with vagal maneuver if AV node-dependent rhythm, diltiazem, esmolol or adenosine.

Table 11.10 Common ECG bradycardia rhythms in dogs and cats with characteristic features and possible treatment options.

Sinus bradycardia – narrow QRS, regular rhythm, P-wave associated with QRS

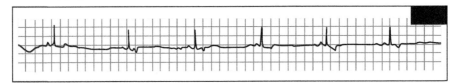

Treat underlying disease (concern for increased intracranial pressure), electrolyte disorders; can treat with atropine, glycopyrrolate, or beta-agonists if poor perfusion persists.

Atrioventricular block 1°: increased P-R interval, narrow QRS, P-QRS still associated

Atrioventricular block 2°: narrow QRS, P without QRS

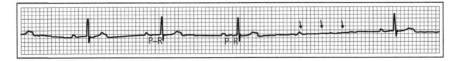

Treatment generally not required; if associated with poor perfusion treat as sinus bradycardia.

Atrioventricular block 3°: wide QRS, P-waves and QRS not associated, independent rates

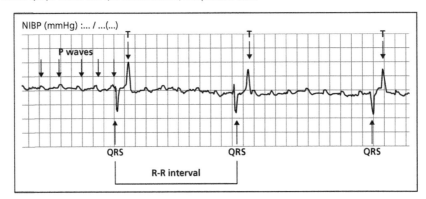

Treat initially as sinus bradycardia, may require pacemaker implantation.

Asystole – no discernible P-QRS-T waveforms, flatline ECG, arrest arrhythmia

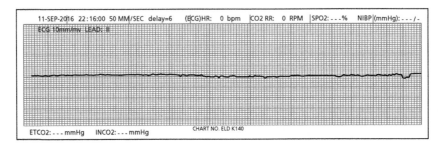

Treat by initiating CPR.

Atrial standstill – wide QRS (ventricular escape beats), no visible P-wave.

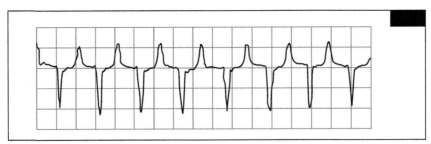

Treat for hyperkalemia (most common cause).

Sick sinus syndrome – paroxysmal bradycardia mixed with paroxysmal tachycardia. Treat temporarily with atropine, glycopyrrolate or beta-agonists; pacemaker implantation if poor cardiac output.

Table 11.11 Common ECG normal heart rate rhythms with characteristic features and possible treatment.

Normal sinus rhythm – narrow QRS, P-wave for each QRS

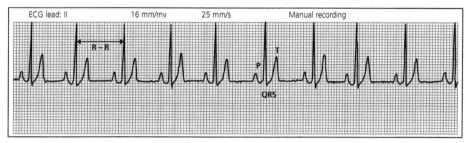

Slow atrial fibrillation – narrow QRS, no associated P-wave, f waves, irregularly irregular rhythm

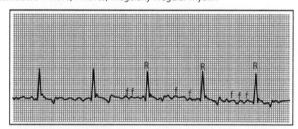

No specific treatment if heart rate and cardiac output are acceptable.

Right bundle branch block – normal rate with wide and negative QRS (deep S-wave) in lead II

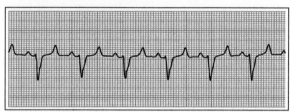

No specific treatment required.

Electrical alternans - normal rate with alternating tall and short R waves, suggestive of pericardial effusion.

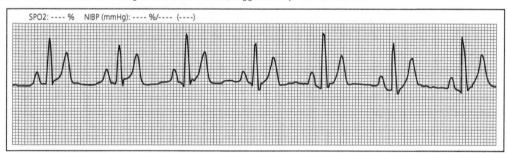

Investigate for pericardial effusion; pericardiocentesis may be warranted.

Left bundle branch block – P for each QRS, wide QRS is positive and bizarre. Complete cardiac evaluation required; cardiac pacing may be required.

stimulation, ventricular arrhythmia, migration of the pulse generator, and skin erosion. A study of permanent transvenous cardiac pacing in 40 dogs found that it is a feasible, less traumatic alternative to epimyocardial pacing. However, successful use requires careful implantation technique and anticipation of the potential complications [28]. Pacemaker pacing rates are typically 60–100 bpm in dogs and 100 bpm in cats.

Antiarrhythmic agents can actually worsen existing arrhythmias. This occurrence is called the proarrhythmic effect of antiarrhythmic drugs. The proarrhythmic effect can be manifested by increasing the duration or frequency of the arrhythmia, increasing the number of

premature complexes or couplets, altering the rate of the arrhythmia or causing new arrhythmias [29]. Arrhythmogenesis in the setting of a long QT interval may be related to marked asynchrony of repolarization. Three types of proarrhythmias have been described: ventricular (torsade de pointes, monophasic and polyphasic ventricular tachycardia, fibrillation), atrial (atrial flutter, increased defibrillation threshold) and abnormal conduction or impulse formation (sinus node dysfunction, AV block, accelerated ventricular rate in atrial fibrillation). An increased incidence has been found in humans with left ventricular systolic dysfunction. Antiarrhythmic drugs that have been associated with this proarrhythmic effect include Class IA

Table 11.12 Common antiarrhythmic drugs used in the dog and cat.

Drug class	Mechanism	Drugs	Indication
I	Na channel blocker (membrane stabilizing) Ia – intermittent association/dissociation, K channel-blocking effect Ib – fast association/dissociation Ic – slow association/dissociation	Procainamide (Ia) Lidocaine (Ib) Mexilitine (Ib) Flecainide (Ic)	Multiform VPC VT
II	Beta-blocker (sympatholytic)	Esmolol Propranolol Sotalol Atenolol Carvedilol	SVT Sympathetically stimulated VT
III	K channel blocker (prolongs repolarization)	Amiodarone Sotalol	SVT VT
IV	Ca channel blocker	Diltiazem	AF SVT
Other	Inhibits Na-K-ATPase pump	Digoxin	SVT Rapid AF

AF, atrial fibrillation; APTase, adenosine triphosphatase; Ca, calcium; K, potassium; Na, sodium; SVT, supraventricular tachycardia; VPC, ventricular premature contraction; VT, ventricular tachycardia.

(quinidine, procainamide), Class IC (flecainide), and Class III (amiodarone, sotalol) drugs. The use of these drugs warrants close monitoring of the ECG for signs of Q-T prolongation [30].

Disorders of cardiac contraction

The heart's ability to pump an adequate amount of blood to peripheral tissues (an adequate forward cardiac output) is determined by at least six factors: the usual four factors taught in cardiovascular physiology that deal with the normal heart (preload, afterload, contractility, and heart rate) and two additional factors that must be considered when cardiovascular disease is present – cardiac hypertrophy and leaks in the cardiovascular system [4]. These factors, their interrelationships, and their effect on cardiac output are depicted in Figure 11.14.

The radius of the systemic arterioles is the primary determinant of resistance and impedance. Consequently, both can be manipulated with vasodilators and vasoconstrictors. Impedance is also influenced by the stiffness of the aorta and several other factors. Heart failure stimulates the constriction of systemic arterioles and stiffening of the aorta by increasing sympathetic tone and increasing the circulating concentration of angiotensin II [1].

Cardiogenic shock

Cardiogenic shock is a life-threatening medical condition resulting from failure of the ventricles of the heart to function effectively, causing inadequate tissue (end-organ) perfusion. This results in decreased oxygen and nutrient delivery to the tissues and, when prolonged, potentially end-organ damage and multisystem failure. Patients with cardiogenic shock have a low cardiac output, elevated filling pressures of the left, right or both ventricles, and a decreased mixed venous oxygen saturation. The systemic vascular resistance is often high in response to the baroreceptor response, but it can be normal or low. Individuals with normal or low systemic vascular resistance often have profound hypoperfusion and an inflammatory response, with an associated worse prognosis.

Causes of cardiogenic shock can be categorized into one of three mechanisms: cardiomyopathic (myocardial dysfunction), mechanical (pericardial tamponade, ruptured chamber, ruptured chordae) or arrhythmias. Cardiogenic shock can be a largely irreversible condition, depending on the cause, and as such is more often fatal than other forms of shock. It is also not uncommon for hypovolemic, distributive, septic or hemorrhagic shock to occur simultaneously with cardiogenic shock.

Numerous studies have demonstrated evidence of myocardial depression during septic syndromes and systemic inflammatory response syndromes. Septic cardiomyopathy has been defined as a global but reversible dysfunction of both the left and right sides of the heart, with left ventricular contractile dysfunction common [31]. The pathogenesis of myocardial depression in sepsis is the result of a complex interaction between genetic, molecular, structural, autonomic, and hemodynamic alterations [32]. Although patients with sepsis have profound myocardial depression, cardiac output is usually maintained because of cardiac dilation and tachycardia [33]. There was no evidence of injury to cardiac myocytes in the patient with myocardial depression. It is speculated that the cardiac dysfunction can be explained by "cell stunning," similar to what occurs during myocardial ischemia [34]. Presumably, sepsis activates defense mechanisms that cause cellular processes reduced to basic "housekeeping" roles with immunostimulated cells experiencing diminished oxygen consumption.

The clinical signs of cardiogenic shock are the same as the signs seen with other causes of shock. Tachycardia (dogs), bradycardia (cats, decompensatory sign in dogs), weak or absent pulses, pale or white mucous membranes and prolonged (>3 seconds) or absent CRT are common physical perfusion parameters found with severe hypotension. Oliguria (<0.5 mL/kg/h) can be evident as well as cool extremities and altered level of consciousness. An arrhythmia, heart murmur or gallop, pulmonary edema or other signs of heart failure might be discovered to direct diagnostic efforts towards a cardiogenic cause of hypotension.

Treatment of cardiogenic shock depends on the cardiac disorder and whether or not other causes of shock are present. Unfortunately, most forms of shock present with similar clinical signs and multiple causes may not be readily apparent. Oxygen supplementation is recommended during the course of resuscitation. The cardiac output in septic shock can be improved by infusing fluids (increasing the preload) and administering vasopressors (supporting systemic vascular resistance). This is not likely to be the case with pure cardiogenic shock.

The heart is an organ that cannot tolerate large volumes of intravenous fluids when it is dysfunctional. An assessment of the patient

Table 11.13 Medications used with cardiac disease in critical care.

Drug	Mechanism/ indication	Dose	Side-effects
Adenosine	Vagomimetic action (negative ino-, chrono- and dromotropic); paroxysmal SVTs, other wide QRS tachycardias	2 mg/kg IV	Hypotension
Aminophylline	Phosphodiesterase inhibitor, bronchodilator, increases epinephrine; clinically significant bradyarrhythmias	10 mg/kg PO q 12 h or 10 mg/kg IV, 4 mg/kg IM (cat)	Tachyarrythmias, CNS stimulation, GI signs
Amiodarone	Class III antiarrhythmic (K channel blocker, although demonstrates Class I, II, and IV effects); SVTs and ventricular tachyarrhythmias	5 mg/kg over 10 minutes; 10–25 mg/kg PO	Hypotension, bradycardia, potentially pulmonary fibrosis
Amlodipine	Smooth muscle calcium channel blocker; hypertension	0.2–0.4 mg/kg PO q 12 h	Hypotension and bradycardia are possible
Amrinone	Phosphodiesterase inhibitor and other venodilating, inotropic properties; second line for CHF	0.75 mg/kg slow IV then CRI of 5–10 μg/kg/min (dog); 1–3 mg/kg slow IV, then CRI of 30–100 μg/kg/min (cat)	Arrhythmias, hypotension, GI effects
Aspirin (acetylsalicylic acid)	Inhibits cyclooxygenase (thromboxane and platelet aggregation); thromboprophylaxis	0.5 mg/kg PO q 12 h or cats ¼ of 81 mg tablet PO q 24 h	GI ulceration, inhibition of normal platelet function
Atenolol	Class II antiarrhythmic (beta-blocker); SVTs, Afib, Aflutter	0.25–1 mg/kg PO q 12–24 h	Contraindicated in AV block, SSS, bronchiolar disease; bradycardia and CHF
Atropine	Parasympatholytic	0.02–0.04 mg/kg IV	Tachycardia, contraindicated with glaucoma; dry mouth and other GI effects
Benazepril	ACE inhibitor; CHF, hypertension and protein-losing disease	0.25–0.5 mg/kg PO q 12–24 h	Transient azotemia, GI effects, hypotension (theoretically)
Carvedilol	Nonselective beta- and alpha-blocker; hypertension and CHF	0.5 mg/kg PO q 12 h	Starting at a low dose and increasing over time; dose must be carefully titrated and monitored; hypotension and bradycardia
Clopidogrel	Thienopyridine (ADP receptor antagonist, antiplatelet drug); thromboprophylaxis	18.75–mg (1/4 of 75–mg tablet) PO q 24 h (cat); 0.5–4 mg/kg PO q 24 h (dog)	Bleeding
Digoxin	Cardiac glycoside (Na/K ATPase antagonist); positive inotrope and used for supraventricular tachyarrhythmias (parasympathomimetic action)	0.003 mg/kg PO q 12 h (cat), 0.2 mg/m² PO q 12 h (dog), adjusted based on blood levels; may be given incrementally IV at ¼ of 0.01–0.03 mg/kg IV q 30–60 min	GI upset, loss of appetite, ECG and electrolyte changes; monitoring ECG and blood pressure with IV administration is necessary; monitoring blood levels recommended due to narrow therapeutic index
Diltiazem	Class IV antiarrhythmic (calcium channel blocker); supraventricular tachyarrhythmias	0.125–0.35 mg/kg IV slowly over 2–3 min; same dose as a CRI/h; 0.5–1 mg/kg PO q 8 h	Hypotension, negative chronotropy, arrhythmias
Dobutamine	Beta-agonist, high-dose alpha-agonist, inotropy, chronotropy, arteriolar vasodilation, vasoconstriction (high); positive inotrope (DCM, severe MVD) with CHF	2–20 μg/kg/min (dog), 1–5 μg/kg/min (cat)	Arrhythmias, hypertension; ECG and blood pressure should be monitored continuously
Dopamine	Dopaminergic agonist (low dose), beta-agonist (mid dose), alpha-agonist (high dose); positive inotropy, chronotropy, vasodilation, vasoconstriction (high); hypotension	2–10 μg/kg/min (dog), 1–5 μg/kg/min (cat)	Arrhythmias, hypertension, ECG and blood pressure should be monitored continuously
Enalapril	ACE inhibitor; CHF and hypertension	0.25–0.5 mg/kg PO q 12–24 h	See Benazepril
Epinephrine	Beta- and alpha-agonist, positive inotrope, chronotrope, vasodilation, vasoconstriction (high); CPR and hypotension	0.01–0.1 μg/kg/min	Excitability, hyper- and hypotension, arrhythmias
Esmolol	Beta-blocker; supraventricular tachyarrhythmias	0.5 mg/kg IV over 1–2 min then 50–200 μg/kg/min CRI	Ultra short-acting; hypotension and bradycardia
Furosemide	Loop diuretic (inhibits Na-K-2Cl co-transporter in thick ascending limb); CHF	1–4 mg/kg IM or IV initially, 0.5–2 mg/kg/h CRI	Hypochloremic alkalemia, dehydration
Glycopyrrolate	See atropine	0.01–mg/kg IV	Tachycardia, dry mouth
Heparin, unfractionated (LMWH, see Chapter 9)	Inhibits action of coagulation factors II, IX, X, XI, XII; thromboprophylaxis	60–100 IU/kg SC q 8 h	Hypocoagulation should be monitored with coagulation tests
Isoproterenol	Beta-agonist, positive inotrope, chronotrope, vasodilation; AV block	0.04–0.09 μg/kg/min	Ultra short-acting, contraindicated in bradyarrhythmias, tachycardia

(Continued)

Table 11.13 (*Continued*)

Drug	Mechanism/indication	Dose	Side-effects
Hydralazine	Vasodilator by altering cellular Ca metabolism; afterload reducer (vasodilator) for CHF or hypertensive crisis	0.5–2.5 mg/kg PO q 12 h or 0.5–3 mg/kg IV; alternatively 0.1 mg/kg loading dose then 1.5–5 µg/kg/min	Emesis, hypotension; monitor blood pressure regularly
Hydrochlorothiazide	Inhibits Na transport in renal tubules; hypertension, CHF	2–4 mg/kg PO q 12 h	Hypokalemia, hypochloremic alkalosis
Lidocaine	Class IB (Na channel blocker), decreases slope of phase 0; ventricular arrhythmias	2–4 mg/kg bolus, then 25–80 µg/kg/min CRI (dog); 0.25–0.75 mg/kg bolus and 10–40 µg/kg/min CRI (cat)	Neurological side-effects (seizures, cats sensitive)
Magnesium sulfate	Magnesium supplementation; hypomagnesemia, torsades des pointes, refractory ventricular arrhythmias	30 mg/kg (0.243 mEq/kg) slow over 5–10 min	CNS side-effects, hypotension, arrhythmias
Metoprolol	Beta-blocker; SVTs, VPCs, hypertension	0.2–1 mg/kg PO q 8 h	See Carvedilol
Mexilitine	Class IB (Na channel blocker), decreases slope of phase 0; ventricular arrhythmias	4–8 mg/kg PO q 8–12 h	GI, CNS side-effects, arrhythmias
Milrinone	Phosphodiesterase III inhibitor, Ca sensitizer, positive inotrope, arteriolar vasodilation; hypertension and CHF	0.275–0.75 µg/kg/min	Hypotension, arrhythmias
Nitroglycerine ointment	Balanced vasodilator, vascular smooth muscle relaxer; CHF	¼ inch of dermal cream on the axillary or aural skin or oral mucous membranes q 6–8 h	Hypotension; staff should wear gloves to apply
Nitroprusside	Arterial and venous vasodilation; CHF and hypertensive crisis	0.5–10 µg/kg/min CRI	Start at low dose and taper up, maintain a mimimum blood pressure of 70–80 mmHg. Hypotension
Norepinephrine	Beta-agonist. Positive inotrope, chronotrope, vasoconstriction; hypotension	0.01–3.0 µg/kg/min	Hypertension, arrhythmias
Oxygen	See Chapter 8	See Chapter 8	
Phenytoin	Class IB (Na channel blocker), decreases slope of phase 0; supraventricular tachyarrhythmias	2–4 mg/kg IV increments to maximum of 10 mg/kg	GI and hepatic side-effects
Pimobendan	Phosodiesterase III inhibitor, Ca sensitizer, postive inotrope, arteriolar vasodilation	0.25 mg/kg PO q 12 h (dog), 1.25 mg/cat PO q 12 h (cat)	GI and cardiac side-effects
Procainamide	Class IA (Na channel blocker), depresses phase 0. Supraventricular tachyarrhythmias (APCs, VPCs, Afib, other atrial and ventricular tachycardias)	6–8 mg/kg IV over 5–10 min; CRI 20–40 µg/kg/min (dog); 1–3 mg/kg slow IV, CRI of 3–8 µg/kg/min (cat)	Cautiously in cats
Propranolol	Class II antiarrhythmic (beta-blocker); SVTs, Afib, Aflutter	0.02–0.06 mg/kg slow IV	Contraindicated in AV block and SSS, bronchiolar disease; monitor blood pressure and ECG
Sildenafil	Phosphodiesterase inhibitor; pulmonary artery hypertension (PAH)	2–3 mg/kg q 8 h PO for PAH	Hypotension
Sodium nitroprusside	Vasodilation	0.5–4 µg/kg/min	Hypotension, continuous blood pressure monitoring required
Sotalol	Beta-blocker and potassium channel blocker (class III antiarrhythmic); ventricular arrhythmias	1–6 mg/kg/day divided q 12 h PO	Arrhythmias, GI side-effects
Spironolactone	ADH receptor antagonist; diuretic for CHF	1–4 mg/kg PO q 12 h	Electrolyte changes (hyperkalemia), dehydration
Terbutaline	Clinically significant bradyarrhythmias; beta-2 agonist	0.2 mg/kg PO q 8–12 h OR 0.01 mg/kg IV or SC	Tachycardia, CNS side-effects (excitement)
Supplements			
Taurine	Amino acid supplement; cardiomyopathies (DCM)	500 mg PO q 12 h	GI upset
Omega-3 fatty acids	Fatty acid supplement; may decrease risk of arrhythmias and progression of chronic heart disease	30–40 mg/kg PO q 24 h (EPA) or 20–25 mg/kg PO q 24 h (DHA)	GI upset
L-carnitine	Amino acid supplement; cardiomyopathies	110 mg/kg PO q 12 h	GI upset

ACE, angiotensin converting enzyme; ADH, antidiuretic hormone; ADP, adenosine diphosphate; Afib, atrial fibrillation; Aflutter, atrial flutter; APC, atrial premature contraction; ATP, adenosine triphosphate; AV, atrioventricular; CNS, central nervous system; CPR, cardiopulmonary resuscitation; CRI, constant rate infusion; DCM, dilated cardiomyopathy; CHF, congestive heart failure; DHA, docosahexaenoic acid; ECG, electrocardiogram; EPA, eicosapentaenoic acid; GI, gastrointestinal; LMWH, low molecular weight heparin; MVD, mitral valve disease; SSS, sick sinus syndrome; SVT, supraventricular tachycardia; VPC, ventricular premature contraction.

history or physical evidence of dehydration or fluid loss into third body fluid spaces can indicate that intravascular fluid replacement would be beneficial to improve the preload and ventricular filling. Small volume resuscitation techniques are used that will carefully titrate small amounts of fluids to reach low normal endpoints (see Chapter 2). Careful monitoring of the physical perfusion parameters, blood pressure, central venous pressure (if central line in place), respiratory rate, lung auscultation, and urine production is required to determine when to modify or terminate fluid therapy.

Cardiogenic shock due to intrinsic heart disease requires rapid evaluation of cardiac rhythm (ECG) and myocardial contractility (FS%). Treatment of diagnosed cardiac arrhythmias is indicated. The EDV demonstrated by echocardiogram has been proven to provide a better indication of recruitable cardiac output (the increase in cardiac output that can be obtained in response to fluids) [35]. Once the optimal right ventricular EDV has been reached, pressors or inotropes should be considered if cardiac output is still deemed inadequate. It has been shown that in the absence of right heart failure or valvular heart disease, the right ventricular EDV correlates well with left ventricular EDV [36,37].

The administration of a positive inotropic agent (such as dobutamine; see Table 11.13) has increased contractility, which has increased the strength of the contraction. This will also decrease end-systolic diameter and end-systolic volume (the ventricle becomes smaller). This means the ventricle can contract further against the same afterload. However, a patient given dobutamine as an inotrope that fails to increase the ejection fraction is less likely to benefit from remaining on this drug, and alternatives such as amrinone could be tried. Inotropes should be used cautiously and only

after adequate volume resuscitation. Hayes et al. showed that the aggressive use of inotropes to reach a predefined target level of cardiac index (cardiac output indexed to body size) resulted in significantly increased mortality in human patients [38].

There is no direct method for measuring myocardial contractility. Monitoring procedures provide a measure of central venous pressure (CVP) or pulmonary capillary wedge pressure (PCWP) or measures of volume (right ventricular EDV) or right ventricular end-diastolic volume index as surrogate markers. Both CVP and PCWP are generally considered poor indicators of preload. These measures are probably best used as indicators of whether an individual patient is likely to tolerate a fluid bolus without developing excessively high venous pressures.

Congestive heart failure

Congestive heart failure most commonly results from myocardial or valvular disease in the dog and cat. Most commonly, signs of respiratory failure result from increased pressure in the left atrium leading to increased venous and lymphatic pressures causing pulmonary edema (dogs and cats) or pleural effusion (cats). This results in clinical signs such as orthopnea, increased respiratory rate and effort, altered breathing patterns (see Chapter 8, Table 8.2, Figure 8.2) and pulmonary crackles (or dull lung sounds and open-mouth breathing). Many patients in a respiratory crisis are not tolerant of manipulative diagnostics (such as radiographs or ultrasound) and immediate intervention is often required.

Guidelines for the initial management of an acute crisis caused by congestive heart failure are listed in Box 11.5. Pharmacological intervention can include one or more of the following: diuretics

---

Box 11.5 General guidelines for the management of acute congestive heart failure.

Intervention may require a step-by-step method to minimize patient stress.

A. Initial stabilization of dog or cat in mild-to-moderate respiratory distress
1. Provide anxiolytic drug (such as butorphanol 0.2–0.4 mg/kg IM or IV).
2. Provide supplemental oxygen via flow-by, nasal prongs, mask, hood or cage.
3. Reduce preload with furosmide (initially at 1–4 mg/kg IM or IV); when an IV catheter is in place, 0.5–2 mg/kg/h CRI can be infused).
4. Place an IV catheter.
5. Consider 2% topical nitroglycerine (wear gloves and cover site on patient).

B. Initial stabilization of dog or cat in severe respiratory distress
1. Administer flow-by oxygen.
2. Place IV catheter.
3. For patients with impending respiratory arrest or severe work of breathing:
   a. administer rapid-acting injectable anesthetic (propofol, alfaxolone, ketamine/diazepam or etomidate/diazepam; see Table 8.12).
   b. Suction airway if necessary.
   c. Place endotracheal tube, confirm, secure and inflate cuff; provide manual ventilation with AMBU bag or therapeutic ventilator with 100% oxygen.
   d. Continue with treatments 4 and 5 below while supporting respiratory functions.
   e. Provide postural drainage by periodically elevating the hind end of the patient (ET tube pointed towards the ground) and firm compression of the thoracic cavity and suction fluid from the large airways.
   f. Place nasal oxygen line(s) while anesthetized to use after extubation.
   g. Allow patient to recover and extubate when spontaneous respiration on flow-by oxygen can maintain SpO$_2$ >93% and effort of breathing is acceptable. Some patients may require short-term mechanical ventilation.
4. Administer sodium nitroprusside (beginning at 0.2–0.5 µg/kg/min), titrate to effect while maintaining a mean arterial pressure ≥70 mmHg. Hydralazine is an alternative.
5. Dobutamine (starting at 2.5 µg/kg/min and increasing by 2.5 µg/kg/min intervals if necessary to a maximum of heart rate ≥180 bpm or dose of 15 µg/kg/min), reduce dose or discontinue if ventricular arrhythmias occur.
6. Monitor total fluid infusion volume and type of fluid to avoid volume overload and hyponatremia if using 5% dextrose in water for CRI administration of drugs.
7. Monitor ECG, blood pressure.

C. Animals with thoracic effusion
1. Perform thoracocentesis (outlined in Box 8.3).

D. Patient with abdominal effusion from right heart failure causing respiratory distress
1. Perform an abdominocentesis (guidelines for the procedure outlined in Box 15.1).
2. Monitor perfusion parameters and blood pressure closely for possibility of decreasing intraabdominal pressure causing a relative hypovolemia.

Continue with diagnostic procedures and specific therapy for underlying problems.

(reduce preload), vasodilators (reduce afterload), positive inotropes (improve contractility), and negative chronotropes when tachycardia is a contributing factor; negative chronotropes must be used with caution as some patients may be rate dependent to maintain CO. Medications used to treat congestive heart failure in the ICU patient are listed in Table 11.13, with dose, indications, and potential side-effects. Once the patient is stabilized, diagnostic testing can be performed to determine whether the heart failure is systolic, diastolic or valvular in origin.

Systolic failure

Systolic dysfunction (or systolic heart failure) occurs when the heart muscle does not contract with enough force, impairing cardiac output and oxygen delivery to the tissues. Systolic failure most commonly occurs in the dog and cat with dilated cardiomyopathy (DCM), but can also occur with sepsis and rarely with myocardial infarction and infection. Signs of DCM may result in systemic signs of shock or signs of pulmonary congestion and respiratory distress (see Chapter 8). When a patient is stable, it may be appropriate to perform diagnostic imaging (radiographs; Table 11.6), with the definitive diagnosis made with echocardiography. Performing an electrocardiogram is usually essential since ventricular arrhythmias are common. Medications that are used to maintain cardiac output (positives inotropes) include dobutamine, amrinone, pimobendan, and digoxin (doses in Table 11.13). Dogs with severe congestive heart failure or evidence of significant decreases in cardiac output may benefit from a constant rate infusion of dobutamine. It is important to also address the impact of preload and afterload on the heart with diuretics and vasodilators (see Box 11.5).

Diastolic failure

Diastolic failure is essentially a loss of preload or diastolic filling of the heart. Common causes of diastolic dysfunction include tachyarrhythmias, hypertrophic cardiomyopathy and cardiac tamponade.

Cardiac tamponade is pressure on the heart that occurs when blood or fluid builds up in the space between the myocardium and the pericardium. The pericardial fluid accumulation can be caused by a ruptured mass, infection, cancer, ruptured atrium or idiopathic causes. Physical examination most commonly notes muffled heart sounds, tachycardia, jugular venous distension and subsequently poor peripheral blood flow. Ultrasound-guided pericardiocentesis is warranted. The guidelines for the procedure to drain the pericardial sac and relieve tamponade are outlined in Box 11.6.

Hypertrophic cardiomyopathy is characterized by concentric hypertrophy of the myocardium and is most common in cats (often secondary to hyperthyroidism). Treatment typically involves furosemide (if pulmonary congestion is present), ACE inhibitors, and antiplatelet drugs to limit the possibility of thromboembolism. Table 11.13 lists the dose, indications, and potential side-effects of the drugs. Pimobendan can be used in the treatment of refractory HCM, with beta-blockers and calcium channel blockers used only if significant arrhythmias are present. Any cardiac disease may result in pleural effusion in cats and a thoracocentesis may be required. The procedure for performing pleurocentesis is provided in Chapter 8, Box 8.3.

Atrioventricular valve failure

Failure of the AV valves (particularly the mitral valve) is the most common type of heart disease in the dog. It leads to increased pressure within the atria, and subsequently increases in central (right atrial) or pulmonary (left atrial) venous pressure, causing an increase in fluid accumulation in the pulmonary or systemic venous

---

Box 11.6 Steps to perform a pericardiocentesis.

1. Place an IV catheter.
2. Administer sedation (such as butorphanol, 0.2–0.4 mg/kg IV).
3. Clip and scrub with chlorhexidine the right or left thoracic region from halfway up the thorax to near ventral midline between rib spaces 2–6.
4. Use the ultrasound to identify the effusion when available. An experienced ultrasonographer may identify masses, clots or tamponade.
5. Monitor the electrocardiogram during the procedure.
6. Administer a local lidocaine block.
7. Insert a 1.5" to 6", 22–14 G needle or catheter cranial to the rib between spaces 3–4 or 4–5.
8. Advance needle slowly until fluid comes out.
9. Advance the catheter and remove the needle if using a catheter.
10. Connect the needle or catheter to an extension set, three-way stopcock, and syringe.
11. Aspirate the pericardial space, observing for movement of the needle if against the heart. A "scratching" sensation and arrhythmias may indicate that the heart is being touched with the tip of the needle.
12. Assess perfusion and administer intravascular volume support if needed to provide adequate preload.
13. Improvement in heart rate and perfusion parameters should occur.
14. Recheck with ultrasound when possible that the fluid is decreased; an experienced ultrasonographer may recognize alleviation of tamponade.
15. Monitor for arrhythmias (ventricular rhythms are common).
16. Assess the pericardial fluid for clotting. Typically the fluid will not clot unless it is a subacute presentation.
17. Monitor the patient for signs of shock and the PCV/TP, blood pressure, electrocardiogram.
18. Recheck for recurrence of accumulation of pericardial fluid with ultrasound (in six hours, 12 hours, 24 hours, one week, and one month post centesis).
19. Perform a systemic work-up and imaging for evidence of primary tumors, metastasis, and coagulopathies.

---

system. Both diseases essentially result in an increase in capillary hydrostatic pressure upstream of the back leak through the valve. Increase of central (vena cava) pressure will result in development of portal hypertension and eventually ascites. Increased pressure of the pulmonary venous system will result in pleural effusion (particularly in cats) or pulmonary edema (both cats and dogs).

Myocardial hypertrophy is an expected compensatory consequence of valvular insufficiency. The FS% may be higher than normal to maintain cardiac output. An echocardiogram is necessary to determine whether contractility is adequate and to guide inotropic therapy. Adjusting the preload and afterload with diuretics and vasodilators is often the mainstay of therapy for mitral regurgitation. Therapy with ACE inhibitors and pimobendan is instituted when the patient is able to tolerate oral medications.

Other heart diseases
Pulmonary hypertension

Pulmonary hypertension (PH) is diagnosed more commonly in veterinary patients with recent advances of echocardiography. As our understanding of the disease and its diagnosis improves, it may become even more prominent. Patients that present with this disease often have a history of coughing or respiratory difficulty and a heart murmur is often present.

There are many potential causes of PH, including idiopathic, chronic alveolar hypoxia, chronic left heart elevated preload, chronic progressive small artery pulmonary thromboembolisms, chronic pulmonary disease (such as fibrosis and bronchitis), neoplasia, heartworm disease, and others [39,40]. Radiographs may identify enlargement of the right side of the heart with PH. The radiographic appearance of the pulmonary fields can be variable, from normal to diffuse or patchy alveolar infiltrates [41]. The value of the vertebral heart scale (VHS) in dogs with PH secondary to myxomatous valvular disease has been evaluated. A VHS short axis of >5.2 vertebrae and a length of sternal contact of >3.3 vertebrae were considered suitable for the detection of PH. The predictive accuracy of this model is 85.9%, and it is judged to be useful to screen for PH due to left heart disease in dogs with myxomatous valvular disease without echocardiography [42].

The diagnosis of PH is most often made with echocardiography. A number of abnormalities on the echocardiogram are supportive of a diagnosis of PH, including small (underloaded) left ventricle, underloaded pulmonary veins, inadequate filling of left atrium, right ventricular dilation with hypertrophy, right atrial dilation, flattening of the interventricular septum, paradoxical septal motion, high-velocity tricuspid or pulmonic regurgitation and upward diastolic billowing of the pulmonic valve leaflets [43].

Therapy involves treating underlying pulmonary or cardiac disease (when present) and initiation of sildenafil (a phosphodiesterase type 5 inhibitor, dose in Table 11.13) to dilate pulmonary blood vessels. Management of this disease by an experienced specialist is advised. Novel therapies for use in dogs with PH are under investigation, such as imatinib, a tyrosine kinase inhibitor [44].

Heartworm disease (dirofilariasis)

Dirofilaria immitis is the heartworm and it can cause clinically significant cardiac and pulmonary disease in dogs and cats, resulting in caval syndrome, right-sided heart disease, and pulmonary embolism, while the patient is infected or during therapy. Prevention is the best course of action with patients tested to ensure they are negative prior to initiating preventative medications lethal to the larval stages (microfilaria). Once *Dirofilaria* infection is confirmed, therapy can be challenging and risky to the patient.

The American Heartworm Society has recently updated the recommended therapy for *Dirofilaria* infection. Therapy for *Dirofilaria* involves three aspects:

- initiation of a preventative agent to minimize development of new microfilaria into adult worms
- prevention of complications of therapy (most notably pulmonary emboli), with anticoagulants, exercise restriction, and possible glucocorticosteroids
- adulticide therapy with the organic arsenical melarsomine (Immiticide®, Merial, Duluth, GA). Treatment with melarsomine will kill the adult worms, but pulmonary parasitic embolization remains a consequence.

Surgical removal of worms is uncommonly performed and associated with high risk.

Wolbachia spp. are gram-negative bacteria that infect filarial nematodes, including *D. immitis*, and elicit an inflammatory response in cats and dogs. Antimicrobial therapy (such as doxycycline, 10 mg/kg/day PO) directed against these bacteria has resulted in decreased microfilarial loads, inhibition of the development of larval worms, female worm infertility, and reduced numbers of *Wolbachia* organisms [45].

Research into the adulticide effects of ivermectin (6 µg/kg PO q 7 days) combined with doxycycline (10 mg/kg/day PO) found the combination to be as effective as melarsomine with a reduced immune regulation toward the parasite [46,47]. An up-to-date and detailed description of the heartworm syndromes and recommendations for treatment provided by the Heartworm Society are available on its website at www.heartwormsociety.org.

Cardiopulmonary arrest and resuscitation

The most catastrophic cardiac disorder that an ICU patient can have is cardiopulmonary arrest. Being prepared for this event involves close monitoring of patients at risk, having a fully stocked "ready area" and CPR crash cart (see Box 20.1) and maintaining a knowledge base on the technique by practicing CPR drills with the staff on a regular basis. Roles should be defined for personnel and charts and medications should be ready. All members of the medical team should be familiar with the ready area and how they can take part in CPR when needed. Recording data during CPR is essential and shown in Figure 20.2. Patients should have a predetermined CPR code noted on their cage and record (or wear a color-coded collar); this will direct the staff regarding the owner's wishes for CPR efforts. These procedures are detailed in Chapter 20.

Respiratory distress, heart failure, severe metabolic derangements, intracranial or high cervical lesions, thromboembolic events, high vagal tone, and ongoing hemorrhage are but a few of the conditions of the small animal ICU patient that can predispose to cardiac arrest. The overall survival rate after CPR is poor in veterinary medicine. The Reassessment Campaign on Veterinary Resuscitation (RECOVER, www.acvecc-recover.org) was created to define guidelines for CPR in veterinary patients and to identify gaps in the current knowledge base to direct further research [48]. These guidelines are updated as new recommendations become available and can be found at www.acvecc-recover.org.

The first signs of cardiopulmonary arrest is apnea or a nonresponsive animal. Recognition of these signs should occur quickly (within only seconds) and Basic Life Support should be initiated. The time it takes to determine if a heart beat or pulse is present wastes valuable seconds in the resuscitation process; in addition, minimal injury to the patient occurs when chest compressions are initiated. An algorithm to guide the decision-making process during Basic Life Support (BLS) and Advanced Life Support (ALS) procedures for CPR is provided in Figure 11.18.

Basic Life Support

Basic Life Support begins by initiating a full two-minute cycle of cardiac compressions at 100–120 compressions per minute. When using the thoracic pump technique, it is important to release the thorax completely in between compressions to optimize blood flow during CPR.

Small dogs (<12 kg body weight) and cats can often be adequately perfused by closed chest cardiac massage. These smaller animals benefit from the thoracic pump technique or the cardiac pump technique (direct cardiac compressions). Medium-sized animals (12–25 kg body weight) have little cardiac compression and benefit primarily form the thoracic pump technique. Large animals (>25 kg body weight) can get some benefit from the thoracic pump but fare best with open chest heart massage.

In small-sized animals, chest compressions are best performed with the cardiac pump technique, placing one hand around the thorax, thumb on one side and fingers on the other to compress the heart; the palm of the other hand may be placed on the back to prevent excessive movement of the patient. Alternatively, compression with both hands directly over the heart may be used. Chest compressions for medium- or large-sized dogs (thoracic pump technique) are best performed with the back of the animal toward the compressor, with the compressor elevated above the animal. The arms are held in extension with locked elbows, bending at the

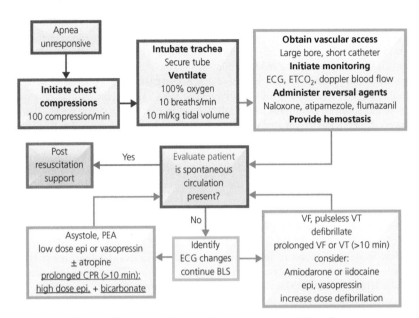

Figure 11.18 An algorithm to guide the decision-making process during cardiopulmonary resuscitation of an unresponsive small animal with apnea. Blue boxes represent Basic Life Support procedures. Green boxes represent Advanced Life Support procedures. At least two minutes should elapse after the administration of a drug or defibrillation before determining the success or failure of the intervention. CPR is considered to be prolonged after 10 minutes of resuscitative efforts. Source: Adapted from Boller MA, Fletcher DJ. RECOVER evidence and knowledge gap analysis on veterinary CPR. J Vet Emerg Crit Care 2012;22(s1):s4–s131 [48]. BLS, Basic Life Support; CPR, cardiopulmonary resuscitation; ECG, electrocardiogram; Epi, epinephrine; $ETCO_2$, end-tidal CO_2; min, minute; PEA, pulseless electrical activity; VF, ventricular fibrillation; VT, ventricular tachycardia.

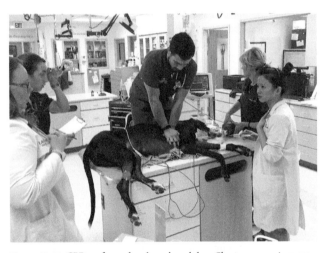

Figure 11.19 CPR performed on large breed dog. Chest compressions are performed with back of the animal toward the compressor and the compressor elevated above the animal. One team member is ventilating while others administer drugs and record the procedures.

Table 11.14 End-tidal CO_2 ($ETCO_2$) readings during cardiopulmonary resuscitation (CPR).

$ETCO_2$ reading (mmHg) during CPR	Significance
35–45	This is a normal value for reference
<8–12	Inadequate CPR efforts, consider changing technique such as hand position, strength of compression, rate of compression, person compressing; ensure ventilation is not excessive and confirm ET tube placement.
8–12	Adequate CPR efforts, continue BCLS in two-minute cycles
15–20	May indicate return of spontaneous circulation
Dramatic rise or >30	Likely indicates a return of spontaneous circulation

waist to perform compressions; the palms of the hands are used to compress the thorax, decreasing the diameter of the thorax approximately 30–50% (see Figure 11.19).

The trachea is rapidly intubated and the endotracheal tube immediately secured and cuff inflated. Ventilation is initiated with 100% oxygen using an AMBU bag or anesthetic machine that has been flushed of anesthetic. The recommendation for the frequency of ventilations is 10 breaths/minute with a tidal volume of 10 mL/kg and an inspiratory time of one second. Overinflation and/or excessive rates of manual ventilation will interfere with venous return and the thoracic pump, potentially cause ruptures of the pulmonary tree resulting in a pneumothorax or pneumediastinum, and interfere with end-tidal CO_2 ($ETCO_2$) monitoring.

When it is difficult or impossible to inflate the lungs, a tension pneumothorax is likely and a large-bore needle or tube is rapidly placed in the pleural space to evacuate the air. If the air leak is severe, open chest CPR should be performed.

Advanced Life Support

Advanced Life Support (see Figure 11.18) begins with establishing vascular access by placing a large-bore, short intravenous or intraosseous catheter for drug and fluid administration. A catheter can be temporarily placed down the endotracheal tube to initially administer the drugs to be absorbed by the pulmonary circulation if the time for successful IV or IO access is prolonged. Monitoring is initiated with an ECG and $ETCO_2$. The $ETCO_2$ values of significance during CPR are listed in Table 11.14. Pulse oximetry and blood

Box 11.7 Outline for open chest CPR.

1. Clip the hair from the chest if time permits. Wear sterile gloves.
2. At the level of the fifth or sixth intercostal space, incise skin, subcutaneous tissues, and thoracic musculature using Mayo scissors (or a scalpel) near to ventral and dorsal midline; guarding the blade with thumb and index finger, apply pressure to penetrate through the intercostal muscles (while ventilation is temporarily discontinued). Use Mayo or Metzenbaum scissors to complete the incision through the intercostal muscles along the cranial aspect of the ribs. Avoid the internal thoracic vessels running parallel to the sternum.
3. Open the pericardial sac with forceps and Metzenbaum scissors, avoiding the phrenic and vagus nerves. Do not sharply elevate or twist the heart, since these movements can cause avulsion of large veins from the heart.
4. Hold the heart in the palm of the hand or by both hands and apply equal compression to both ventricles of the heart simultaneously. Cutting the rib cranial and caudal at the costochondral junction or using Finochietto retractors will improve visualization.
5. Begin the compressions at the apex and move upward toward the base of the heart.
6. Apply compression of the descending aorta (modified Rommell tourniquet, pictured below) passing curved hemostats around the aorta (blunt dissection), pulling a red rubber tube around and applying the hemostat to the tube; this should stay in place for a maximum of 10 minutes and will improve distribution of the blood to the myocardium and brain.

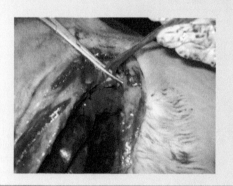

pressure monitoring are not helpful during CPR; some may consider placing a Doppler flow transducer on the cornea or in the esophagus, but patient movement during CPR may give a false positive for blood flow. If narcotics or other anesthetic or sedative agents have been administered prior to cardiac arrest, the administration of reversal medications (such as naloxone for opioids, atipamezole for medetomidine, flumazenil for benzodiazepines) is recommended. Inhaled gas anesthetics (such as isoflurane, sevoflurane) should be immediately discontinued and the anesthesia circuit flushed with fresh oxygen.

Ventilations and chest compressions are continued throughout the ALS procedures. Open chest CPR may be necessary in patients with any of the following: unwitnessed arrest, trauma, suspected or known pleural, pericardial, thoracic wall or diaphragmatic disease, in large animals (>10 kg), those with recent surgery, or poor response to closed chest CPR for 10 minutes. A brief outline of the procedure for rapid entry into the thorax and cardiac massage is presented in Box 11.7.

The ECG should be evaluated to identify the heart conduction rhythm (not more frequently than every two-minute cycle of CPR

efforts), and personnel performing chest compression and ventilation are rotated to remain fresh. There are four major arrhythmias associated with cardiac arrest.

1. Asystole appears as a flat line and suggests complete absence of electrical activity. However, many arrhythmias that appear to be asystole are, in fact, fine ventricular fibrillation. For this reason, open chest heart massage and direct observation of myocardial activity are warranted early with this arrhythmia. Hyperkalemia should be ruled out as a cause.
2. Pulseless electrical activity (PEA) can demonstrate waveforms, but there is no cardiac no muscular activity; no contractions mean no cardiac output. With PEA, the ECG will have a normal or slow rate and there will be no heart sounds or pulse activity. However, inability to auscultate the heart may not necessarily mean PEA; severe hypovolemia, pericardial effusion and significant accumulation of fluid or air in the pleural cavity may prevent detection of heart sounds. The ECGs associated with these "beating heart" conditions will have tachyarrhythmias in contrast to the usually normal or slow rate of PEA.
3. Ventricular fibrillation (VF) demonstrates multiple foci within the ventricles firing rapidly and independently, resulting in no coordinated mechanical activity. There are no ventricular contractions and no cardiac output. The goal of therapy is to abruptly stop the electrical activity and allow one strong focus to take over.
4. Pulseless ventricular tachycardia (pulseless VT) has electrical activity originating from an ectopic ventricular focus producing insufficient pressure to generate a peripheral pulse.

Other arrhythmias resulting in cardiopulmonary arrest are possible.

When the patient has VF or pulseless VT, electrical defibrillation is the treatment of choice. The doses for both the monophasic or biphasic defibrillators and for external and internal defibrillation are provided in Figure 11.20. The defibrillator is charged and electrical conduction gel applied while BLS continues. Ensure no one is touching the patient or the table, then yell "CLEAR" in a loud and clear voice. Discharge the defibrillator and immediately resume BLS for two minutes prior to evaluation of the ECG. If a defibrillator is not present, a precordial thump may be administered, but this is considered less effective. When the pulseless ventricular tachycardia or fibrillation has been present for more than 10 minutes, administering amiodarone or lidocaine (see Table 11.13 and Figure 11.20 for doses) or increasing the defibrillator dose by 50% may be warranted.

If the patient is suffering asystole or PEA, a low dose of epinephrine (0.01 mg/kg IV every 3–5 minutes) or vasopressin (0.8 U/kg IV every 3–5 minutes) alone or with low-dose epinephrine can be given. Atropine may be considered every other two-minute cycle for patients with bradyarrhythmias or with diseases associated with high vagal tone. With prolonged cardiopulmonary arrest, a high dose of epinephrine (0.1 mg/kg IV) or bicarbonate (1 mEq/kg (1 mmol/kg) IV) therapy may be warranted. High-dose epinephrine is associated with an improved return of spontaneous circulation, but a lower survival to discharge. Every drug that is administered should be flushed with 5–20 mL of normal saline IV or IO to promote entry into the central circulation. Dosages for drugs used during CPR are listed in Figure 11.20.

CPR emergency drugs and doses

		Weight (kg)	2.5	5	10	15	20	25	30	35	40	45	50
		Weight (lb)	5	10	20	30	40	50	60	70	80	90	100
	DRUG	**DOSE**	ml	ml	ml	ml	ml	ml	ml	ml	ml	ml	ml
Arrest	Epi low (1:1000)	0.01 mg/kg	0.03	0.05	0.1	0.15	0.2	0.25	0.3	0.35	0.4	0.45	0.5
	Epi high (1:1000)	0.1 mg/kg	0.25	0.5	1	1.5	2	2.5	3	3.5	4	4.5	5
	Vasopressin (20 U/ml)	0.8 U/kg	0.1	0.2	0.4	0.6	0.8	1	1.2	1.4	1.6	1.8	2
	Atropine (0.54 mg/ml)	0.05 mg/kg	0.25	0.5	1	1.5	2	2.5	3	3.5	4	4.5	5
Anti-arrhyth	Amiodarone (50 mg/ml)	5 mg/kg	0.25	0.5	1	1.5	2	2.5	3	3.5	4	4.5	5
	Lidocaine (20 mg/ml)	2–8 mg/kg	0.25	0.5	1	1.5	2	2.5	3	3.5	4	4.5	5
Reversal	Naloxone (0.4 mg/ml)	0.04 mg/kg	0.25	0.5	1	1.5	2	2.5	3	3.5	4	4.5	5
	Flumazenil (0.1 mg/ml)	0.01 mg/kg	0.25	0.5	1	1.5	2	2.5	3	3.5	4	4.5	5
	Atipamezole (5 mg/ml)	50 µg/kg	0.03	0.05	0.1	0.15	0.2	0.25	0.3	0.35	0.4	0.45	0.5
Defib biphasic	External defib (J)	2–4 J/kg	6	15	30	50	75	75	100	150	150	150	150
	Internal defib (J)	0.2–0.4 J/kg	1	2	3	5	6	8	9	10	15	15	15

Figure 11.20(a) Drug and biphasic defibrillation doses based on weight for CPR. *Source*: Boller MA, Fletcher DJ. RECOVER evidence and knowledge gap analysis on veterinary CPR. J Vet Emerg Crit Care 2012;22(s1):s4–s131 [48]. Used with permission from Wiley.

CPR emergency drugs and doses

		Weight (kg)	2.5	5	10	15	20	25	30	35	40	45	50
		Weight (lb)	5	10	20	30	40	50	60	70	80	90	100
	DRUG	**DOSE**	ml	ml	ml	ml	ml	ml	ml	ml	ml	ml	ml
Arrest	Epi low (1:1000)	0.01 mg/kg	0.03	0.05	0.1	0.15	0.2	0.25	0.3	0.35	0.4	0.45	0.5
	Epi high (1:1000)	0.1 mg/kg	0.25	0.5	1	1.5	2	2.5	3	3.5	4	4.5	5
	Vasopressin (20 U/ml)	0.8 U/kg	0.1	0.2	0.4	0.6	0.8	1	1.2	1.4	1.6	1.8	2
	Atropine (0.54 mg/ml)	0.05 mg/kg	0.25	0.5	1	1.5	2	2.5	3	3.5	4	4.5	5
Anti-arrhyth	Amiodarone (50 mg/ml)	5 mg/kg	0.25	0.5	1	1.5	2	2.5	3	3.5	4	4.5	5
	Lidocaine (20 mg/ml)	2–8 mg/kg	0.25	0.5	1	1.5	2	2.5	3	3.5	4	4.5	5
Reversal	Naloxone (0.4 mg/ml)	0.04 mg/kg	0.25	0.5	1	1.5	2	2.5	3	3.5	4	4.5	5
	Flumazenil (0.1 mg/ml)	0.01 mg/kg	0.25	0.5	1	1.5	2	2.5	3	3.5	4	4.5	5
	Atipamezole (5 mg/ml)	50 µg/kg	0.03	0.05	0.1	0.15	0.2	0.25	0.3	0.35	0.4	0.45	0.5
Defib Monophasic	External defib (J)	2–10 J/kg	20	30	50	100	200	200	200	300	300	300	360
	Internal defib (J)	0.2–1 J/kg	2	3	5	10	20	20	20	30	30	30	50

Figure 11.20(b) Drug and monophasic defibrillation doses based on weight for CPR. Source: Fletcher DJ, Boller M, Brainard BM, et al. RECOVER evidence and knowledge gap analysis on veterinary CPR. Part 7: Clinical Guidelines. J Vet Emerg Crit Care 2012;22(S1):S102–31.Used with permission from Wiley.

Intravenous fluids may be administered to patients who are known or suspected to have hypovolemia (10–30 mL/kg crystalloid and/or 2–5 mL/kg colloid). Patients with a normal fluid volume, however, can have a decrease in cerebral and myocardial perfusion pressures when excessive fluids are administered during CPR [49].

Dextrose can be administerd to patients with suspected or known hypoglycemia. Steroids should not be administered during CPR unless hypoadrenocorticism or anaphylaxis is a suspected underlying problem. Patients with hyperkalemia may benefit from calcium gluconate and/or regular insulin with dextrose administration.

Once electrical and mechanical cardiac activity has been established and associated with a peripheral pulse, postresuscitation care is essential. A schematic of factors of concern after the return of spontaneous circulation post CPR is presented in Figure 11.21. If the chest was opened, the animal must be moved to the operating room. The wound is converted to a surgical wound, the thoracic cavity is thoroughly lavaged, any problems (either underlying or iatrogenic from the resuscitation) are corrected, a thoracostomy tube is placed, and the thoracic cavity is closed. Oxygen and ventilator support are usually required for an extended period of time post resuscitation. It may become necessary to do a tracheotomy to allow ventilatory support in the awake animal, should long-term support be required.

Acid–base, glucose, and electrolyte abnormalities should be corrected. Systemic inflammatory response syndrome should be anticipated and the blood pressure, coagulation status, cardiac contractility, and major organ function monitored and supported (follow the Rule of 20). The reason for the arrest must be investigated and the underlying cause corrected. Unfortunately, rearrest is common, requiring that the animal be monitored closely. Patients are often kept sedated while diagnostics and further stabilization are being performed.

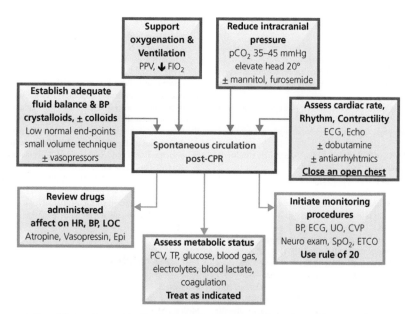

Figure 11.21 Schematic representation of factors to consider for the immediate support of the patient with return of spontaneous circulation post cardiopulmonary resuscitation. Problems such as hypovolemia, hypotension, hypoxemia, hypercarbia, cerebral edema, poor cardiac contractility, cardiac arrhythmias, hypoglycemia, hyperkalemia, oliguria, and disseminated intravascular coagulation should be anticipated. The timely initiation of supportive, diagnostic, and monitoring procedures can play a vital role in patient survival during this immediate postresuscitation period. BP, blood pressure; CPR, cardiopulmonary resuscitation; CVP, central venous pressure; ECG, electrocardiogram; Echo, echocardiography; Epi, epinephrine; ETCO$_2$, end-tidal CO$_2$; FIO$_2$, fraction of inspired oxygen; HR, heart rate; LOC, level of consciousness; pCO$_2$, partial pressure of oxygen; PCV, packed cell volume; PPV, positive pressure ventilation; SpO$_2$, pulse oximeter reading; TP, total protein; UO, urine output.

References

1. Kittleson MD, Kienle RD, eds. Normal clinical cardiovascular physiology. In: Small Animal Cardiovascular Medicine. St Louis: Mosby, 1998.

2. Berne RM, Levy NL, eds. Cardiovascular Physiology, 7th edn. St Louis: Mosby, 1992.

3. Schlant RC, Sonnenblick EH. Normal physiology of the cardiovascular system. In: The Heart, 7th edn. Hurst JW, Schlant RC, eds. New York: McGraw-Hill, 1990.

4. Braunwald E, Sonnenblick EH, Ross JJ. Contraction of the normal heart. In: Heart Disease: A Textbook of Cardiovascular Medicine. Braunwald E, ed. Philadelphia: WB Saunders, 1980.

5. Jacob R, Dierberger B, Gulch RW, et al. Geometric and muscle physiological factors of the Frank–Starling mechanisms. Basic Res Cardiol. 1993;88(1):86–91.

6. 6.ter Keurs HE, de Tombe PP, Backx PH, et al. Rheology of myocardium: the relation between force, velocity, sarcomere length and activation in rat cardiac muscle. Biorheology 1991;28(3–4):161–70.

7. Jacob R, Dierberger B, Kissling G. Functional significance of the Frank–Starling mechanism under physiological and pathophysiological conditions. Eur Heart J. 1992;13(suppl E):7–14.

8. Westerhof N, Elzinga G, Sipkema P, et al. Quantitative analysis of arterial system and heart by means of pressure flow relations. In: Cardiovascular Flow Dynamics and Measurements. Hwan NHC, Norman NA, eds. Baltimore: University Park, 1977.

9. Hall AC, Guyton JE, eds. Textbook of Medical Physiology, 11th edn. Philadelphia: WB Saunders, 2005: pp116–22.

10. Betts JG. Anatomy & Physiology. Houston: Openstax, 2013: pp 787–846.

11. Spratt DP, Mellanby RJ, Drury N, Archer J. Cardiac troponin I: evaluation of a biomarker for the diagnosis of heart disease in the dog. J Small Anim Pract. 2005;46(3):139–45.

12. Polizopoulou ZS, Koutina CK, Eron JJ, et al. Correlation of serum cardiac tropnin I and acute phase protein concentrations in clinical staging in dogs with degenerative mitral valve disease. Vet Clin Pathol. 2015;44(3):397–404.

13. Prosek R, Sisson DD, Oyama MA, Solter PF. Distinguishing cardiac and non cardiac dyspnea in 48 dogs using plasma atrial natriuretic peptide, B-type natriuretic factor, endothelin and cardiac troponin-I. J Vet Intern Med. 2007;21(2):238–42.

14. Fox PR, Rush JE, Reynolds CA, et al. Multicenter evaluation of plasma N-terminal probrain natriuretic peptide (NT-pro BNP) as a biochemical screening test for asymptomatic (occult) cardiomyopathy in cats. J Vet Intern Med. 2011;25(5):1010–20.

15. Oyama MA. Using cardiac biomarkers in veterinary practice. Clin Lab Med. 2015;35(3):555–66.

16. Fox PR, Oyama MA, Hezzell MJ, et al. Relationship of plasma N-terminal probrain natriuretic peptide concentrations to heart failure classification and cause of respiratory distress in dogs using a 2nd generation ELISA assay. J Vet Intern Med. 2015;29(1):171–9.

17. Fox PR, Oyama MA, Reynolds C. Utility of plasma N-terminal pro-brain natriuretic peptide (NT-proBNP) to distinguish between congestive heart failure and non-cardiac causes of acute dyspnea in cats. J Vet Cardiol. 2009;11:S51–S61.

18. Polizopoulous ZA, Koutinas CK, Dasopoulou A, et al. Serial analysis of serum cardiac troponin I changes and correlation with clinical findings in 46 dogs with mitral valve disease. Vet Clin Pathol. 2014;43(2):218–25.

19. Noszczyk-Nowak A. NT-pro-BNP and troponin I as predictors of mortality in dogs with heart failure (in dilated cardiomyopathy). Pol J Vet Sci. 2011;14(4):551–6.

20. Linklater A, Lichtenberger MK, Thamm D, et al. Serum concentration of cardiac troponin I and cardiac troponin T in dogs with class IV congestive heart failure due to mitral valve disease. J Vet Emerg Crit Care 2007;17(3):243–9.

21. De Francesco TC, Atkins CE, Keene BW, et al. Prospective clinical evelution of serum cardiac troponin T in dogs admitted to a veterinary teaching hospital. J Vet Intern Med. 2002;16(5):553–7.

22. Smith KF, Quinn RL, Rahilly LJ. Biomarkers for differentiation of causes of respiratory distress in dogs and cats: Part 1 Cardiac Diseases and Pulmonary Hypertension. J Vet Emerg Crit Care 2015;25(93):311–29.

23. Fox PR, Oyama MA, Reynolds C, et al. Utility of plasma NT-pro BNP to distinguish between congestive heart failure and non-cardiac causes of acute dyspnea in cats. J Vet Cardiol. 2009;11:S51

24. Connolly DJ, Soares Magalhaes RJ, Fuentes VI, et al. Assessment of the diagnostic accuracy of circulating natriuretic peptide concentrations to distinguish between cats with cardiac and non cardiac causes of respiratory distress. J Vet Cardiol. 2009;11:S41.

25. Keinle RD, Thomas WP. Echocardiography. In: Veterinary Diagnostic Ultrasound. Nyland T, Mattoon J, eds. Philadelphia: WB Saunders, 1995.

26. Mazzaferro EM. Monitoring the critical patient. Proceedings of the Latin American Veterinary Emergency and Critical Care Society (LAVECCS), Leon, MX, 2009.

27. Sanders RA, Ralph AG, Olivier NB. Cardioversion of atrial fibrillation in a dog with structural heart disease using an esophageal–right atrial lead configuration. J Vet Cardiol. 2014;16(4):277–81.

28. Sisson D, Thomas WB, Woodfield JP, et al. Permanent transvenous pacemaker implantation in forty dogs. J Vet Intern Med. 1991;5(6):322–31.

29. Zipes DP. Proarrhythmic effects of antiarrhythmic drugs. Am J Cardiol. 1987;59(11):26E–31E.

30. Roden DM. Mechanisms and management of proarrhythmia. Am J Cardiol. 1998;82(4A):49I–57I.

31. Repesse X, Charron C, Vieillard-Baron A. Evaluation of left ventricular systolic function revisited in septic shock. Crit Care 2013;17:164–7.

32. Antonucci E, Fiaccadori E, Donadella K, et al. Myocardial depression in sepsis: from pathogenesis to clinical manifestations and treatment. J Crit Care 2014; 29:500–11.

33. Parrillo JE. Pathogenetic mechanisms of septic shock. N Engl J Med. 1993; 328:1471–7.

34. Hotchkiss RS, Karl IE. The pathophysiology and treatment of sepsis. N Engl J Med. 2003;348:138–50.

35. Diebel LN, Wilson RF, Tagett MG, et al. End-diastolic volume. A better indicator of preload in the critically ill. Arch Surg. 1992;127:817–22.

36. Mellema M. Cardiac output, wedge pressure and oxygen delivery. Vet Clin North Am Small Anim Pract. 2001;31:1175–205.

37. Huemer G, Kolev N, Kurz A, et al. Influence of positive end-expiratory pressure on right and left ventricular performance assessed by Doppler two-dimensional echocardiography. Chest 1994;106:67–73.

38. Hayes MA, Timmins AC, Yau EH, et al. Elevation of systemic oxygen delivery in the treatment of critically ill patients. N Engl J Med. 1994;330:1717–22.

39. Stepien RL. Pulmonary arterial hypertension secondary to chronic left-sided cardiac dysfunction in dogs. J Small Anim Pract. 2009;50(suppl 1):34–43.

40. Henik RA. Pulmonary hypertension. In: Kirk's Current Veterinary Therapy XIV. Bonagura JD, Twedt DC, eds. St Louis: Elsevier Saunders, 2009: pp 697–703.

41. Kellihan HB, Waller KR, Pinkos A, et al. Acute resolution of pulmonary alveolar infiltrates in 10 dogs with pulmonary hypertension treated with sildenafil citrate: 2005–2014. J Vet Cardiol. 2015;17(3):182–91.

42. Miyagawa Y, Toda N, Tominaga Y, Takemura N. Predictive model for the detection of pulmonary hypertension in dogs with myxomatous mitral valve disease. J Vet Med Sci. 2015;77(1):7–13.

43. Pyle RL, Abbott J, MacLean H. Pulmonary hypertension and cardiovascular sequelae in 54 dogs. Int J Appl Res Vet Med. 2004;2(2):99–109.

44. Arita S, Arita N, Hikasa Y. Therapeutic effect of low-dose imatinib on pulmonary arterial hypertension in dogs. Can Vet J. 2013;54(3):255–61.

45. Frank K, Heald RD. The emerging role of Wolbachia species in heartworm disease. Comp Contin Educ Vet. 2010;32(4): E4.

46. Bazzocci C, Mortarino M, Grandi G, et al. Combined ivermectin and doxycycline treatment has microfilaricidal and adulticidal activity against Dirofilaria immitis in experimentally infected dogs. Int J Parasitol. 2008;38(12):1401–10.

47. Passeri B, Vismarra A, Cricri G, et al. The adulticide effect of a combination of doxycycline and ivermectin in Dirofilaria immitis-experimentally infected dogs is associated with reduction in local T regulatory cell populations. Vet Parasitol. 2014;205(1–2):208–10.

48. Boller MA, Fletcher DJ. RECOVER evidence and knowledge gap analysis on veterinary CPR. J Vet Emerg Crit Care 2012;22(s1):s4–s131.

49. Ditchey RV, Lindenfeld J. Potential adverse effects of volume loading on perfusion of vital organs during closed-chest resuscitation. Circulation 1984;69(1): 181–9.

Further reading

Kittleson MD, Kienle RD, eds. Small Animal Cardiovascular Medicine. St Louis: Mosby, 1998.

Mellema M. Cardiac output, wedge pressure and oxygen delivery. Vet Clin North Am Small Anim Pract. 2001;31:1175–205.

Noble WH, Kay JC. Cardiac catheterization in dogs. Can Anesth Soc J. 1974;21: 616–20.

Tilley LP, Smith FWK Jr, Oyama MA, Sleeper MM, eds. Manual of Canine and Feline Cardiology, 4th edn. St Louis: Elsevier Saunders, 2008.

CHAPTER 12
Neurological status

Christine Iacovetta
BluePearl Veterinary Partners, Queens, New York

Introduction

Seizures, coma, paraplegia, quadriplegia, and generalized tremors are four of the most devastating neurological problems that necessitate early recognition and immediate therapeutic intervention for ICU patients (Figure 12.1). The end-result of successful therapy is not just patient survival, but includes recovery from neurological dysfunction after injury. Whether the patient presents to the ICU with neurological signs or develops neurological signs later as a consequence of disease outside the nervous system, there is little room for error in diagnosis and administering treatments.

Neurological injury occurs in two phases. Primary injury occurs immediately and directly from the initial effects of the insult (e.g. mechanical tissue damage, contusion, infarction). Secondary injury occurs minutes to days later and results from intracranial and extracranial factors secondary to the primary insult.

Respiratory rate and effort, cardiac output, blood pressure, endocrine regulation, and basal organ functions depend upon the integrity of the brain and spinal cord. As the control center of the body, the nervous system requires a consistent amount of oxygen and glucose to preserve life-sustaining metabolic functions. Metabolic and homeostatic changes such as hypotension, hypoxia, hypoglycemia or fever contribute to secondary damage (Table 12.1). Hypoxia and hypoglycemia are the two most devastating systemic abnormalities. Neural tissues become damaged due to lack of the energy source adenosine triphosphate (ATP). Cell membrane channels and pumps become dysfunctional, and ultimately, there is an intracellular influx of calcium and sodium ions. The resultant osmotic effect causes cellular and extracellular swelling. Edema of the nervous tissue occurs due to the release of inflammatory mediators, reactive oxygen species, and enzyme systems, each leading to cell death. Brain edema and swelling within an intact cranium can progress to life-threatening brain herniation with coma and respiratory paralysis. It is therefore essential to monitor the neurological status of all ICU patients, giving particular attention to clinical signs of brain swelling, spinal cord compression, and systemic influences that may affect nervous tissue function.

Monitoring methods

Appropriate diagnostic tests and therapy can be initiated while working to minimize or eliminate the impact of systemic disorders on the nervous system. Important information is gained from the patient history, followed by thorough physical, orthopedic, and neurological examinations. Serial assessments of neurological function are important since patient status can rapidly change or deteriorate. Additional diagnostic and monitoring tools include routine and ancillary clinicopathological testing, neuroimaging, electrodiagnostic testing, and more invasive procedures such as cerebrospinal fluid (CSF) collection or intracranial pressure (ICP) monitoring. The choice of tests and the sequence in which they are performed will vary depending on patient status.

History

A review of the recent and past patient history should include signalment (age, breed, sex), prescribed medications (Table 12.2), recent or past seizures, head or spinal trauma, past loss of consciousness, known neurological diseases, liver, renal and thyroid function, environment, potential exposure to toxins, gagging or regurgitation, presence of other animals, past problems with anesthesia, known allergies, and diet. Information is gathered from other clinicians (neurologist, radiologist, and/or surgeon) interacting with the patient for details regarding previous patient history, examination and diagnostic findings, recent treatment, drugs or contrast agents administered, complications to anticipate and treatment recommendations.

Physical and orthopedic examinations

Basic physical parameters to monitor begin with temperature, pulse, and respiration, which reflect central nervous system (CNS) energy demands, CNS perfusion capabilities, and brain control of ventilation. Changes in the breathing pattern may occur with disease of the cerebrum or one of the four parts of the brainstem (diencephalon, midbrain, pons, and medulla). Cheyne–Stokes respirations are cycles where respiration becomes increasingly deeper then increasingly shallower with possible apneic periods. Severe cerebral or diencephalic (cranial brainstem) lesions can result in Cheyne–Stokes respirations. Hyperventilation can occur with severe midbrain disease, but must be differentiated from hyperventilation associated with acidosis or pain. An apneustic breathing pattern is characterized by deep gasping inspirations held for 30–90 seconds then expelled. Irregular and apneustic breathing is often associated with caudal pontine or medulla oblongata lesions due to loss of the vagal nerve and pneumotaxic center function. Loss of consciousness and changes in posture and pupils discussed below usually accompany abnormal respirations. High cervical lesions can result in respiratory paresis or paralysis due to loss of intercostal and diaphragm motor function from compression, edema or hemorrhage and immediate ventilatory assistance may be required.

Careful examination for evidence of trauma, systemic disease, pain, bleeding or bruising should be performed to detect systemic problems that can impact the nervous system. Evaluation of the

Monitoring and Intervention for the Critically Ill Small Animal: The Rule of 20, First Edition. Edited by Rebecca Kirby and Andrew Linklater.
© 2017 John Wiley & Sons, Inc. Published 2017 by John Wiley & Sons, Inc.

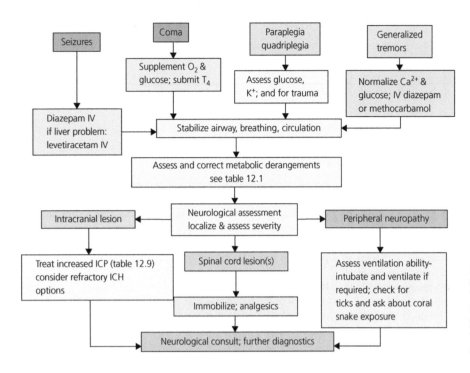

Figure 12.1 Prioritization and approach to severe neurological signs in the ICU patient. The four most critical presentations or changes in neurological signs in the ICU patient are listed at the top of the algorithm with guidelines for immediate patient stabilization.

eyes may reveal chorioretinitis suggestive of infectious disease or neoplasia, papilledema suggestive of increased ICP, or scleral hemorrhage. Orthopedic examination is performed to detect bone, tendon, joint, or muscular disorders that can influence the response to neurological testing or contribute to further neurological injury. Neck or back pain is noted and affected animals are handled little until analgesics are given and vertebral fracture or dislocation is ruled out. Pain on manipulation of the neck or back can provide an initial localization of a spinal cord lesion.

Neurological examination

Goals of the neurological examination are to:
- determine if there are neurological deficits present
- localize the lesion(s)
- determine lesion severity
- monitor for changes over time.

An attempt should be made to explain all neurological deficits by a single lesion. If that is impossible then a multifocal neurological disorder is most likely present. It is best to perform the initial neurological examination prior to administration of sedatives or analgesics when possible, unless seizures, delirium or pain warrants medication sooner.

The neurological examination usually begins with an assessment of seizures, mentation, level of consciousness, cranial nerves, and basic body posture to identify and localize intracranial problems. Lesions of the brainstem have a poorer overall prognosis than those in the cerebrum and cerebellum. Asymmetrical neurological deficits suggest a more focal disorder, such as mass, infarct or hemorrhage. Multifocal lesions are more typical of inflammation or metastatic neoplasia. A guide for localization of intracranial lesions by neurological and clinical signs is provided in Table 12.3.

Seizures

Past or present seizures indicate a primary disease of the cerebrum or diencephalon or secondary effects of metabolic disease. The majority of seizures in dogs are generalized with loss of consciousness and tonic clonic movements. However, focal seizures may occur with or without the loss of consciousness and can have a wide variety of manifestations. Patients will often present with focal facial seizures that may progress to a more generalized seizure. A list of common toxins known to cause seizures or tremors is provided in Box 12.1. Prolonged seizures result in hypoxia, hypoglycemia, hyperthermia, and lactic acidosis and constitute a neurological emergency. The seizure must be stopped immediately to reduce the amount of secondary brain damage (see Seizure treatment and complications below).

Mentation and level of consciousness

The patient should be observed at rest and wandering around the examination room if ambulatory, noting their basic movements and response to the environment. Animals with lesions of the cerebrum and diencephalon may have a blank stare, wander aimlessly, compulsively pace, press their head against a corner or wall or circle (with no head tilt) or turn the head toward the side of the lesion.

Alterations of mentation and consciousness may be graded from 1 to 18 using a modified Glasgow Coma Scale (Table 12.4). A defined grading system provides a more objective means to determine the initial severity of intracranial disease and monitor for changes. The mentation can be classified as conscious with normal, hysterical, inappropriate, or obtunded behavior. Changes in levels of consciousness include stupor (laterally recumbent responsive only to noxious stimuli) or coma (unconscious, unresponsive to any stimuli) (Table 12.5). Stupor or coma can occur with lesions anywhere in the cerebrum or brainstem, due to dysfunction of the ascending reticular activating system (ARS). Input to the ARS normally alerts the brain, resulting in consciousness. Stimulation of sensory peripheral and cranial nerves projects impulses into the reticular formation within the medulla, pons, and midbrain, which then projects through the diencephalon to alert the cerebral cortex. Common causes of alterations in mentation and consciousness include brain trauma, neoplasia, and inflammation as well as systemic metabolic or inflammatory disease, intoxication or prescribed medications (see Table 12.2).

Table 12.1 Systemic disorders that influence CNS function.

Parameter	Neurological derangement	Mechanism of effect on CNS	Treatment goal	Note
Oxygen $PaO_2 \leq 80$ mmHg $PaO_2 \leq 60$ mmHg = severe hypoxemia	Anxiety Dull mentation Seizures	Inadequate energy production	Oxygen support $PaO_2 > 60$ mmHg	Avoid nasal cannula if causes sneezing or agitation
Carbon dioxide Hypocarbia $PCO_2 < 35$ mmHg Hypercarbia $PCO_2 > 45$ mmHg	Anxiety Dull mentation Dull mentation Coma	Cerebral vasoconstriction Cerebral vasodilation, sympathetic stimulation	Normalize $PCO_2 = 35–45$ mmHg	Mechanical ventilation may be required to maintain normal PCO_2
pH Acidemia pH <7.35 Alkalemia pH >7.45	Dull mentation Dull mentation	Alterations in cerebral blood flow, cardiovascular effects, ROS	Normalize pH 7.34–7.40	Correct fluid deficits, ventilation and other abnormalities Administer sodium bicarbonate only if refractory metabolic acidemia
Glucose Hypoglycemia Hyperglycemia	Weakness Seizures Stupor Coma Weakness Stupor Coma Neuropathy	Alterations in cerebral blood flow, altered Na/K ATPase, increased intracellular calcium, ROS Lactate production, edema, excitatory amino acid release, ROS, altered cerebral blood flow	Euglycemia – <180 mg/dL	Supplementation with solutions greater than 7.5% dextrose should not be administered in a peripheral catheter. Monitor often to titrate needs
Potassium Decreased	Generalized weakness Paralysis Ventral flexion of neck in cats	Depressed muscle excitability causing severe weakness or paralysis	Normalize 3.5–5 mEq/L	Ventilation can be needed if paralysis of diaphragm; may be seen with chronic renal disease in cats. Replace no faster than 0.5 mEq/kg/h
Magnesium Increased Decreased	Lethargy Weakness Hyporeflexia Respiratory depression Arrhythmia Weakness Ataxia Tremors Seizures	Decreased acetylcholine release and neuromuscular blockade Increased acetylcholine release	Normalize Dogs: 1.9–2.5 mg/dL total or 0.4–0.6 mmol/L Cats: 1.8–2.9 mg/dL total or 0.4–0.7 mmol/L	Correct any potassium or calcium abnormalities as well as magnesium
Phosphorus Increased Decreased	Weakness Seizures Ataxia Seizures	Signs usually secondary to calcium sequestration leading to hypocalcemia Decreased cellular energy and 2,3-DPG	Normalize 2.5–5.5 mg/dL Supplementation with KH_2PO_4	Treat primary disease to correct Make sure to take into account the K amount given to avoid overdosing
Blood pressure Hypotension Hypertension	Weakness Ataxia Dull mentation Blindness Disorientation Seizures Head tilt	Decreased oxygen and energy supply Vascular inflammation and injury, altered blood flow	Systolic pressure: 100–150 mmHg	Patients with severe hypertension should have a stepwise decrease in pressure while hospitalized to avoid signs of hypotension

(Continued)

Table 12.1 (Continued)

Parameter	Neurological derangement	Mechanism of effect on CNS	Treatment goal	Note
Thiamine Deficiency (B_1)	Bilateral vestibular signs Mydriasis Ventral flexion of neck in cats Lethargy Seizures	Deficiency in carbohydrate metabolism leading to energy depletion and neuronal necrosis	Supplement: 12.5–50 mg/dog 12.5–25 mg/cat IM, SC or PO daily	Seen with diets mainly of raw fish or diets heated to excessive temperatures
Thyroid Hypothyroidism	Peripheral neuropathy Myxedema coma	Not completely understood – possibly depletion in energy metabolism and altered cerebral blood flow	Supplementation to normal levels	An association also exists with: Peripheral vestibular signs Facial nerve paralysis Laryngeal paralysis Megaesophagus
Hyperthyroidism	Hypertensive signs Thyroid storm Agitation Seizures Thyrotoxic periodic paralysis	Increased stimulation of the cardiovascular and sympathetic systems	Normalize with drug therapy or radioactive iodine	Treatment of thyroid storm will necessitate rapid reduction in hormone production and release as well as cardiovascular support
Body temperature Hypothermia	Lethargy Dull mentation	Decreased metabolic demand and altered blood flow	Normalize body temperature 100–102.5 °F	Warming should be performed slowly with careful attention to blood pressure Cooling efforts should be stopped around 103 °F to avoid overshooting If a true fever exists, treatment should be aimed at the underlying disease, not active cooling
Hyperthermia	Dull mentation Seizures	Increased metabolic demand and altered blood flow		
Coagulation Hypocoagulation	Dull mentation Seizures	Hemorrhage directly into or around nervous tissue leading to dysfunction and potential increased intracranial pressure	Monitor coagulation factor parameters and platelet numbers	Plasma is not recommended unless clinical risk of bleeding is high or there is active hemorrhage
Hypercoagulation	Dull mentation Seizures	Ischemia/infarct to nervous tissue, vascular effects altering blood flow		
Calcium Decreased	Tremors Facial scratching Stiff gait Seizures	Decreased cell membrane threshold potential	Normalize ionized calcium levels	Always measure ionized levels as other factors can affect total calcium levels
Increased	Lethargy Weakness Ataxia Twitching Seizures	Increased cell membrane threshold potential		
Sodium Decreased	Dull mentation Seizures Coma	Osmotic swelling of cells	Normalization of sodium levels	Do not change serum sodium level faster than 0.5 mEq/L/h unless the disease is acute to avoid worsened neurological insult
Increased	Dull mentation Seizures Coma	Osmotic shrinkage of cells		

ROS, reactive oxygen species generation.

Table 12.2 Potential CNS side-effects of drugs frequently used in the ICU.

CNS signs	Drug	Therapy
Vestibular	Metronidazole	Discontinue – diazepam
	Aminoglycosides	Discontinue if possible
Seizures	Enrofloxacin IV	Discontinue or change route of administration
	Lidocaine	Discontinue, reduce dose, intralipid
	Dobutamine	Discontinue, reduce dose
	Iohexol contrast	Stop administration
		*For all cases, diazepam can be given to stop the immediate seizure
Depression/	Acepromazine	Discontinue, reduce dose
sedation	Chlorpromazine	Discontinue, reduce dose
	Benzodiazepines	Discontinue, reduce dose, flumazenil
	Opiates	Discontinue, reduce dose, naloxone
	Anticonvulsants	Wait for signs to improve, change drug
	Dexmedetomidine	Discontinue, reduce dose, atipamezole
	Mirtazapine	Discontinue, reduce dose, decrease frequency
	Tramadol	Discontinue, reduce dose
Agitation/	Opiates	Discontinue, reduce dose, naloxone, change drug
disorientation	Benzodiazepines	Discontinue, reduce dose, flumazenil
	Metoclopramide	Discontinue, reduce dose
Ataxia	Any sedative drug	Discontinue, reverse drug if possible
	Epidural/local block	Wait for effects of drug to wear off
Tremors	Avermectins	Discontinue, intralipid
	Isoproterenol	Discontinue, reduce dose
	Epinephrine	Discontinue, reduce dose

Box 12.1 Common toxins associated with seizures and generalized tremors.

Toxins associated with seizures

Ivermectin
Chocolate
Bromethalin
Baclofen
Tricyclic antidepressants
Amphetamines
Cocaine
Serotonin
Organophosphates
Carbamates
Ethylene glycol
Lead
Strychnine
Xylitol
Insulin overdose
Neurotoxic mushrooms
Salt poisoning
Moth balls

Toxins primarily associated with tremors
(may progress to seizures)

Pyrethroids/permethrin
Tremorgenic mycotoxins
Metaldyhyde

Table 12.3 Localization of neurological lesions in the brain by clinical signs.

Lesion location	Clinical signs	Note
Cerebrum and diencephalon CN I CN II	Seizures, behavior change, dementia, delirium, depression, stupor or coma with normal or miotic pupils; head pressing; pacing; circling; loss of smell (CN I); blind with dilated pupils (CN II) or normal pupils; Cheyne–Stokes breathing pattern	Acute lesions may have transient contralateral hemiparesis or quadriparesis; spinal reflexes normal or exaggerated
Midbrain CN III CN IV Rubronuclei (main flexor tract)	Stupor, coma, dilated (CN III) or midrange fixed pupils; ventrolateral strabismus (CN III); absent pupil light response (CN III); pupil rotation (CN IV)	Quadriparesis with bilateral lesion; decerebrate rigidity with severe lesion; spinal reflexes normal or exaggerated in all four limbs
Pons CN V	Depression, stupor, coma; miotic pupils with normal mentation; atrophy of temporal and masseter muscles or decreased facial sensation or hyperesthesia of face (CN V)	Ipsilateral hemiparesis; spinal reflexes normal or exaggerated in all four limbs
Cranial medulla oblongata CN VI CN VII CN VIII Reticulospinal tract (extensor tract) Vestibulospinal tract (extensor tract)	Depressed or normal mentation; stupor or coma; medial strabismus (CN VI); reduced blink, lip and ear reflex (CN VII); nystagmus and disequilibrium (CN VIII)	Ipsilateral hemiparesis; spinal reflexes normal or exaggerated in all four limbs
Caudal medulla oblongata CN IX CN X CN XI CN XII	Depressed or normal mentation; stupor or coma; hyperventilation; apneustic breathing; heart rate and blood pressure alterations; dysphagia (CN IX or X); megaesophagus (CN X); laryngeal paresis (CN X); tongue atrophy or paralysis (CN XII)	Ipsilateral hemiparesis; spinal reflexes normal or exaggerated in all four limbs
Cerebellum	Intention tremors and ataxia of the head; head tilt away from lesion; nystagmus; loss of menace response; ipsilateral or bilateral dysmetria; normal limb strength	Normal reflexes all four limbs unless opisthotonus or decerebellate rigidity (conscious animal)

CN, cranial nerve.

Table 12.4 Modified Glasgow Coma Scale. Within each category a score of 1–6 is assigned. A score of 18 is normal; as the score decreases from this, the severity of neurological injury increases [3]. A score of 8 at admission is associated with a 50% probability of survival [4].

Motor activity	Score
Normal gait, normal spinal reflexes	6
Hemiparesis, tetraparesis, or decerebrate activity	5
Recumbent, intermittent extensor rigidity	4
Recumbent, constant extensor rigidity	3
Recumbent, constant extensor rigidity with opisthotonus	2
Recumbent, hypotonia of muscles, depressed or absent spinal reflexes	1
Brainstem eflexes	
Normal pupillary reflexes and oculocephalic reflexes	6
Slow pupillary reflexes and normal to reduced oculocephalic reflexes	5
Bilateral unresponsive miosis and normal to reduced oculocephalic reflexes	4
Pinpoint pupils with reduced to absent oculocephalic reflexes	3
Unilateral, unresponsive mydriasis and reduced to absent oculocephalic reflexes	2
Bilateral, unresponsive mydriasis and reduced to absent oculocephalic reflexes	1
Level of consciousness	
Occasional periods of alertness and responsive to environment	6
Depression or delirium, responsive, but response may be inappropriate	5
Semicomatose, responsive to visual stimuli	4
Semicomatose, responsive to auditory stimuli	3
Semicomatose, responsive only to repeated noxious stimuli	2
Comatose, unresponsive to repeated noxious stimuli	1
Total score	

Source: Platt SR, Radaelli ST, McDonnell JJ. The prognostic value of the Modified Glasgow Coma Scale in head trauma in dogs. J Vet Med. 2001;15(6):581–4. Open Access License, Wiley.

Table 12.5 Levels of consciousness in the cat and dog.

Level of consciousness	Definition
Normal	Exhibits a response typical of the "normal" temperament of the patient
Demented	Response is not typical of the "normal" temperament of the patient or is different from what is a normal expected response
Delirium	Irrational or uncontrollable emotional response
Obtunded	Decreased conscious response to external nonnoxious stimuli – subjectively is graded as mild, moderate or severe
Stupor	Conscious response only with the application of a noxious stimulus
Unconscious	Lack of any conscious response to any external stimuli limited to a brief period of time (seconds or minutes)
Coma	Prolonged lack of any conscious response to any external stimuli – spinal and cranial nerve reflexes may or may not be present depending on the location of the lesion

Mentation changes caused by systemic metabolic disorders should improve markedly as the systemic abnormalities are corrected unless secondary damage has occurred.

Cranial nerves

The functions of the cranial nerves (Table 12.6) are assessed to evaluate the health of the peripheral nerve and the area of the brainstem containing the nucleus of that nerve. Normal cranial nerve function reduces the likelihood of a lesion in a specific region of the brainstem. A change in mentation or level of consciousness with normal cranial nerve functions suggests cerebral and diencephalic disease.

The eyes are examined for direct and indirect pupillary light responses (cranial nerve (CN) II and III), eyeball position, and the vestibuloocular reflex. Normal responsive pupils or small but reactive pupils are typically found with cerebral or diencephalic lesions. Dilated unresponsive pupils (unilateral or bilateral) or midrange fixed unresponsive pupils occur with midbrain lesions. Miotic unresponsive pupils suggest a lesion within the pons or medulla. Eyeball position (CN III, IV, and VI) can also reflect midbrain and medulla function. Ventrolateral strabismus indicates CN III or midbrain disease. Dorsolateral rotation of the pupil can be observed in cats with CN IV or midbrain disease. Medial strabismus indicates CN VI or cranial medulla disease.

The vestibuloocular reflex is done only when no cervical injury is suspected. This is not performed in patients comatose from head trauma until cervical fracture or dislocation has been ruled out radiographically, as head and neck trauma may occur simultaneously. The head is slowly moved from side to side while observing for normal physiological nystagmus. Loss of normal physiological nystagmus can occur with CN III, IV, VI, and VIII disease or the corresponding brainstem nuclei. Asymmetrical atrophy of the muscles of mastication can occur with unilateral ipsilateral CN V and pontine lesions. Bilateral atrophy of the muscles of mastication is most commonly associated with masticatory myopathy or generalized cachexia.

Loss of the palpebral response in a conscious patient occurs in CN VII or cranial medulla lesions. The palpebral response will often fatigue and disappear upon repeated testing in patients with myasthenia gravis. Head tilt (ear closer to the ground on one side), spontaneous nystagmus, and disequilibrium occur with CN VIII, rostral medulla or cerebellar lesions. The head tilts toward the side of the lesion in CN VIII and medulla lesions, but away from the side of the lesion in cerebellar or other medulla lesions. Loss of the swallowing reflex in a conscious patient can occur with lesions of CN IX and X or the caudal medulla. Loss of consciousness can result in loss of the palpebral and swallowing reflexes due to the release of a descending inhibitory pathway from the higher brain centers suppressing the normal reflex.

Basic body posture and involuntary movements

Abnormal body postures can aid in localizing neurological lesions. With decerebrate rigidity, an animal is unconscious with extension of the head, neck, and limbs and a midbrain lesion is suspected. With decerebellate rigidity, the animal is conscious and has extension of the head, neck, and thoracic limbs with flexion of the pelvic limbs and a lesion of the rostral lobe of cerebellum is suspected. A transient increase in extensor tone in the neck and limbs can occur when moving unconscious or conscious patients with cervical lesions. This is the result of unopposed stimulation of postural muscles (extensor) in response to impulses from the vestibular system. Animals with acute T3–L3 spinal cord lesions from

Table 12.6 Cranial nerve localization and evaluation.

Cranial nerve	Location of nuclei	Function	Testing	Note
I Olfactory	Diencephalon	Olfaction	Cover eyes and present food under nose	Not usually tested. Irritating substances should not be used to avoid stimulation of other nerves
II Optic	Diencephalon	Vision	Menace response Visual tracking of cotton ball/object	Note any anisocoria
III Oculomotor	Mesencephalon (midbrain)	Motor to extraocular muscles (lateral, medial, ventral rectus)	Look for strabismus – resting and positional	Deficit results in ventrolateral strabismus
		Motor to levator palpebrae superioris	Look for drop of the upper eyelid	
		Parasympathetic control to pupil	Look for mydriasis and response to light	
IV Trochlear	Mesencephalon (midbrain)	Motor to extraocular muscle (dorsal oblique)	Look for strabismus – resting and positional	Deficit results in medial strabismus
V Trigeminal	Metencephalon (pons)	Sensory to the face Three branches: maxillary nerve mandibular nerve ophthalmic nerve Motor to muscle of mastication	Corneal reflex – touch surface of cornea and look for withdrawal of head/globe	Motor response is due to CN VI and VII
			Palpebral reflex – touch medial and lateral palpebral fissures and look for closure of the eyelid	Motor response is due to CN VII
			Facial sensation – pinch both sides of the rostral upper and lower lip and look for withdrawal of the lip and blinking; if there is no response insert a small blunt-ended object into each nostril to evoke withdrawal of the head Palpate masseter and temporal muscle for symmetry and size. Mouth should be in a closed position	Motor response is due to CN VII and neck muscles
VI Abducens	Myelencephalon (cranial medulla)	Motor to extraocular muscles (retractor bulbi and lateral rectus)	Look for strabismus – resting and positional	Deficit results in top of eye rotated laterally – not obvious on dogs due to circular pupil
			Corneal reflex – touch surface of cornea and look for withdrawal of the globe backwards	Sensory response is due to CN V
VII Facial	Myelencephalon (cranial medulla)	Motor to muscle of facial expression	Look for facial symmetry Palpebral reflex – touch medial and lateral palpebral fissures and look for closure of the eyelid	Sensory response is due to CN V
			Facial sensation – pinch both sides of the rostral upper and lower lip; look for withdrawal of the lip and blinking	Sensory response is due to CN V
		Parasympathetic supply to lacrimal gland and sublingual and submandibular salivary gland Sensory and taste to rostral 2/3 of tongue	Schirmer's tear test can be used to test lacrimal innervation	
VIII Vestibulocochlear	Myelencephalon (cranial medulla)	Vestibular function and hearing	Ataxia with wide-based stance Circling, head tilt Resting nystagmus Positional ventrolateral strabismus Vestibuloocular reflex – slowly move the nose to one side, the eyes should move in the opposite direction to stabilize the visual field forward (physiological nystagmus)	Usually toward lesion Fast phase away from lesion Same side as lesion Positional nystagmus should also be assessed by laying the patient on its back and looking for rapid eye movements Bilateral disease will not have a head tilt or nystagmus of any kind (including physiological) Cerebellar lesions will cause paradoxical vestibular signs, proprioceptive deficits used to decipher side of lesion

(Continued)

Table 12.6 (*Continued*)

Cranial nerve	Location of nuclei	Function	Testing	Note
IX Glossopharyngeal	Myelencephalon (caudal medulla)	Motor to larynx and pharynx Sensory supply to pharynx Sensory and taste to caudal 1/3 of tongue Parasympathetic supply to parotid and zygomatic salivary gland	Gag reflex	It is important to question the owner about changes in voice, or any dysphagia/regurgitation at home
X Vagus	Myelencephalon (caudal medulla)	Motor to larynx and pharynx Sensory supply to pharynx Parasympathetic supply to viscera	Gag reflex	Same for CN IX
XI Accessory	Myelencephalon (caudal medulla)	Motor to trapezius muscle	Look for trapezius atrophy	Difficult to assess
XII Hypoglossal	Myelencephalon (caudal medulla)	Motor to tongue muscles	Look for atrophy, asymmetry or deviation of the tongue	In chronic cases tongue will deviate to the affected side
Horner's syndrome	Sympathetic fibers in the hypothalamus course through the cervical spinal cord to the T1–3 region and via the sympathetic trunk pass to the cranial cervical ganglia. From here they continue to the middle ear and ophthalmic nerve (CN V branch) to smooth muscle of the face	Motor to dilator muscle of the pupil and smooth muscle of the orbit/lid Vascular tone to blood vessels in the head	Look for ptosis, miosis, and enophthalmos with third eyelid elevation. Miosis is most commonly seen Loss of vascular tone on ipsilateral side of the head leading to the skin feeling warm Should prompt evaluation of cervical, thoracic or middle ear disease along with primary intracranial disease	1% phenylephrine applied to the eye and wait for pupil dilation Time it takes to dilate corresponds with lesion location; the shorter the time, the closer the lesion is to the eye

CN, cranial nerve.

intervertebral disk herniation or vertebral trauma may exhibit Schiff-Sherrington syndrome manifested as extension of the thoracic limbs and paralysis of the pelvic limbs. Animals with focal spinal cord lesions are conscious with normal mentation. Abnormal involuntary movements such as myoclonus, tremors, and head bobbing are noted. If an animal has rolling to one side worsened with handling accompanied by a head tilt then a lesion of the vestibular system (CN VIII, medulla or cerebellum) is suspected.

Gait, limb strength and sensation, and postural reactions

The gait, limb strength, and postural reaction tests may be affected by lesions anywhere in the central or peripheral nervous systems. Acute cerebral and diencephalic disease can cause contralateral hemiplegia or hemiparesis (weakness or paralysis of the limbs on one side of the body), but recovery occurs within 24–48 hours. High unilateral midbrain disease causes contralateral hemiparesis or hemiplegia, whereas caudal unilateral midbrain disease causes ipsilateral signs. Unilateral lesions of the rest of the brainstem, spinal cord, and peripheral nerves produce ipsilateral deficits. Animals with gait and limb deficits associated with focal brainstem disease will also have ipsilateral cranial nerve deficits that correspond to that brainstem segment.

Nonrecumbent animals can be observed walking, trotting, going up and down stairs, and turning in circles. A conscious recumbent animal with no history of trauma can be supported to assess limb strength, tone, and motor function. An animal experiencing pain from irritation of spinal nerves may be lame or hold a limb flexed, referred to as a "root signature." A "root signature" is most commonly seen in a thoracic limb.

Gait and limb function can be assigned a number grade on a scale from 0 to 5 as follows: 0 = normal; 1 = ataxia, no paresis; 2 = paresis but ambulatory; 3 = nonambulatory, voluntary movement and deep pain still present; 4 = nonambulatory, no voluntary movement, but deep pain still present; and 5 = nonambulatory, no voluntary movement and deep pain absent. The lower the number initially or the reduction of the number over time, the better the prognosis. However, as much as 50% of animals with acute grade 5 (paralysis and no deep pain) injuries initially can recover function over time so serial neurological examinations are essential.

Ataxia is the lack of coordination of voluntary movements manifested by hypermetria (exaggerated flexion), hypometria (exaggerated extension), crossing over of the limbs or taking disjointed strides. If head bobbing with or without a head tilt accompanies ataxia, then cerebellar disease is suspected. Ataxia manifested by falling to each side during ambulation (drunken gait) may also be associated with bilateral CN VIII (vestibular) disease. This is differentiated from cerebellar disease, as there is no hypermetria, hypometria or head bobbing. Ataxia can be associated with spinal cord lesions that affect the superficial sensory tracts going to the cerebellum. Spinal ataxia can affect all four limbs or only the pelvic limbs.

Paresis is weakness of one or more limbs. Paralysis is loss of all voluntary motor activity. Animals with paresis have weak voluntary movement and muscle strength and tone. If ambulatory, a short stride or trembling while standing may be observed in paretic animals. Lowered neck or hips while walking and dragging of the toes may be a manifestation of thoracic and pelvic limb paresis respectively. Some paraparetic animals lean slightly forward to bear weight on the thoracic limbs, but this is more commonly observed in orthopedic disease of the hips and knees. Paralyzed (plegic) animals have absence of any voluntary movement in one or more limbs.

Hemiparesis or hemiplegia is paresis or paralysis of thoracic and pelvic limbs on one side respectively. Quadriparesis or quadriplegia (tetraparesis or tetraplegia) is paresis or paralysis of all four limbs respectively. Paraparesis or paraplegia is paresis or paralysis of pelvic limbs respectively. In general, nonambulatory patients (grades 3–5) with acute spinal cord signs require immediate imaging (often in anticipation of surgery) as soon as anesthesia can be tolerated. Immediate surgical decompression, where indicated, can improve the prognosis of return of neurological function.

Deep pain is tested by pinching the bones of the digits with hemostatic forceps (not just the fingers) and observing the animal for a behavioral response. The animal must turn and look or cry when the digit is tightly compressed. Deep pain is not pronounced absent until all the digits of a limb have been compressed and no response is observed. Withdrawing the limb does not mean deep pain is present, only that the spinal reflex to the tested limb is present.

Postural reaction assessment involves evaluation of conscious proprioception, hopping, hemiwalking, wheelbarrowing, extensor postural thrust, and visual and tactile placing. These tests are helpful to detect subtle neurological abnormalities of the cerebrum, brainstem or spinal cord and may be abnormal even if the gait appears normal. Conscious proprioception testing is a highly sensitive indicator of neurological lesions. Conscious proprioceptive deficits are demonstrated when the animal fails to return the foot to the normal position when made to bear weight on the dorsum of the paw.

Spinal reflexes and cutaneous trunci responses

The brain orchestrates limb movements and spinal reflexes via ascending sensory pathways to the cerebellum and descending upper motor neurons (UMN) from the cerebrum and brainstem. The UMN synapse on the lower motor neuron (LMN) reflex arc and both are needed for normal limb strength and reflexes. Interruption of the UMN pathways outside the brachial or lumbosacral intumescences will result in exaggerated or spastic spinal reflexes in the limbs caudal to the site of the lesion. Interruption of the LMN in the brachial or lumbar intumescence results in depressed or absent spinal reflexes in the affected limbs.

Spinal reflexes can be useful to localize a lesion to specific spinal cord segments (Table 12.7). The neural pathway for most limb reflexes includes the sensory receptors of muscles and tendons, afferent (sensory) nerves, usually an internuncial neuron in the spinal cord, efferent nerves (LMN), the myoneural junction, and effector muscle(s). Any interruption in the reflex pathway will result in one or more reduced or absent limb reflexes. The thoracic limb reflexes (triceps, biceps, extensor carpi radialis, and withdrawal reflexes) are associated with the C6–T1 peripheral nerves and spinal cord segments (brachial intumescence). The pelvic limb reflexes (patellar, cranial tibial, gastrocnemius, and withdrawal reflexes) require integrity of the peripheral nerves and spinal cord

Table 12.7 Lesion localization to a spinal segment based on limb reflexes.

Spinal segment	Thoracic limb reflexes	Pelvic limb reflexes
C1–C5	Exaggerated to spastic (UMN)	Exaggerated to spastic (UMN)
C6–T2	Depressed or absent (LMN)	Exaggerated to spastic (UMN)
T3–L3	Normal or Rigid extension with Schiff-Sherrington syndrome	Exaggerated to spastic (UMN)
L4–L6	Normal	Depressed to absent (LMN) L4–L5 Patellar L6–S2 Cranial tibial, gastrocnemius, and withdrawal reflexes
L6–S3	Normal	Decreased to absent pelvic limb withdrawal; decreased to absent perineal or perianal reflexes; patellar reflexes may appear increased due to loss of flexor tone

LMN, lower motor neuron; UMN, upper motor neuron.

segments of L3–S1 (lumbosacral intumescence). The anal and micturition reflexes require integrity of the cauda equina (S1–S3). The results from testing spinal reflexes are recorded as normal, depressed or absent (LMN), and exaggerated or spastic (UMN) reflex activity.

The cutaneous trunci response is manifested as twitching of the superficial thoracolumbar paravertebral muscles, when the skin is pinched. Loss of the cutaneous trunci muscle response localizes a T3–L3 spinal cord lesion within three segments.

Quadriparesis or quadriplegia with depressed or absent spinal reflexes and loss of the cutaneous trunci muscle response indicates a generalized peripheral nerve or myoneural junction disorder. Weakening of the patellar reflex with repetitive tapping may be indicative of the decremental response as seen in myasthenia gravis, warranting further clinicopathological and electrodiagnostic testing. The findings from the physical and neurological examinations are used to direct clinicopathological testing, neuroimaging, and monitoring procedures.

Point of care (POC) testing

The minimum database (POC testing) should include the hematocrit, total protein, blood urea nitrogen, blood glucose, electrolytes, and venous blood gas to rapidly search for systemic factors that can affect the CNS (see Table 12.1). Evidence of anemia or increased blood viscosity from polycythemia or hyperproteinemia can cause inadequate delivery of oxygen to nervous tissues. High blood glucose, hypernatremia, and hyponatremia can significantly alter blood osmolarity and result in fluid shifting out of or into the brain cells. Elevated blood glucose can cause increased cerebral blood flow in patients with elevated ICP and has been associated with a negative outcome in humans with brain trauma. Low blood glucose brings concern for inadequate substrate for CNS energy production. Hypokalemia can cause ventral neck flexion and generalized paresis or paralysis, with weakness of the diaphragm potentially causing life-threatening hypoventilation. Seizures, muscle tremors, and profound weakness can occur with both hypoglycemia and hypocalcemia. Alterations in CO_2 will affect cerebral blood flow, potentially contributing to increased ICP and hypoxia of nervous tissues.

Blood profiles

For all patients, a complete blood count, biochemistry profile, ammonia level, coagulation profile, and acid–base status are performed to detect any metabolic abnormalities that can contribute to or result from a CNS disease. Thyroid, adrenal, and hepatic function testing may also be warranted. Toxicology screening might include assays for lead, ethylene glycol, and other potential medication overdoses. Measuring serum anticonvulsant levels to assess therapeutic and potentially toxic concentrations might be appropriate for phenobarbital and bromide if indicated. Acetylcholine receptor antibody testing and tensilon testing to diagnose myasthenia gravis or genetic testing for diseases such as exercise-induced collapse of Labradors should be submitted for patients with compatible clinical signs. Immunoassays for toxoplasmosis, neosporosis, fungal diseases, distemper, and other organisms might demonstrate an underlying etiology.

Neuroimaging

Radiographs of the thorax and abdomen and abdominal ultrasound are recommended to evaluate for pneumonia and megaesophagus, masses, metastasis, and abscesses. The vertebrae and long bones may be radiographed for fractures, luxation or lytic lesions if not done previously. An open fontanelle may allow ultrasound examination of the brain but other neuroimaging is usually required. Traditionally, imaging of the spinal cord was performed with a myelogram and radiographs; with advances and availability of advanced imaging, these techniques are used less frequently.

Computed tomography (CT) or magnetic resonance imaging (MRI) can demonstrate intracranial lesions and changes of the meninges, intervertebral disk spaces, spinal cord, nerve roots, vertebrae or surrounding soft tissues. CT provides excellent bone and blood detail with moderate soft tissue detail, and can be performed more rapidly than MRI, frequently making it the imaging choice immediately post trauma. MRI provides exceptional soft tissue and moderate bone detail, making it the primary choice for imaging the parenchyma of the brain and spinal cord. General anesthesia is normally necessary for both imaging modalities, requiring prior patient stabilization. Contrast agents (e.g. diatrizoate (MD76) IV for CT and gadodiamide IV for MRI) may be given intravenously or with a myelogram (e.g. iohexal) to enhance visualization of lesions. Patients should be monitored and treated for seizures after myelography.

Electrodiagnostic testing

Electroencephalography (EEG) is a recording of the electrical activity of the brain. The EEG is abnormal during seizures, following brain trauma and in the presence of inflammation, edema, neoplasia, and hydrocephalus. An EEG can be useful to differentiate seizures from sedation recovery.

Brainstem auditory evoked responses (BAER) are a recording of the electrical pathway for hearing generated by a click stimulus in the ear canal. Neurologists routinely use the BAER to screen puppies and geriatric animals for unilateral or bilateral deafness associated with CN VIII (auditory portion) lesions. In the ICU, the BAER is useful to determine brainstem function in the comatose patient as waveforms appear at various points along the brainstem auditory pathway. Brain death is defined as no electrical activity on the EEG and no BAER.

Electromyography (EMG) is a recording of the electrical activity of muscle and is most useful in generalized and focal neuropathies. Muscle denervation produces fibrillation potentials and runs of positive sharp waves on EMG and can localize which spinal nerves are dysfunctional. Motor and sensory nerve electrical stimulation and calculation of the nerve conduction velocity (NCV) is a usual part of the EMG examination. In peripheral nerve injuries such as brachial plexus trauma, the EMG with NCV can be useful to determine which nerves are affected and if there is nerve integrity.

Cerebrospinal fluid analysis

Cerebrospinal fluid analysis is especially important to detect inflammatory etiologies of CNS disease (meningitis). The CSF usually does not help identify neoplasia other than occasionally CNS lymphoma if abnormal lymphocytes are observed. CSF collection is performed after CT or MRI imaging when possible to identify patients that should not be sampled and to limit alterations of images from iatrogenic hemorrhage. CSF collection is contraindicated in patients with imaging evidence of brain herniation or known increased ICP from trauma, neoplasia or other causes, spinal fracture, atlantoaxial subluxation, or coagulopathy.

The CSF collected should be immediately submitted for cytology, specific gravity, protein, and glucose. Cellular contents will begin to deteriorate within an hour of collection. Patient serum can be added to the CSF to preserve any cells (1 drop of serum to 0.25 mL CSF) and the CSF refrigerated prior to submission. A separate aliquot of CSF without serum is maintained for protein analysis. When the CSF cell number is increased, paired serum and CSF immunoassays for pathogens such as *Toxoplasma gondii*, *Neospora caninum*, distemper virus, and fungi may be indicated.

Risks encountered with CSF collection include brain herniation through the foramen if increased ICP is present, introduction of infection, hemorrhage, and puncture of cerebellar, brainstem or spinal cord parenchyma. Mild hyperventilation ($pCO_2 = 30\text{–}40\,mmHg$) prior to the tap can reduce ICP if necessary.

Intracranial pressure monitoring

Direct monitoring of ICP can be obtained when a special probe that records pressure is inserted through a small hole in the skull and a few centimeters into the brain. Direct recordings of ICP can be extremely useful to ensure early therapeutic interventions and avoid unnecessary therapy in comatose patients. Expertise and equipment costs and availability limit the use of direct ICP monitoring in most veterinary ICUs. However, without direct ICP measurement, a diagnosis of intracranial hypertension relies upon detecting the clinical signs associated with increased ICP: deterioration in mentation or level of consciousness, pupil abnormalities, abnormal respiratory patterns, and pathological change in heart rate and blood pressure.

Systemic monitoring

Each parameter of the Rule of 20 can have an impact on the CNS, requiring careful assessment 1–2 times per day. Monitoring of oxygenation (arterial blood gas or pulse oximetry), ventilation (blood gas, end-tidal CO_2), acid–base balance (blood gas), perfusion parameters (blood pressure, heart rate, pulse intensity, capillary refill time), glucose, electrolytes, urine output, body weight, body temperature, and osmolarity allows early intervention to prevent secondary injury to the nervous tissues.

Disorders of the neurological system

Management of critical problems of the brain

The identification and treatment of neurological problems of the brain are a priority in the ICU patient. There should be immediate concern that continuation or progression of the underlying problems could cause permanent impairment of neurological function or that the consequences of the neurological activity (e.g. seizures) could lead to systemic problems. In addition, systemic disorders can impact and worsen neurological signs and lesions. Seizures, generalized tremors, acute vestibular signs, stupor, and coma are the most critical signs of brain disease that must be addressed immediately. Cerebral blood flow (CBF) must be maintained at optimal levels and brain edema and herniation recognized and treated in the early stages for the best long-term outcomes.

Seizures

Seizures are caused by paroxysmal discharges from groups of neurons in the brain. There is excessive excitation or loss of inhibition of the affected neurons due to abnormal neurotransmission at the synapse and ion channels. Primary (intracranial) etiologies of seizures include epilepsy (inherited or acquired), brain tumors, traumatic brain injury, encephalitis, hydrocephalus, and cerebrovascular accident. Secondary etiologies (outside the brain) include toxins (e.g. lead, organophosphates), metabolic disorders (e.g. hypoglycemia, hypoxemia, hepatoencephalopathy, uremia), and thiamine deficiency.

There are three basic types of seizures: generalized seizures, partial seizures (to include psychomotor seizures), and partial seizures that secondarily generalize. In generalized seizures, neuronal discharges begin bilaterally and produce symmetrical tonoclonic motor activity and usually loss of consciousness. Partial or focal seizures are caused by abnormal neuronal discharges in one part of the cerebrum or diencephalon and have clinical signs dependent upon which area is affected. Most animals with partial seizures are conscious, but may have compulsive behavior or mentation alterations. The neuronal discharges can begin in one area then spread and result in more generalized activity and are then referred to as partial seizures that secondarily generalize. Partial seizures that secondarily generalize are the most common seizure type in animals. During the seizure, the patient should be carefully examined for asymmetrical involvement of face and limbs. Asymmetry means

the seizure is originating from a focus within the brain (e.g. acquired epilepsy, tumor or encephalitis) and a primary toxic, metabolic or nutritional disorder is unlikely. Recognition of seizures in a recumbent animal can be difficult when tonoclonic activity is not apparent. Persistently dilated pupils and facial muscle twitching can be evidence of mild seizure activity, but an EEG is necessary to confirm seizure activity in comatose or anesthetized patients.

Seizure activity can lead to increases in ICP, blood pressure, oxygen delivery, and neurotransmitter release, making seizures potentially harmful in critical ICU patients [1]. Immediate IV anticonvulsant therapy is required to stop the seizure activity, taking precedence over completing a physical or neurological examination [2]. Benzodiazapines provide first-line anticonvulsant therapy except for seizures due to hepatocencephalopathy for which levetiracetam can be administered. Diazepam has higher lipid solubility and may cross the blood–brain barrier faster than midazolam. A continuous infusion of diazepam or midazolam may be started for patients with cluster seizures or status epilepticus. Levetiracetam is the anticonvulsant of choice and is administered preoperatively as an adjunct to medical management in patients undergoing portosystemic shunt surgery [2].

Continued anticonvulsant therapy may be warranted for cluster seizures, status epilepticus, primary intracranial disease with seizures or the critical patient with unstable seizure control. The choice of maintenance anticonvulsant drug will depend on the individual patient, concurrent illnesses, side-effects, cost, frequency of administration, availability, and clinician preference, and options are listed in Table 12.8. An algorithm for the treatment of status epilepticus is given in Figure 12.2. For the critical patient, a loading dose of IV or IM phenobarbital can be administered to achieve therapeutic levels quickly.

Patients at risk for seizures are kept in a highly visible cage and continuously monitored for seizure activity. Bells may be placed on the collar of the animal that will ring if seizure activity occurs. The dose of the prescribed anticonvulsant should be calculated and posted on the cage or treatment sheet in advance with the drug

Table 12.8 Medications used during acute-onset seizures.

Drug	Dose	Comments
Diazepam	0.5 mg/kg IV or 1 mg/kg rectally	For acute active seizures
		For rectal administration use a short soft catheter, do not place into the distal colon; cautious use for patients with suspect portovascular anomaly
Diazepam or midazolam	CRI: 0.2–1 mg/kg/h	CRI should be tapered: reduce dose by 25–50% every 4–6 hours as long as no seizures occur
		Midazolam is preferred due to reduced plastic absorption, drug precipitation, and accumulation of metabolites
Phenobarbital	Loading: 4–mg/kg IV q 0.25–4 h up to 16–20 mg/kg IV total dose	During loading, if the patient looses their gag reflex due to sedation, the next dose is delayed
	Maintenance: 2.5–3 mg/kg IV or PO q 12 h	For patients already on phenobarbital with break through seizures you may increase the dose by 25–50% while pending drug levels
Levetiracetam	Load: 40–60 mg/kg IV	May be effective rectally (5)
	Maintenance: 20 mg/kg IV or PO q 8 h (30 mg/ kg for extended release PO q 12 h)	An extended release product is available to be given Q 12 hr
Propofol	2–8 mg/kg IV bolus followed by CRI at 0.1–0.6 mg/kg/min as needed	Note occult seizure activity may still occur. Patient may need to be intubated and ventilated.
		CRI should be tapered.
Isoflurane	0.5–2% for 1–6 h	Uncommonly used, patient will require oxygen and ventilation
Bromide	KBr: 400–600 mg PO or per rectum divided over 1–5 days	Rectal administration is irritating to the mucosa and may cause diarrhea
		NaBr is an IV alternative, bit it is not commonly available and may cause hypernatremia. Dose must be reduced by 15%

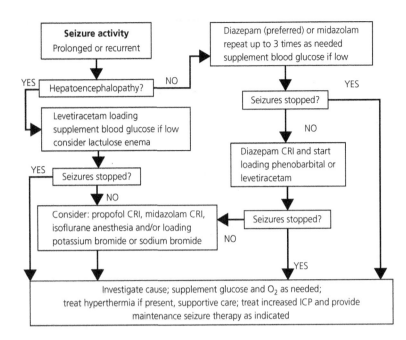

Figure 12.2 Algorithm presenting decision-making guidelines for stabilizing seizure activity in the ICU patient. See Table 12.8 for doses.

readily available. Glucose supplementation, temperature control, intravenous fluid infusion and endotracheal intubation with oxygen may be required. The effect of sedation and postictal activity must be recognized during patient evaluation. Prolonged or vigorous seizure activity can result in brain edema and increased ICP that requires treatment (Table 12.9).

Head and body tremors

Generalized tremors will increase oxygen and glucose consumption, elevate body temperature, cause patient discomfort, and interfere with normal functions such as eating and walking. The differential diagnosis of common causes of generalized tremors in mature animals includes toxicity, metabolic disorder (hypocalcemia and hypoglycemia), side-effects of specific drugs, steroid-responsive encephalomyelitis, and idiopathic tremor syndrome in dogs. Dysmyelinogenesis has been described in Chows and several other purebred dogs with head and body tremors beginning at 2–8 weeks of age. Most recover over the next few months. Tremors from metabolic disturbances tend to be episodic and irregular in frequency. Disorders of calcium, glucose, sodium, and acid–base are investigated and treated when discovered. Hepatoencephalopathy can cause tremors in conjunction with changes in mentation and seizures. A complete review of all medications and side-effects is essential as some prescribed drugs such as epinephrine, isoproterenol, and avermectins can cause tremors. Toxins to consider include mycotoxins, organophosphates, and hexachlorophene.

Therapy is directed towards managing the inciting cause and supporting the patient. Hypocalcemia and hypoglycemia are the more likely causes of acute onset of tremors in ICU patients and are evaluated with supplementation provided as needed. Generalized tremor syndrome of dogs and feline encephalomyelitis may be associated with mild inflammation of the CNS, and diazepam and corticosteroids (prednisolone 1–2 mg/kg q 12 h orally) usually improve clinical signs. Patient support can include IV glucose and fluid infusion, padded cages, assistance with ambulation, hand feeding or feeding tubes, temperature control, and analgesics as needed.

Vestibular disease

Animals with acute vertigo (a spinning sensation) from vestibular disease may be presented with violent flailing of the limbs and rolling that can initially appear similar to a seizure. On closer inspection, nystagmus is usually present and the animal is conscious, although disoriented from the vertigo. Attempts to handle the animal for closer inspection usually stimulate more violent rolling and flailing and sedation is required. Vomiting associated with vertigo is rare in animals as compared to humans. The differential diagnosis of common causes of acute vestibular signs includes inner ear infections or other inner ear disease, head trauma, hypothyroidism, idiopathic congenital or geriatric vestibular disease, and side-effects of drugs. The latter can be ruled out with a thorough history. Inner ear infections are diagnosed with otoscopic examination and MRI and treated with the appropriate antibiotic. Monitoring and management of head trauma are described below. Hypothyroidism is ruled out with normal serum T4 and thyroid stimulating hormone (TSH) levels. Idiopathic vestibular disorders are a diagnosis of exclusion.

The tendency might be to anticipate a guarded prognosis and erroneously suggest euthanasia for geriatric dogs with acute severe vestibular signs, but most recover function over time, retain only mild head tilt and lead quality lives.

Delirium, stupor or coma

Delirium is usually associated with primary or secondary cerebral or diencephalic disease. A neurological examination is performed to detect evidence of other cerebrum or brainstem signs or limb paralysis before sedation is administered.

Stupor or coma is due to either cerebral or brainstem lesions, with brainstem lesions carrying a worse prognosis. The pupil size and reactivity, examination of other cranial nerves, observation of body posture, and assessment of the respiratory pattern are used to localize the lesion (see Table 12.3). Normal cranial nerve responses and a Cheyne–Stokes breathing pattern support cerebral disease. Dilated or midrange unresponsive pupils and decerebrate rigidity

Table 12.9 Guidelines and options for treating intracranial hypertension. A combination of the treatment options can be selected based upon the severity of the neurological signs and whether the clinical signs are deteriorating or improving.

Recommendations	Treatment	Monitoring	Notes
Maintain fluid balance	Intravenous crystalloid and/or colloid support	Body weight, physical perfusion parameters, heart rate, blood pressure, CVP, lactate	Colloids may help maintain intravascular volume retention compared to crystalloids
Maintain $PaO_2 \geq 80$–100 mmHg	O_2 supplementation by flow-by, hood, mask, O_2 cage, or nasal cannula (avoid sneezing)	Arterial blood gas, pulse oximetry, respiratory rate, and effort	May require intubation and mechanical ventilation; treat any underlying respiratory problems
Maintain $PaCO_2$ between 35 and 45 mmHg	O_2 supplementation, pain control if concurrent thoracic trauma, thoracocentesis for pleural fluid/air, or mechanical ventilation	Arterial blood gas, end-tidal CO_2, care with sedative or NMB drugs and thoracic bandages	Consider IV lidocaine (0.75 mg/kg) prior to endotracheal intubation as an attempt to minimize gagging, coughing
Maintain systolic arterial blood pressure ≥ 90 mmHg	Intravenous crystalloid and/or colloid support, blood products as indicated, supplement electrolytes and glucose as indicated, positive inotropes and vasopressors	Indirect or direct arterial blood pressure; trends in central venous pressure may be helpful to assess fluid volume status but can be misleading; monitor electrolytes and blood glucose	Echocardiography and ECG can assess cardiac function; vasopressors should be used in conjunction with maintaining fluid balance, not as a substitute
Treat problems causing increasing CMRO$_2$, (i.e., hyperthermia, seizures, thrashing, or tremors, pain)	Hyperthermia: cold pack, fan, or NSAIDS if safe to do so. Seizures: antiepileptics Thrashing/tremors: sedatives, muscle relaxants Pain: analgesics (see below)	Body temperature, seizure watch, pain scale	Any abnormalities should be rapidly addressed; if naturally occurring hypothermia is present, can allow patient to warm passively but must avoid shivering
Elevate head, neck, shoulders (maintain normal head position)	20–30° head elevation over body on slant; keep head at normal angle to body	Neurological examination, ICP	Head elevation promotes cerebral venous drainage; abnormal head position can contribute to ICH
Consider hyperosmolar therapy if GCS <8, deteriorating patient, prolonged seizure activity	Mannitol (0.5–1.5-g/kg IV) administer over 20 min; onset 15–30 min, duration 2–8 h; a filter must be used or 7.5% hypertonic saline (4–7 mL/kg dogs; 2–4 mL/kg cats); administer at 1 mL/kg/min	Neurological examination, urine output, blood pressure, fluid balance, ICP	Avoid if already hyperosmolar from disease or anuric. Maintain hydration. Repeat doses as necessary but can cause osmotic diuresis, dehydration, hypotension, and ischemia; no evidence that mannitol is contraindicated with hemorrhage; no strong evidence to recommend giving furosemide with mannitol
Consider glucocorticoid therapy (only for brain tumors or inflammatory cerebral diseases Not for head injury)	Antiinflammatory or immunosuppressive dosing depends on underlying disease; oral or injectable based on patient factors	Neurological examination, urine output, body temperature, gastrointestinal signs	No benefit for head trauma; side-effects include immunosuppression, GI signs, hyperglycemia; consider GI protectants
Control pain	Pure mu-agonist opiates (fentanyl CRI 2–6 μg/kg/h IV); NSAIDs may be used in certain cases as long as cardiovascular status is stable and no contraindications	Pain scale, neurological examination, blood pressure, respiratory rate and effort	Reassess frequently; if refractory pain, may consider additional receptor targets; ketamine (2–20 μg/kg/min) and/or lidocaine (10–50 μg/kg/min, not cats) CRI
Maintain nutritional balance	Target 100% RER over 2–3 days, route of administration will be dictated by patient neurological status	Body weight, hydration, (intravenous fluid needs may be reduced), blood glucose, electrolytes	Head injury results in hypermetabolic and catabolic state; nasally placed feeding tube only if does not cause sneezing
Maintain blood glucose between 100 and 180–mg/dL (glycemic control)	Supplement with 50% dextrose if hypoglycemic (0.5–1 mL/kg bolus diluted to 25% then continue on 1.25–5% CRI) If significant and sustained hyperglycemia, regular insulin 0.2 U/kg IV q 1–4 h based on blood glucose or CRI at 0.05–0.2 U/kg/h, beginning at low dose and titrated based on blood glucose	Blood glucose q 1 h initially; if glucose ≤180 mg/dL, stop insulin administration and monitor closely; be prepared to supplement with dextrose	Hypoglycemia must be avoided to prevent further neurological injury. Initiate nutritional support simultaneously. Hyperglycemia potentiates neurological injury, increases free radical production and glutamate release, alters cerebral vasculature

CMRO$_2$, cerebral metabolic rate of oxygen consumption; CRI, continuous rate infusion; CVP, central venous pressure; ECG, electrocardiogram; GI, gastrointestinal; GSC, Glasgow Coma Score; ICP, intracranial pressure; ICH, intracranial hemorrhage; NMB, neuromuscular blocking, NSAID, nonsteroidal antiinflammatory drug; RER, resting metabolic rate.

indicate midbrain disease. The use of the Modified Glasgow Coma Scale can assist the clinician in determining the initial severity and monitor response to therapy (see Table 12.4).

The differential diagnosis of common causes of stupor and coma include traumatic brain concussion or contusion, meningoencephalitis, hydrocephalus, neoplasia, metabolic disorders, toxicities, and thiamine deficiency. It is critical to identify the inciting cause and initiate appropriate therapeutics as quickly as possible. Oxygenation, ventilation, glucose, blood pH, blood pressure, cardiac output, sodium concentration, and low thyroid levels are rapidly assessed and treatment plans initiated if abnormalities are found. Hepatopathy, renal disease, coagulopathies (causing brain hemorrhage), embolism (causing brain infarction), and sepsis (causing brain abscessation) are examples of systemic disease that can result in altered levels of consciousness. An investigation of drugs and dosages recently administered, with particular attention to anesthetics, analgesics, and sedatives, may reveal a reason for sudden mental depression, stupor or coma. Brain edema and increased ICP should be anticipated as a component of any cause of stupor or coma, with management of increased ICP as part of the treatment plan.

Clinical signs of traumatic brain injury can include mild mental confusion, depression, stupor, coma or seizures. The result of the primary injury can be concussion, hemorrhage, laceration, contusion, and skull fractures. Secondary injury commonly causes changes in CBF, increased ICP or intracranial hemorrhage with the potential for brain herniation. Serious systemic problems from trauma, such as shock, hemorrhage or impaired respiration, can initially mask neurological abnormalities. Therefore, the level of consciousness and voluntary limb movement should be assessed multiple times throughout the initial resuscitation period. The presence of head wounds, epistaxis, blood in the ear canal and facial or cranial abrasions or fractures can provide an initial indication of traumatic head injury. Dogs with hydrocephalus are at a high risk for traumatic brain injury due to the thin calvarium and open fontanelles.

Dogs with head trauma have an increased rate of developing seizures while in the hospital compared to the general population [6]. Cats with head trauma appear to be less at risk [7]. The neurological examination might need to occur in stages, depending upon concurrent traumatic injuries requiring resuscitation. Since animals with cerebral and diencephalic trauma are often able to compensate quite well, the long-term prognosis might be good even when presented initially in a coma [8]. Neuroimaging with CT or MRI is needed to definitively diagnose intracranial hemorrhage, brain swelling and herniation, skull fractures, and hydrocephalus. Serial neurological examinations can provide a trend of change in the Modified Glasgow Coma Score to evaluate response to therapy over time. Changes in CBF and ICP should be anticipated and treatment for increased ICP provided as warranted by the clinical signs.

Cerebral neoplasia and secondary edema can usually be seen on an MRI so immediate therapy as described below can be instituted to control edema progression. Meningitis, meningoencephalitis, and encephalitis can usually be seen on the MRI also. If edema and brain swelling are not obvious, CSF collection and analysis are performed to obtain a diagnosis of meningoencephalitis prior to administration of antiinflammatory drugs. Consultation with a neurologist may be needed to provide a long-term treatment plan and prognosis for cerebral neoplasia, meningoencephalitis, and hydrocephalus.

Cerebral blood flow

The brain has high requirements for oxygen and glucose, few recruitable capillaries, and consumes oxygen at a consistent rate. Cerebral blood flow is regulated by neuronal stimulation, PaO_2, $PaCO_2$, and pressure autoregulation. Pressure autoregulation keeps the CBF consistent over a mean arterial pressure (MAP) range of 50–150 mmHg. Injured areas of the brain lose the ability to autoregulate blood flow so that cerebral perfusion pressure (CPP) becomes dependent upon systemic MAP and is impaired by elevations in ICP (CPP = MAP – ICP). The CBF affects the cerebral metabolic rate of oxygen consumption ($CMRO_2$). Local $CMRO_2$ increases with neuronal activity, such as seizures or fever, and decreases with decreased activity, such as hypothermia and anesthesia. When CBF decreases below autoregulation levels, oxygen extraction will increase in an attempt to maintain $CMRO_2$ for as long as possible. Seizure activity and increased ICP will increase the metabolic demands of normal as well as damaged brain tissue. Cerebral blood flow can be inadequate due to hypotension from shock or exaggerated due to hypertension from catecholamine release. A decline in oxygen delivery and an increase in intracranial volume can worsen brain tissue injury.

Increased intracranial pressure and brain edema

Vasogenic and cytoxic mechanisms are two main causes of brain edema (Figure 12.3). Vasogenic edema is caused by an increase in pore size of the capillary endothelium of the blood–brain barrier. This results in the movement of water and protein into the brain interstitium, increasing intracranial volume and pressure. Cytotoxic edema occurs due to disruption of brain cell metabolism and impaired function of sodium and potassium pumps. There is intracellular retention of sodium and water causing cell swelling. Interstitial edema occurs due to altered osmolarity and changes in the ability of the brain cell to handle water and electrolytes. Volume buffering begins by displacing CSF into the subarachnoid space, followed by shunting of CBF into the jugular veins. Thereafter,

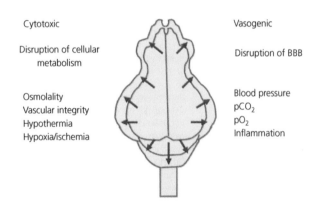

Figure 12.3 Causes of brain edema. In cytotoxic edema, the blood–brain barrier remains intact but a disruption in cellular metabolism impairs the sodium and potassium pump. Sodium and water retention leads to brain cell swelling. Cytotoxic edema is seen with various toxins, severe hypothermia, early ischemia, encephalopathy, stroke, and hypoxia. Contributing factors are listed above. Vasogenic edema occurs due to a breakdown in the tight junctions of the endothelial blood–brain barrier. Fluids and proteins can leak into the brain tissue, causing interstitial edema. This type of edema can occur as a result of trauma, ischemia, focal inflammation, neoplasia, and intracranial hypertension. Factors contributing to vasogenic edema are listed above. BBB, blood–brain barrier; pCO_2, partial pressure of carbon dioxide; pO_2, partial pressure of oxygen.

small increases in intracranial volume result in a marked increase in ICP. Slow elevation of ICP is better tolerated than acute elevation.

Depression, stupor, and coma are the usual clinical signs associated with brain edema and increased ICP. The severity of clinical signs varies with the cause, rate of onset, and ability of the brain to compensate. With severe elevations of ICP, central sympathetic stimulation will cause systemic vasoconstriction (Cushing's response) with subsequent systemic hypertension and reflex bradycardia. Patients with these clinical signs are at high risk for brain herniation and benefit from immediate therapy to reduce ICP. If the cranium is intact, a swelling cerebrum expands caudally under the tentorium cerebelli (a band of bone and soft tissue that separates cerebral and cerebellar compartments). Tentorial herniation causes compression of the midbrain with stupor and coma and dilated or midrange pupil size. If untreated at this stage, the cerebellum then swells and shifts caudally through the back of the skull to compress the medulla and cranial spinal cord, causing respiratory paralysis and death. Tentorial herniation can be reversed with treatment of increased ICP so it is critical to recognize this and treat aggressively.

Options for the medical management of increased ICP are directed at making conditions optimal for natural volume buffering, reducing $CMRO_2$, treating systemic metabolic abnormalities, and reducing brain edema (see Table 12.9). It is important to avoid compression of the jugular veins, warranting removal of collars, and avoiding neck leads to assist in volume buffering. Hyperosmolar medications may be warranted for patients with Glasgow Coma Scale <8, deteriorating clinical signs or brainstem involvement. Mannitol or 7.5% hypertonic saline can reduce cellular swelling. Mannitol decreases blood viscosity, potentially increasing CBF and nutrient delivery. Hypertonic saline may have antiinflammatory and cardiac benefits while reducing endothelial cell swelling. The administration of osmotic agents can cause dehydration and administration site phlebitis and is used with caution. Corticosteroid administration can be useful to reduce brain swelling secondary to brain tumors and inflammatory diseases of the brain. Glucocorticoids have not been shown to be beneficial in traumatic brain injury.

Critical patients refractory to initial therapeutics for increased ICP will require more aggressive therapy. Tracheal intubation and hyperventilation to maintain the PCO_2 at 30–35 mmHg can induce cerebral vasoconstriction. This is recommended only for short periods of time due to the potential for hypoxemia. Induction of a barbiturate coma to lower the $CMRO_2$ has been described, but a 2012 Cochrane review in human medicine reports no benefit due to concurrent hypotension [9]. Induced hypothermia can be an option to lower $CMRO_2$ in humans, but the benefit in veterinary patients has not been confirmed. Careful monitoring is required since hypothermia can lead to serious metabolic derangements [10].

Decompressive craniotomy can be done when skilled neurosurgeons and advanced imaging are available. Creating a window in the cranium will reduce the caudal expansion of cerebral parenchyma and hematomas, masses or bone fragments can be removed. This procedure has been reported to be associated with decreased ICP and improved CPP in humans [11]. Ventriculotomy catheters can be placed to drain CSF to assist in volume buffering, but require advanced neuroimaging and an experienced surgeon. Clinical evidence in human medicine indicates that progesterone may improve neurological outcomes in patients suffering from traumatic brain injury [12]. However, no treatment recommendations currently exist for progesterone administration for brain injury in veterinary medicine [13].

Hyperbaric oxygen therapy has been described to improve oxygenation, reducing vasogenic edema through vasoconstriction, modulation of inflammation, and promotion of angiogenesis after head injury [14]. The role of hyperbaric oxygen therapy in veterinary medicine appears promising.

Disorders of the spinal cord and peripheral nerves
Acute quadriplegia or quadriparesis
Acute quadriplegia or severe quadriparesis from cervical spinal cord or generalized peripheral nerve or myoneural junction lesions is life threatening and requires immediate treatment. Immediately establishing a patent airway and providing ventilator assistance is essential to prevent hypoxia, anoxia, hypercarbia and death. The minimum database as described above is obtained on all patients and treatment initiated to correct abnormal findings.

The differential diagnosis of common causes of acute cervical spinal cord disease includes intervertebral disk herniation, external trauma, atlantoaxial subluxation, and fibrocartilaginous embolisms. Once pain is managed and the patient is stabilized, CT or MRI is essential as surgical decompression of the spinal cord, within the first 24 hours after onset of signs, can greatly improve the chances of functional recovery. With early surgical intervention and good postoperative management and rehabilitation therapy, many animals with quadriparesis from cervical intervertebral disk herniation, trauma and atlantoaxial subluxation will again become functional. Dogs with spinal cord fibrocartilaginous embolisms are usually nonpainful and asymmetrically affected (hemiplegic on one side and hemiparetic on the other side) and have intraparenchymal spinal cord abnormalities on MRI. Most dogs with cervical fibrocartilaginous infarction have a good long-term prognosis and show signs of improvement within a few days.

The differential diagnosis of common causes of neuromuscular disease includes tick paralysis, coral snake envenomation, acute polyradiculoneuritis (coonhound paralysis, Guillain–Barré syndrome), botulism, and myasthenic crisis. Most animals are presented with a nonpainful flaccid paralysis. There is generalized loss of muscle tone and loss of spinal reflexes and the cutaneous trunci response. Superficial and deep pain sensations are often normal, except in coral snake envenomation. The animal should first be thoroughly examined for a tick, as a single engorged female tick can completely paralyze the animal. Removal of the tick can lead to resolution of the paralysis within a few hours. Coral snakebite wounds are usually not obvious, but a history of potential exposure in specific geographic locations can increase the likelihood of envenomation. With supportive care, most animals with coral snake envenomation begin to recover in a few days and make a full recovery within 1–2 weeks, even without antivenom administration.

Electromyography can be useful to differentiate acute polyradiculoneuritis from the other neuromuscular diseases, as neuromuscular transmission is blocked in tick paralysis, coral snake envenomation and botulism but not in acute polyradiculoneuritis. Most animals with acute polyradiculoneuritis also recover with nursing care over several weeks. Most animals with botulism die within the first 24 hours. Dogs that present collapsed in a myasthenic crisis will greatly improve and become ambulatory for a few minutes following 0.1–0.2 mg edrophonium IV (tensilon test). Once the patient is stabilized, a neurologist should be consulted for long-term management of animals with myasthenia gravis.

Managing the animal with quadriplegia or quadriparesis from any cause is a challenge since secondary problems can contribute significantly to patient comfort and prognosis. The level of pain should be assessed and appropriate analgesics prescribed. Paresis or paralysis of the chest and diaphragm can cause hypoventilation and hypoxemia, requiring careful monitoring of respiratory rate and effort. An appropriately sized endotracheal tube and laryngoscope should be available cage side to rapidly access the airway and provide ventilatory support should it become necessary. Urinary bladder and bowel control may be affected, requiring manual emptying, attention to patient hygiene, and concern for urinary tract infections. Appropriate padding, physical therapy, and limb massage can lower the incidence of pressure sores and reduce the likelihood of blood clots associated with immobilization. Megaesophagus and aspiration pneumonia are common complications of myasthenia gravis. Since nutritional support is essential, feeding tubes and promotility drugs provide an excellent option for minimizing regurgitation. Patients that have lost their blink response or tear production will require lubrication of the corneas.

Acute paraplegia or paraparesis
Although acute paraplegia and paraparesis (grades 3–5) do not constitute the life-threatening situation that acute quadriplegia and quadriparesis do, immediate evaluation and surgical management are critical to provide the best possible chance for functional recovery where indicated. The differential diagnosis of common causes of acute paraplegia or paraparesis includes vertebral fracture dislocation, intervertebral disk herniation, fibrocartilaginous embolism, meningomyelitis, and aortic thromboembolism.

Spinal cord trauma from vertebral fracture requires immediate patient immobilization and rapid stabilization of airway, breathing, circulation, and pain. If a patient also has stupor or coma, signs of spinal cord trauma may not be evident at the time of initial presentation. This can set the stage for secondary neurological injury if systemic problems are not quickly treated or if the animal is moved without being immobilized.

Animals with aortic thromboembolism have flaccid paraplegia (no spinal reflexes), painful limbs, and evidence of cardiac disease. Emergency and ICU management of aortic thromboembolism is discussed in Chapter 9. Once the patient is stable and aortic thromboembolism is not considered likely, survey radiographs of the entire spine are taken to examine for vertebral fractures, luxations or lysis and narrowed intervertebral disk spaces. When no obvious survey radiographic abnormalities are found in an acute nonambulatory paraparetic or paraplegic dog then immediate neuroimaging with CT or MRI is essential to prepare the dog for emergency surgery, if indicated.

Medical treatment of spinal cord lesions is aimed at minimizing secondary injury, managing pain and ensuring optimal spinal cord perfusion and oxygenation. Stable spinal fractures can be managed by placing an external splint to immobilize the spine. Animals with vertebral instability or compression from vertebral dislocation or intervertebral disk herniation should undergo surgical decompression and stabilization as soon as possible [13].The use of methylprednisolone sodium succinate is controversial, with no clear benefit shown in canine models of external trauma or acute disk herniation [15].

Confirmation of the diagnosis is paramount; although several studies have favored the use of nonsteroidal antiinflammatory drugs (NSAIDs) for disk herniation over steroids when medical or surgical management is employed, controversy still exists; both NSAIDs and steroids have been associated with adverse effects [16–18].

However, corticosteroids at antiinflammatory doses can be of benefit for animals with meningomyelitis.

Postoperative patients with intervertebral disk herniation or external trauma should have cage rest and be housed in small kennels close to the ground. Appropriate analgesics, padded cages, urinary and bowel hygiene, physical therapy, massage, and proper nutritional support are important adjuncts to surgical treatment. Acupuncture, laser therapy or treadmill hydrotherapy (after any incisions are healed), as part of rehabilitation, may be initiated within the ICU to reduce pain and maintain muscle strength during the recovery process. Once stabilized, patients can be sling walked and encouraged to stand with support. Even when spinal cord damage appears severe initially on the neurological examination, with early surgical intervention, physical therapy and nursing care, the long-term prognosis for recovery in animals that have deep pain preserved is excellent. It has been estimated that even 50% of patients that initially have no deep pain recover function.

Neck and back pain
Acute neck and back pain in ambulatory animals is always considered a humane emergency for both the patient and their caretakers, even though the possibility of life-threatening complications is low. Analgesics and muscle relaxants are often administered to relieve suffering and so that the animal can be examined more closely. The differential diagnosis of common causes of neck and back pain includes vertebral fracture, intervertebral disk disease, diskospondylitis, meningitis, and neoplasia.

Localized pain of the neck and back most often localizes the lesion to that site and may be one of the earliest signs of irritation or inflammation of the meninges or nerve roots. Intracranial disease can occasionally cause referred neck pain associated with increased ICP, but cerebral or brainstem signs are evident. An animal with a history or evidence of trauma should have immediate immobilization of the site as once muscle relaxation occurs, fractured vertebrae may dislocate and damage the spinal cord.

Once stable and the minimum database evaluated, the patient may be anesthetized for survey radiographs and CT or MRI if indicated. Vertebral fractures may be seen on survey radiographs, but a CT scan will be important to evaluate the patient for vertebral stabilization surgery. Intervertebral disk disease, diskospondylitis, and vertebral neoplasia may be seen on survey radiographs, but CT or MRI will best demonstrate the extent of lesions and potential for the development of quadriparesis or paraparesis. CSF collection and analysis will be necessary to diagnose causes of meningitis.

Supportive care is provided in the ICU and periodic analgesic therapy is continued. Specific therapy and long-term prognosis will vary with each disorder. Vertebral fractures may heal without surgery, but the development of paresis in the ICU usually indicates emergency surgery. Dogs with intervertebral disk disease may recover with analgesics, NSAIDs, and acupuncture and not require surgery. Diskospondylitis requires long-term antibiotic or antifungal medications. Recovery from bacterial diskospondylitis is usually very good, but animals with fungal diskospondylitis usually require long-term or constant antifungal drugs to maintain an acceptable quality of life. Bacterial meningitis will require long-term antibiotics once the offending organism is identified, but most meningitis is of the steroid-responsive type and may require long-term corticosteroid therapy. Some extrameduallary spinal cord tumors can be removed and treatment with chemotherapy or radiation is initiated to improve the long-term prognosis. Vertebral tumors generally have a grave prognosis.

References

1. Bratton SL, Chestnut RM, Ghajar J, et al. Brain Trauma Foundation, American Association of Neurological Surgeons, Congress of Neurological Surgeons, Joint Section on Neurotrauma and Critical Care, AANS/CNS. Guidelines for the management of severe traumatic brain injury. J Neurotrauma 2007;24(S1):S83–6.

2. Fryer KJ, Levine JM, Peycke LE, et al. Incidence of postoperative seizures with and without levetiracetam pretreatment in dogs undergoing portosystemic shunt attenuation. J Vet Intern Med. 2011;25(6):1379–84.

3. Risio L. Structural epilepsy. In: Canine and Feline Epilepsy: Diagnosis and Management. Risio L, Platt S, eds. Wallingford: CABI, 2014: pp 153–4.

4. Platt SR, Radaelli ST, McDonnell JJ. The prognostic value of the modified Glasgow Coma Scale in head trauma in dogs. J Vet Intern Med. 2001;15(6):581–4.

5. Peters R, Schubert T, Clemmons R, Vickroy T. Levetiracetam rectal administration in healthy dogs. J Vet Intern Med. 2014;28(2):504–9.

6. Friedenberg SG, Butler AL, Wei L, Moore SA, Cooper ES. Seizures following head trauma in dogs: 259 cases (1999–2009). J Am Vet Med Assoc. 2012;241:1479–83.

7. Grohmann KS, Schmidt MJ, Moritz A, Kramer M. Prevalence of seizures in cats after head trauma. J Am Vet Med Assoc. 2012;241:1467–70.

8. Sande A, West C. Traumatic brain injury: a review of pathophysiology and management. J Vet Emerg Crit Care 2010;20(2):177–90.

9. Roberts I, Sydenham E. Barbiturates for acute traumatic brain injury. Cochrane Database Syst Rev. 2012;12: CD000033.

10. Polderman KH. Mechanisms of action, physiological effects, and complications of hypothermia. Crit Care Med. 2009;37(Suppl):S186–S202.

11. Bor-Seng-Shu E, Figueiredo EG, Amorim RLO, Teixeira MJ. Decompressive craniectomy; a meta-analysis of influences on intracranial pressure and cerebral perfusion pressure in the treatment of traumatic brain injury. J Neurosurg. 2012;117:589–96.

12. Junpeng M, Huang S, Qin S. Progesterone for acute traumatic brain injury. Cochrane Database Syst Rev. 2011;19(1): CD008409.

13. Platt S, Olby N, eds. BSAVA Manual of Canine and Feline Neurology, 4th edn. Gloucester: British Small Animal Veterinary Association, 2013.

14. Edwards ML. Hyperbaric oxygen therapy. Part 2: application in disease. J Vet Emerg Crit Care 2010;20(3):289–97.

15. Coates JR, Sorjonen DC, Simpson ST, et al. Clinicopathologic effects of a 21-aminosteroid compound (U74389G) and high-dose methylprednisolone on spinal cord function after simulated spinal cord trauma. Vet Surg. 1995;24(2):128–39.

16. Levine JM, Levin GJ, Johnson SI, et al. Evaluation of the success of medical management for presumed thoracolumbar intervertebral disk herniation in dogs. Vet Surg. 2007;36(5):482–91.

17. Levin GJ, Boozer L, Schatzberg SJ, et al. The effects and outcome associated with dexamethasone administration in dogs with thoracolumbar intervertebral disk herniation: 161 cases (2000–2006). J Am Vet Med Assoc. 2008;232(3):411–17.

18. Rossmeisl JH, White C, Pancotto TE, et al. Acute adverse events associated with ventral slot decompression in 546 dogs with cervical intervertebral disc disease. Vet Surg. 2013;42(7):795–806.

Further reading

De Lahunta A, Glass EN, Kent M. Veterinary Neuroanatomy and Clinical Neurology, 4th edn. St Louis: Elsevier Saunders, 2014.

Platt S, Garosi L. Small Animal Neurological Emergencies. London: Manson Publishing/Veterinary Press, 2012.

Platt S, Olby N, eds. BSAVA Manual of Canine and Feline Neurology, 4th edn. Gloucester: British Small Animal Veterinary Association, 2013.

CHAPTER 13

The renal system

Lee Herold

DoveLewis Emergency Animal Hospital, Portland, Oregon

Introduction

The urinary tract consists of the kidneys, ureters, urinary bladder, and urethra. Insult to this system can be attributed to prerenal (blood flow to the kidneys), intrinsic renal (renal parenchyma) or postrenal (ureteral, urinary bladder or urethral) lesions (Table 13.1). Many critically ill patients will have a combination of insults [1,2].

The responsibilities of the kidneys are diverse and proper function is required for homeostasis [3]. Renal functions include but are not limited to the maintenance of water, electrolyte and acid–base balance, production of hormones (such as erythropoietin and vitamin D3), excretion of toxic metabolites, and production of energy through gluconeogenesis [3]. The functioning unit of the kidney is the nephron, which consists of a tuft of capillaries called the glomerulus surrounded by Bowman's capsule that leads to the renal tubules (Figure 13.1) [1,3]. The glomerulus and Bowman's capsule are collectively referred to as the renal corpuscle which is the site of plasma ultrafiltration [1,3]. The volume of ultrafiltrate produced at the glomerulus is dependent on hydrostatic pressures within the glomerular capillaries, determined by systemic blood pressure and by the relative degree of dilation or constriction of the afferent and efferent arterioles. The pressure within the glomerular tuft is often referred to as transglomerular capillary pressure. Bowman's capsule is composed of interdigiting cells called podocytes, surrounded by a specialized glomerular basement membrane. The degree of interdigitation of podocytes and the negative electric charge of the glomerular basement membrane serve to exclude plasma proteins from being ultrafiltered and lost in the urine in the healthy patient.

Diseases that limit renal blood flow or lower transglomerular capillary pressure can contribute to alterations in volume of the glomerular filtrate or the glomerular filtration rate (GFR) [1–3]. Additionally, pathological changes in the glomerular basement membrane can lead to plasma components such as albumin being leaked in the urine.

The renal tubules are divided into proximal tubules, the loop of Henle, distal convoluted tubules, and connecting segment and collecting tubules. These tubular segments are differentiated by their physiological function [3]. The proximal tubule consists of convoluted and straight segments and is the site of active resorption of sodium and isoosmotic resorption of water and filtered solutes. Distinguishing characteristics of the proximal tubular cells include extensive surface area for resorption provided by brush border microvilli, large quantity of mitochrondria providing energy for the high resorption function, and intercellular junctions that allow paracellular transport. The loop of Henle is the site of sodium and chloride resorption in excess of water. Its ability to absorb sodium and water and change the osmolality of urine is due to different permeability characteristics of cells along the loop as well as the countercurrent exchange mechanism. The distal convoluted tube, connecting ducts, and collecting tubules are the final sites of fine and qualitative changes to the urine. The distal nephron is responsive to hormones such as parathyroid hormone and calcitriol to maintain calcium homeostasis, and antidiuretic hormone and aldosterone for fine adjustments in sodium, potassium, and water handling [3].

Azotemia is defined as an increase in serum or blood urea nitrogen (BUN) and creatinine while uremia is the clinical syndrome (pathological manifestations) that develops from severe or prolonged renal azotemia [1,2]. Azotemia can be prerenal, renal or postrenal in origin, with the differentiation being important when planning the stabilization, diagnostic, and therapeutic plan for the critical patient. Acute kidney injury (AKI) implies an abrupt deterioration in renal function [1,2,4]. Chronic kidney disease (CKD) implies kidney damage that has been present for at least three months and is common in our veterinary species [1].

Urinary tract problems can be the presenting concern in the small animal ICU patient, can develop as a consequence of an unrelated systemic illness, or can complicate the progression or response to therapy of an unrelated condition [1,2,4]. The presence of CKD can also cause the animal to be more susceptible to further renal insult, whether prerenal, intrinsic renal or postrenal in origin.

A systematic approach to the diagnosis and monitoring of urinary tract problems in the critically ill veterinary patient is essential for early detection of alterations and to provide a basis for early intervention.

Initial assessment

An abnormality in any portion of the urinary tract can potentially have life-threatening consequences. Evaluation begins with a thorough history and physical examination. Rapid initial assessment is available with cage-side point of care (POC) testing and can identify many important metabolic alterations. This is followed by more thorough clinicopathological testing and imaging. The diagnostic approach to urinary tract disorders is determined by the specific risk characteristics of the patient. Careful patient monitoring is required throughout the diagnostic and treatment period.

Monitoring and Intervention for the Critically Ill Small Animal: The Rule of 20, First Edition. Edited by Rebecca Kirby and Andrew Linklater.
© 2017 John Wiley & Sons, Inc. Published 2017 by John Wiley & Sons, Inc.

Table 13.1 Selected causes of prerenal, renal, and postrenal azotemia.

Prerenal	Renal	Postrenal
Reduced effective circulating volume:	**Infections:**	**Renal tubular obstruction:**
Hypovolemia	Pyelonephritis	Pyelonephritis
Hemorrhage	Leptospirosis (C)	Obstructive casts
Hypotension	Lyme nephropathy (C)	**Ureteral obstruction:**
Vasodilation	Rocky mountain spotted fever	Ureteroliths
Vasculitis	Ehrlichiosis	Ureteral strictures
Decreased cardiac output	**Glomerular disease:**	Ureteritis
Congestive heart failure	Glomerulonephritis/sclerosis	Ureteral cysts
Pericardial effusion	Amyloidosis	Ectopic ureters
Severe anemia	**Renal neoplasia:**	Urinary bladder trigone masses or
Hypoadrenocorticism	Renal lymphoma	neoplasia
Reduced renal blood flow:	Renal adenocarcinoma	Ureteral compression with neoplasia
Renal artery thrombosis or	**Pigment nephropathies:**	**Urethral obstruction:**
infarction	Myoglobinuria	Uroliths
Renal artery avulsion or trauma	Hemoglobinua	Urethral strictures
	Renal trauma:	Urethral trauma
	Crush injuries	Obstructive hematomas
	Renal lacerations	Crystalline plugs
	Renal infarcts	Feline lower urinary tract disease (F)
	Renal tubular disease/interstitial nephritis	**Functional urinary retention:**
	Toxins	Upper motor neuron urinary bladder
	Environmental toxins:	Urethral spasm
	Arsenic/other heavy metals	**Urinary tract leakage:**
	Cholecalciferol or vitamin D containing rodenticides	Urinary bladder rupture/trauma
	Ethylene glycol	Urethral tears
	Grapes or raisins (C)	Ureteral tears or trauma
	Lilium and Hemerocallus plant species (F)	Renal pelvic tears
	Pharmaceuticals:	
	ACE inhibitors	
	Acyclovir	
	Aminoglycosides	
	Amphotericin B	
	Azathioprine	
	Calcipotriene topical creams	
	Cisplatin and carboplatin	
	Cyclosporine	
	Diuretics	
	Nonsteroidal antiinflammatory drugs	
	Oxytetracycline	
	Diagnostic agents:	
	Gadolinium (high dose)	
	IV iodinated contrast	
	Supplements or dietary contaminants:	
	Alpha-lipoic acid	
	Melamine	
	Vitamin D supplements	

C, canines; F, felines.

History

Clinical history is essential to the diagnosis and assessment of risk for renal injury. The signalment can direct diagnostic efforts to breed-related (such as Fanconi's syndrome in Basenjis, Samoyed hereditary glomerulopathy) or congenital and hereditary disorders such as polycystic kidneys. Intact male and female patients may show signs of urinary tract disorders secondary to vaginal, uterine or prostatic disease. Past medical history, including preexisting renal disease, as well as chronic medication history is assessed. Queries are particularly made regarding any medications that may alter renal hemodynamics or have the potential to be nephrotoxic, such as nonsteroidal antiinflammatory drugs (NSAIDS), angiotensin converting enzyme (ACE) inhibitors (ACEi), antihypertensive drugs, and chemotherapeutic agents. Potential exposure to environmental nephrotoxins, including lilies (toxic to cats), raisins or grapes (toxic to dogs), ethylene glycol or dietary supplements such as alpha-lipoic acid, vitamin D-containing toxins, supplements or medications should be identified. Environmental and housing history may highlight the risk of infection with leptospirosis [1,2].

Patients with uremia may have shown signs of hyporexia to anorexia, nausea, vomiting, weight loss, and blood in vomitus (suggestive of gastrointestinal (GI) ulcerations) [1,2,5,6]. The history pertaining to water intake (polydipsia or adipsia) and urination of the animal is essential. Information regarding the estimated amount of urine passed with each effort, the frequency of urination and presence of pain or straining during urination provides essential clues to the underlying disorder. Pollakiuria (increased frequency

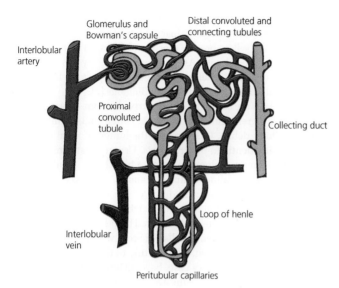

Figure 13.1 The functional unit of the kidneys: a nephron.

of urination), polyuria (increase in quantity of urine), and oliguria (reduced urine quantity) are signs of urinary tract problems that the owner has likely observed [7]. The appearance of the urine may direct diagnostic efforts as well; cloudy urine suggests infection, blood in the urine is possible with stones, trauma, hemoglobin or infection, and dark-colored urine suggests bilirubin, hemoglobin or myoglobin [7,8].

Physical examination

Establishing a baseline for temperature, pulse, and respiratory rate can provide important information regarding any systemic effects of urinary tract disorders. A high body temperature may be present with infectious or inflammatory causes of renal dysfunction. Hypothermia is a common consequence of endogenous renal toxins causing a reset of the thermoregulatory center. Heart or pulse rate can be affected by poor perfusion (tachycardia in dogs, normal rate or bradycardia in cats) or significant hyperkalemia (bradycardia in dogs, tachycardia or bradycardia in cats) secondary to renal failure or urinary tract obstruction or disruption. Severe metabolic acidosis can cause Kussmaul type breathing, while uremic pneumonitis or fluid overload can cause tachypnea and labored breathing.

Physical evaluation of effective circulating volume includes heart rate, pulse quality, mentation, mucous membrane color, and capillary refill time to allow stratification of patients into the categories of compensatory, early decompensatory, and late decompensatory shock [9]. The physical assessment of hydration will include skin turgor, mucous membranes, and corneal moisture [9]. Additional physical examination findings that may indicate the presence of renal disease include oral mucosal ulcerations, decreased body condition in patients with chronic renal failure, and uremic odor to the breath. Special focus should be placed on renal palpation during abdominal palpation to note renal size, symmetry, or the presence of pain. Urinary bladder palpation should be performed to detect pain or a turgid urinary bladder that may suggest obstructive disease. If the urinary bladder is empty of urine and urinary stones are large, they may be palpable on transabdominal palpation. Digital rectal examination can detect some urethral masses, stones, or urethral distension. In male dogs and cats, the penis should be extruded to evaluate for discharge, discoloration, penile or distal urethral masses. In female dogs, digital vaginal exam can be performed if the

clinical history warrants it. Fundic examination should be performed to evaluate for signs of hypertensive retinopathy, including tortuous retinal vessels, retinal hemorrhage, or detachment [1,2].

Point of care testing

The initial POC testing begins with the minimum database consisting of packed cell volume (PCV), total protein (TP), blood urea nitrogen (BUN), glucose, electrolytes, blood gas for acid–base analysis, coagulation profile with buccal mucosal bleeding time (BMBT), and urinalysis (UA). Hemoconcentration may indicate dehydration. Anemia indicated by a low PCV can be a result of bleeding or CKD. Hypoproteinemia (low TP) can be present due to albumin loss through the urine (glomerular disease) or concurrent liver disease.

Urea nitrogen is a byproduct of endogenous and exogenous protein metabolism by the liver. Since urea nitrogen is freely filtered from the blood at the glomerulus, the BUN can be useful as a marker of renal glomerular filtration rate (GFR). However, the BUN level will also elevate due to a reduction in renal blood flow in an adequately functioning kidney. Extrarenal influences should be considered when renal function and renal blood flow are adequate [1,2,10]. The BUN can also be elevated due to an increased rate of urea production (postprandial from dietary protein) or GI bleeding. A low BUN warrants assessment of hepatic function.

The blood glucose is evaluated and correlated with the presence or absence of urine glucose. The renal threshold for glucose in the cat is 300 mg/dL (17 mmol/L) and 180 mg/dL (10 mmol/L) in dogs. Glucose found in the urine when the blood glucose is below the renal threshold localizes the problem to a renal proximal tubular disorder [7].

Acid–base and electrolyte abnormalities in patients with renal failure contribute to the clinical manifestations of uremia and are potential therapeutic targets. A high anion gap metabolic acidosis is the most common acid–base derangement in patients with renal failure [2]. However, metabolic alkalosis may be present in patients with renal failure that are experiencing severe vomiting. The acid–base status should be monitored at least daily in any critically ill patient (see Chapter 7) [2].

Serum electrolytes may be abnormal due to kidney failure or postrenal obstruction or disruption. Of emergent interest is serum potassium since it can increase with a relative decrease in urine output. The presence of hyperkalemia warrants evaluation of the electrocardiogram and urine output, and may require immediate intervention to stabilize myocardial conduction. In contrast, patients with chronic renal failure often have low potassium levels due to chronic polyuria, chronically decreased potassium intake and total body potassium depletion (see Chapter 6) [11].

Hypercalcemia can be the cause of acute renal failure or the result of chronic renal failure. The clinical signs associated with hypercalcemia are dependent on the rate and magnitude of rise in serum calcium. Acute, severe increases or long-standing increases in serum calcium are more likely to result in kidney injury and resultant clinical signs of polyuria, polydipsia, uremia, and lab-detected azotemia. Differentials for hypercalcemia include hyperparathyroidism, neoplasia including osteolytic processes, hypoadrenocorticism, vitamin D toxicities, some types of granulomatous infections, and chronic renal failure [1,2]. Mild increases in serum calcium do not require specific therapy except to treat the underlying cause. However, severe hypercalcemia resulting in azotemia may require specific interventions, discussed under the acute kidney injury section below. Mild hypocalcemia is a common result of chronic renal failure as renal secondary hyperparathyroidism progresses [11,12]. Hypocalcemia can occur with severe hypoalbuminemia in patients with protein-losing nephropathies. Clinical signs of hypocalcemia including tremors, tetany, and seizures are uncommon in patients with hypocalcemia associated with renal insufficiency (see Chapter 6).

The BMBT measures the ability to form an initial platelet plug after capillary injury with a lancet. The components of the coagulation system assessed during BMBT measurement are the endothelial and vascular response to injury, including contribution to the platelet plug by platelets and functional von Willebrand factor. The BMBT can be prolonged with severe thrombocytopenia so results of BMBT should be evaluated in conjunction with a platelet count. Uremic coagulopathy is characterized by platelet dysfunction and BMBT may be useful as a screening tool for uremic coagulopathy (see Chapter 9).

The UA provides results that are integral in the diagnosis and monitoring of urinary tract disorders [4]. The testing is best performed on urine that is collected by aseptic methods of cystocentesis or urinary bladder catheterization. The gross character of urine can indicate the presence of hematuria/hemoglobinuria (red urine), bilirubinuria (bright yellow or greenish urine), methemoglobinuria or myoglobinuria (brown to black urine) [7,8].

Differentiating from hemoglobinuria and myoglobinuria can be challenging but because hemoglobin binds tightly to haptoglobin and does not clear as readily from the serum as myoglobin, a patient with a dark pigmented urine *and* a red coloration to the serum is more likely to have hemoglobinuria, whereas a patient with dark pigmented urine but with clear serum is more likely to have myoglobinuria. Evaluation of urinary and serum pigments in the face of urinary tract disease is important because excretion of an excess of serum pigments can contribute to nephropathy and renal failure [7,8].

Isosthenuria, demonstrated by a urine specific gravity of 1.008–1.020, concurrently with elevation of the BUN and creatinine, is the classic diagnostic criterion for intrinsic renal disease. Urine that is highly concentrated (>1.035) may indicate a prerenal component to the azotemia. Hyposthenuria (<1.008) can narrow the differential list to problems such as psychogenic polydipsia, iatrogenic medullary washout, or nephrogenic or central diabetes insipidus. The UA results beyond urine specific gravity are valuable in determining some etiologies of intrinsic renal insult. The urinary dipstick has test pads for qualitative or semiquantitative assessment for urine protein, glucose, bilirubin, red cells, and leukocytes. The finding of glucosuria without serum hyperglycemia can suggest renal proximal tubular injury [8]. The presence of proteinuria with non-inflammatory urinary sediment usually localizes the problem to the glomerulus and is further tested with the urine protein:creatinine ratio [13,14].

Examination of the urine sediment for the presence of casts, crystals, cells, and bacteria provides a reflection of the urine contained in renal tubules and the urinary bladder. The presence of inflammatory cells combined with bacteria supports urinary tract infection and possibly pyelonephritis (white cell casts). Urine cytology can be diagnostic of urinary tract neoplasms if there is exfoliation of neoplastic cells. The finding of crystalluria may assist in the diagnosis of urolithiasis. The presence of calcium oxalate crystals (octahedral or envelope shaped) can be a normal finding in dogs or cats but may also be the result of ethylene glycol toxicity, or indicative of calcium oxalate urolithiasis. Triple phosphate crystals, also called magnesium ammonium phosphate, or struvite crystals

("coffin lid" shaped) can be present in alkaline urine associated with stone formation or bacterial urinary tract infections. Ammonium biurate crystals (yellow-brown "thorn-apple" shaped) can be found with portosystemic shunts. Ammonium biurate crystals may also be the result of a genetic defect of the urate transporter, a finding in some normal Dalmations and English Bulldogs [7].

Urinary casts are composed of a matrix of Tamm–Horsfall protein secreted by renal tubular cells, which often contain imbedded cells or cellular debris. Casts mirror the lumen of renal tubules, and are easily identified on urinalysis. Urinary casts are categorized as cellular (red blood cell, white blood cell, tubular cell), granular, waxy or hyaline. Cellular, granular, and waxy casts represent different states of breakdown of the cellular component imbedded in the cast mucoprotein matrix. Cellular casts contain intact and discernible cells including red blood cells, renal tubular epithelial cells or white blood cells. The cells within granular casts have partially broken down, contributing to the granular appearance. The cells within waxy casts have disintegrated and are not discernible, contributing to the waxy appearance. Small quantities of hyaline or waxy casts may be a normal finding on urinalysis. The presence of cellular or granular casts represents tubular pathology. Tubular necrosis and tubular cell sloughing will contribute to tubular casts. Severe hematuria with trauma, coagulopathy, or idiopathic renal hemorrhage may result in red blood cell casts. White blood cell casts may be seen in severe pyelonephritis [7].

In addition to being a diagnostic aid, urinalysis can also be a valuable monitoring tool for the ICU patient. A high urine specific gravity during fluid therapy indicates that dehydration is still present. A lower urine specific gravity during fluid diuresis is appropriate. A daily examination of the urine sediment for tubular casts is a sensitive indicator of tubular injury and is of particular utility when monitoring for nephrotoxicity associated with aminoglycoside or other drug therapy [1,2,4].

Initial clinicopathological testing

A complete blood count (CBC) and serum biochemistry should be performed in patients with azotemia. Red blood cell (RBC) levels should always be interpreted in light of the patient's fluid balance. Chronic renal failure is associated with normochromic, normocytic nonregenerative anemia secondary to decreased erythropoietin production [11]. If GI bleeding is contributing to anemia, the red cells are typically microcytic and hypochromic because of iron deficiency. Chronic anemia of renal failure can be mild to moderate in severity (see Chapter 10). The presence of leukocytosis may indicate an infectious or inflammatory component to the urinary tract injury.

The serum biochemistry results will assist in the diagnosis of renal failure and, when interpreted with urinalysis, may help with localization to specific parts of the kidney. Creatinine elevation is the most widely used clinical marker of renal function, providing the most rapid and readily available surrogate for GFR [10]. Because serum creatinine is influenced by fewer extrarenal factors than BUN, changes in creatinine can be interpreted as proportional to the degree of renal insult and a reflection of the GFR and rate of tubular flow [1,2,10]. The serum biomarker symmetric dimethylarginine (SDMA) has been evaluated in dogs and cats [15–17]. SDMA has been shown to have a linear and reciprocal relationship to GFR and may be more sensitive than serum creatinine for the detection of chronic kidney disease in cats [15–17]. When the BUN and creatinine are interpreted in conjunction with UA results (such as abnormal specific gravity, proteinuria, renal casts), they remain the standard for the diagnosis of renal failure [1,2,4,10,18].

Increases in serum BUN and creatinine during therapy may signify progressive or ongoing renal injury, may be a warning for the development of oliguria, or may be a marker of inadequate fluid therapy. Decreases in BUN and creatinine during therapy can indicate improved hydration, improved GFR and tubular flow, renal recovery or a combination of these factors [1,2,4,10]. Monitoring the trend of change of BUN and creatinine in hospitalized patients could facilitate early detection of AKI as well as assessing the response to treatment.

Serum phosphorus levels are the result of dietary intake of phosphorus balanced with renal excretion. Hyperphosphatemia is common in patients with acute and chronic renal failure due to decreases in GFR [4]. However, postrenal obstruction or disruption can also cause hyperphosphatemia. Elevations in serum phosphorus can cause a decrease in ionized calcium through renal secondary hyperparathyroidism (rHPTH). Renal secondary hyperparathyroidism has been demonstrated to occur early in renal disease. Calcium-phosphorus changes have been associated with an increased mortality in CKD in humans, cats, and dogs. When the total calcium and phosphorus product exceeds 60–70, there is an increased risk of malignant calcification of tissues [11].

Evaluation of hepatic function is important when assessing for problems that affect both renal and hepatic function (such as leptospirosis or life-threatening hepatorenal syndrome). Hepatorenal syndrome is characterized by renal failure as a consequence of end-stage cirrhotic liver failure. Evidence of hepatic failure such as hypoalbuminemia, alterations in serum cholesterol, low BUN, high blood ammonia, and prolonged clotting times, in association with evidence of renal failure, supports the hepatorenal syndrome diagnosis. Hypoalbuminemia may occur as a consequence of albumin loss secondary to glomerulopathies. Since antithrombin may also be lost through the diseased glomerulus, patients with severe hypoalbuminemia should be assessed for hypercoagulability or for evidence of thrombus formation.

The presence of proteinuria with an active urinary sediment including the presence of red blood cells, white blood cells ± bacteria on the initial urinalysis warrants submission of a urine sample for culture and susceptibility testing. The presence of proteinuria without a reactive sediment directs the submission of urine for a urine protein:creatinine (UPC) ratio to identify potential glomerular sources of urine protein [13,14].

Diagnostic imaging

Urinary tract imaging modalities from plain to contrast radiographs and abdominal ultrasound are complementary in the diagnosis and management of patients with urinary tract pathology. No single imaging technique is preferred as the gold standard of evaluation. Patients with renal failure often undergo several imaging modalities to fully evaluate the upper and lower urinary tract, and to assist in therapeutic recommendations [19].

Radiographic studies

Abdominal radiographs will allow assessment of the size and symmetry of the kidneys and retroperitoneal space, the size of the urinary bladder, the size and position of reproductive organs associated with the urinary tract and the location and shape of other abdominal organs. Canine kidneys will appear as bean-shaped on radiographs and measure 2.5–3.5 times the length of the second lumbar vertebra. The right kidney is usually one-half length cranial

to the left kidney. Renal size in the cat as measured on the VD radiograph varies from 2.4 to 3.0 times the length of the second lumbar vertebral body (L2). However, it is fairly common for older cats (over 10 years of age) to have kidneys that range from 2.0 to 2.4 times the length of L2, without biochemical changes indicative of renal disease [19].

Abdominal radiographs remain the standard of care for evaluation of the presence of radiopaque urolithiasis (such as calcium phosphate, calcium oxalate, silicate, struvite) anywhere in the urinary tract. Urate and occasionally cysteine uroliths may be radiolucent [19].

Excretory urography is an intravenous (IV) contrast radiographic study that can provide a subjective assessment of renal function [20]. It also detects the presence of pyelectasia or hydronephrosis and can demonstrate urine leakage from the level of the kidneys to the urethra. Table 13.2 provides guidelines for performing urinary contrast studies. The risk of the procedure must be evaluated due to the potential for contrast-induced renal failure from IV iodinated contrast agents. The patient undergoing the procedure must be well hydrated with adequate perfusion prior to the administration of any contrast agent [20].

Positive contrast and double-contrast cystourethrograms can be performed to detect bladder and urethral lithiasis caused by radiolucent calculi (see Table 13.2). Positive contrast placed into the urinary bladder can also be used to demonstrate urinary bladder rupture (Figure 13.2). Urinary bladder wall thickness, mural and luminal masses, strictures and polypoid diseases can be highlighted with a double-contrast cystourethrogram [21].

Ultrasound

Abdominal ultrasound is used to detect radiolucent uroliths and assess renal architecture, perinephric tissues, and the retroperitoneal space. Changes within the urinary tract that may be seen on ultrasound include renal cysts, renal infarcts, renal parenchymal echogenic changes suggestive of toxic injury, infiltrative disease or neoplasia, renal pelvic dilation, ureteral dilation, urinary bladder wall thickness, bladder luminal masses, and the detection of free peritoneal or retroperitoneal fluid from urine leakage [19]. Table 13.3 provides imaging and abdominal fluid analysis criteria for the diagnosis of uroabdomen [22,23]. Monitoring the trends of change over time with ultrasound (such as renal pelvic size for pyelonephritis or ureteral dilation for obstructive disease) may demonstrate therapeutic success or structural deterioration which may necessitate more aggressive intervention, such as surgery.

Advanced imaging

Computed tomography (CT) and magnetic resonance imaging (MRI) are planar imaging modalities that provide sensitive morphological evaluation of the kidneys and urinary bladder [19]. CT or MRI technology is limited by the requirement for anesthesia and their diagnostic benefits in urinary tract disease should be compared carefully due to the wide availability and utility of abdominal radiographs and ultrasound. When CT or MRI is chosen, images and diagnostic yield are complementary to the information obtained with radiographs and ultrasound.

Uroscopic imaging

Video urethrocystoscopy allows for direct visualization of the vaginal, urethral, and bladder mucosa for diagnosis of many lower urinary tract abnormalities, including cystitis, ectopic ureter,

Table 13.2 Urinary contrast studies.

Contrast study	Indications	Patient preparation	Procedure	Notes
Excretory urogram	Subjective evaluation of GFR Determination of renal size and position Evaluation of size, and shape of renal pelvis Evaluation for ureteral patency Evaluation for ectopic ureter Evaluation for patency or leaks from the level of the bladder to the ureters and urinary bladder	12–24-hour fast Serial enemas as needed to clear the colon of fecal material Place IV catheter for contrast injection Sedation as needed to achieve radiographs	1. Obtain survey lateral and VD abdominal radiographs to ensure clearance of fecal material 2. Administer undiluted iodinated contrast at 400–800 mg/kg IV single bolus 3. Take immediate lateral and VD abdominal radiograph and then timed radiographs at 5, 20, and 40 minutes 4. Oblique radiograph views may be taken to evaluate for ectopic ureter	Iodinated contrast should not be administered to patients who are dehydrated Allergic reactions to iodinated contrast are uncommon and anaphylactic reactions rare Contrast-induced vomiting is transient and treated with supportive care Contrast-induced renal failure is uncommon but use of nonionic contrast is advocated to minimize complications IV fluid administration post contrast is recommended to maintain hydration and induce diuresis
Negative-contrast cystogram or pneumocystogram	Identify size, shape, and location of urinary bladder	12–24-hour fast Serial enemas as needed to clear the colon of fecal material Sedation as needed to achieve urinary catheter placement and radiographs Sterile urinary catheter placement for contrast injection	1. Obtain survey lateral and VD abdominal radiographs 2. Pass a urinary catheter with aseptic technique 3. Inject 10 mL/kg of negative contrast 4. Take lateral and VD abdominal radiographs immediately post injection 5. Remove negative contrast from the bladder post procedure for patient comfort	Radiographs can be taken with urinary catheter in place or removed The negative contrast used can be air or medical carbon dioxide Vascular air embolism from diseased urinary bladder wall is a rare but possible complication Use of carbon dioxide may reduce the risk of air embolism
Positive contrast cystourethrogram	Identify size, shape, and location of urinary bladder Evaluate for urinary bladder or urethral diverticula Evaluate for urinary bladder or urethral patency or leakage Evaluate for filling defects for urolith detection or hematomas Evaluate for some bladder mucosal filling defects such as polyps or masses	Same patient preparation as a negative-contrast cystogram	1. Obtain survey lateral and VD abdominal radiographs 2. Pass a urinary catheter with aseptic technique 3. Inject 10 mL/kg of sterile iodinated contrast solution 4. Take lateral and VD abdominal radiographs immediately post injection 5. For the urethrogram, pull the catheter back to the distal urethra and take a lateral caudal abdominal radiograph while simultaneously injecting contrast to achieve good filling of the urethra 6. Alternatively a voiding urethrogram can be performed by removing the urinary catheter and taking a radiograph while the patient is voiding or when the bladder is actively being expressed	Iodinated contrast can be diluted with sterile saline (1:2 or 1:5 depending on the original concentration of iodinated contrast agent) and still achieve good opacification of urinary bladder and urethra Radiographs with the pelvic limbs of the patient moved to different positions (pulled cranially or caudally) may be needed for good evaluation of the entire urethra Contrast agent can be removed from the urinary bladder post procedure or the patient can be allowed to void the contrast
Double-contrast cystogram	Identify size, shape, and location of urinary bladder Evaluate for urinary bladder diverticula Evaluate for urinary bladder leakage Evaluate for filling defects for urolith detection or hematomas Increased resolution for detection of bladder mucosal filling defects such as polyps, masses, and thickenings compared to positive contrast cystogram	Same patient preparation as a negative-contrast cystogram	1. Obtain survey lateral and VD abdominal radiographs 2. Pass a urinary catheter with aseptic technique 3. Inject 10 mL/kg of negative contrast 4. Inject sterile iodinated contrast (most have a concentration >/= 200 mg/mL) at a dose of 1 mL/cat, 1–3 mL for dogs <25 lbs, or 3–6 mL for dogs >25 lbs 5. Take lateral and VD abdominal radiographs post injection of positive contrast 6. Remove positive and negative contrast from the bladder post procedure for patient comfort	Undiluted iodinated contrast provides a better study than diluted contrast The negative contrast used can be air or medical carbon dioxide Vascular air embolism from diseased urinary bladder wall is a rare but possible complication Use of carbon dioxide may reduce the risk of air embolism

GFR, glomerular filtration rate; IV, intravenous; VD, ventrodorsal.

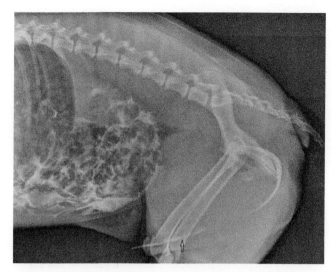

Figure 13.2 Lateral radiograph of a positive-contrast cystourethrogram demonstrating abdominal extravesicular location of contrast medium in a patient with traumatic bladder rupture. There is no urethral leakage of contrast. At surgery, a large tear was found at the apex of the urinary bladder. The open arrow demonstrates the tip of the urinary catheter within the distal urethra that was used to inject the contrast medium.

Table 13.3 Supportive and diagnostic criteria for uroabdomen.

Finding	
Diagnostic imaging	
Radiography	Loss of abdominal detail and free peritoneal fluid (S)
	Abdominal extravasation of contrast in urinary contrast studies (D)
Ultrasound	Free peritoneal fluid (S)
	Observation of fluid flow directly from a urinary tract (D)
Fluoroscopy	Free peritoneal fluid (S)
	Abdominal extravasation of contrast in urinary contrast studies (D)
Computed tomography	Free peritoneal fluid pockets (S)
	Abdominal extravasation of contrast in urinary contrast studies (D)
Paired fluid and serum testing	
Creatinine	Peritoneal fluid creatinine ≥2× serum creatinine (D)
	Peritoneal fluid creatinine > serum creatinine (S)
Potassium	Peritoneal fluid potassium ≥1.4× serum potassium (D)
	Peritoneal fluid potassium > serum potassium (S)

(S) is supportive of the diagnosis of uroabdomen; (D) is diagnostic for uroabdomen. Multiple criteria are usually combined to achieve a diagnosis.

urethral and bladder masses, urolithiasis, and urethral diverticula. Urethrocystoscopy can be used to direct the collection of diagnostic samples including cytology, biopsy, and samples for culture of the lower urinary tract. Urethrocystoscopy is used for interventional procedures such as intracorporeal lithotripsy for breakdown and removal of urinary bladder calculi [24].

Table 13.4 Endogenous creatinine clearance.

Requirements	• Accurately timed and complete urine collection (24-hour urine collection is ideal, but 4-hour urine collection can be used)
	• Body weight
	• Simultaneous urine and serum creatinine concentrations in mg/dL
Equation	**Creatinine clearance in mL/kg/min = (Ucr × Vurine/ Scr × T)/BWkg**
	Where: Ucr = urine creatinine concentration in mg/ml, Vurine = total volume of urine collected in mL, Scr = Serum creatinine concentration in mg/mL, T = time in minutes of urine collection, BWkg = body weight in kilograms
Reference interval	• 2–5 mL/kg/min
Interpretation notes	• Creatinine clearance may overestimate GFR by 10–20%

Glomerular filtration rate

Methods to measure GFR are feasible in clinical practice and include nuclear scintigraphy (using radionucleotides and gamma camera) and iohexol clearance measurements. Iohexol is an iodinated contrast agent that was found to be a suitable marker for GFR. After IV injection, iohexol is eliminated in the urine by glomerular filtration, with no tubular secretion or reabsorption. Plasma iohexol clearance can be calculated with collection and measurement of iohexol in serial blood samples. Laboratory quantitation of iohexol is required by liquid chromatography or x-ray absorption [25]. Nuclear scintigraphy and iohexol clearance methods of GFR measurement, though accurate, are unable to assess ongoing changes in GFR, and with the time and equipment needed for results, this gives them little clinical utility over the endogenous creatinine clearance in the veterinary ICU [10].

While the standard in human medicine for measuring GFR is the iohexol clearance test, the endogenous creatinine clearance can provide a reasonable estimation. A decrease in clearance indicates a decrease in GFR [25]. When performed correctly, a creatinine clearance test provides the benefit of detecting approximately 20% decrease in renal function, compared to the 75% functional loss that is necessary before elevations in BUN and creatinine concentrations are detected. In order to increase the diagnostic accuracy of creatinine clearance for GFR assessment, this test should only be performed in well-hydrated, nonazotemic animals. The procedure for performing and calculating the endogenous creatinine clearance is provided in Table 13.4. Inaccuracies with the endogenous creatinine clearance test are possible due to incomplete evacuation of the bladder, tubular secretion of creatinine in some male dogs, possible increased extrarenal secretion of creatinine (such as in the GI tract), and measurement of noncreatinine chromagens in the serum. Creatinine clearance is useful to rule in or out kidney disease in patients with polyuria and polydipsia but without azotemia [25].

The fractional excretion of urinary electrolytes is the fraction of the filtered electrolyte that is then excreted in urine. This urine parameter has been used to assess the appropriateness of renal electrolyte handling by the kidney and aids in localizing the cause of renal azotemia in humans. The fractional sodium excretion is used most commonly [10]. Fractional excretion is easy to measure clinically with spot urine and serum electrolyte measurements normalized by simultaneous urine and serum creatinine measurement [26]. The formula is:

$$FE(\%) = 100 \times \left[Na_{urine} \times Cr_{plasma} \right] \div \left[Na_{plasma} \times Cr_{urine} \right]$$

where FE = fractional excretion, Na = sodium, Cr = creatinine. In humans, the results are used to help differentiate prerenal disease (FE <1%) from acute tubular necrosis or other kidney disease (FE >2–3%) [10,26]. Interpretation of fractional sodium excretion in veterinary medicine is challenged by lack of normal reference intervals and due to large intra- and inter-patient variability reported in fractional excretion [10]. Fractional excretion measurement has not been shown to be of additional value over monitoring BUN and creatinine trends in the veterinary ICU [10,26].

Urine biomarkers

The field of urinary biomarkers is rapidly expanding and there are likely to be significant advancements to guide clinicians over the next decade [27,28]. Acknowledging the insensitivity of BUN and creatinine in detecting kidney injury, researchers have been working on identifying urinary biomarkers that may improve diagnostic sensitivity in renal failure [27]. The biomarker can be a specific urinary protein that indicates structural loss of either tubular or glomerular cells, a marker of inflammation or indicator of loss of cellular function [27]. The ideal biomarker would fulfill the criteria of being "an easy to measure early indicator of renal injury that could localize the injury as prerenal, renal, post renal injury, and localize injury within the nephron (glomerular or tubular) as well as be a prognostic marker" [27]. It is unlikely that a single biomarker will meet all of these criteria, but several urinary enzymes show promise as a guide for clinical decision making [27–29].

The urinary enzyme N-acetyl-b-D-glucosaminidase (NAG) is located within tubular cell lysosymes. The urinary enzyme gamma-glutamyl transferase (GGT) is located in the tubular luminal brush border. The appearance of these enzymes in urine supports tubular cell injury. Urinary GGT and NAG values are normalized for alterations in urine specific gravity by assessing a ratio with urine creatinine in spot urine samples [28]. There is no established reference interval for urine GGT or NAG and baseline values vary widely between individuals [28]. The monitoring of trends of urine GGT and NAG is most useful when compared to a baseline for the patient [28]. As an example, the urinary GGT:creatinine ratio is more sensitive than creatinine alone for detecting the onset of renal injury in the patient undergoing prophylactic diuresis for acute nephrotoxin ingestion [28]. Urinary GGT:creatinine ratios may have a role in monitoring patients on aminoglycoside therapy in the future. The utility of clinic monitoring of urinary NAG and other urinary biomarkers is limited because commercial, easily accessible testing is not currently available.

Additional testing

Additional clinicopathological diagnostic testing performed in patients with the potential for the diagnosis of renal failure might include serological or polymerase chain reaction (PCR) testing for leptospirosis and *Borrelia burgdorferi*, assays to detect ethylene glycol, analysis and culture of uroliths and urinary tract cytological or histological sampling.

Urinary tract cytological and histological sampling

The technique for urinary tract sampling will vary with the anatomical location to be sampled. Ultrasound-guided renal aspirates may be performed easily under mild sedation and assist in the diagnosis of some renal neoplasms. Renal biopsy can be achieved with ultrasound-guided true-cut biopsy, laparoscopically assisted, or obtained during open abdominal surgery. Renal biopsy provides a histological diagnosis and is of particular value in the diagnosis of amyloidosis and protein-losing glomerular lesions [13,14]. Renal biopsy may assist in prognosis for renal recovery with a histological assessment of the presence of intact tubular basement membrane. However, the risks of renal biopsy, including hemorrhage and worsening renal function, often outweigh the diagnostic benefit in patients with AKI.

Sampling of the urinary bladder wall, polyps or masses can be achieved by traumatic urethral/urinary bladder catheterization or under direct uroscopic visualization. Ultrasound-guided aspiration of urinary bladder abnormalities can be performed but transabdominal aspiration of possible neoplastic urinary bladder abnormalities is not recommended because of the potential risk of abdominal seeding of neoplastic cells.

Surgery can be a diagnostic tool and both palliative or curative in the treatment of many urinary tract disorders. It is often necessary to perform a contrast study or other advanced imaging to determine urine flow or production of the affected and unaffected kidneys and ureters or to assist in localization of the problem. Some problems that may be addressed surgically include nonchemotherapy-responsive neoplasms, progressive urinary system obstruction due to stones, neoplasia or strictures, and infections such as renal abscessation or renal parasitism. The details of urinary surgical management can be found in veterinary texts addressing surgery of the urinary tract [30,31].

Equipment-based monitoring

Body weight measurements during the course of rehydration and throughout fluid therapy will provide technically simple and early indicators of fluid balance, fluid retention or third space fluid losses. Body weight trends are of particular importance in cats and small dogs where the margin for overhydration is smaller and body weight increases most often precede the development of overt signs of fluid overload. Body weight changes should be trended every 4–6 hours in animals with potential for fluid intolerance.

The effective circulating volume is more challenging to monitor than hydration but also combines information from physical monitoring with measured values. These physical parameters (heart rate, pulse intensity, CRT, mucous membrane color) are combined with trends in blood pressure (BP) and central venous pressure (CVP) [9]. Blood pressure monitoring for the presence of hypotension and hypertension is essential in the small animal ICU patient with potential for renal damage or disease (see Chapter 3). Hypotension causes prerenal azotemia which progresses to renal injury if not rapidly corrected. The kidneys are able to preserve their perfusion through autoregulation at mean arterial pressures greater than 60 mmHg. This is a reasonable minimal target for blood pressure when treating hypotension, acknowledging that "normal" blood pressure does not necessarily equate with adequate organ perfusion [9]. Mild hypertension may result from overhydration or excessive volume loading. However, hypertension can be secondary to chronic renal disease due to abnormal sodium and water excretion and abnormalities in the intrarenal renin-angiotensin-aldosterone system. Hypertension can be a cause of kidney damage or failure due to impaired renal blood flow [32].

With normal right heart function, CVP measurement provides additional information about the status of the intravascular volume.

The CVP targets should be higher (5–10 cmH₂O (3.7–7.4 mmHg)) when systemic inflammatory response syndrome disorders are present. Higher than normal CVP targets in this patient population will ensure adequate intravascular volume to meet the demands for a high cardiac output. However, animals with trauma, bleeding or significant heart disease may need resuscitation to a more normal CVP (3–5 cmH₂O (2.2–3.7 mmHg)). Recent evidence has shown a positive correlation between changes in CVP values and changes in the diameter (measured with B-mode ultrasound) and flow velocity (assessed with v-wave Doppler) of the caudal vena cava and hepatic veins during acute intravascular fluid administration [33]. Focused sonography of the caudal cava may provide a noninvasive assessment of the adequacy of fluid resuscitation [33].

Quantitative urine output is the standard of care and is technically simple to perform with the placement of indwelling urinary catheters connected to closed collection systems. Strict aseptic technique is required to reduce the risk for bacterial urinary tract colonization from environmental contamination. The entire urinary collection system should be kept clean and changed or replaced when soiled. The placement of soft, flexible red rubber, silicone, latex or polyvinyl chloride catheters is important to patient comfort. Rigid polypropylene urinary catheters are not recommended as indwelling urinary catheters. Additionally, placement of a catheter with a diameter large enough to avoid urine leakage around the catheter will improve accuracy of urine output measurements. For this reason, Foley urinary catheters, with an inflatable balloon tip designed to reside within the trigone of the urinary bladder and minimize leakage around the catheter, are preferred as indwelling catheters for urine output measurement.

Urinary quantitation allows the clinician to compare the fluid input through fluid therapy and nutritional support to fluid output through the urine. The difference between "ins and outs" can reflect whether the fluid therapy plan is appropriate and often provides an early indication of renal injury by detecting polyuria, oliguria, or anuria. Polyuria is defined as urine production >2 mL/kg/h and its presence allows more aggressive IV fluid infusions. The assessment of oliguria and anuria should only be made in a patient that has adequate blood pressure (mean arterial pressure (MAP) >60 mmHg), adequate hydration, and a patent urinary collection system (no kinks in catheters or obstructions). Oliguria is defined as urine output <0.5 mL/kg/h. Relative oliguria occurs when an increase in urine output is expected but does not occur (such as after rapid, large-volume crystalloid infusion) and is quantitated as 0.5–2 mL/kg/h. Anuria is defined as urine output <0.03 mL/kg/h [1,2]. Oliguria and anuria are indicators of severe renal injury [2,4] and associated with a high risk for volume overload. Treatment is directed toward converting oliguria or anuria to polyuria to allow further diuresis. When medical therapy to convert the patient to oliguria is unsuccessful, dialysis or renal replacement therapy should be pursued.

Semiquantification of urine output can be achieved by measuring urine collected from the cage floor or nonabsorbent litter pellets (for cats), combined with weighing bedding. While this method avoids urinary bladder catheterization, it provides only an estimation of urine production.

The greatest monitoring information is gained by combining trends in serum BUN and creatinine, the quantity of urine output relative to fluid input, and physical signs and measured parameters that assess fluid balance. One value or number taken alone out of context with the other parameters could lead to erroneous assumptions and clinical decisions. Figure 13.3 provides a clinical algorithm for guiding the assessment of renal values in association with changes in urine output.

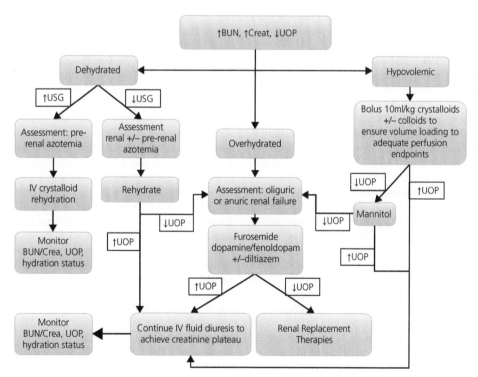

Figure 13.3 Clinical algorithm for the assessment, treatment, and monitoring of patients with kidney injury. BUN, blood urea nitrogen; Crea, serum creatinine; UOP, urine output; USG, urine specific gravity.

Disorders of the urinary tract

Insults to the kidneys should be localized to prerenal, intrinsic renal or postrenal problems, with the acknowledgment that many critically ill small animals will have a combination of insults [1,2]. Prerenal contributions to azotemia and AKI are caused by a decrease in effective renal blood flow. Renal injury or failure is due to abnormalities within the kidney structure or function that prevent filtering of waste products from the blood. Postrenal contributions to azotemia are caused by obstruction or disruption of the urinary outflow tract.

Prerenal azotemia

The renal arteries provide oxygenated blood to the kidneys for the production of energy by the renal cells and receive 20–25% of the cardiac output. These arteries branch into the interlobar and interlobular arteries within the kidney and further branch to become the arterioles and glomerular capillary tufts of the nephron. The arterial blood then flows through the peritubular capillaries providing oxygen and nutrients to the cells of the nephron and absorbing waste products emitted by the cells. These capillaries empty into the renal venous system for transport of deoxygenated blood and waste products from the kidney.

Anything that affects the blood flow through the kidney will impact renal function. These prerenal insults will result in a reduction of the GFR and will decrease the oxygen supply to the renal tissues [2,3,34]. A decrease in effective circulating blood volume is one of the most common causes of prerenal azotemia in the ICU patient and can be caused by problems such as hypovolemia, hemorrhage, cardiac disease, arrhythmias, hypotension, hypertension or maldistribution of blood flow. Renal arterial or venous thrombosis or occlusion will also significantly alter renal blood flow and provide a source of prerenal injury. As GFR declines, autoregulation within the nephron causes alterations in the level of vasoconstriction and vasodilation of the afferent and efferent arterioles of the glomerulus, which can alter peritubular capillary oxygen delivery to renal cells, contributing to prerenal causes of kidney injury.

In the absence of intrinsic renal disease, prerenal azotemia is characterized by normal or elevated urine specific gravity [1,2]. The BUN and creatinine are typically elevated but should return to normal after correction of fluid balance and renal blood flow. Physical signs of poor perfusion (tachycardia, weak or absent pulses, prolonged CRT, pale mucous membranes) or dehydration (dry mucous membranes and cornea, skin tenting) will provide evidence of prerenal contributions. Hemoconcentration (elevated PCV and TS) may be demonstrated on the minimum database.

In the critically ill patient, establishing an effective fluid balance becomes the primary therapeutic target when correcting prerenal azotemia. The hemodynamic causes of AKI can often be avoided by early intervention. While a decrease in effective circulating volume and dehydration are known to be detrimental to renal function, intravascular volume overload and overhydration of interstitial tissues can also be detrimental. Fluid overload can lead to renal cell swelling and increased interstitial fluid. The consequences can include reduced oxygen and nutrient delivery to the cells, cellular dysfunction, and eventually cell death [34,35].

Deficits in effective circulating volume can be corrected with IV isotonic replacement crystalloid infusion, combined with hydroxyethyl starch (colloid) to enhance intravascular retention of fluid volume and promote tissue perfusion. Colloid solutions have been associated with renal injury in humans but adverse renal effects have not been demonstrated in veterinary species and 6% colloid solutions remain a viable option for intravascular volume expansion in critically ill veterinary patients. Low normal resuscitation endpoints (normal physical perfusion parameters, MAP BP >60 mmHg, CVP 3–5 cmH$_2$O) should be targeted in critical patients with problems that predispose to fluid intolerance, such as pulmonary trauma, traumatic brain injury, intracavitary hemorrhage, confirmed oliguric renal failure, and brain or lung edema. High normal resuscitation endpoints (normal physical perfusion parameters, MAP BP >80 mmHg, CVP 8–10 cmH$_2$O) are targeted for most other underlying disorders [9]. Refractory hypotension requires examination of cardiac function and support with positive inotropes (such as dobutamine) if poor contractility is present with adequate vascular volume. Vasopressor drugs (such as dopamine, norepinephrine) can be used if blood pressure targets cannot be achieved or maintained when cardiac contractility and blood volume are adequate. However, an improvement in systemic blood pressure does not necessarily equate with a sufficient renal blood flow (see Chapter 2).

Patient hydration is reassessed once the perfusion has been restored. The remaining dehydration is corrected with IV isotonic replacement crystalloid therapy at a rate determined by the fluid tolerance of the patient and the rate at which the dehydration developed. Rapid onset of dehydration warrants a more rapid correction (2–6 hours) in patients that can tolerate the fluids. However, animals with problems such as heart disease, hypoalbuminemia, vasculitis, organ or peripheral edema or oliguric renal failure can require a slower rate of rehydration to avoid tissue edema. Chronic dehydration may need to be corrected over a longer period of time (12–24 hours). Physical parameters of hydration should be assessed after the period of rehydration and at least twice daily thereafter. Body weight is monitored as well as the PCV and TS trends [9]. More complete guidelines for monitoring of fluid balance are provided in Chapter 2.

Renal artery occlusion secondary to thrombosis, trauma, or ligation can contribute to renal failure that is localized to prerenal origin. The renal artery may sustain thrombosis in hypercoagulable states or may be occluded by intravascular invasion with neoplasms. The renal artery may be compressed by extraluminal enlargement of local masses. All of these etiologies cause a reduction in renal arterial flow, decreasing oxygen delivery to the kidneys and resulting in hypoxic and ischemic renal injury, accelerated apoptosis, and acute tubular necrosis. Examples of conditions in veterinary species predisposing to hypercoagulability, which may lead to thrombosis, include patients with hyperadrenocorticism, protein-losing nephropathy or enteropathy, immune-mediated hemolytic anemia, systemic inflammatory response syndrome, and others. Heart diseases, including hypertrophic cardiomyopathy in cats, can predispose to thromboembolic disease. Patients with renal artery laceration present with acute hemorrhagic shock and signs referable to trauma. Diagnostics for the stable patient in which renal artery thrombosis is suspected is the same as the recommendations for all patients with renal failure [1]. However, ultrasound imaging with Doppler color flow interrogation of the renal arteries and/or contrast CT images of the kidneys may highlight renal artery thrombi for definitive diagnosis.

Renal azotemia

Intrinsic renal failure is caused by lesions that alter the structure or function of any component of the nephron or interstitium. Acute tubular necrosis (ATN) is a common histological finding in hospitalized humans with AKI. Though ATN does not specifically identify an etiology, it is usually seen in ischemic or nephrotoxic renal injury. A glomerular localization of renal pathology can be the result of glomerulonephritis secondary to systemic illness and inflammation, idiopathic, immune or vascular glomerulopathies. Interstitial disease can be an end-stage result of chronic infection, inflammation, or degeneration. Congenital and inherited renal lesions such as renal dysplasia and polycystic kidney disease can contribute to intrinsic renal failure. In addition to direct renal insults, intrinsic renal failure can be secondary to prolonged pre- or post-renal insults. Unlike prerenal azotemia, intrinsic renal failure cannot be readily corrected with just restoration of fluid volume and blood flow. When the etiology of renal failure is known, specific therapy targeted at the cause of kidney failure is warranted as well as general supportive care [1,2,4].

Acute kidney injury

Acute kidney injury, previously termed acute renal failure, is diagnosed in humans by an abrupt decrease in renal function. It is manifested by increasing trends in serum creatinine, with or without decreasing trends in urine output [36,37]. To underscore the importance of AKI in human ICUs, the Acute Dialysis Quality Initiative (ADQI) group published a consensus definition of human AKI [38]. These recommendations came to be known as the RIFLE classification which identified three severity categories (**R**-risk, **I**-injury, **F**-failure) based on change in serum creatinine from baseline or reduction in GFR and urine output measurements [38]. The RIFLE scheme also identified two outcome categories of **L**oss, defined as persistent renal failure requiring renal replacement greater than four weeks, and End-stage kidney disease requiring dialysis for >3 months (Table 13.5) [38]. The Acute Kidney Injury Network (AKIN) modified the RIFLE criteria (Table 13.6) to include not just a percentage change from baseline but an absolute change in creatinine of ≥0.3 mg/dL to highlight the importance of small changes in serum creatinine as a marker of AKI [36].

Both the human RIFLE and AKIN criteria have been modified for the diagnosis and staging of AKI in veterinary patients (Table 13.5 and Table 13.7) [18,39]. As in the human RIFLE and AKIN categories, the veterinary AKI (VAKI) criteria highlight that AKI can be diagnosed with small changes in creatinine from baseline, with values often remaining within the normal reference interval [18]. Both the human and veterinary RIFLE and AKIN criteria are intended to improve the sensitivity for detection of AKI since it has been shown to be an independent risk factor for

mortality in critically ill humans and dogs [40,41]. The retrospective application of the veterinary modified RIFLE and veterinary acute kidney injury (VAKI) in dogs has confirmed that increasing RIFLE or VAKI grade is associated with poorer prognosis [18,39].

Fluid diuresis for azotemia relies on the ability of the kidneys to produce urine and ideally induce polyuria. The presence of oliguria or anuria significantly limits the ability of fluid therapy alone to be used to correct azotemia and uremia. The etiologies and mechanism of oliguria mirror the mechanisms of renal injury in general and can be localized to prerenal, renal or postrenal as well as localized within

Table 13.6 Classification of acute kidney injury according to the Acute Kidney Injury Network (AKIN) in humans.

Stage	Serum creatinine	Urine output
1	Increase in creatinine ≥0.3 mg/dL (≥26.4 µmol/L) or increase by 150–200% (1.5–2-fold increase) of baseline creatinine	<0.5 mL/kg/h >6 h
2	Increase by 200–300% (>2–3-fold increase) of baseline	<0.5 mL/kg/h >12 h
3	Increase by >300% of baseline or serum creatinine ≥4 mg/dL (354 µmol/L) with an acute increase of at least 0.5 mg/dL (44 µmol/L) or the need for renal replacement	<0.3 mL/kg/h >24 h or anuria >12 h

Source: Mehta RL, Kellum J, Shah SV, et al. Acute Kidney Injury Network: report of an initiative to improve outcomes in acute kidney injury. Crit Care 2007;11(2):R31. Used with permission of Lippincott, Williams and Wilkins.

Table 13.7 Criteria for veterinary acute kidney injury (VAKI) staging for dogs.

Stage	Creatinine
0	Increase <150% of baseline creatinine (up to 1.5-fold increase)
1	Increase >0.3 mg/dL (26.5 µmol/L) from baseline or increase 150–199% of baseline creatinine (1.5–1.9-fold increase)
2	Increase of 200–299% of baseline creatinine (2–2.9-fold increase)
3	Increase of ≥300% of baseline creatinine (>3-fold increase) or an absolute creatinine value >4 mg/dL (354 µmol/L)

Source: Thoen ME, Kerl ME. Characterization of acute kidney injury in hospitalized dogs and evaluation of a veterinary acute kidney injury staging system. J Vet Emerg Crit Care 2011;21(6):648–57. Used with permission of Wiley.

Table 13.5 Acute Dialysis Quality Initiative RIFLE (risk, injury, failure, loss, and end-stage renal failure) [38] criteria and modification for application in dogs [39].

RIFLE severity category	RIFLE crea and GFR criteria	RIFLE UOP criteria	Veterinary modified crea criteria
Risk	≥1.5-fold increase crea from baseline or >25% decrease in GFR	<0.5ml/kg/hr x 6 hours	1.3–2.0 mg/dL (116–174 µmol/L)
Injury	≥2.0-fold increase in crea from baseline or >50% decrease in GFR	<0.5ml/kg/hr x 12hrs	2.0–3.9 mg/dL (175–347.9 µmol/L)
Failure	≥3.0-fold increase in crea from baseline or >75% decrease in GFR or absolute serum crea ≥4 mg/dL (>354 µmol/L) or acute rise ≥0.5 mg/dL	<0.3 ml/kg/hr X 24hrs or anuria x 12hrs	≥3.9 mg/dL (≥347.9 µmol/L)
RIFLE outcome category			
Loss	Persistent ARF or complete loss of kidney function requiring renal replacement >4 weeks		Not evaluated
ESKD	End-stage kidney disease requiring hemodialysis >3 months		Not evaluated

ARF, acute renal failure; crea, serum creatinine; GFR, glomerular filtration rate; UOP, urine output.

the nephron. Abrupt decreases in renal artery and glomerular blood flow decreasing glomerular filtration are intuitive contributors to oliguria. Oliguria can occur at the level of the renal tubular cells as well. Ischemia resulting in loss of cellular adenosine triphosphate (ATP) causes energy-dependent cell wall pumps that maintain the normal intra- and extracellular ion gradients to fail, with the ultimate consequence of tubular cellular swelling and death. These renal tubular cells will slough into the tubular lumen as they die and can contribute to tubular obstruction. Functional tubular obstruction can occur with postrenal obstructive diseases that increase tubular pressure. Direct toxic injury to kidney cells also causes cellular swelling, and cell death. Nephrons can be progressively destroyed in renal diseases such as interstitial nephritis and amyloidosis where they are replaced with fibrosis and amyloid [1,2].

A high priority is placed on restoring any perfusion and hydration deficits (eliminating prerenal contributions) while ensuring that there is a patent urinary outflow tract (eliminating postrenal contributions). It is critical to maintain perfusion and hydration while avoiding volume overload. Intravenous crystalloid fluid therapy is the mainstay of treatment. The type of crystalloid may be selected based upon specific patient electrolyte status (see Chapter 2). Replacement IV crystalloid fluid therapy restores perfusion and hydration, promotes diuresis for excretion of uremic toxins, replaces ongoing fluid losses from vomiting and diarrhea and provides maintenance fluid requirements in patients that are not drinking. Careful monitoring of fluid infusion rates, urine output through a patent closed collection system, CVP, BP, PCV/TP, and body weight are essential to avoid fluid overload associated with oliguria or anuria [9].

Because drug therapy and renal excretion of drugs are altered in AKI, a review of all prescribed medications is performed in patients with suspected renal azotemia. Special attention should be given to drugs that require renal metabolism or excretion, or may have ongoing nephrotoxicity. Adjustments in medication dose or interval must be made where appropriate (see Chapter 18) [2]. A list of nephrotoxic medications and drugs is given in Table 13.8.

Hyperkalemia due to reduced potassium excretion can be a life-threatening consequence of AKI, especially during oliguria or anuria. Potassium-induced cardiac arrhythmias can affect perfusion and can be initially managed by administering calcium gluconate (50–150 mg/kg slowly over 10–15 minutes IV) while monitoring the ECG. Other therapies for hyperkalemia can include insulin (regular insulin: 0.5 U/kg IV dogs; 1 unit/cat IV cats) and dextrose (500 mg/U of regular insulin given, followed by 1.25–2.5% dextrose in IV fluids); sodium bicarbonate therapy is occasionally indicated (1–2 mEq/kg IV over 10–15 minutes) to promote intracellular shifting of potassium. Table 13.9 lists medications and doses used to treat patients with renal insufficiency. The frequency of potassium monitoring (ECG, blood levels) can vary. However, the more acute and severe the clinical signs are, the more frequent the reassessment should be. The goal is to stabilize the cardiovascular system and allow time to establish urine production [1,2].

Medical strategies are available to try to increase urine production, with the knowledge that this allows more aggressive intravenous fluid therapy and diuresis but might not improve the prognosis for recovery of renal function. Mannitol (0.25–1 g/kg IV) is an osmotic diuretic that is freely filtered at the glomerulus and, when given to patients with oliguric renal failure, may increase urine flow [2,4]. Mannitol should not be administered to patients that have volume overload or severe vasculitis. Furosemide is a loop diuretic working at the thick ascending loop of Henle [2,4].

Table 13.8 Examples of nephrotoxins.

Environmental toxins
  Arsenic and other heavy metals
  Cholecalciferol or vitamin D-containing rodenticides
  Ethylene glycol
  Grapes or raisins (canine)
  Lilium and Hemerocallis plant species (feline)
Pharmaceuticals
  ACE inhibitors
  Acyclovir
  Aminoglycosides
  Amphotericin B
  Azathioprine
  Calcipotriene topical creams
  Cisplatin and carboplatin
  Cyclosporine
  Diuretics
  Nonsteroidal antiinflammatory drugs
  Oxytetracycline
  Thiacetarsemide
Diagnostic agents
  Gadolinium (high dose)
  IV iodinated contrast
Supplements or dietary contaminants
  Alpha-lipoic acid
  Melamine
  Vitamin D supplements

The dose of furosemide administered by continuous rate infusion (CRI) (0.1–0.5 mg/kg/h IV) is recommended in AKI since it results in greater diuresis and natriuresis than when given as intermittent IV injections (1–2 mg/kg IV) [42]. Care must be taken to avoid drug-induced hypokalemia, hypovolemia or dehydration.

Dopamine has been used in humans and veterinary patients with renal failure to increase urine production [43,44]. At renal doses (0.5–3 μg/kg/min IV by CRI), dopamine is a renal dopaminergic receptor agonist that increases renal blood flow and GFR, resulting in natriuresis [43,44]. However, dopamine therapy should be carefully considered given the potential side-effects of hypertension and cardiac arrhythmias and the lack of veterinary studies documenting effects in small animal patients with AKI [43]. Large multicenter trials in humans receiving dopamine therapy for renal failure did not decrease the dialysis requirement [44]. Fenoldopam (0.1–0.5 μg/kg/min IV by CRI) is a selective dopaminergic receptor agonist that has been shown to increase urine production in cats and dogs [43,45]. This selective dopaminergic (DA1) receptor agonist may avoid the adverse effects associated with dopamine, and shows promise as an alternative to dopamine for increasing urine production in oliguric or anuric renal failure [43,46]. Diltiazem (0.1–0.5 mg/kg IV slowly, then 1–5 μg/kg/min IV by CRI) is a calcium channel blocking agent reported to facilitate increase in urine production by decreasing renal vasoconstriction [1,2,47]. In a series of dogs with leptospirosis-induced renal failure, the use of diltiazem improved renal recovery as measured by improvements in creatinine [47]. The dogs receiving diltiazem had a trend toward increasing urine production after 24 hours; although this did not reach statistical significance, it may be considered in leptospirosis cases [47].

When the etiology of AKI is known, targeted medical, surgical or interventional therapies aimed at elimination of the underlying cause should be pursued. Nephrotoxin-induced AKI can include

Table 13.9 Therapies and drugs used to treat patients with renal and urinary tract disease.

Therapy	Rationale	Dose	Special considerations in renal disease
Furosemide	Loop diuretic that can increase urine production and allow continued IV fluid diuresis	1–2 mg/kg IV single dose or 0.1–0.5 mg/kg/h IV CRI	An increase in urine production does not necessarily equate with improved renal function. Furosemide can worsen dehydration or volume depletion. Hypokalemia can be a significant side-effect. CRI infusions have been shown to be more effective at increasing urine production than intermittent dosing.
Mannitol	An osmotic diuretic may increase urine production after it is filtered at the glomerulus allowing for continued IV fluid diuresis	0.25–1 g/kg IV single dose	Mannitol should not be used in patients that are volume overloaded or dehydrated
Dopamine	As a dopaminergic agonist, it is thought to increase urine production by differential effects on afferent and efferent arteriolar constriction	0.5–3 µg/kg/min CRI	Dopamine is less effective at increasing urine production in cats. In humans with renal failure, dopamine therapy has not decreased the requirement for renal replacement despite increases in urine production. Dopamine can contribute to hypertension and arrhythmias due to adrenergic effects
Fenoldopam	As a more selective DA-1 receptor agonist, it may increase urine production similar to dopamine but without adrenergic side-effects	0.1–0.5 µg/kg/min CRI	Fenoldopam has been reported to result in greater increase in urine production in cats compared to dopamine. Avoids the adrenergic side-effects of dopamine
Diltiazem	A calcium channel blocker that may increase urine production	0.1–0.5 mg/kg IV slow bolus followed with IV CRI of 1–5 µg/kg/min	Can cause hypotension and bradyarrhythmias. Often used for leptospirosis-induced AKI
H2 histamine antagonists	Used to improve gastric fluid pH and treat mucosal ulcerations associated with uremic gastritis	Famotidine 0.5–1 mg/kg IV q 12–24 h Ranitidine 0.5–2 mg/kg IV or PO q 24 h	Cats and dogs with renal failure have been demonstrated to have gastric fibrosis and mineralization rather than gastric necrosis and ulcers as a manifestation of uremic gastritis. Ranidtine may have some prokinetic activity
Proton pump inhibitors	Used to decrease gastric fluid pH and treat mucosal ulcerations associated with uremic gastritis	Pantoprazole 0.5–1 mg/kg IV q 24 h	Takes several days to reach maximal therapeutic effect. Cats and dogs with renal failure have been demonstrated to have gastric fibrosis and mineralization rather than gastric necrosis and ulcers as a manifestation of uremic gastritis
Sucralfate	Used to coat mucosal ulcerations associated with uremic gastritis	0.5–1 g/PO q 8 h (C) 0.2–0.5 g/PO q 8 h (F)	Cats and dogs with renal failure have been demonstrated to have gastric fibrosis and mineralization rather than gastric necrosis and ulcers as a manifestation of uremic gastritis. Must be given orally separate from other oral medications or food
Maropitant	A neurokinin receptor antagonist and central antiemetic	1 mg/kg SC q 8 h 2 mg/kg PO q 24 h	Maximum duration of treatment has been reported to be up to 5 days
Serotonin antagonists	Central antiemetic	Ondansetron 0.5–1 mg/kg IV q 12–24 h Dolasetron 0.5–1 mg/kg IV q 12–24 h	No special considerations in renal failure
Metoclopramide	Central antiemetic effects via dopaminergic antagonism and peripheral prokinetic effects	0.4 mg/kg SC q 8 h or 1–2 mg/kg/day CRI in IV fluids	Due to dopaminergic antagonist activity, may have effects to promote afferent arteriolar constriction and therefore reduce glomerular filtration. Dose reduction may be considered
Chlorpromazine	Broad-spectrum phenothiazine antiemetic	0.2–0.5 mg/kg SC q 8–12 h	Hypotension and sedation can be significant side-effects

(Continued)

Table 13.9 (*Continued*)

Therapy	Rationale	Dose	Special considerations in renal disease
Erythropoietin analogs	Stimulate red blood cell production	Epogen® 100IU/kg SC 3 times a week until target PCV reached then 50–100IU/kg SC once- to twice-weekly maintenance Darbopoeitin® 0.45–1 µg/kg SC q 7d until target PCV reached then 0.45–1 µg/kg SC every 2nd or 3rd week	Iron supplementation may be needed at the start of therapy For both Epogen and Darbopoeitin therapy target PCV in dogs=30%, cats=25% Risk of pure red cell aplasia is ~25% with Epogen and 10% with Darbopoeitin
ACE inhibitors	Decrease renal proteinuria	Benazepril 0.25–0.5 mg/kg PO q 12–24h (C, F) Enalapril 0.5–1 mg/kg PO q 12–24h (C), 0.25–0.5 mg/kg PO SID-BID (F)	Benazepril may be preferred over enalipril as it relies less on renal elimination All ACE inhibitors may cause a worsening of azotemia
Losartan	Angiotensin receptor antagonist that may decrease hypertension secondary to protein-losing nephropathy, may decrease proteinuria	In azotemic dogs: initial dose of 0.125 mg/kg/day PO escalating to 0.5 mg/kg/day (C) In nonazotemic dogs: initial dose of 0.5 mg/kg/day, escalating to 1 mg/kg/day (C)	There is little published information on the use of losartan in dogs. There are no dosing recommendations for cats Can be used in combination with ACE inhibitors for refractory hypertension and proteinuria
Amlodipine	Calcium channel blocker. Reduces hypertension	0.05–0.1 mg/kg PO q 24h (C) 0.625–1.25 mg/PO q 24h (F)	Can be used in combination with ACE inhibitors. Monitor for hypotension
Nitroprusside	Vascular smooth muscle relaxant, vasodilator to treat hypertensive crisis	Initial infusion rate of 0.5 µg/kg/min CRI, titrated upward to a maximum of 10 µg/kg/min until target blood pressure is achieved	Blood pressure should be monitored continuously with invasive arterial blood pressure monitoring or every 1–2 minutes with noninvasive Doppler during therapy
Hydralazine	Arteriolar dilator to treat hypertension or hypertensive crisis	0.5–3 mg/kg PO q 12h; start at low dose and escalate dosing until target BP is reached; injectable available	Can be titrated at 1 mg/kg hourly in a hypertensive crisis to achieve blood pressure target more rapidly. Maximum cumulative dose with titration is 3 mg/kg then it can be administered BID
Calcitriol	Vitamin D analog to reduce renal secondary hyperparathyroidism	2–2.5 ng/kg/day PO, monitor PTH and calcium levels to establish dosing. Dose should not exceed 5 ng/kg/day	Usually requires compounding to achieve adequate dosing. Goal with calcitriol therapy is to reduce PTH levels without inducing hypercalcemia
Potassium gluconate	Oral potassium supplement for chronic hypokalemia	0.5–1 mEq/kg PO in food once to twice daily	Monitor potassium levels to adjust dosing
Aluminum hydroxide	Phosphate binder	30–100 mg/kg/day PO	Monitor phosphorus levels every 1–2 weeks to titrate dosing. Sucralfate is an alternative
Calcium gluconate	Cardioprotective to reduce arrhythmias associated with hyperkalemia	5–15 mg/kg IV slow injection once	Monitor ECG during slow infusion
Regular insulin	Emergency treatment of severe hyperkalemia	0.5 U/kg IV once (C) 1 U/IV once (F)	Administration of regular insulin for the treatment of hyperkalemia should be followed by administration of dextrose at a dose of 500 mg dextrose/unit of insulin that was administered. Patients may require dextrose CRI at 1.25–2.5% for 1–4 h after insulin administration to avoid hypoglycemia
Sodium bicarbonate	Emergency treatment of severe hyperkalemia	0.5–1 mEq/Kg IV slow injection	No special considerations in renal disease
Prazosin	Alpha-1 antagonist used as a urethral smooth muscle relaxant	0.5–2 mg/PO q 12–24h (C) 0.5–1 mg/PO q 12–24h (F)	Monitor for hypotension
Phenoxybenzamine	Alpha-antagonist used as a urethral smooth muscle relaxant	0.25 mg/kg PO q 12h (C) 2.5–7.5 mg/PO q 12–24h (F)	Monitor for hypotension

ACE, angiotensin converting enzyme; BID, twice a day (bis in die); C, canine; CRI, continuous rate infusion; F, feline; IV, intravenous; PO, orally (per os); PTH, parathyroid hormone; SID, once a day (semel in die); SQ, subcutaneous; TID, three times a day (ter in die).

ingested toxins (ethylene glycol, lilies), pigment-induced (hemolysis, rhabdomyolysis) toxicity or medications (contrast agents, aminoglycosides, NSAIDS). Ethylene glycol has a specific antidote available and early treatment with 4-methylpyrazole (canine protocol 20 mg/kg IV initial dose, followed by 15 mg/kg 12 and 24 hours after initial dose, then 5 mg/kg 36 hours after initial dose; feline protocol 125 mg/kg initial dose, then 31.25 mg/kg at 12, 24, and 36 hours) or ethanol (as a 20% ethanol solution – administer 2 mL/kg IV bolus, followed by a CRI of 0.5–1 mL/kg/h until a negative ethylene glycol test or for 48 hours) may prevent progression to renal failure. Dialysis can support patients with toxin-induced renal failure and can also eliminate dialyzable nephrotoxins [48–50]. Glomerular disease and pyelonephritis can cause AKI and require specific management strategies or intervention which are described below. Chemotherapy-responsive renal neoplasms such as lymphoma should be treated with protocols to induce remission. Hypercalcemia can cause AKI requiring specific interventions including IV fluid therapy, furosemide (1–2 mg/kg IV) and/or prednisone (1–2 mg/kg/day) to promote calciuresis, and bisphosphonates (pamidronate 1–2.2 mg/kg IV over 1–2 hours) to more rapidly reduce hypercalcemia and prevent ongoing renal damage; Table 6.6 contains further information.

The AKI criteria for veterinary patients have put monitoring renal health and injury in the forefront of ICU patient management [18,39]. The mainstay of effective clinical monitoring incorporates the widely available BUN and creatinine trends of change, urine output, and physical monitoring parameters for perfusion and hydration. Should oliguria or anuria develop that cannot be converted to a sufficient urine output, the only available treatment options are intracorporeal (peritoneal dialysis) or extracorporeal renal replacement therapies (intermittent hemodialysis (IHD), continuous renal replacement therapy (CRRT)). Increasing availability of renal replacement centers has the potential to dramatically improve the success of managing veterinary patients with AKI in the future [50].

Pyelonephritis

Pyelonephritis is the inflammation of the renal tissues, calyces, and pelvis from either an ascending urinary tract or blood-borne infection (usually bacterial). Underlying diseases such as diabetes mellitus or immune compromise may make the patient more susceptible to kidney infection. Clinical signs can range from mild depression and anorexia to significant systemic signs such as fever, nausea, vomiting, renal pain, and painful urination [51]. Renal failure in pyelonephritis is caused by a combination of interstitial infiltrates with inflammatory cells and tubular occlusion with purulent exudate [1,2]. A presumptive diagnosis of pyelonephritis can be made on the basis of azotemia with inflammatory urinary sediment (red blood cells, white blood cells, bacteria, and protein). Diagnosis is confirmed with positive culture and susceptibility of a urine sample collected by cystocentesis [7]. Urine collected from the urinary bladder is sufficient for diagnosis in most cases of pyelonephritis but in rare instances a urine sample will need to be collected from the renal pelvis by ultrasound-guided pyelocentesis to confirm a diagnosis [7].

Pyelonephritis should be treated with antibiotics that have no nephrotoxicity. Intravenous rather than oral therapy is warranted to establish therapeutic concentrations more quickly and bypass a potentially abnormal GI tract. Long-term therapy is guided by culture and susceptibility. Prior to obtaining urine culture results, empirical antibiotic selection should be based on the most common uropathogens as well as specific tissue penetration of the antibiotic(s). The most common organism cultured from the urinary tract in dogs and cats is *Escherichia coli*, accounting for one-third to one-half of all uropathogens [52,53]. The second most common group of organisms affecting the urinary tract is gram-positive cocci [52]. First-line antibiotics in urinary tract infection include aminopenicillins, beta-lactamase inhibitor penicillins, and trimethoprim sulfadiazine. Fluoroquinolones should be considered as second-tier antibiotics in cases of uncomplicated lower tract infection but can be selected as first tier in cases of pyelonephritis or where tissues such as prostate need to be penetrated [52].

Leptospirosis

Leptospirosis is a zoonotic disease of mammals, including dogs and humans, caused by the *Leptospira* spp. spirochete bacteria. There are few reports of leptospirosis in cats. Infection with different leptospirosis serovars contributes to clinical syndromes in dogs, including acute febrile illness, acute renal failure, hepatopathy or hepatic failure, pulmonary hemorrhage, and death. Leptospirosis is contracted from water sources which have been contaminated with urine from infected wildlife or domestic mammals. Patients presenting with any of the clinical syndromes, especially acute renal failure and history of access to stagnant water sources in a geographic region known to have endemic leptospirosis, should raise the index of suspicion for leptospirosis [54].

In addition to the minimum database described above for evaluation of all patients with renal failure, patients with suspected leptospirosis should undergo specific testing to support a diagnosis. Titers performed via the microscopic agglutination test (MAT) remain the standard for diagnosis of leptospirosis. Demonstration of high acute and fourfold rise in convalescent titers improves the diagnostic accuracy of MAT. Previously vaccinated animals can make interpretation of mild elevations in MAT difficult because vaccinated animals may show positive titers and cross-reactivity with vaccinal serovars. Blood and urine PCR tests can be used to support the diagnosis. PCR requires bacterial DNA to be present and can be falsely negative if therapy has already been instituted. Bacterial cultures for leptospirosis are rarely indicated or required to achieve a diagnosis. Dark field microscopy for direct detection of leptospires in urine can be performed although, with the ready availability of MAT and PCR tests, dark field microscopy is rarely performed [54].

In addition to standard therapy for acute renal failure, patients with leptospirosis should undergo antibiotic therapy targeted at elimination of leptospiremia and elimination of leptospires from the renal tubules. Leptospiremia and renal carrier state of leptospirosis are eliminated with doxycycline (tetracycline) alone or in combination with aminopenicillin (beta-lactam) therapy. Antibiotic therapy should continue for two weeks [54]. Patients with leptospirosis treated in hospital may benefit from diltiazem infusion as it has been shown to improve renal outcomes with a trend of increasing urine production in a case series of dogs with leptospirosis [47].

Leptospirosis is a zoonotic disease and both in hospital and at home precautions should be taken to prevent zoonotic spread or spread to other dogs in the same household. In the hospital setting, placement of indwelling urinary catheters to contain the infectious urine is recommended. A protocol for adherence to barrier protocols and personal protective equipment for staff when handling the patient should be implemented, including gloves, gowns and goggles when disposing of infected urine. Clients should be educated on the zoonotic risk, with advice to wear gloves when cleaning up urine spills and disinfecting with 10% bleach solutions where possible for urine spills. Clients should be encouraged to seek medical attention via their family physician at the first signs of illness. Two-way (*Icterohaemorrhagiae* and *Canicola*) and four-way (*Icterohaemorrhagiae, Canicola, Pomona, Grippotyphosa*) leptospirosis vaccines for dogs have been shown to be protective against sero-group specific infection with some cross-protection to heterologous serogroups. Vaccination is recommended for canine patients based on their individual environmental risk for exposure [54].

Glomerulonephropathy

Glomerular diseases are a wide spectrum of conditions affecting the glomerulus characterized by persistent proteinuria. Glomerulopathy is not a specific diagnosis and can be caused by hereditary glomerulopathies, glomerular lesions as a consequence of chronic or systemic infections or inflammation, amyloid deposition, neoplasia or of idiopathic origin. Glomerulonephritis (GN) is the term often assigned in the clinical diagnosis of glomerulopathies. GN and other glomerular lesions can be histologically characterized by renal biopsy. Irrespective of the underlying cause, moderate and persistent glomerular proteinuria is a marker of glomerular disease [13,14].

Proteinuria does not always indicate a glomerular lesion and when proteinuria is diagnosed, the clinician should consider the differentials for localization for proteinuria. Prerenal proteinuria caused by the presence of plasma proteins (typically hemoglobin or myoglobin) does not require specific therapy to treat the proteinuria, and diagnostics and therapy are targeted at the underlying cause. Postrenal proteinuria is usually suspected when there is an active urinary sediment or contamination by proteins from the vagina, prepuce or penis. When proteinuria is determined to be renal, it does not necessarily indicate a pathological process that requires treatment. Functional proteinuria caused by fever, stress, or strenuous exercise is expected to resolve readily without specific treatment for the proteinuria. When renal proteinuria is considered pathological, it can be further localized to pathological tubular and pathological glomerular. The differentiation between pathological tubular and pathological glomerular proteinuria is often difficult but glomerular proteinuria is suspected when UPC is persistently greater than 2.0 [13,14].

Proteinuria is a marker of progressive CKD and can also contribute to worsening renal function. This makes lowering proteinuria a therapeutic target that can slow the progression of CKD and be renal protective. Recognizing the importance of proteinuria in evaluating CKD patients, the International Renal Interest Society (IRIS) has published proteinuria substaging guidelines for CKD (Table 13.10) with recommendations for monitoring and treatment based on proteinuria substage combined with CKD stage (Table 13.11), and blood pressure substage (Table 13.12) [55]. Any medications that could worsen proteinuria, such as glucocorticoids, should be avoided in glomerular disease unless an immune-mediated etiology has been documented. Therapeutic interventions for renal proteinuria include dietary management that reduces the quantity of dietary protein but enhances the quality, combined with omega-3 fatty acid supplementation and finally administration of ACE inhibitors [11].

Table 13.10 IRIS chronic kidney disease proteinuria substage.

Substage	Nonproteinuric	Borderline proteinuric (BP)	Proteinuric (P)
UPC	<0.2 (C, F)	0.2–0.5 (C) 0.2–0.4 (F)	>0.5 (C) >0.4 (F)

Source: Modified from www.iris-kidney.com/guidelines/staging.shtml.
C, canine; F, feline; IRIS, International Renal Interest Society; UPC, urine protein:creatinine ratio.

Table 13.11 IRIS chronic kidney disease (CKD) staging.

CKD stage	At risk	1	2	3	4
Creatinine μmol/L	<125 (C) <140 (F)	<125 (C) <140 (F)	125–180 (C) 140–250 (F)	181–440 (C) 251–440 (F)	>440 (C) >440 (F)
Creatinine mg/dL	<1.4 (C) <1.6 (F)	<1.4 (C) <1.6 (F)	1.4–2.0 (C) 1.6–2.8 (F)	2.1–5.0 (C) 2.9–5.0 (F)	>5.0 (C) >5.0 (F)
Comments	History indicative of increased risk for CKD such as breed predisposition, age, history of nephrotoxin exposure	Nonazotemic with other indicators of renal insufficiency (isosthenuria, palpation or imaging abnormalities)	Mild azotemia – clinical signs mild or absent	Moderate azotemia – clinical signs may be present	Severe azotemia with high risk for uremic crisis and severe clinical signs

Source: Modified from www.iris-kidney.com/guidelines/staging.shtml.
C, canine; F, feline; IRIS, International Renal Interest Society; UPC, urine protein:creatinine ratio.

Table 13.12 IRIS chronic kidney disease (CKD) blood pressure (BP) substaging.

BP substage	Normotensive	Borderline hypertensive	Hypertensive	Severely hypertensive
Systolic BP (mmHg)*	<150	150–159	160–179	≥180
Risk of future target organ damage	Minimal	Low	Moderate	High

Source: Modified from www.iris-kidney.com/guidelines/staging.shtml.
C, canine; F, feline; IRIS, International Renal Interest Society.
* If available, breed-specific reference ranges for blood pressure should be used for substaging.

The ACEi drugs can restore the charge and permeability selectivity of the glomerular basement membrane to reduce proteinuria. While ACE inhibitors are generally considered poor drugs for treating hypertension, they provide a benefit in glomerular proteinuria by decreasing glomerular hypertension through postcapillary vasodilation and exhibiting antiplatelet and antiinflammatory effects [11]. ACEI drug therapy is recommended in dogs with IRIS stage I CKD and UPC >2.0, IRIS stage II and III CKD with UPC >0.5, and IRIS stage IV CKD with UPC = 0.2–0.5 [56]. The clinical implications of proteinuria in cats are less well defined and true glomerular proteinuria in cats is uncommon [13]. IRIS recommendations in cats include treatment with ACEi in those with IRIS stage I CKD and UPC >1, IRIS stage II, III, IV CKD with UPC >0.4 [57]. ACEi can reduce GFR by their differential effect on afferent and efferent arteriolar dilation so any dosage increase should occur slowly, with careful monitoring of BUN, creatinine, BP, UPC, and physical parameters.

Chronic kidney disease

Renal compensatory hypertrophy and improvement of function can occur for up to 3 months after AKI. Therefore, CKD, also referred to as chronic renal failure and chronic renal insufficiency, is defined as kidney damage that has been present for at least 3 months or a reduction in GFR >50% for at least 3 months. There are many causes of CKD, and by the time the animal shows signs, the cause may not be apparent. Diagnostic criteria to support CKD include the presence of anemia, azotemia, hyperphosphatemia, + hypercalcemia, and isosthenuria. The presence of CKD can complicate the treatment plan of any ICU patient and must be considered when assigning fluid therapy, prescribing drugs and planning the nutritional supplementation. The presence of proteinuria and hypertension becomes important when assigning therapy and categorizing the stage of CKD for monitoring response to treatment [1,11,32]. Table 13.11 presents the International Renal Interest Society (IRIS) criteria for staging CKD in the dog and cat. Though IRIS CKD staging is based on serum creatinine values, recommendations for incorporation of SDMA values into IRIS staging and treatment guidelines acknowledge the increased sensitivity of SDMA. Patients with creatinine values <1.4 mg/dl (dog) or 1.6 mg/dl (cat), but persistently documented SDMA values >14 ug/dl may be categorized at IRIS CKD stage I. Patients with low body condition and creatinine values that place them in IRIS II CKD stage but have SDMA ≥25 ug/dl should be treated with IRIS CKD stage III recommendations. Patients with IRIS CKD stage III creatinine values but with SDMA ≥45 ug/dL should be treated with IRIS CKD stage IV recommendations. Complete IRIS treatment recommendations based on CKD stage are available at http://www.iris-kidney.com/guidelines/recommendations.html [55–57].

In the acute setting, hypertension can be the result of fluid overload which should be ruled out by critical assessment of fluid balance. When fluid overload is the cause, therapy will target reducing fluid retention (furosemide 1–2 mg/kg IV) and reduction of fluid infusion rates and volumes. However, hypertension is a common consequence of kidney disease unassociated with intravascular volume changes. While the normal range for indirect systolic blood pressure is variable, repeatable (2–3 separate episodes at least 30 minutes apart) indirect SBP > 150 mmHg confirms hypertension. Table 13.12 presents the IRIS substaging for hypertension associated with CKD in small animals. A systolic BP > 180 mmHg is consistent with arterial pressure substage severely hypertensive, with detrimental consequences to the kidneys and other target organ (commonly the eyes, brain, cardiovascular system) damage anticipated [11,32].

Antihypertensive therapy should be initiated if there is evidence of end-organ damage or if reliable BP measurements categorize the patient in BP substages hypertensive (systolic pressure 160–179 mmHg) or severely hypertensive (systolic pressure >180 mmHg). The targets for BP reduction with therapy should be conservative. For BP substage severely hypertensive, initial target blood pressure with treatment are systolic/diastolic pressures of < 160/100 mmHg [2,4,58]. If glomerular protein loss is a component of the renal disease, then ace-inhibitor (ACEi) drug therapy is the first line treatment for hypertension. Benazepril (0.25–1.0 mg/kg q 12–24h PO cats; 0.25–0.5 mg/kg q 12–24h PO dogs) is the drug of choice since it does not require renal excretion like enalapril. If the ACEi drugs are insufficient to reduce hypertension, then the calcium channel blocker, amlodipine (cats: 0.625–1.25 mg/cat PO q 24h; dogs: 0.1–0.4 mg/kg PO q 12h) is started at the lower dose and titrated to effect. If the anti-hypertensive response is not complete with initiation of one medication, it is recommended to first increase the dosage and then add a second drug if necessary. In most cases, the hypertension is not an emergency and 3–4 weeks can be allowed between drug dosage adjustments [11,32].

Emergency intervention may be required for the animal that is severely hypertensive with progressive or severe neural or ocular target organ damage. A combination of ACEi and calcium channel blocker may be initiated simultaneously in the dog at the onset of treatment. Cats appear to respond rapidly to the calcium channel blocker amlodipine alone in many instances. To facilitate faster reductions in blood pressure, arteriolar and venous vasodilators, including hydralazine (0.5–3 mg/kg PO BID- start at low dose and escalate dosing until target BP is reached; see Table 13.9) and nitroprusside (Initial infusion rate of 0.5 ug/kg/min CRI, titrated upward to a max of 10 ug/kg/min until target blood pressure is achieved) may be required if the patient is severely hypertensive and deteriorating rapidly. Drug dosages must be titrated with vigilant monitoring to prevent too rapid and too much of a decline in the BP [11,32].

Managing uremia

Irrespective of the inciting cause or localization of renal injury, the clinical syndrome of uremia is predictable and results from a combination of retention of uremic toxins and alterations in the homeostatic functions of the kidneys. All organs in the body are targets for uremia (Table 13.13). Pain in patients with renal failure can be the result of ulcerations or secondary to renal visceral pain, depending on the etiology of renal failure. Pyelonephritis, hydronephrosis, and obstructive renal diseases can all contribute to varying levels of pain and should be treated accordingly. Opioid analgesics are appropriate to use in patients with renal failure to manage varying levels and sources of pain. Opioids have the benefit of being titratable, and reversible in the ICU patient (see Chapter 19). Nonsteroidal antiinflammatory medications are not recommended as analgesics in patients with acute or chronic renal injury.

The majority of critically ill veterinary patients, including those with renal failure, will be anorexic or hyporexic. Nutritional support and early nutritional intervention should not be overlooked in these fragile patients. Chapter 16 gives guidelines on the approach to nutrition in critically ill patients. Anemia, hypertension, osteomalacia, malnutrition, weight loss, muscle catabolism, pneumonitis, immune suppression, and systemic inflammation can all contribute

Table 13.13 Organ system targets of uremia.

Target rgan	Clinical effect	Mechanism/cause	Potential interventions
Gastrointestinal	Gastritis and gastrointestinal ulceration Stomatitis Uremic halitosis Pancreatitis Inappetance and anorexia Nausea Vomiting	Excess gastrin Central and peripheral effects of other uremic toxins	Histamine antagonists Proton pump inhibitors Sucralfate Antiemetics Appetite stimulants Feeding tubes and nutritional support Analgesia
Neurological	Lethargy and depression Weakness Muscle twitching Peripheral neuropathy Uremic Encephalopathy Seizures	Chronic dehydration Hypo- or hyperkalemia Hypo- or hypercalcemia Cerebral edema Vasculitis	Rehydration and fluid therapy Parenteral or oral potassium supplementation for hypokalemia Correction of electrolyte abnormalities Calcitriol therapy Nutritional support Mannitol or osmotic agents if cerebral edema is suspected Antiepileptic drugs
Hematological	Anemia Platelet dysfunction Hemorrhagic diathesis Thrombosis	Decreased erythropoietin production Loss in GI ulceration Uremic toxin effects on platelet function Vasculitis Bone marrow suppression Glomerular antithrombin loss	Recombinant erythropoietin or Darbopoietin Treat uremic gastritis and ulcerations Antiplatelet drugs for thromboprophylaxis ACE inhibitors to reduce glomerular antithrombin loss
Respiratory	Uremic pneumonitis Pulmonary edema	Uremic toxins Vasculitis Secondary to oliguria/anuria combined with fluid therapy	Supplemental oxygen support Careful fluid therapy Medical therapy to convert to polyuria Diuretics for pulmonary edema Renal replacement therapies to address overhydration
Nutrition	Malnutrition Weight loss	Impaired glucose and carbohydrate metabolism Altered insulin secretion and degradation Increased muscle catabolism Uremic toxins	Renal diets with reduced but high-quality protein sources Omega fatty acid supplementation Appetite stimulants Feeding tubes Antidiarrheal medications to reduce GI nutrient losses
Skeletal	Osteomalacia	Renal secondary hyperparathyroidism Chronic metabolic acidosis	Calcitriol therapy Fluid therapy to reduce uremia and metabolic acidosis Nutritional support
Immunological	Increase infection rates Chronic inflammation	Increases in C-reactive protein, TNF, and oxidative stress	Attention to monitoring for development of urinary tract infection Antibiotics for infections of the urinary tract and other systems guided by culture and sensitivity Fatty acid supplementation to reduce oxidative stress
Cardiovascular	Hypertension Thrombosis Hypovolemia Arrhythmias secondary to hyperkalemia	Activation of renal and systemic RAAS Glomerular antithrombin loss Decreased urine concentrating ability Chronic dehydration Decreased fluid intake Malnutrition Urethral obstruction, anuria or oliguria	Antihypertensive medications Antiplatelet drugs or anticoagulants for thromboprophylaxis Maintain hydration, fluid, and nutritional intake Correction of hyperkalemia by relieving obstructions, or treatment of uroabdomen Medical correction of hyperkalemia with insulin, dextrose, bicarbonate Calcium gluconate for arrhythmia secondary to hyperkalemia

ACE, angiotensin converting enzyme; RAAS, renin-angiotensin-aldosterone system; TNF, tumor necrosis factor.

to the lethargy, weakness, and general malaise of CKD. Supportive care measures for complications associated with uremia are important in the treatment of the ICU patient with AKI or CKD. Therapeutic targets include the management of uremic gastropathy, uremic encephalopathy, acid–base and electrolyte abnormalities, anemia, and nutritional support [4,11].

Uremic gastropathy, in the dog and cat, is the result of reduced gastrin elimination and the presence of circulating uremic toxins. The gastric histological lesions include edema, vasculopathy, fibrosis or mineralization [5,6]. Clinical manifestations of uremic gastropathy include oral mucosal ulcerations, hypersalivation, anorexia, vomiting, nausea, and abdominal pain, each providing a therapeutic target (see Tables 13.9 and 13.13) [1,2,4]. Anorexia, nausea, and vomiting are the result of local gastrin effects in addition to the central effect of uremic toxins at the level of the chemoreceptor trigger zone. Medications commonly used to support uremic gastropathy include H2-antihistamines (famotidine 0.5–1.0 mg/kg IV or PO q 12–24 h), proton pump inhibitors (pantoprazole 0.5–1.0 mg/kg IV q 24 h, omeprazole 1 mg/kg PO q 12 h), and sucralfate (0.5–1 g/dog PO q 8 h; 0.2–0.5 g/cat PO q 24 h) to coat gastric ulcers. Antiemetics to target central and peripheral emetogenesis include serotonin receptor antagonists (ondansetron 0.5–1 mg/kg IV q 12–24 h, dolasetron 0.5–1 mg/kg IV q 12–24 h), neurokinin receptor antagonist (maropitant 1 mg/kg SC q 24 h), and dopaminergic antagonists (metoclopramide 0.4 mg/kg SC q 8 h or 1–2 mg/kg/day IV by CRI). Chlorpromazine (0.2–0.5 mg/kg SC q 18–12 h) and other phenothiazines are highly effective antiemetics but are used with caution in patients with renal failure due to their hypotensive effects [2].Chapter 15 provides additional information.

Neurological manifestations of uremia result from uremic toxins as well as the hyperosmolality, acidosis, and electrolyte abnormalities that accompany AKI or CKD. Mild neurological signs include depression, lethargy, and weakness. In severe instances, problems such as severe obtundation, tremors, seizures, and coma can occur. Altered mentation, generalized weakness, and peripheral neuropathy may be long-term neurological consequences of uremia. Treatment is supportive and symptomatic. Other primary neurological disorders should be ruled out (see Chapter 12). Supplementation of vitamins and ensuring appropriate nutrition can minimize changes associated with thiamine or other nutritional deficiencies. It is important to review the medications the animal is receiving with the goal of minimizing or eliminating their impact on the nervous system. Ensuring adequate glucose, electrolyte, and acid–base status is critical. If the neurological status deteriorates, dialysis may be required.

Metabolic alterations of uremia can include hyperphosphatemia, alterations in serum calcium and potassium, and metabolic acidosis. Hyperphosphatemia is a result of reduced phosphate excretion due to decreased GFR. Therapy for hyperphosphatemia in the ICU patient should focus on improvement of GFR and urine production. Patients with chronic renal disease may need dietary phosphorus restriction and dietary phosphate binders (see Table 13.9). Serum calcium can be either low, as a consequence of high serum phosphorus, or elevated secondary to renal hyperparathyroidism. Controlling the serum phosphorus concentrations is critical to correcting hypocalcemia. Severe hypocalcemia manifesting as weakness, arrhythmias or tremors, though uncommon in patients with renal failure, may require short-term supplementation with IV calcium gluconate (100 mg/kg IV slowly while monitoring ECG) [11].

Calcitriol (initially 2.5 ng/kg/day in dogs) is indicated in dogs with chronic kidney disease stages 3 and 4 to slow the progression of rHPTH and extend survival. However, do not begin calcitriol

therapy until the patient's serum phosphorus concentration is 6 mg/dL or less. Unfortunately, evidence for or against calcitriol therapy in cats with chronic kidney disease is weak. The dose of calcitriol may be adjusted to achieve a treatment endpoint of normalizing PTH concentrations without inducing hypercalcemia. An alternate approach is to attempt to provide two or three days total dose of calcitriol every second or third day. This dosage may mitigate the hypercalcemia and increase the effect on parathyroid hormone (PTH) concentrations. When treating with calcitriol, monitor ionized calcium and PTH concentrations weekly until a treatment endpoint is reached. Patients receiving calcitriol should have their serum calcium, ionized calcium, and phosphorus concentrations monitored at least every two to three months [11].

Despite acidosis being common in patients with renal failure, specific alkaline therapy for severe acidosis (pH <7.1 or $HCO_3 < 12$ mmol/L) with bicarbonate administration is rarely required in the ICU. Refer to Chapter 7 for specific acid–base monitoring and intervention points.

Alterations in serum potassium are anticipated. Both hypokalemia and hyperkalemia can have a negative impact on the patient. The renal consequences of hypokalemia include renal afferent arteriolar constriction, decreased GFR, and interstitial fibrosis. Clinical signs of hypokalemia can range from mild depression to severe weakness, ventral flexion of the head and neck, or impaired respiratory efforts due to weakness of the diaphragm and other muscles of respiration. Intravenous potassium supplementation (maximum rate of 0.5 mEq/kg/h), often combined with oral potassium (potassium gluconate 0.5–1 mEq/kg PO twice a day) is necessary to correct potassium depletion and maintain adequate serum potassium levels during diuresis.

Anemia is a component of CKD that can result from multiple factors including:

- blood loss from GI tract, blood sampling, and platelet function defects
- decreased erythropoietin production by the kidney
- uremic toxin and inflammation-induced bone marrow suppression
- decreased red blood cell survival.

Acute, severe anemia can manifest as weakness, tachypnea, tachycardia, pale gums, and bounding pulses. Patients showing these signs can require transfusion of packed red blood cells in order to restore the oxygen-carrying components necessary for continued therapy. However, most patients with CKD have chronic anemia and their clinical signs are much less severe. Therapy in these chronic patients is primarily targeted at reducing any blood loss and providing erythropoietin replacement therapy (see Table 13.9). The risk of forming antierythropoietin autoantibodies and hypertension in response to the drug therapy warrants reserving these drugs for patients with severe nonregenerative anemia associated with CKD, generally considered at a PCV <19% [4,11].

Postrenal disorders

Postrenal azotemia is caused by a reduction in the excretion of urine from the body due to obstruction or disruption at the level of the renal distal tubules, ureters, urinary bladder or urethra. Within the kidney, the distal tubules can be obstructed by cellular debris, inflammatory debris, nephroliths or crystals. Ureteral obstruction can be caused by ureteroliths, ureteral strictures, and ureteritis. At the level of the urinary bladder or urethra, obstruction occurs due to urolithiasis, urinary neoplasia, as a result of feline lower urinary tract disease (FLUTD) and urethral spasms in cats, neurogenic bladder, and less commonly due to obstructive hematomas or accumulation of inflammatory debris. Renal failure from postrenal obstruction occurs as a consequence of renal pelvic dilation and progressive increase in backpressure in the renal tubules with decreased capillary filtration pressure.

While urine flow may be adequate with a disruption in the urinary tract, urine leakage into the abdominal, retroperitoneal space or tissues will cause postrenal azotemia [1,2]. Disruption of the urinary tract allows the flow of excreted molecules and electrolytes into the tissues or body cavity where reabsorption back into the bloodstream can produce toxic levels [23]. Tissues are also damaged by prolonged contact with the urine. With urinary leakage, an infection that had been localized to the urinary tract can become systemic. Monitoring for a rupture of the urinary tract should be instituted in any ICU patient that has experienced abdominal or pelvic trauma with a consideration that urinary tract leakage in trauma patients may not be apparent until fluid resuscitation restores urine flow [23].

Indwelling urethral catheters serve as a monitoring tool to assess urine output and can also be used for urinary contrast studies to confirm a diagnosis of uroabdomen (see Table 13.3) [22,23]. In patients with confirmed uroabdomen surgical intervention is recommended to achieve abdominal lavage, and for removal and/or repair of the site of urinary leakage. In cases of uroabdomen in which surgery needs to be delayed, placement of an abdominal catheter to remove urine from the abdomen and facilitate peritoneal lavage can assist in stabilizing the patient in preparation to pursue general anesthesia and surgery [23].

Obstructive uropathies will require placement of indwelling urethral catheter or urinary diversion with percutaneous cystostomy tubes until definitive therapy is achieved. Any patient who has undergone relief of a postrenal obstructive process will be expected to have a postobstructive diuresis and their fluid requirements should be closely titrated with monitoring urine output. With the advent of interventional radiology techniques, many obstructive uropathies now have options for specific and targeted therapy to restore urine flow beyond surgical interventions. Urethral stents are indicated for urethral obstruction secondary to urethral masses or strictures. Ureteral stents, percutaneous nephrostomy tubes, or subcutaneous ureteral bypass systems can be placed to establish urine flow or for urinary diversion in cases of ureteral obstruction [59]. Intracorporeal laser lithotripsy can be performed for breakdown and removal of urinary stones in selected cases.

Renal replacement therapies

When therapies aimed at increasing urine production fail in oliguric or anuric renal failure, the only medical therapeutic options remaining are renal replacement therapies. Renal replacement can be achieved with intracorporeal peritoneal dialysis (PD) [48,49]. As with all replacement therapies, peritoneal dialysis is labor intensive and requires expertise for success. The advantage of peritoneal dialysis is that it does not require highly specialized equipment. PD requires the aseptic placement of a peritoneal dialysis catheter. In PD the peritoneum is used as a dialysis membrane. Warmed dialysate (10–20 mL/kg) is infused into the abdominal cavity. Dialysate composition can be formulated with patient-specific factors in mind. The dialysate contains dextrose (1.5%, 2.5% or 4.25%) at concentrations chosen to create the osmotic gradient that will draw the desired amount of water, electrolytes, and other substances through the peritoneal membrane into the dialysate at the rate desired. The higher the dextrose concentration, the

more rapid the movement of water and subsequent solute drag of molecules into the dialysate. The size, charge, and concentration of the molecule in the plasma will determine whether it will pass into the dialysate. The dialysate is allowed to equilibrate within the abdomen for a period of time (dwell time is usually 45 minutes), and the fluid is then drained from the abdomen. The process is immediately repeated during the acute phase of PD until the desired results have occurred. Less frequent exchanges are made once the patient has been stabilized to maintain control of uremic or toxic effects. Common complications of peritoneal dialysis include mechanical obstruction or dislodging of the catheter, dehydration due to rapid fluid shifts, abdominal discomfort, and infection. Dialysis disequilibrium, a neurological syndrome resulting from rapid correction of azotemia, is uncommon from peritoneal dialysis [48,49].

Intermittent hemodialysis and continuous renal replacement therapies are extracorporeal therapies that can be used to manage oliguric or anuric renal failure. Additionally, IHD can be used for long-term management of patients with CKD. Both IHD and CRRT require vascular access with vascular dialysis catheters and anticoagulation of the patient or the extracorporeal circuit. Blood is drawn out of the patient through an external dialysis filter or membrane for blood purification then returned to the patient. The dialysis prescription or mode of continuous renal replacement will determine how quickly patient BUN and creatinine values change. Dialysis prescriptions and CRRT modes can be programmed to facilitate fluid removal in patients that are volume overloaded. Dialysis disequilibrium syndrome is an important complication, resulting in neurological signs attributed to the development of cerebral edema. Infection, bleeding, and thrombosis are other potential complications. The utility of IHD and CRRT for most veterinary patients is limited by availability of a dialysis center and the cost [50,60].

References

1. Lunn KF. The kidney in critically ill small animals. Vet Clin North Am Small Anim Pract. 2011;41(4):727–44.
2. Ross L. Acute kidney injury in dogs and cats. Vet Clin North Am Small Anim Pract. 2011;41(1):1–14.
3. Rose BD, Post TW. Clinical Physiology of Acid-Base and Electrolyte Disorders, 5th edn. New York: McGraw-Hill, 2001.
4. Cowgill L, Langston C. Acute kidney insufficiency. In: Nephrology and Urology of Small Animals. Bartges J, Polzin D, eds. Oxford: Wiley-Blackwell, 2011: pp 472–523.
5. McLeland SM, Lunn KF, Duncan CG, Refsal KR, Quimby JM. Relationship among serum creatinine, serum gastrin, calcium-phosphorus product, and uremic gastropathy in cats with chronic kidney disease. J Vet Intern Med. 2014;28(3):827–37.
6. Peters RM, Goldstein RE, Erb HN, Njaa BL. Histopathologic features of canine uremic gastropathy: a retrospective study. J Vet Intern Med. 2005;19(3):315–20.
7. Reine NJ, Langston CE. Urinalysis interpretation: how to squeeze out the maximum information from a small sample. Clin Tech Small Anim Pract. 2005;20 (1 Spec. Iss.):2–10.
8. Hamilton PRW, Hopkins MB, Shihabi ZK, Hamilton DRW, Shlhabi ZK. Myoglobinuria, hemoglobinuria, and acute renal failure. Clin Chem. 1989;35(8):1713–20.
9. Rudloff E, Kirby R. Colloid and crystalloid resuscitation. Vet Clin North Am Small Anim Pract. 2001;31(6):1206–27.
10. Lefebvre H. Renal function testing. In: Nephrology and Urology of Small Animals. Bartges J, Polzin D, eds. Oxford: Wiley-Blackwell, 2011: pp 91–8.
11. Polzin D. Chronic kidney disease. In: Nephrology and Urology of Small Animals. Bartges J, Polzin D, eds. Oxford: Wiley-Blackwell, 2011: pp 433–71.
12. Talavera J, Bayo A, Cortadellas O, Ferna MJ. Calcium and phosphorus homeostasis in dogs with spontaneous chronic kidney disease at different stages of severity. J Vet Intern Med. 2010;24:73–9.

13. Lees G, Brown SA, Elliot J, Grauer GF, Vaden S. Assessment and Management of Proteinuria in Dogs and Cats: 2004 ACVIM Forum Consensus Statement (Small Animal). J Vet Intern Med. 2005;19:377–85.

14. Littman M, Gaminet S, Grauer G, Lees G, van Dongen A. Consensus recommendations for the diagnostic investigation of dogs with suspected glomerular disease. J Vet Intern Med. 2013;27:S19–26.

15. Hall J, Yerramilli M, Obare E, Yerramilli M, Jewell DE. Comparison of serum concentrations of symmetric dimethylarginine and creatinine as kidney function biomarkers in cats with chronic kidney disease. J Vet Intern Med. 2014;28(6):1676–83.

16. Braff J, Obare E, Yerramilli M, Elliott J, Yerramilli M. Relationship between serum symmetric dimethylarginine concentration and glomerular filtration rate in cats. J Vet Intern Med. 2014;28(6):1699–701.

17. Hall J, Yerramilli M, Obare E, Yerramilli M, Melendez LD, Jewell DE. Relationship between lean body mass and serum renal biomarkers in healthy dogs. J Vet Intern Med. 2015;29:808–14

18. Thoen ME, Kerl ME. Characterization of acute kidney injury in hospitalized dogs and evaluation of a veterinary acute kidney injury staging system. J Vet Emerg Crit Care 2011;21(6):648–57.

19. Johnston G, Feeney D. Comparative organ imaging lower urinary tract. Vet Radiol Ultrasound. 1984;25(4):146–53.

20. Heuter KJ. Excretory urography. Clin Tech Small Anim Pract. 2005;20(1 Spec. Iss.):39–45.

21. Essman SC. Contrast cystography. Clin Tech Small Anim Pract. 2005;20(1 Spec. Iss.):46–51.

22. Schmiedt C, Tobias KM, Otto CM. Evaluation of abdominal fluid: peripheral blood creatinine and potassium ratios for diagnosis of uroperitoneum in dogs. J Vet Emerg Crit Care 2001;11(4):275–80.

23. Stafford JR, Bartges JW. A clinical review of pathophysiology, diagnosis, and treatment of uroabdomen in the dog and cat. J Vet Emerg Crit Care. 2013;23(2):216–29.

24. Messer JS, Chew DJ, McLoughlin M. Cystoscopy: techniques and clinical applications. Clin Tech Small Anim Pract. 2005;20(1 Spec. Iss.):52–64.

25. Von Hendy-Willson VE, Pressler BM. An overview of glomerular filtration rate testing in dogs and cats. Vet J. 2011;188(2):156–65.

26. Prowle J, Bagshaw SM, Bellomo R. Renal blood flow, fractional excretion of sodium and acute kidney injury: time for a new paradigm? Curr Opin Crit Care 2012;18(6):585–92.

27. De Loor J, Daminet S, Smets P, Maddens B, Meyer E. Urinary biomarkers for acute kidney injury in dogs. J Vet Intern Med. 2013;27(5):998–1010.

28. Goldstein R. Urinary enzyme activity for detection of acute kidney injury. In: Nephrology and Urology of Small Animals. Bartges J, Polzin D, eds. Oxford: Wiley-Blackwell, 2011: pp 70–2.

29. Sasaki A, Sasaki Y, Iwama R, et al. Comparison of renal biomarkers with glomerular filtration rate in susceptibility to the detection of gentamicin-induced acute kidney injury in dogs. J Comp Pathol. 2014;151(2-3):264–70.

30. Tobias K, ed. Veterinary Surgery: Small Animal. Philadelphia: Saunders. 2011.

31. Fossum T, ed. Small Animal Surgery, 4th edn. St Louis: Mosby, 2012: pp 1640.

32. Acierno MJ, Labato MA. Hypertension in renal disease: diagnosis and treatment. Clin Tech Small Anim Pract. 2005;20(1 Spec. Iss.):23–30.

33. Nelson NC, Drost WT, Lerche P, Bonagura JD. Noninvasive estimation of central venous pressure in anesthetized dogs by measurement of hepatic venous blood flow velocity and abdominal venous diameter. Vet Radiol Ultrasound 2010;51(3):313–23.

34. Brienza N, Giglio MT, Dalfino L. Protocoled resuscitation and the prevention of acute kidney injury. Curr Opin Crit Care 2012;18(6):613–22.

35. Ragaller MJ, Theilen H, Koch T. Volume replacement in critically ill patients with acute renal failure. J Am Soc Nephrol. 2001;12(Suppl 1):S33–9.

36. Mehta RL, Kellum J, Shah SV, et al. Acute Kidney Injury Network: report of an initiative to improve outcomes in acute kidney injury. Crit Care 2007;11(2):R31.

37. Mandelbaum TA, Scott DJ, Lee J, et al. Outcome of critically ill patients with acute kidney injury using the AKIN criteria. Crit Care Med. 2011;39(12):2659–64.

38. Bellomo R, Ronco C, Kellum J, Mehta RL, Palevsky P. Acute renal failure – definition, outcome measures, animal models, fluid therapy and information technology needs: the Second International Consensus Conference of the Acute Dialysis Quality Initiative (ADQI) Group. Crit Care 2004;8(4):R204–12.

39. Lee YJ, Chang CC, Chan JPW, Hsu WL, Lin KW, Wong ML. Prognosis of acute kidney injury in dogs using RIFLE (Risk, Injury, Failure, Loss and End-stage renal failure)-like criteria. Vet Rec. 2011;168(10):264.

40. Harison E, Langston C, Palma D, Lamb K. Acute azotemia as a predictor of mortality in dogs and cats. J Vet Intern Med. 2012;26(5):1093–8.

41. Lai CF, Wu VC, Huang TM, et al. Kidney function decline after a non-dialysis-requiring acute kidney injury is associated with higher long-term mortality in critically ill survivors. Crit Care 2012;16(4):R123.

42. Adin DB, Taylor AW, Hill RC, Scott KC, Martin FG. Intermittent bolus injection versus continuous infusion of furosemide in normal adult greyhound dogs. J Vet Intern Med. 2003;17(5):632–6.

43. Sigrist NE. Use of dopamine in acute renal failure. J Vet Emerg Crit Care 2007;17(2):117–26.

44. Kellum JA, Unruh ML, Murugan R. Acute kidney injury. Clin Evidence 2011;1–36.

45. Simmons JP, Wohl JS, Schwartz DD, Edwards HG, Wright JC. Diuretic effects of fenoldopam in healthy cats. J Vet Emerg Crit Care. 2006;16(2):96–103.

46. Bloom CA, Labato MA, Hazarika S, Court MH. Preliminary pharmacokinetics and cardiovascular effects of fenoldopam continuous rate infusion in 6 healthy dogs. J Vet Pharmcol Ther. 2012;35(3):224–30.

47. Mathews K, Monteith G. Evaluation of adding diltiazem therapy to standard treatment of acute renal failure caused by leptospirosis: 18 dogs (1998–2001). J Vet Emerg Crit Care 2007;17(2):149–58.

48. Bersenas AME. A clinical review of peritoneal dialysis. J Vet Emerg Crit Care. 2011;21(6):605–17.

49. Ross L, Labato MA. Current techniques in peritoneal dialysis. J Vet Emerg Crit Care 2013;23(2):230–40.

50. Cowgill LD, Guillaumin J. Extracorporeal renal replacement therapy and blood purification in critical care. J Vet Emerg Crit Care 2013;23(2):194–204.

51. Smee N, Loyd K, Grauer G. UTIs in small animal patients: part 1: etiology and pathogenesis. J Am Anim Hosp Assoc. 2013;49(1):1–7.

52. Boothe DM. Treatment of bacterial infections. In: Small Animal Clinical Pharmacology and Therapeutics, 2nd edn. Boothe DM, ed. St Louis: Elsevier Saunders, 2012: pp 270–363.

53. Smee N, Loyd K, Grauer GF. UTIs in small animal patients: part 2: diagnosis, treatment, and complications. J Am Anim Hosp Assoc. 2013;49(2):83–94.

54. Sykes JE, Hartmann K, Lunn KF, Moore GE, Stoddard R, Goldstein RE. 2010 ACVIM Consensus Statement on Leptospirosis: Diagnosis, Epidemiology, Treatment and prevention. J Vet Intern Med. 2011;25:1–13.

55. IRIS Staging of CKD (modified 2013). 2013;1–8. Available at: http://www.iris-kidney.com/guidelines/(accessed 30 May 2016).

56. Treatment Recommendations for CKD in Dogs (2013). 2013;1–13. Available at: http://www.iris-kidney.com/guidelines/(accessed 30 May 2016).

57. Treatment Recommendations for CKD in Cats (2013). 2013;1–14. Available at: http://www.iris-kidney.com/guidelines/(accessed 30 May 2016).

58. Brown S, Brown C, Jacobs G, Stiles J, Hendi RS, Wilson S. Effects of the angiotensin converting enzyme inhibitor benazepril in cats with induced renal insufficiency. Am J Vet Res. 2001;62(3):375–83.

59. Berent AC. Ureteral obstructions in dogs and cats: a review of traditional and new interventional diagnostic and therapeutic options. J Vet Emerg Crit Care 2011;21(2):86–103.

60. Eatroff AE, Langston CE, Chalhoub S, Poeppel K, Mitelberg E. Long-term outcome of cats and dogs with acute kidney injury treated with intermittent hemodialysis: 135 cases (1997–2010). J Am Vet Med Assoc. 2012;241(11):1471–8.

CHAPTER 14

White blood cells, immune status, and antimicrobial stewardship

Carol E. Haak

Milwaukee, Wisconsin

Introduction

Life or death in the critically ill small animal patient is often the result of the host's ability to mount a rapid and aggressive immune response. Both primary pathogens and secondary invaders can cause disease. Etiologies include bacteria, viruses, rickettsia, fungi, protozoa, parasites, and foreign material. The primary immune response should occur at the first exposure of the tissues or blood to the pathogen. A schematic of the basic mechanisms involved in this primary immune response (both innate and acquired) is illustrated in Figure 14.1.

The first immune response is dictated by the innate portion of the immune system. This response is nonspecific and does not require previous exposure to the antigen. The skin, gastrointestinal (GI) mucosal barrier, and mucous membranes form some of the innate physiochemical barriers to antigen invasion. Chemicals such as lysozymes, antiproteases, and complement present in bodily fluids can block replication or lyze the outer membranes of invading organisms. Phagocytic and cytotoxic myeloid cells including polymorphonuclear cells (PMNs) or neutrophils, macrophages, natural killer (NK) cells, and mast cells are recruited to the area of antigen deposition to destroy the pathogen. This approach can be very effective against many extracellular viruses and bacteria. However, many extracellular and most intracellular pathogens require a more sophisticated defense.

After the initial innate response comes the acquired portion of the immune response. This is antigen specific and creates immunological memory through dedicated lymphoid cells. T- and B- lymphocytes are exposed to antigen, then proliferate and migrate back to the site of injury. Cytokines released attracts other effector cells. Activated B-cells will synthesize and release immunoglobulins. Immunoglobulins (circulating) become bound to cell surfaces (antibodies), thus marking invaders and activating complement. Thus myeloid cells are recruited and the antigen is then neutralized or destroyed.

The immune system of the ICU patient is constantly challenged by a multitude of internal and external factors. It is important to consider patient-specific, disease-specific, and hospital-specific factors in the critically ill patient. Most commonly, we consider disease-specific factors in our patients: open fracture, wounds, infectious agent, disease-specific immunosuppression, chemotherapeutics, etc. However, patient-specific factors such as retroviral status, GI function, risk of GI bacterial translocation, co-infection due to aspiration, malnutrition, immune dysfunction or drug suppression often make a significant contribution to morbidity and mortality. At the other end of the spectrum, an abnormally active or improperly stimulated immune system may result in autoimmune or allergic disorders that can be equally life threatening. Additional factors are introduced in a hospital environment such as contamination of wounds or fractures, indwelling medical devices (IV and urinary catheters, suture material, implants), and nosocomial infections, which must all be considered. All of these may result in activation of the systemic inflammatory response syndrome (SIRS), multiple organ dysfunction syndrome (MODS), and death (Figure 14.2).

When a bacterial infection is part of the underlying disease or a consequence of critical illness, antibiotics will have an important role in the therapeutic plan. Choosing the best antibiotic regimen requires guidance from a bacterial culture and susceptibility test. This information will not be immediately available so the initial choice is typically made based on the most likely pathogen(s). Initial treatment with inappropriate or insufficient antimicrobial therapy increases both morbidity and mortality [1–3].

Antibiotic stewardship is the practice of minimizing bacterial resistance. The importance of responsible antibiotic stewardship in today's ICU cannot be overemphasized. This responsibility necessitates that protocols and guidelines be established for the ICU facility and personnel regarding antibiotic selection, environmental surveillance, patient isolation, and monitoring culture results from the clinical laboratory.

Diagnostic and monitoring procedures

The potentially catastrophic impact that infection can have on patient survival requires early and effective intervention to optimize recovery. Appropriate patient diagnostic and monitoring procedures can provide insight into the status of the immune system and presence of likely pathogen(s). This information is vital to guide appropriate therapy and antibiotic selection.

Currently, there is no routine laboratory test that will demonstrate specific problems with the immune response. Data collection begins with a thorough history and physical examination, followed by cage-side point of care (POC) laboratory testing, clinicopathological laboratory testing, and diagnostic imaging. Careful assessment of the leukogram and each component of the white blood cell (WBC) line can provide a window into the status of the patient's immune capabilities. Diligent monitoring is necessary to identify occult infections or failed antibiotic response.

Monitoring and Intervention for the Critically Ill Small Animal: The Rule of 20, First Edition. Edited by Rebecca Kirby and Andrew Linklater.
© 2017 John Wiley & Sons, Inc. Published 2017 by John Wiley & Sons, Inc.

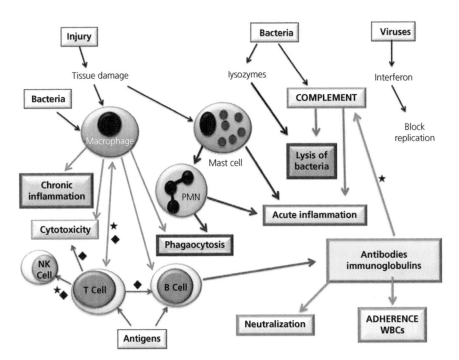

Figure 14.1 Schematic of the primary immune response to antigens or injury. The innate immune system is the first line of defense against pathogens. Efficacy does not require previous exposure to a specific invader. This nonspecific immune response includes physicochemical barriers, molecules normally present in body fluids (such as lysozyme, complement, antiproteases) and phagocytic and cytotoxic cells (such as PMNs, macrophages, NK cells, mast cells). This first-line response protects the host from many extracellular organisms, but not all intracellular organisms (protozoa, viruses, certain bacteria). The acquired immune system is specific and has immunological memory through dedicated immune cells (lymphoid cells). Antibodies and immunoglobulins are produced that specifically counteract the antigens (viral, bacterial, fungal, foreign bodies). The T- and B-cells recognize the antigen, proliferate in response to it, and migrate back to the site of injury. There they release cytokines that attract effector cells (cytotoxic T-cells, activated macrophages, and committed B-cells). Cytokines include interferons, interleukins, colony stimulating factors, and tumor necrosis factors. Antigen specificity is mediated by lymphocytes. This is the most important aspect of the acquired immune system. T-cells typically respond to surface-bound antigens (usually cell associated) and the B-cells typically respond to soluble, extracellular antigens. The immune response is called "humoral" when antibodies are involved in removing antigen and "cell mediated" when T-cells and macrophages are involved. ◆, cytokine release; ★, activation; NK, natural killer cell; PMN, polymorphonuclear cell; WBCs, white blood cells.

History and physical examination

The history begins with the signalment (age, sex, breed) to identify any possible age, sex, or breed predispositions to immune disorders. Very young animals may have poor innate immunity due to failure of passive antibody transfer from the mother. Older animals are more likely to have renal or hepatic dysfunction leading to excessive or toxic drug concentrations at standard doses. Purebred animals may be at increased risk for genetic immune dysfunction, including IgA deficiency in Chinese Sharpeis, IgM deficiency in Doberman Pinschers, IgG deficiency in Weimaraners, and Chédiak–Higashi syndrome in Blue Smoke Persian cats.

The patient's past medical history can provide insight into concurrent disease states that might compromise the immune response (such as diabetes mellitus, hyperadrenocorticism) or medications that cause immunosuppression (glucocorticoids, chemotherapy drugs). Recurrent urinary tract or skin infections and chronic GI dysfunction may be important pathogen sources. A list of drugs that cause immunosuppression in the dog and cat is provided in Box 14.1.

The history can also suggest likely exposure to pathogens, such as recent boarding, removal of ticks, vaccination history, exposure to endemic areas (such as leptospirosis or systemic fungi), or trauma. Known or suspected drug allergies (such as penicillin, cephalosporin or sulfa drugs) or intolerances (vomiting, diarrhea) should be noted and the offending agent(s) posted on the cage card and record. Past antibiotic treatment regimens should be recorded and evaluated when making the current antibiotic selection. Chronic history of recurrent infections (skin, urogenital, pulmonary) should be evaluated for indication of an inadequate immune response.

Patient-specific factors such as age, pregnancy, and preexisting conditions should all be discovered during anamnesis (history taking). These will have direct relevance when choosing appropriate antibiotic therapy. For example, it may be prudent to avoid certain drugs in animals with nervous system disorders. Imipenem can initiate seizures, aminoglycosides will worsen neuromuscular blockage in myesthenics, and beta-lactams at high dosages can cause toxicity within the central nervous system (CNS). Pregnant animals have altered physiology, including larger plasma volume, increased renal blood flow, and hormonal influences on hepatic microsomal enzymes. There are no antibiotics approved for pregnant or lactating animals nor for most animals under 12 weeks of age. Blood flow to the placenta will limit fetal drug delivery, but ultimately the drug will pass across the placenta by passive diffusion.

The physical examination begins with the temperature, pulse rate and intensity, respiratory rate and effort, capillary refill time (CRT), mucous membrane color, and skin turgor. Fever or hypothermia can be an indication of systemic inflammation. The pulse rate and intensity, CRT, and mucous membrane color are used to assess the perfusion status of the patient. Skin turgor, eye position in the orbits, and mucous membrane and corneal moisture are used to

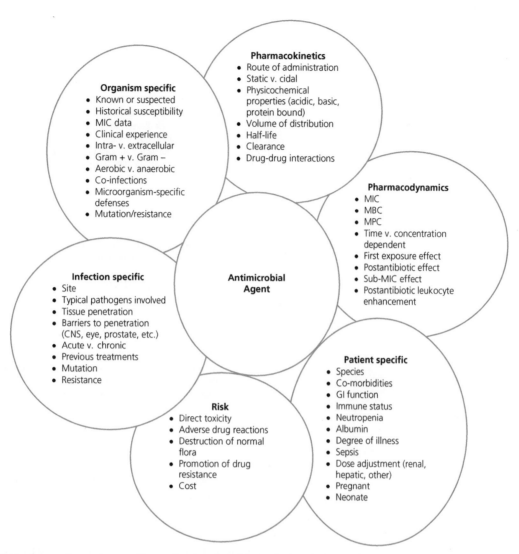

Figure 14.2 Patient-, drug-, and organism-specific considerations in antibiotic selection. CNS, central nervous system; GI, gastrointestinal; MBC, minimum bactericidal concentration; MIC, minimum inhibitory concentration; MPC, mutant prevention concentration. Source: Adapted from Giguère S, Prescott JF, Dowling PM. Principles of antimicrobial drug selection and use. In: Antimicrobial Therapy in Veterinary Medicine, 5th edn. Ames: John Wiley & Sons, 2013 [1]. Used with permission of Wiley.

assess hydration. Pertinent physical examination findings suggestive of obvious or occult bacterial infection include purulent discharge; profuse and/or bloody diarrhea; heart murmur in a febrile patient; redness, pain, heat or swelling in any location; phlebitis or vasculitis; open contaminated wounds; and abdominal pain.

Point of care testing

The minimum laboratory database should include the packed cell volume (PCV), total protein (TP), blood glucose (BG), blood urea nitrogen (BUN), electrolytes, blood gas, coagulation profile, and urinalysis. A complete blood count (CBC) should be performed and a blood smear should be made to assess the WBCs (Box 14.2).

The PCV and TP are evaluated for evidence of anemia, hypoproteinemia or severe dehydration. These can all result from systemic inflammation and may impact antiobiotic therapy. A microhematocrit tube buffy coat layer that is less than 1% or more than 3% may indicate an altered leukogram. Hypoglycemia may be present with sepsis. Hyperglycemia can be associated with a stress response or

diabetes mellitus that can affect immune responses and predispose to infections. An elevation in BUN is concerning for concurrent renal disease which may affect the antibiotic selection and dose regimen. A low BUN brings concern for hepatic dysfunction and antibiotic metabolism. Electrolyte and acid–base status may influence antibiotic efficacy.

Point of care ELISA tests may identify the presence of a specific pathogen. Diagnoses such as parvovirus, feline leukemia virus or feline immunodeficiency virus all have a negative impact on the immune response in an infected dog or cat. ELISA tests for *Ehrlichia*, *Dirofilaria*, *Anaplasma*, and borreliosis (Lyme disease) are available to identify sources of inflammation and guide treatment.

The urinary tract can be a source of systemic bacterial entry. Identification of bacteria and WBCs on routine urinalysis may provide insight into a source of infection. The presence of casts could indicate renal tubular damage from antibiotic use (such as aminoglycosides) or worsening renal injury (see Chapter 13). Patients treated with aminoglycosides should have their urine sediment examined prior to administration of the drug each day.

Box 14.1 Examples of drugs that cause immunosuppression.

Glucocorticoids

Prednisone, prednisolone
Dexamethasone
Hydrocortisone
Cortisone
Methylprednisolone
Betamethasone
Triamcinolone

Cytostatics

Alkylating agents
Cyclophosphamide
Chlorambucil

Antimetabolites

Methotrexate
Hydroxyurea
5-Fluorouracil
Gemcitabine
Azathioprine
Mercaptopurine
Dactinomycin

Antibodies

Polyclonal antibodies
Monoclonal antibodies

Treatment of graft rejection

Cyclosporine
Tacrolimus
Sirolimus

Other drugs

Interferons
Opioids – chronic use
Adalimumab
Etanercept
Mycophenolic acid

Box 14.2 Steps in evaluation of a peripheral blood smear.

1. Make an appropriate blood smear and stain with Romanowsky or Diff-Quik stain.
2. First scan at low power (10×).
   - Evaluate the overall quality of the film. There are three zones (feathered edge, monolayer, thick area near the drop).
   - Identify the monolayer – the area where the RBCs are close together, but do not overlap.
   - Check that the WBCs are well distributed throughout the monolayer. If not, the differential count will not be accurate.
   - Check the RBCs for rouleaux or autoagglutination (see Chpater 10).
   - Check the feathered edge for platelet clumping and abnormal large cells.
3. Using 20× power, obtain a WBC estimate.
   - Count the number of WBCs in 10 50× fields in the monolayer.
   - Divide by 10 to get the average per field
   - Multiply by 500 to get the number of WBCs × 10³/µL.

4.
$$\text{WBC estimate} = \frac{\text{\# leukocytes counted in ten } 50\times \text{ fields}}{10} \times 500$$
$$= \text{\# WBC} \times 10^3 / \mu L \text{ of blood}$$

5. Evaluate cells more closely at 100× (oil immersion) (see also Box 14.3).
   - Check for morphological detail, neutrophil toxicity, reactive lymphocytes, cellular inclusions, atypical cells or organisms.
   - Perform a differential cell count.
   - Evaluate any abnormal cells you found on the initial scan.
   - Obtain a platelet estimate.

$$\text{Platelet estimate} = \text{average} \frac{\text{\# platelets in ten } 100\times \text{ fields}}{10}$$
$$\times 15000 \text{ to } 20000 = \text{\#PLT} \times 10^3 / \mu L \text{ of blood}$$

Source: Adapted from Allison RW, Meinkoth JH. Hematology without the numbers: in-clinic blood film evaluation. Vet Clin North Am Small Anim Pract. 2007;37(2):245–66 [5]. Used with permission from Elsevier.

Clinicopathological testing

Blood is submitted for a CBC and serum biochemical profile. The biochemical profile is examined for evidence of renal or hepatic dysfunction. These are important in selection of antibiotics and dosing regimens. Dose adjustment may be appropriate in cases of renal disease for fluoroquinolones and other antibiotic metabolites that require renal excretion. Vancomycin is excreted by renal glomerular filtration while aminoglycosides are excreted by tubular diffusion, and cephalosporins and penicillins by tubular secretion. Metronidazole, macrolides, clindamycin, and tetracyclines require hepatic metabolism and dose adjustment may be appropriate in hepatic disease (see Chapter 18).

Fluid or tissue samples are collected for cytology, specific antigen or polymerase chain reaction (PCR) testing, histopathology (when indicated), and culture and susceptibility testing. Blood can be tested for titers (antibody levels) for specific pathogens, such as *Leptospira* spp., rickettsial diseases, toxoplasmosis, and fungal diseases, although detectable levels may require convalescent titers performed at a later date. Table 14.1 lists sites and techniques for culture and sensitivity sample collection.

Cytological examination of collected fluid or cells may allow identification of the infectious organism, and provide insight into the type of inflammation present. A gram stain is helpful in bacterial identification and to guide initial antibiotic selection. The presence of a large number of neutrophils (neutrophilic inflammation) is most commonly associated with bacterial infection or tissue necrosis. Mixed inflammation or pyogranulomatous inflammation (neutrophils and macrophages) is more commonly associated with fungal infection, foreign bodies, and mycobacterial infections. An abundance of eosinophils is often associated with allergic disease or parasites.

The quantification of glucose in abdominal cavitary fluids is a useful diagnostic test. If the abdominal fluid glucose is >20 mg/dL lower than the patient's peripheral blood glucose, a septic source is likely and surgical exploration of the abdomen is recommended [4]. Fluid collected directly from the abdomen or from a drain for analysis of glucose or lactate in postoperative patients does not provide the same diagnostic information [5,6].

Diagnostic data suggestive of bacterial infection include unexplained hypoglycemia; neutropenia or neutrophilia with left shift; degenerative or toxic neutrophils and bacteria seen on cytological examination of discharge, sputum, or sampled fluid; bacteriuria or pyuria; hyperbilirubinemia; hypoalbuminemia; moderate thrombocytopenia; and alterations in coagulation tests without obvious cause. Additional specific testing may demonstrate abnormalities compatible with the site of bacterial infection. These include valvular heart lesions on echocardiogram in febrile animal; free

Table 14.1 Sites and techniques for culture and susceptibility testing sample collection.

Site	Technique
Tissue aspirate	Clean intact skin, air dry, 22 G needle aspirate from several areas, remove needle with hemostat, discard needle, and recap
Swabs (eyes, ears, uterus ONLY)	Moisten swab with preservative-free solution, collect without touching skin, rotate swab over 1 cm area for 4 sec, place in transport sleeve
Skin/wound	DO NOT use swabs, DO NOT collect pus, instead aspirate or collecte macerated tissue or biopsy. For superficial skin, scrape cleaned skin and allow to air dry. Transport in liquid media
Bone	Collected aseptically, keep moist with saline
Drain site	Treat as contaminated wound, DO NOT culture tube as biofilm may misrepresent sample, collect tissue at site of infection
Urine	Cystocentesis after surgical scrub, keep sample cold and submit within 24 hours
Blood culture	Using liquid media (1 part blood:10 parts media), collect from at least three sites at three different time points, ideally when a fever is present
Cerebrospinal fluid/joints	Collect into blood culture media, collect aseptically.
Gastrointestinal tract	Fecal specimens may be collected for *Campylobacter, Shigella, Salmonella, Clostridium, Yersinia, Vibrio, Aeromonas,* and some *E. coli* spp.

Table 14.2 Criteria for the diagnosis of the systemic inflammatory response syndrome (SIRS) in the dog and cat. The patient must have two or more criteria.

SIRS criteria dogs	SIRS criteria cats
• Tachycardia (HR >120 beats/min)	• Bradycardia (HR <140 beats/min) or tachycardia (HR >225 beats/min)
• Tachypnea (RR >20 breaths/min)	• Tachypnea (RR >40 breaths/min)
• Fever (>104 °F) or hypothermia (<100.4 °F)	• Fever (>104.0 °F) or hypothermia (<100.4 °F)
• Leukopenia (<5000 WBC/µL) or leukocytosis (>18 000 WBC/µL)	• Leukopenia (<5000 WBC/µL) or leukocytosis (>18 000 WBC/µL)

HR, heart rate; RR, respiratory rate; WBC, white blood cell.

abdominal fluid or cavitary lesion(s) on radiographs or ultrasound; and purulent exudate on bronchoalveolar lavage or transtracheal wash. The criteria for diagnosing SIRS in the dog and cat are listed in Table 14.2. When present, these signs should prompt the clinician to intervene with early and appropriate antibiotic therapy as soon as possible and long before culture and sensitivity or bacterial titer results are available.

The leukogram

Evaluation of the immune status begins by interpreting the leukogram portion of the CBC results. This includes the total WBC count, complete differential, and WBC morphology. Leukocyte counts are relatively constant in health but will increase in response to infection, inflammation, tissue trauma or injury, stress, and immune stimulation.

All leukocytes are derived from common hematopoietic stem cells in the bone marrow. The differentiation of progenitor cells into the various cells lines is signaled by various cytokines (Table 14.3). This process takes approximately six days – three days for proliferation and three days for maturation of the WBCs.

The total WBC count on the leukogram is used to calculate the absolute numbers of WBCs found in the differential count. Normal leukogram reference ranges are typically 5.3–19.8 k/µL for dogs and 4–19 k/µL for cats and will vary by laboratory (Table 14.4). The total WBC count should consist primarily of PMNs and lymphocytes. However, presence of a leukocytosis does not automatically equate with infection. Inflammation, pain, stress, and trauma can all cause a stress leukogram. A stress leukogram is denoted by neutrophilia, lymphopenia, eosinopenia, and monocytosis. The most consistent of these findings is a lymphopenia. These changes occur due to the influence of catecholamines and/or glucocorticoids. The general patterns of the leukocyte response are shown in Table 14.5.

A total WBC count can be estimated based on a cytology slide (Box 14.3) [7] or hand-counted with a hemocytometer. When using an automated machine, be aware that other cells such as nucleated red blood cells and large platelets may alter total WBC counts and give inaccurate readings.

Various diseases can interfere with normal leukocyte function. Glycosylation of granulocytes in chronic diabetes mellitus patients will decrease oxidative burst and phagocytic killing. Cushing's patients may have a relative lymphopenia or decreased ligand affinity [8]. Hereditary diseases involving neutrophil function defects have been reported in Doberman Pinschers and Weimeraners [9,10]. Hereditary lysosomal storage diseases are reported in dogs and cats [11].

Leukocyte function testing is available only at research laboratories. These techniques allow specific testing of *in vitro* chemotaxis, oxidative burst, phagocytosis, killing, and activation marker expression in granulocytes. Lymphocytes are tested for proliferative response, B- or T-cell receptor, and expression of other markers. Disorders of neutrophil function include canine leukocyte adhesion defect and cyclic hematopoiesis of Gray Collies [12,13].

White blood cell lines

Evaluation of a peripheral blood smear provides vital information regarding the cell populations and morphology (Figure 14.3). A systematic scan is required to obtain accurate and consistent results. The leukogram is interpreted in light of patient-specific clinical information. The absolute cell counts are evaluated, not the percentages. Abnormal leukocyte morphology, presence of a left shift, monocytosis or persistent eosinophilia can each indicate an inflammatory response.

There are several pathogens that may be diagnosed from a peripheral blood smear (Figure 14.4). Specific inclusion bodies in neutrophils and red blood cells (RBCs) can be found in canine distemper virus infections. *Anaplasma phagocytophilum* morulae can be found in canine neutrophils while *Hepatozoon americanum* gamonts are found in canine monocytes. Intracellular organisms may be identified in circulating granulocytes during bacterial or fungal infections. A review of cell morphology by a pathologist can provide valuable information and should be requested when there is a high index of suspicion for WBC abnormalities.

Automated blood cell counters can often provide more consistent results and decreased inherent errors by approximately 5% [14]. However, the clumping of leukocytes or breakage of fragile cells can result in inaccurate counts. An automated hemocytometer

Table 14.3 White blood cells and their contribution to immunity.

Cell type	Description	Function	Dysfunction
Lymphocytes	Large single pink-staining nucleus. Produced in lymph nodes and other lymphoid tissues. Include B-cells, T-cells, memory cells, plasma cells, and natural killer cells	Responsible for cell-mediated and humoral immunity	Severe combined immunodeficiency. Congenital disorders. May have normal lymphocyte numbers with abnormal function
B-cells	Responsible for humoral immunity. Produce immunoglobulins after differentiation into plasma cells. 12% of total lymphocytes. Mature and proliferate in lymph nodes	Produce antibodies. Combat pyogenic bacteria. Prevent blood-borne infections. Neutralize toxins. Usually require T-cell assistance to respond to antigen. Can also recognize antigen directly through surface Ig. Responses are antigen specific while effects are mainly through complement	
T-cells Helper T-cells CD4+ CD8+	Responsible for cell-mediated immunity; 70–80% of total lymphocytes Recognize antigen within presenting cells. Release cytokines to control development of immune response Recognize and kill cells infected with virus	Especially important against intracellular organisms including protozoa and fungi. Role in graft rejection and immune surveillance of neoplasia. Long-lived memory cells. Activity by cytokine production	
Memory cells	T- and B-cells that are antigen specific or Ig secreting	Part of secondary immune response. Recruited after second exposure to Ag	
Plasma cells	These are fully differentiated B-cells. Role in innate and adaptive immune response	Secrete antibodies. Kill virus-infected cells. Role in antigen presentation	
Natural killer cells	Also called large granular lymphocytes. Part of lymphoid system, have no differentiating cell surface markers	Efficacy against virus-infected and neoplastic cells	
Monocytes/ macrophages	Blood-borne monocytes will replenish tissue-specific macrophage populations. These are long-lived cells with widespread distribution. Stem cell differentiation via monocyte-colony stimulating factor	Responsible for phagocytosis and killing of microorganisms; activation of T-cells, innate immunity, and antigen presentation. Surface receptors for Ig and activated complement allow cells to take up immune complexes. Major source of colony stimulating factors and cytokines	
Dendritic cells	Found mainly in lymphoid tissue	Function as antigen-presenting cells. Initiate adaptive immune response. Most potent stimulators of T-cell activation	
Mast cells	Allergic reactions	Release granules containing histamine, leukotrienes, chemokines, and cytokines	
Neutrophils (granulocytes)	Also called polymorphonuclear cells (PMNs). Short-lived (12 h in blood, 12 h in tissues). Circulating and marginated pools. Granulocyte-colony stimulating factor triggers cell differentiation during production in bone marrow	Responsible for phagocytic clearing of bacterial infections. Role in innate immunity. Circulating PMNs interact with endothelial surface via selectins, then form firm adhesion with integrins for final margination at site of infection or inflammation	Neutropenia can be caused by increased margination, peripheral destruction or decreased bone marrow production. Inappropriate neutropenia may indicate immune dysfunction or incompetence in critically ill patients. Lysosomal storage disorders can cause dysfunction. Congenital disorders include Chédiak–Higashi Syndrome and Pelger–Hüet anomaly
Eosinophils (granulocytes)	Cells with double-lobed nucleus, orange cytoplasmic granules containing toxic compounds. Interleukin-5 triggers stem cell differentiation	Kill antibody-coated antigens through degranulation. Prominent in allergic inflammation	
Basophils	Blue granules containing toxic and inflammatory compounds. Stem cell factor triggers differentiation	Cell-killing cells. Important in allergic reactions and parasitic infections	

may also incorrectly classify abnormal cells such as lymphoblasts and nucleated red blood cells. A WBC estimate on a stained blood smear should be compared to the automated count to identify cell or cell fragments that might change the count. Performing a manual differential as a POC test allows severe neutropenia or abnormal cell populations to be identified and addressed early. As the patient improves, the leukogram should show resolution of abnormalities such as a left shift and toxic changes. Recovery of lymphopenia or eosinopenia may precede clinical recovery.

The basic characteristics of the individual WBC lines and their role in the immune response are listed in Table 14.3. Common causes of high and low cell counts in specific WBC cell lines in the dog and cat are listed in Table 14.6. A bone marrow aspirate or core biopsy is indicated when there is a persistent moderate-to-severe neutropenia without a left shift or toxic change, particularly when there is no evidence of a septic source; pancytopenia with nonregenerative anemia; monocytosis with depressed numbers in other cell lines; myelophthisis; myeloid or lymphoid leukemia; and subleukemic or aleukemic leukemia.

Neutrophils

The normal immune response to an antigen or pathogen should increase the number and enhance the function of neutrophils at sites of injury and inflammation. Neutrophils (or PMNs) exist in the body in two pools of approximately equal size: circulating and marginated. Cytokine release will stimulate neutrophil release from the bone marrow. Marginated neutrophils roll along the endothelial surfaces of capillaries and interact with low-affinity selectin. Firm adhesion occurs through integrins, with the PMN ultimately migrating through the capillary toward sites of infection or inflammation by chemotaxis. The immune stimulation of neutrophils by

cytokines enhances antimicrobial cell function and phagocytic killing. The presence of lipopolysaccharides from gram-negative bacteria will also increase neutrophil oxidative burst and adhesion to the endothelium, but will decrease the ability of neutrophils to marginate across vascular endothelium.

The presence of a neutrophilia can imply infection, inflammation, or a stress response due to endogenous or exogenous corticosteroids. An extreme neutrophilic leukocytosis (leukemoid response) or a marked lymphocytosis requires further diagnostic testing to rule out granulocytic leukemia, lymphocytic leukemia,

Table 14.4 Laboratory reference ranges for canine and feline complete blood cell counts.

Test	Reference range		Units
	Canine	**Feline**	
WBC	4.9–17.6	3.9–19.0	K/µL
RBC	5.39–8.70	7.12–11.46	M/µL
HGB	13.4–20.7	10.3–16.2	g/dL
HCT	38.3–56.5	28.2–52.7	%
MCV	59–76	39–56	fL
MCH	21.9–26.1	12.6–16.5	pg
MCHC	32.6–39.2	8.5–37.8	g/dL
Reticulocyte	10–110	3–50	K/µL
Platelet	143–448	155–641	K/µL
Neutrophil	2940–12670	2620–15170	/µL
Lymphocyte	1060–4950	850–5850	/µL
Monocyte	130–1150	40–530	/µL
Eosinophil	70–1490	90–2180	/µL
Basophil	0–100	0–100	/µL

fL, femtoliters; g/dL, grams per deciliter; HCT, hematocrit; HGB, hemoglobin; K/µL, thousand per microliter; M/µL, million per microliter; MCH, mean corpuscular hemoglobin; MCHC, mean corpuscular hemoglobin concentration; MCV, mean corpuscular volume; pg, picograms; RBC, red blood cell; WBC, white blood cell;/µL, microliter.

Box 14.3 How to perform a manual WBC differential.

1. Obtain a total WBC using your in-house machine.
2. Perform a manual differential.
   - Using 100× magnification
     - Identify 100–200 leukocytes
     - Count and classify by type:
       - Segmented neutrophil
       - Band neutrophil
       - Monocyte
       - Eosinophil
       - Basophils
       - Lymphocyte.
     - Skip damaged, broken, smudged or unidentifiable cells. If large numbers of metamyelocytes, myelocytes, or other precursor cells are noted, it is appropriate to count these as a category. This may indicate leukemia.
   - Count the number of nucleated red blood cells (nRBC) per 100 leukocytes.
     - WBC must be corrected for the number of nRBCs per 100 leukocytes.
     - Corrected WBC count = (initial WBC × 100) ÷ (100 + #nRBC).
   - Calculate the absolute numbers for cellular components.
     - # Neutrophils you counted out of 100 leukocytes = % neutrophils
     - % Neutrophils × total WBC = absolute number neutrophils per microliter (µL) of blood.
     - Repeat for other cell lines.
     - Immature cell types within a line should be counted separately, but included in the total for that cell line (i.e. 10% bands added to number of segmented neutrophils; 12% atypical/reactive lymphocytes added to the number of mature lymphocytes).
   - To cross-check, total the absolute counts for the leukocyte subtypes. This should equal the total WBC count.

Source: Allison RW, Meinkoth JH. Hematology without the numbers: in-clinic blood film evaluation. Vet Clin North Am Small Anim Pract. 2007;37(2):245–66 [5]. Used with permission of Elsevier.

Table 14.5 General patterns of leukocyte response.

Condition	WBC	Seg	Band	Lymph	Mono	Eos
Acute inflammation	↑	↑	↑	↓, or no change	Variable	Variable
Chronic inflammation	↑, or no change	↑, or no change	↑, or no change	↑, or no change	↑	Variable
Overwhelming inflammation	↓, or no change	↓, or no change	↑	↓, or no change	Variable	Variable
Excitement leukocytosis	↑	D – ↑ C – ↑, or no change	No change	D – no change C – ↑	No change	No change
Stress leukogram	↑	↑	No change	↓	↑, or no change	↓, or no change

C, cats; D, dogs; Eos, eosinophils; Mono, monocytes; Seg, segmented neutrophils; WBC, white blood cells. *Source*: Adapted from Rebar AH, MacWilliams PS, Feldman BF, et al. A Guide to Hematology in Dogs and Cats. Jackson Hole: Teton NewMedia, 2002 [33].

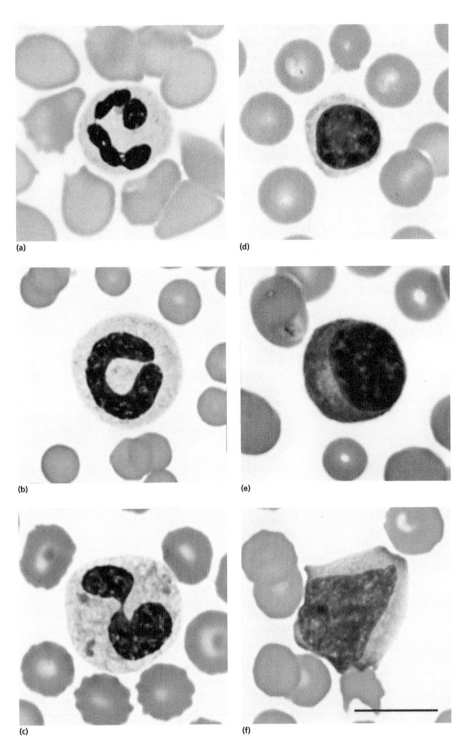

Figure 14.3 Peripheral blood cells. (a) Normal canine neutrophil. (b) Feline band neutrophil. (c) Toxic canine neutrophil. (d) Normal canine small lymphocyte. (e) Reactive canine lymphocyte. (f) Neoplastic canine lymphocyte. Aqueous Romanowsky stain. Scale bar = 10 microns. *Source*: courtesy of Dr Robin Allison.

and lymphoma. An abnormally low number of neutrophils may be due to sequestration or consumption due to acute overwhelming inflammation or infection, peripheral destruction or decreased central marrow production. Neutropenia in critically ill patients suggests dysfunction or incompetence of the immune response.

Neutropenia with a left shift further indicates that the inflammation is acute or overwhelming and that the bone marrow has not yet responded or cannot keep up with demand for neutrophil response to tissue damage or infection. A left shift is identified if immature or band neutrophils make up greater than 3% of the

total neutrophil population. Band neutrophils have a horseshoe-shaped nucleus with smooth, parallel sides that lack the typical segmental constrictions seen in nuclei of mature neutrophils. A left shift may be further characterized as "degenerative" if the number of band neutrophils is greater than 10% of the total neutrophil count, the total segmental neutrophil count is within or below the reference interval, or the total number of bands (with metamyelocytes and myelocytes included) is greater than or equal to the total number of segmented neutrophils [14,15]. The presence of a degenerative left shift indicates that the tissue

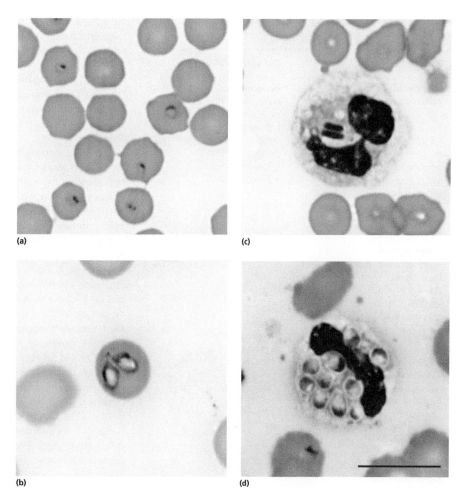

Figure 14.4 Infected peripheral blood cells. (a) Circulating *C. felis* piroplasms in feline red blood cells. (b) Circulating large *Babesia* piroplasms in canine red blood cells. (c) Bacterial rods in a neutrophil from a septic cat. (d) *Histoplasma capsulatum* yeasts in neutrophil from a dog with disseminated histoplasmosis. Aqueous Romanowsky stain. Scale bar = 10 microns. Source: courtesy of Dr Robin Allison.

demand for WBCs is surpassing the rate of bone marrow production and is associated with a poor prognosis.

Evaluation of neutrophil morphology is important for accurate interpretation of the leukogram and neutrophil count and may also provide prognostic information. Abnormal neutrophil morphology can represent increased bone marrow recruitment or band release, accelerated neutrophil development or aging. Certain morphological changes (inclusions) are pathognomonic for intracellular infection or particular infectious etiologies.

Toxic change in neutrophils is identified by cytoplasmic basophilia with vacuoles. Circulating toxins, infection or accelerated neutrophil production by the bone marrow can cause these morphology changes. The altered cytoplasmic appearance is due to the presence of remnants of organelles and ribosomes from early cellular development. Giant neutrophils, aberrant nuclear shapes (such as ring forms), and Dohle bodies also indicate toxicity. Dohle bodies are leftover precipitates of rough endoplasmic reticulum that appear as 1–3 μm light blue-gray oval inclusions near the periphery of the neutrophil. They are frequently seen in the neutrophils of healthy cats, so the presence of Dohle bodies in canine neutrophils is of much greater significance. Neutrophil hypersegmentation may result from sample aging or drugs such as corticosteroids.

Several hereditary diseases can affect neutrophil morphology. In Chédiak–Higashi syndrome of Blue Smoke Persian cats, the neutrophils and other nucleated cells often contain large peroxidase-positive cytoplasmic granules filled with lysosomal enzymes [16]. Lysosomal storage disorders are characterized by a lack of

mobilization of the lysosomal granule contents, resulting in PMN dysfunction and an increased susceptibility to infections. In the neutrophil anomaly of Birman cats, reddish-purple cytoplasmic granules can be seen within the neutrophils [17]. Pelger–Hüet anomaly seen in both dogs and cats is characterized by hyposegmented nuclei with coarse, clumped chromatin [18,19]. Because the cells appear hyposegmented, they may be inadvertently classified as band neutrophils and misinterpreted as a severe left shift consistent with inflammation.

Lymphocytes

Lymphocytosis, while infrequent in critically ill patients, can be seen with chronic antigenic stimulation, recent vaccination, or neoplasia. A transient epinephrine-induced lymphocytosis is common in fractious cats. Critically ill dogs and cats should have a stress-induced lymphopenia, making the presence of lymphocytosis cause to test for hypoadrenocorticism (Addison's disease) or relative adrenal insufficiency.

A leukocytosis with a marked lymphocytosis could be indicative of lymphoid leukemia and warrants evaluation of lymphocyte morphology. The neoplastic lymphocytes appear larger than normal cells and have increased basophilia to the cytoplasm, large round nuclei, coarse granular chromatin, and nucleolar whorls. Due to abnormal size and morphology changes, these cells may not be accurately recognized or classified as lymphocytes by in-house analyzers, requiring examination of a blood film. Occasionally patients with leukemia will have marked increases in normal-appearing

Table 14.6 Common causes of high and low white blood cell line numbers in dogs and cats.

Increased WBCs	Decreased WBCs
Neutrophilia	**Neutropenia**
Inflammation	Acute, severe inflammation
Infection	Increased peripheral destruction
Tissue necrosis, ischemia	Immune-mediated destruction
Corticosteroids (endogenous or exogenous)	Decreased bone marrow production
Rebound neutrophilia	• Marrow necrosis
Hemorrhage or hemolysis	• Drug reactions
Primary neoplasia (myelogenous leukemia)	• Viral infections
Functional defects affecting adhesion	• Toxicity
	• Myelopthesis
	Hereditary (Gray Collies)
Lymphocytosis	**Lymphopenia**
Reactive lymphocytes	Stress response (750–1500 K/µL)
Hypoadrenocorticism	Acute infection
Epinephrine induced (cats)	Lymphedema
Glucocorticoid deficiency	
Lymphoid leukemia	
Monocytosis	**Monocytopenia**
Inflammation	Bone marrow disorder
Immune-mediated hemolytic anemia	Folate and B12 deficiencies
Tissue necrosis	Endotoxemia
Foreign body reactions	Chemotherapy
Pyogranulomatous inflammation	
Organisms such as fungi, filamentous bacteria, *Mycobacteria*, *Pythium*, *Toxoplasma*	
Erythrophagocytosis	
Hemophagocytic syndrome	
Monocytic neoplasia	
Chronic infection	
Eosinophilia and basophilia	**Eosinopenia and basopenia**
Allergic reactions	*Esosinophils*
Parasitic infections	Hyperadrenocorticism
Inflammation	Glucocorticoids
Ongoing systemic hypersensitivity	Stress response
Hypoadrenocorticism	
Neoplasia	*Basophils*
Paraneoplastic diseases	Thyrotoxicosis
Systemic mastocytosis	Acute hypersensitivity reactions
Idiopathic hypereosinophilia	Infection

small lymphocytes. Special stains can be used to help differentiate acute myelogenous leukemia from lymphoblastic leukemia. A concurrent nonregenerative anemia is common due to bone marrow crowding of red blood cell precursors. The granulocyte and platelet lines may also be decreased.

Lymphopenia (750–1500 k/µL) is the most reliable and consistent clue to making the diagnosis of a stress leukogram. Unfortunately, this is indistinguishable from lymphopenia of acute viral or bacterial infection. Marked lymphopenia warrants consideration of other differential causes such as lymphoma, chylous effusion, and lymphedema. Declining lymphocyte counts in an apparently healthy patient may indicate impending illness but cannot be distinguished from a corticosteroid effect. Persistent lymphopenia can suggest ongoing disease.

Lymphocyte morphology should be assessed on a blood smear. Reactive lymphocytes are larger in size, have increased basophilic cytoplasm, and have larger nuclei with finely granular chromatin. The presence of reactive lymphocytes indicates immune system reactivity. Large granular lymphocytes may represent the presence of circulating natural killer, cytotoxic T-lymphocytes, or neoplastic lymphoblasts.

Diseases of abnormal lymphocyte function include severe combined immunodeficiency and other rare congenital disorders [20–22]. These patients may have normal lymphocyte numbers with abnormal function.

Monocytes

While a mild increase in monocytes can accompany normal endogenous stress response, a more marked monocytosis is suggestive of inflammation. Monocytosis is expected in diseases with high phagocytic activity, including immune-mediated hemolytic anemia, tissue necrosis, foreign body reactions, and organisms associated with pyogranulomatous or granulomatous inflammation. These organisms include fungi, filamentous bacteria (*Nocardia*, *Actinomyces*, *Dermatophilus*), mycobacteria (tuberculosis, leprosy, atypical mycobacteriums), *Pythium*, *Toxoplasma*, and others. When evaluating a peripheral blood smear or cytology sample, it is important to check the monocytes carefully for inclusions or intracellular organisms. When a monocytosis is seen concurrently with other WBC line deficiencies, several differential diagnoses, including erythrophagocytosis, hemophagocytic syndrome, and monocytic neoplasia, should be considered.

Monocytes are of low frequency in the bone marrow and circulating blood and are the major source of colony stimulating factors and cytokines. They are less effective than neutrophils at microbial defense. Once they enter the tissues, monocytes transform into macrophages that contain more granules and proteolytic enzymes. Their function is to digest foreign material and dead cells. Macrophages are important for antigen processing and presentation to T-lymphocytes. These tissue macrophages may survive for prolonged periods. Monocyte-derived macrophage populations include the macrophages and histiocytes found in exudates, pleural and peritoneal macrophages, pulmonary alveolar macrophages, connective tissue histiocytes, and also the Kupffer cells of the liver. The macrophages of the spleen, lymph nodes, and bone marrow are collectively referred to as the reticuloendothelial system. There are several organisms that can survive and replicate within macrophages including *Mycobacteria* spp., *Rickettsia* spp., *Leishmania* spp., and *Toxoplasma* spp.

Eosinophils and basophils

Like monocytes, eosinophils are typically of low frequency in the bone marrow and circulating blood. These are primarily tissue-dwelling cells and can accumulate in tissues without a circulating eosinophilia. Eosinophilias may be seen in allergic reactions, parasitic infections (GI, heartworm, larval migrans), and inflammation (feline asthma, allergic gastroenteritis). A persistent eosinophilia is typically associated with an ongoing systemic hypersensitivity. Patients with hypoadrenocorticism often have a persistent eosinophilia and lack a mature neutrophila. Other less common causes of eosinophila include neoplastic and paraneoplastic conditions, hypoadrenocorticism, systemic mastocytosis, and idiopathic hypereosinophilic syndrome.

Basophils also exist in small numbers in the bone marrow and circulating blood. Basophilia can be seen in similar conditions as eosinophilia.

Bacterial culture and susceptibility testing

Choosing the appropriate sample, collection technique, and timing is important for obtaining the most accurate bacterial culture and susceptibility information. Common sample sites and techniques for sample collection are provided in Table 14.1. If a "dirty" site is to be sampled, the area should be aseptically prepared and sterile technique used for sample collection. Any exudate or necrotic debris should be cleared away prior to sample collection. While it is ideal to collect samples for culture prior to treating, rational antimicrobial therapy should *not* be delayed in order for samples to be collected [1]. Appropriate broad-spectrum antimicrobial therapy should be instituted as soon as possible to avoid increased mortality [2].

Diagnostic imaging

Radiographs of the chest and abdomen and abdominal ultrasound may help to identify sources of infection. Particular attention is given to the genitourinary tract, GI tract, and respiratory tract since these nonsterile sites provide common sources of bacterial colonization. The presence of free air in the closed abdomen is indicative of an anaerobic pathogen or rupture of a hollow viscus and either scenario necessitates exploratory surgery of the abdomen. Echocardiogram will identify valvular lesions compatible with bacterial endocarditis and can help identify cardiac systolic dysfunction consistent with SIRS. Focused ultrasound of the thorax may be helpful for pleural space disease and sample collection. Free fluid or loculated fluid pockets should be tapped and the fluid evaluated. Advanced imaging, such as computed tomography (CT) and nuclear magnetic resonance imaging (nMRI), may be used to better define pathology in bone and in the soft tissue structures of the CNS and other difficult-to-assess areas of the body.

Monitoring procedures

The Rule of 20 provides an important checklist of monitoring priorities for the patient with infection or immune compromise. A single leukogram provides the clinician with a snapshot of the immune status of the patient at one moment in time, but does not provide information about chronicity or trend of change. Serial assessment of the leukogram (every 48–72 hours) is needed to determine improvement or deterioration of the WBC response to immune stimulation.

Physical parameters (such as body temperature, body weight, peripheral perfusion parameters, hydration status, and mentation) and POC minimum database parameters are monitored several times daily to assess response to therapy and identify new clinical problems. The discovery of a new fever or infection or a failed antibiotic response necessitates a careful review of the antibiotic and environmental protocols established by the antimicrobial stewardship program of the facility.

Antimicrobial stewardship

Antimicrobial Stewardship is the practice of minimizing the emergence of antimicrobial resistance. Antibiotics are used only when there is evidence from a positive culture result or a high index of suspicion (Table 14.7) that bacterial infection is an important component of the disease process.

The three Ds are three simple steps to follow: decontaminate, design, and deescalate [23]. Decontaminate is to reduce bacterial exposure, particularly to resistant bacteria. This includes treating patients in order of least risk to most risk and appropriate early discharge of patients from the hospital to minimize exposure. Removing resistant microbes from the environment is paramount.

Table 14.7 Patient and laboratory factors commonly associated with bacterial infection. The presence of two or more of these factors supports the presence of a bacterial pathogen as a component of the underlying disease process.

Patient factors	Diagnostic factors
Fever, hyperthermia	Leukocytosis with left shift
Severe prolonged hypotension	Leukopenia
	Hypoglycemia
Severe gastrointestinal signs	Thrombocytopenia
	Hypoalbuminemia
Open wound	Bacteria seen on cytology (tissue aspirate, sputum, bronchial fluid, urine, purulent exudate, abdominal fluid, etc.)
Hot, swollen joints, tissues	
Bone pain on deep palpation	Bacteriuria/pyuria
Acute abdominal pain	Hyperbilirubinemia
Purulent exudate	Abnormal coagulation
Abscessation or pustules	Free abdominal gas on radiographs
Cough	Positive bacterial culture results
Vasculitis	Enlarged uterus on imaging
Enlarged painful prostate	Glucose lower in abdominal fluid than in blood
Sudden-onset or new heart murmur	Cardiac valvular lesions (with fever)

Proper hand washing, barrier nursing techniques (such as gloves, gowns; see Box 20.9), and use of bandages for wounds are important to prevent horizontal transmission.

Design means to select the most appropriate drug, drug dose, and dosing interval for the infection. This will require identification of the site or body system and the most likely bacterial pathogen(s) involved (Table 14.8). It is important to select appropriate empirical antibiotics before culture results are available. The decision to use antibiotics is made based on information obtained from history, physical examination, laboratory data, imaging, and sample analysis.

Finally, deescalate starts with *not* using antimicrobials when alternate therapy is equally effective. Other components of deescalation include decreasing hospital length of stay, length of antimicrobial therapy, and decreasing the use of invasive devices (such as catheters) whenever possible. When culture results are available, antibiotic therapy should be deescalated to the most appropriate narrow-spectrum or first-line antibiotic(s). Individual hospital policies providing guidelines for the use of antimicrobial agents should be designed to minimize development of multiresistant bacteria. Patients infected with resistant bacteria are likely to experience ineffective treatment, recurrent infection, delayed recovery, or even death. Antibiotic use to prevent infection is called *chemoprophylaxis*, and has been employed in humans to:

- protect healthy individuals who have had specific exposure to pathogenic bacteria
- prevent secondary infection in a patient who is weakened from a primary infection or therapeutic intervention
- prevent infection resulting from surgery and the risk of bacterial contamination.

The risks of infection must be weighed against the potential side-effects of the drug and the development of resistant bacteria. The institution of antibiotic prophylaxis in the first situation is based on the likelihood that the exposed animal will be infected by the known pathogen. It is ideal to prevent infection by utilizing aseptic technique during procedures rather than administering chemoprophylaxis.

The goal of antimicrobial therapy is to assist the patient in containing and eliminating infection without causing toxicity, adverse

Table 14.8 Common bacterial pathogens associated with various organ systems in the dog and cat.

Infection site/organ	Common pathogens
Skin	*Staphylococcus pseudointermedius* is the primary organism in pyoderma. Secondary bacteria include *Escherichia coli*, *Proteus*, *Pseudomonas* [34]
Urinary tract	*Escherichia coli*, *Staphylococcus*, *Streptococcus*, *Enterococcus*, *Proteus*, *Pseudomonas*, *Klebsiella*, *Enterobacter*, *Corynebacterium*, and more [35,36]
Gastrointestinal	Small bowel: *E. coli*, *Staphylococcus*, *Clostridium perfringens*, *Bacteroides*, *Salmonella*, *Shigella*, *Campylobacter jejuni*, *H. pylori*
Hepatobiliary	*Escherichia coli*, *Enterococcus*, *Staphylococcus pseudintermedius*, *Streptococcus*, *Klebsiella pneumoniae*, *Enterobacter*, *Pseudomonas*, *Citrobacter*, *Clostridium* spp., *Propionibacterium acnes*, *Actinomyces*, *Corynebacterium*, *Bacteroides*, *Peptostreptococcus* and others [37]
Reproductive	Pyometra: *E. coli* is the most common, others include streptococci, staphylococci, *Proteus*, *Klebsiella*, *Serratia*, *Salmonella*, *Pseudomonas*, *Clostridium* [38],*Pasteurella*, and *Moraxella* [36]
	Prostate: *E. coli*, *Staphylococcus*, *Streptococcus*, *Klebsiella*, *Proteus*, *Mycoplasma*, *Pseudomonas*, *Enterobacter*, *Pasteurella*, *Hemophilus* [39]
	Mastitis: *Staphylococcus*, *Escherichia coli*, *Streptococcus*, *Klebsiella*
Central nervous system	*Staphylococcus*, *Streptococcus*, *Pasteurella*, *E. coli*, *Klebsiella* spp., *Proteus* spp., *Salmonella* spp., *Actinomyces* spp., *Nocardia* spp. Anaerobes have been identified as well [40]
Respiratory (pneumonia)	*Bordatella*, *Mycoplasma*, *Streptococcus*, *E. coli*, *Klebsiella*, *Pseudomonas* spp., *Yersinia pestis*, *Mycobacteria*, *Pasteurella*, *Neisseria*, *Staphylococcus*, *Moraxella* [41]
Respiratory (pyothorax)	Dogs: *Bacteroides*, *Pasteurella*, *Peptostreptococus*, *Fusobacterium*, *E. coli*, *Actinomyces*, *Streptococcus canis*, *Staphylococcus pseudintermedius*, *Prevotella*, *Nocardia nova*
	Cats: *Pasteurella*, *Bacteroides*, *Fusobacterium*, *Clostridium*, *Peptostreptococcus*, *Actinomyces*, *Porphyromonas*, *Prevotella*
Cardiovascular (endocarditis)/ hematogenous	*Staphylococcus pseudintermedius* or coagulase-positive spp., *Streptococcus*, *Enterococcus*, *Corynebacterium*, *E. coli*, *Salmonella*, *Enterobacter*, *Klebsiella pneumoniae*, *Pseudomonas aeruginosa* (cats), *Proteus* (cats), *Bartonella*, *Clostridium perfringens*, *Propionibacterium acnes*, *Bacteroides* spp., *Fusobacterium* spp. [42]
Bone/joint	Osteomyelitis: primarily *Staphylococcus*; other organisms may include *E. coli*, *Klebsiella*, *Pasteurella*, *Serratia*, *Proteus* as well as some anaerobic bacteria: *Bacteroides*, *Fusobacterium*, *Clostridium* and others [36]

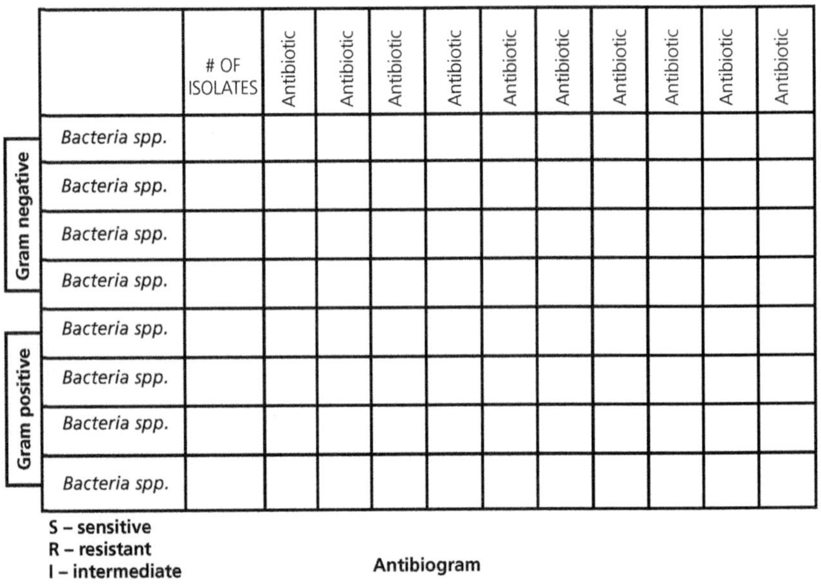

Figure 14.5 Antibiogram. This is one example format for charting bacterial isolates and their antibiotic susceptibilities. Results from each culture submitted from ICU patients in a specific facility should be entered into the antibiogram. The antibiotics available and tested are listed on the horizontal upper axis and the bacteria species isolated and tested are listed along the vertical axis. There are several options for recording results. If there are few results available, put an S, R or I in the appropriate square to indicate whether that bacteria was sensitive, resistant or had an intermediate response to the antibiotics tested. If there were multiple culture results for the one bacterial species, the % of isolates sensitive to the antibiotics can be noted under the antibiotic column, with the number of isolates noted by the bacterial identification.

side-effects or drug interactions, or increasing antimicrobial resistance. Factors to consider when selecting the "best" initial antibiotic regimen include infection location and likely pathogens, patient (host) status, other drugs being administered, and specific characteristics of the selected drug. A schematic of drug and patient factors to consider during antimicrobial selection is shown in Figure 14.2 [24]. Reviewing the list of common bacterial pathogens in the dog and cat (see Table 14.8), as well as the antibiogram (see Figure 14.5) specific for the ICU facility, will provide insight into which bacteria to target with a particular antibiotic.

Common parenteral antibiotics used to treat critically ill dogs and cats are listed in Table 14.9, along with the spectrum, mechanism

Table 14.9 Antibiotics commonly used in the veterinary ICU, arranged by class. Side-effects, mechanism of action, and spectrum of activity are noted [24,43,44].

Drug class	Mechanism of action (MOA) and spectrum of activity		Adverse effects
Penicillins	MOA: binding to penicillin-binding proteins to cross-link peptidoglycans. This inhibits bacterial cell wall synthesis. Bactericidal Spectrum: Gram +, Gram − and anaerobic bacteria. Ticarcillin combinations will have increased activity against *Pseudomonas*		GI distress, hypersensitivity reactions
Amoxicillin	20–30 mg/kg IV, IM, SC q 6–12 h (d)		
Ampicillin	20–40 mg/kg IV, IM, SC q 6–8 h (d,c)		
Ampicillin-sulbactam	22–30 mg/kg IV q 6–8 h (d,c)		
Ticarcillin-clavulanate	50 mg/kg IV q 6–8 h (d,c)		
Cephalosporins	MOA: binding to penicillin-binding proteins to cross-link peptidoglycans. This inhibits bacterial cell wall synthesis. Bactericidal Spectrum: varies by generation of drug. Not interchangeable. General rule of thumb is increased gram-negative coverage with higher number generations. Anaerobic coverage varies		GI distress, hypersensitivity reactions
Cefazolin	22–30 mg/kg IV, IM, SC q 6–8 h (d,c)	First generation	
Cefoxitin	30 mg/kg IV q 6–8 h	Second generation	
Ceftazidime	20–30 mg/kg IV q 6–12 h (d,c)	Third generation	
Cefovecin	8 mg/kg SC q 7 days	Third generation	
Cefotaxime	25–50 mg/kg IV q 6–8 h (d,c)	Third generation	
Carbapenems	MOA: binding to penicillin-binding proteins to cross-link peptidoglycans. This inhibits bacterial cell wall synthesis. Bactericidal Spectrum: Gram +, Gram − and anaerobic bacteria. Not effective against methicillin-resistant organisms		GI distress, hypersensitivity reactions. These are broad spectrum. Recommend use only if indicated by culture and sensitivity results. Cilastatin is used to slow renal drug clearance
Imipenem-cilastatin	5–10 mg/kg IM, IV q 6–8 h (d,c)		
Meropenem	8–12 mg/kg IV q 8–12 h (d,c)		
Aminoglycosides	MOA: binding to 30S ribosomal subunit. Bactericidal Spectrum: primarily Gram − organisms, some Gram +, aerobes *only*		Nephrotoxicity, ototoxicity, neuromuscular paralysis PAE allows q 24 h dosing Synergistic with beta-lactams
Amikacin	15–30 mg/kg IV, IM, SC q 24 h (d), 10–15 mg/kg IM, SC q 24 h (c)		
Gentamicin	6–10 mg/kg IV q 24 h (d), 6 mg/kg IV q 24 h (c)		
Macrolides	MOA: reversible binding to 50S ribosomal unit. Cidal or static depending on organism Spectrum: Gram +, *Mycoplasma* spp., *Bartonella, Borrelia, Campylobacter, Chlamydia, Leptospira, Campylobacter*. Anaerobes except *Bacteroides*		GI distress (esp. severe with erythromycin) Concentration in macrophages will achieve high concentration at site of infection
Azithromycin	5–10 mg/kg IV q 24 h (d,c)		
Erythromycin	10–20 mg/kg IV q 8–12 h (d,c)		
Phenicols	MOA: inhibits 50S ribosomal unit. Bacteristatic Spectrum: Gram +, Gram −, anaerobes, spirochetes, *Rickettsia, Chlamydia, Bordatella, Mycoplasma, Hemobartonella*		In patients: reversible and irreversible bone marrow suppression; GI distress. In human caretakers: risk of idiosyncratic irreversible bone marrow suppression
Chloramphenicol	25–50 mg/kg IV, IM, SC q 8 h (d), 15–20 mg/kg IV, IM, SC q 6–12 h (c)		
Lincosamides	MOA: inhibit 50S ribosomal subunit, at a site separate from macrolides. Bacteriostatic Spectrum: Gram + cocci and anaerobes, *Toxoplasma gondii, Neospora caninum, Hepatozoon, Babesia*. Concentrated in phagocytic leukocytes. May have cidal or static effect depending on concentration and site		GI distress, esophageal injury (oral administration)
Clindamycin	10–15 mg/kg IV q 12 h (d,c)		
Tetracyclines	MOA: bind to 30S ribosomal unit. Bacteriostatic Spectrum: Gram +, Gram −, *Mycoplasma, Hemobartonella, Leptospirosis, Pasteurella, E. coli, Klebsiella, Salmonella*		GI distress; collapse if administered quickly; esophageal injury (oral administration); discoloration of teeth in juvenile patients
Doxycycline	5–10 mg/kg IV q 12 h (d,c)		
Fluoroquinolones	MOA: directly inhibits DNA synthesis by action on topoisomerases Spectrum: primarily Gram −, some Gram +		GI distress, cartilage defects, blindness (cats) Long postantibiotic effect
Enrofloxacin	10–15 mg/kg IV q 24 h (d), 5 mg/kg IV q 24 h (c)		
Glycopeptides	MOA: inhibit cell wall synthesis. Bactericidal Spectrum: Gram + aerobes and anaerobes. Resistant strains of *Staphylococcus* spp., *Streptococcus* spp., anaerobes		Histamine release (hypotension tachycardia), potentiates nephrotoxicity, GI distress Ethical use in veterinary patients remains under debate. Use only as last resort. Typically superior choices exist
Vancomycin	15 mg/kg IV q 8 h (d), 10–15 mg/kg IV q 8–12 h (c)		

(Continued)

Table 14.9 (Continued)

Drug class	Mechanism of action (MOA) and spectrum of activity	Adverse effects
Nitroimidazoles Metronidazole	MOA: metabolite inhibits nucleic acid synthesis. Bactericidal Spectrum: metabolite produced primarily in anaerobic cells, so major effect is on anaerobic bacteria. *Clostridium difficile.* Gram +, Gram −, anaerobes, some protozoa. Some antiinflammatory effect 10–15 mg/kg IV q 12 h (d,c)	Neurotoxicity (central vestibular signs, seizures, cerebellar dysfunction); hepatotoxicity; urine discoloration
Antifolates Trimethoprim-sulfamethoxazole or sulfadiazine	MOA: block DNA and RNA synthesis by inhibition of purine metabolism. Bacteristatic. Spectrum: Gram − staphylococci, some streptococci, *Nocardia*, *Protozoa*, *Mycobacteria*, *Pneumocystis*, unpredictable against streptococci, *no activity against enterococci or obligate anaerobes* 30 mg/kg IV q 12 h (d,c)	Hypersensitivity reactions; bone marrow suppression; dysuria; inhibition of thyroid hormone synthesis; keratoconjunctivitis sicca; idiosyncratic reactions; polyarthropathy

(c) cat; (d) dog; GI, gastrointestinal; PAE, postantibiotic effect.

of action, dosage, and a few precautions for each category of agent. It is important to review the drug insert prior to prescribing any antibiotic. For companion animals, most antibiotic use is extra-label and subject only to scientific justification. The cost of ongoing therapy can also be a factor when selecting antimicrobial agents, particularly in patients who will require prolonged therapy.

Antibiotic selection

The characteristics of specific antibiotics(s) must be considered when making an initial empiric selection. Is the antibiotic bactericidal or bacteriostatic? What is its spectrum of activity against gram-positive, gram-negative, aerobic, anaerobic or facultative bacteria? Will the drug reach appropriate concentrations in the target tissue? What will be the route, frequency, and cost of administration? All of these as well as any potential adverse effects or drug interactions are important to consider (see Figure 14.2).

The concentration of the antimicrobial drug in the targeted tissues will depend on the drug solubility, ionization, protein binding, and pKa. Additional drug characteristics to consider when prescribing a drug and dosing regimen for the ICU small animal patient are presented in Chapter 18. Antimicrobial penetration into barrier-protected sites such as the eye, prostate, and brain requires selection of drugs that are lipid soluble, nonprotein bound, and transported by a transcellular route. Antibiotics such as chloramphenicol and trimethoprim-sulfa can penetrate these barriers. If there is inflammation of the blood–brain, blood–aqueous, or blood–prostate barriers, then additional drugs may penetrate. Liposome-entrapped antimicrobial drugs have enhanced activity against facultative intracellular pathogens, and in some cases (amphotericin B) have decreased systemic toxicity.

In general, bactericidal antimicrobials cause interference of bacterial cell function that is lethal to the bacteria (*in vitro*). These drugs can target the cell wall biosynthesis (beta-lactams, polyene antifungals), cause cell membrane leakage (polymyxin), damage DNA (fluoroquinolones) or damage multiple bacterial ribosomal subunits (macrolides: erythromycin, azithromycin). The major classes of bactericidal antibiotics, regardless of drug–target interaction, stimulate the production of highly deleterious hydroxyl radicals. This occurs in both gram-positive and gram-negative bacteria, and ultimately contributes to cell death [25]. Bactericidal antibiotics are preferred for life-threatening infections when host defense

mechanisms or vital organs are at risk and when patients are immunosuppressed.

Bacteriostatic drugs inhibit cell growth by damaging a single ribosomal subunit (tetracyclines) or disrupting a metabolic pathway (sulfonamides). Bacteriostatic drugs have not been shown to produce hydroxyl radicals. The action of the antibiotic, however, will ultimately be dependent on the concentration of the drug in the target tissue. Bactericidal and bacteriostatic antibiotics should not be combined because the bacteriostatic drug may neutralize effects of the cidal drug. However, combination of two bacteriostatic drugs that act synergistically can result in a bactericidal effect.

Culture and susceptibility (also called sensitivity) results will be used to determine which specific antibiotic is more likely to be effective in treating the infection *in vivo*. Several different parameters may be reported. The minimum inhibitory concentration (MIC) is a measure of the lowest drug concentration inhibiting bacterial growth (10^5 cfu/mL). Should the amount of drug required to inhibit growth exceed what can be safely administered, the bacterium is labeled as "resistant" to that drug. These measures are often based on tissue levels, but in some tissues or fluid (example, urine), the concentration of the antibiotic may be much higher, resulting in clinically therapeutic levels. The minimum bactericidal concentration (MBC) measures bactericidal activity of the antibiotic. Unfortunately, bactericidal and bacteriostatic activity are determined *in vitro* and do not always translate to *in vivo* situations. It may be difficult to safely achieve a bactericidal concentration of a drug at the site of infection in a particular patient. If the MBC is not achieved at the site of infection, even a bactericidal drug can be bacteriostatic *in vivo*.

More recently, the mutant prevention concentration (MPC) has been described as a novel measurement of *in vitro* susceptibility or resistance and is based on the testing of larger bacterial inocula (>/= 10^9 cfu/mL) [26]. The MPC defines the lowest drug concentration required to block the growth of the least susceptible cell present in high-density bacterial populations. MPC testing is assessed on microorganisms considered susceptible to the drug by MIC testing. Doses that achieve a concentration that is higher than the MIC but lower than the MPC are described as falling within the mutant selection window (MSW). This is undesirable because it will encourage the emergence of resistant strains (mutants). Failure to achieve the MPC *in vivo* may allow emergence of resistant microbes,

Table 14.10 Clinically useful antimicrobial drug combinations.

Indication	Drugs	Note
Peritonitis	Gentamycin + clindamycin	Broad-spectrum activity
	Cefuroxime + metronidazole	Broad-spectrum activity
Coliform meningitis	Trimethoprim + sulfamethoxazole	Synergistic with good cerebrospinal fluid penetration
Cryptococcal meningitis	Amphotericin + flucytosine	Synergistic, decreased toxicity
Severe undiagnosed infection	Beta-lactam + aminoglycoside	Broad spectrum, synergistic
	Cefoxitin + clindamycin	Broad spectrum, synergistic

Source: Adapted from Giguère S, Prescott JF, Dowling PM. Principles of antimicrobial drug selection and use. In: Antimicrobial Therapy in Veterinary Medicine, 5th edn. Ames: John Wiley & Sons, 2013 [1].

especially in at-risk or immunosuppressed patients, ultimately leading to treatment failure.

The range of bacteria affected by the antibiotic is termed the spectrum and describes the effect of the antibiotic against gram-positive (Gram +) or gram-negative (Gram −) bacteria. Antibiotics that kill or inhibit a wide range of Gram + and Gram − bacteria are said to be *broad spectrum*. If effective mainly against Gram + **or** Gram − bacteria, they are *narrow spectrum*. If effective against a single organism or disease, they are referred to as *limited spectrum*.

Bacteria can be classified into aerobes and anaerobes. Aerobic bacteria require oxygen to remain alive, while anaerobic bacteria do not rely on oxygen for survival and may die in its presence. This anaerobic type of bacteria does have a growth advantage in areas of the body unexposed to oxygen, and may be a source of infection associated with leakage or absorption of GI bacteria, deep wounds, open fractures, and surgery (abdominal or implant orthopedics).

Facultative bacteria can make adenosine triphosphate (ATP) by aerobic respiration if oxygen is present, but are capable of switching to fermentation or anaerobic respiration if oxygen is absent. Mixed infections involve complex interactions between facultative bacteria and strict anaerobes, many of which possess intrinsic pathogenicity. The best therapeutic results are realized with antimicrobial drugs that are active against both types of microorganisms. This emphasizes the importance of culture and susceptibility testing. For example, the facultative bacterium *Escherichia coli* is often responsible for acute peritonitis and sepsis associated with bowel perforation. However, anaerobes, particularly *Bacteroides fragilis*, play the seminal role in subsequent abscess formation. Treatment of only the facultative bacteria, without adequate antibiotic coverage for anaerobic bacteria, leads to clinical failures with complications of abscess formation. Such therapeutic misadventures have been witnessed in the treatment of mixed infections with cephalosporins and penicillins that lack significant activity against anaerobes. Similarly, use of metronidazole or clindamycin as a single agent is associated with failures caused by infection with facultative bacteria.

Antimicrobial drug combinations are often indicated in critical patients with compromised defenses or immune impairment. Infections such as peritonitis, pyothorax, aspiration pneumonia, and urogenital infections often have mixed bacterial populations. Combining drugs that have different mechanisms of action can widen the target for bacterial destruction and reduce the likelihood of microbial resistance during treatment. In some cases, combining two agents can decrease dose-related toxicity (flucytosine + amphotericin B). Keep in mind that not all drugs work synergistically and not all drug combinations are desired. Some combinations can have added or synergistic toxicity. Combinations that destroy normal GI

flora may promote superinfection, a second infection superimposed upon the first. Synergistic antibiotic combinations used in dogs and cats are listed in Table 14.10.

The most appropriate route of administration for antimicrobial agents in the ICU is by IV injection, providing 100% bioavailability of the drug. Factors such as poor perfusion, dehydration, overhydration, and abnormal GI function can affect the antibiotic plasma drug concentration (PDC) after subcutaneous, intramuscular or oral administration (see Table 18.1, Chapter 18). Administration of a loading dose by IV injection, as directed by drug insert, can be used to rapidly achieve therapeutic PDC. Constant rate infusions may be indicated to maintain therapeutic drug levels throughout the dosing interval for antimicrobials, requiring frequent administration to maintain PDC above MIC (also called time-dependent antibiotics). Suboptimal antibiotic concentrations increase the likelihood of treatment failures, antibiotic resistance, and patient toxicity. As patients recover and transition to step-down wards or discharge to home care, they will be transitioned to oral medications. Adequate GI function must be achieved prior to this transition.

Whenever possible, drugs with a large therapeutic index should be chosen. This means there is a large window between the amount of drug that causes therapeutic effect and the amount of drug that causes toxicity. Knowledge of possible adverse drug reactions for the selected agent(s) should be reviewed and orders established for monitoring and intervention, should it become necessary. Idiosyncratic reactions are independent of dose and duration and cannot be predicted.

Critically ill dogs and cats are typically on multiple medications including IV fluids, antimicrobials, and nutrition. It is important to consider how these may interact with one another both before and after administration. Tetracyclines mixed with calcium-containing fluids and enrofloxacin combined with magnesium-containing fluids will chelate, thus reducing drug delivery. Cephalosporins and aminoglycosides provide a synergistic antibacterial combination *in vivo*, but will precipitate when mixed in solution together. Some drug interactions can be used to advantage. The drug probenecid has been used to block renal excretion of ampicillin, thereby increasing the PDC of ampicillin. Antibiotics, antifungals, and other drugs can alter hepatic microsomal systems. This may put patients at risk for hepatic damage, or may alter drug metabolism and excretion. The administration of antacids, corticosteroids, immunosuppressants, and p450 enzyme inhibitors or promoters will also alter drug efficacy.

Corticosteroids can delay healing, reduce fever, suppress inflammation, impair phagocytosis, and impair the normal immune response. Concurrent administration of corticosteroids with antimicrobials, while poorly investigated in companion animals, is typically not recommended. Exceptions to this rule exist. Patients that have immune-mediated disease and a bacterial infection will require antibiotic and immunosuppressive therapy. In addition, when the inflammatory response to the bacterial infection is potentially life threatening (such as bacterial meningitis or fungal pneumonitis), the combination of corticosteroids and antibiotics is often recommended. The administration of short-term high doses of corticosteroids has been shown to be harmful in humans and animals with septic shock [27]. The administration of long-term low-dose corticosteroid therapy (with hydrocortisone) has shown some promise in human patients but there is no evidence to support this in companion animals at this time [28].

Some antibiotics will have a postantibiotic effect (PAE), meaning they continue to act after the drug has been removed. Proposed mechanisms by which the PAE occurs include nonlethal damage induced by the antimicrobial agent and a limited persistence of the antimicrobial agent at the bacterial binding site [29]. The specific microorganism-antimicrobial combination is the most important factor to influence the presence and duration of the PAE. Additional factors include the antimicrobial concentration and the length of antimicrobial exposure. Most antimicrobial agents produce a PAE when tested against Gram + cocci. However, against Gram − bacilli, beta-lactam antibiotics (except for imipenem) have a minimal, or even a negative, PAE. Aminoglycosides, inhibitors of protein and nucleic acid synthesis, and fluoroquinolones have PAEs against Gram − bacteria that range from one to four hours. Extending the dosing interval of an antimicrobial agent (such as an aminoglycoside) that produces a PAE has several possible advantages, most notably in decreasing undesirable effects of the drug.

Perioperative antibiotics

The concern for surgical bacterial contamination during "clean" surgical procedures (such as clean, clean with prosthesis, and clean with contamination) has lead to the use of perioperative antibiotics in surgical procedures. Short-term therapeutic doses of antibiotics appropriate for the potential pathogens have been recommended for clean procedures, such as intraabdominal surgery or surgical insertion of implants. The antibiotics need to be in the tissues at the time of the surgery and potential contamination, requiring antibiotic administration before and often during surgery. There is no apparent benefit of antibiotic administration in these patients after the surgical wound has been closed, with continued antibiotic administration often causing resistance among bacteria.

A typical perioperative antibiotic regimen would incorporate the IV administration of either a first-generation cephalosporin or beta-lactam antibiotic at the time of patient induction. The antibiotic dose is repeated every 1–2 hours during the surgical procedure. Clean or clean contaminated wounds are given 1–2 doses of antibiotic postoperatively.

Adequate lavage will minimize bacterial colonization. Submission of tissue cultures will rapidly identify persistent flora. Contaminated or dirty surgical procedures will have an existing established infection at the time of surgery and should already be receiving antibiotic therapy prior to and during surgical intervention.

Hospital antibiotic surveillance

Restricting the use of certain antibiotics or classes of antibiotics has been shown in human ICUs to reduce the appearance of nosocomial and resistant bacterial populations [30]. Additional advantages include decreased pharmacy expense and avoidance of adverse drug reactions. It is important to create an antibiotic protocol for the ICU and ensure that personnel adhere to the guidelines of antibiotic selection, utilization, and environmental bacterial surveillance.

Creating an antibiotic protocol

Available antibiotics and their action, spectrum, potential toxicity, and other specific notes are presented in Table 14.9. First-line antibiotics include ampicillin and amoxicillin with or without potentiating agents; first-generation cephalosporins; trimethoprim-sulfonamide combinations; doxycycline; and metronidazole. When co-infection with Gram − aerobes and/or anaerobes is suspected, additional antibiotics should be combined with first-line agents until culture results are available. Appropriate choices may include amikacin, gentamicin, clindamycin, and metronidazole. For aggressive anaerobic coverage, metronidazole is given IV. The addition of an aminoglycoside is strongly recommended for serious infection from Gram − organisms. Third generation cephalosporins can be used if renal function is compromised. Appropriate doses and dosing intervals for all agents is emphasized.

There is some evidence in human ICUs that combination therapy with narrow-spectrum agents over prolonged periods may help curb resistance to broad-spectrum antibiotics while still providing effective treatment of serious infections. Treatment with potent, broad spectrum drugs (imipenem, meropenem, third-generation cephalosporins) should be reserved for life threatening infections. Therapy should be deescalated as soon as possible. The culture and sensitivity will direct this final antibiotic choice, with the safest, most effective narrow-spectrum drug chosen whenever possible.

The antibiogram

Active charting of bacterial cultures and susceptibilities will create an antibiogram. This is used to identify emerging resistance to first-line antibiotics and assist in making any changes in the hospital antibiotic protocol deemed necessary. It is also examined for an indication of probable nosocomial pathogens in hospitalized patients. An example of a format for an antibiogram is presented in Figure 14.5. Though all cultures are tracked, the bacteria that most commonly develop resistance (*Klebsiella pneumoniae*, *Enterobacter* spp., *Pseudomonas aeruginosa* and *Staphylococcus* spp.) are closely monitored for evidence of resistance to the first-line antibiotics recommended by the hospital protocol. The frequency of charting may depend on the patient population of the facility, with higher populations warranting more frequent charting (such as 6–12-month intervals).

When resistance is found, the origin of the infection and the antibiotic prescribed should be investigated. A pattern of resistance found in infections treated recently at a veterinary facility or bacterial isolates atypical of naturally occurring infections in small animals (such as *Morexella* spp., *Acinetobacter* spp., *Serratia* spp., *Enterococcus* spp.) suggest that the infection may be nosocomial. The first animal that presented to the hospital with the identified resistant infection most likely did not develop the resistance to that first-line antibiotic within your hospital environment. Persistent resistance patterns for previously susceptible bacteria suggest that resistance has occurred to the first-line antibiotics in your hospital. The hospital antibiotic protocol should be amended to direct prescribing of a different first-line agent or agents. Carbapenems, third-generation cephalosporins, and fluoroquinolones are avoided as first-line agents due to the high incidence and rapid onset of resistance. Potent antimicrobial agents such as vancomycin, tigecycline, and imipenem should be reserved for resistant infections, with their use guided by culture and susceptibility testing. The reservation of life-saving antimicrobial agents (vancomycin, tigecycline) for use in resistant human infections is an ongoing ethical debate. In veterinary medicine, we are fortunate in that we do not routinely face infections with this degree of antimicrobial resistance. Only continued ethical and appropriate antimicrobial stewardship will prevent escalation of this problem.

Antibiotic rotation is the strategy used in human ICUs where a class of antibiotic or a specific antibiotic is withdrawn from use for a defined period of time and reintroduced at a later point in an attempt to limit bacterial resistance. There is limited clinical data available as to its effectiveness, with the rotation reserved for facilities with a high incidence of resistance or nosocomial infections. Limited antibiotic rotation has been employed at some veterinary facilities with success.

Nosocomial infections

Nosocomial infections are defined as infections acquired from the hospital environment that develop more than 48 hours after admission to hospital. These infections are generally more serious and difficult to treat because the patient is weaker and less able to combat an infection. The bacteria are likely antibiotic resistant and more virulent. Conditions in busy veterinary facilities are conducive to the development of nosocomial infections and include patient crowding, frequent broad-spectrum antibiotic usage, inappropriate use of barrier techniques, and inadequate hand hygiene. Sources of patient contamination are plentiful, including cages, work surfaces, examination tables, sinks, floor drains, and equipment (clippers, pulse oximeter probes, blood pressure cuffs, endotracheal tubes, etc.). Identification, treatment, and containment of nosocomial bacterial infections are challenging and expensive.

A *complicated infection* is a bacterial or fungal infection associated with a structural or functional abnormality. These abnormalities may be congenital (e.g. patent urachus), functional (e.g. dialysis dependent), or iatrogenic (e.g. orthopedic implant). Animals in the ICU may have multiple catheters (such as intravenous, urinary, central lines), tubes (such as chest tubes, feeding tubes, oxygen cannulas), and life-saving invasive procedures (such as peritoneal dialysis, mechanical ventilation, surgical cutdown) that predispose them to complicated infections. The causative bacteria are often antibiotic resistant, residing in fibrin tags or biofilms formed around the tips of the catheters or tubing. While appropriate antibiotic therapy is vital to a successful outcome, the indwelling device must be removed to achieve effective decontamination.

Bacterial resistance

Bacterial resistance is acquired when antibiotic-resistant bacterial strains develop from formerly antibiotic-susceptible bacteria. This can result from a mutant gene or altered DNA sequence. Plasmids are small molecules of altered DNA that can be transferred between bacteria for the rapid spread of antibiotic resistance among bacterial populations. Stimuli for the development of bacterial resistance include repeated antibiotic exposure, widespread antibiotic use (such as with fluoroquinolones), incorrect antibiotic dosing, or insufficient duration of antibiotic therapy. The importance of bacterial resistance has been demonstrated in human medicine, with the development of methicillin-resistant and

vancomycin-resistant *Staphylococcus aureus*, enterococci, and Gram − bacteria. Isolation of methicillin-resistant *Staphylococcus aureus* from small animals has been reported and causes similar therapeutic concerns for the veterinarian and facility as experienced in human medicine.

Hygiene and environmental surveillance

Each hospital should have a structured antibiotic stewardship program, to include hospital hygiene, barrier nursing techniques, staff educational programs, patient isolation area, and a strict antibiotic policy for restricting and guiding antibiotic use. Hand washing is the single most important way to reduce microorganism transfer and hospital-acquired infection. Hands can be washed with soap and water, or alcohol-based hand rinses (70% ethanol). Noncompliance with hand-washing protocols is the greatest obstacle to reducing pathogen transfer from patient to patient. Other barrier nursing techniques are discussed in Chapter 20. Exam gloves are primarily to keep the staff's hands clean and do not provide an adequate barrier to prevent transmission of bacteria or viruses between animals. The use of gloves *does not* replace hand washing.

Strict aseptic techniques must be applied when inserting indwelling catheters, performing venipuncture, aspirating cells or fluids, or performing invasive procedures such as mechanical ventilation, bone marrow sampling, or peritoneal dialysis. Surgical suites, ward and ICU cages, scrub sinks, tables, and treatment surfaces should have a regular routine of cleaning with bactericidal cleansers. Typically, the most appropriate products are quaternary ammonium compounds or accelerated hydrogen peroxide cleaners. Drains in the wards and runs must be cleaned and sanitized on a routine basis. Items such as hair clippers, thermometers, stethoscopes, and otoscopes must be carefully cleaned and monitored for contamination. Mop buckets and cleaning solutions must be changed frequently. Routine cultures of the environment can be monitored in hospital areas where nosocomial infections may originate, such as common surfaces (surgical suites or prep tables, cage surfaces) and common equipment (such as surgical ventilator and radiology tables). However, careful hospital-wide surveillance of the resistance patterns of cultured organisms will be more effective for identification of nosocomial and resistant infections.

Patient isolation

Patients should be placed into isolation when they have a contagious infectious disease, or when they are known or suspected to have a multiresistant pathogen (such as open surgical wounds). The list of possible pathogens or problems requiring patient isolation includes, but is not limited to, the following: *Salmonella, Campylobacter,* parvovirus, *Giardia, Cryptosporidium,* psittacosis, canine distemper virus, influenza, methicillin-resistant *Staphycoccus* infections, plague, rabies, tularemia, infectious canine tracheobronchitis, infectious feline upper respiratory diseases, feline distemper, and resistant bacterial strains.

Isolation units are separated from the general ICU or hospital population and should have separate ventilation and filtered air. Ideally, the personnel are dedicated to the area and do not work with the general ICU population during their shift. Alternately, staff may handle these patients at the end of their shift. Hand washing and gloves are mandatory, as are protective gowns, masks, caps, and booties. Footbaths may be appropriate to clean the shoes of personnel when entering and leaving the isolation facility.

Patients should be minimally handled or moved within the isolation unit to reduce surface contamination. Whenever possible, diagnostic, surgical, and other procedures should be performed within the unit, avoiding common patient areas in the general hospital environment. When the procedure can only be performed in the main patient areas, precautions must be taken to avoid fecal, urine, or secretion contamination of the area, and proper cleaning and disinfection should be performed immediately afterward.

All instruments and equipment used to monitor and treat isolation patients is dedicated to that area and should be thoroughly cleaned between patients. Disposable items should not be reused. Ideally, patients should have a separate entrance and a separate elimination area or be allowed to eliminate in their cages to avoid contamination of common areas. Surfaces and equipment contaminated by feces, secretions or blood must be cleaned and disinfected immediately by personnel in charge of the patient. All laundry and waste material should be properly cleaned or disposed of and contaminated surfaces cleaned and disinfected.

A separate mop and bucket must be provided for the isolation area. Discarded protective wear, treatment materials, and waste matter should be discarded in waste bags and directly taken to the trash. Label all laundry from the area for disinfection. Any visitors to the isolation unit must adhere to all infection control policies and procedures.

Similar protocols and procedures are employed for patients that are immune deficient. These patients should be housed in the general ICU area, but separated from other animals. They should not be placed in the isolation unit utilized for contagious disease. Reverse barrier isolation techniques should be used including dedicated nursing personnel that adhere to strict hand-washing procedures and protective wear. Minimal movement within the common area will minimize patient exposure to pathogens from the general hospital population or personnel.

Failed response to antibiotic therapy

There are many reasons why antibiotic therapy can fail to improve the clinical condition or outcome in a critical patient (Box 14.4). When this occurs, the history, physical examination findings, laboratory data, and advanced diagnostics should be reexamined. Different types of bacteria, such as anaerobes or *Mycoplasma*, should be considered along with the possibility that the pathogen is not bacterial at all. The wrong antibiotic may have been chosen or the wrong drug or dose administered to the specific patient. Consider drug dose miscalculation, inappropriate administration, and failure of the drug delivery or penetration as causes of poor response. Antibiotics are ineffective within abscesses or septic exudates and medical therapy is no replacement for appropriate debridement and drainage. Unfortunately, bacteria can rapidly develop antibiotic resistance to even the most appropriate drug regimen. Inappropriate drug choice, dosage, dosing interval, length of therapy, and repeated antibiotic exposure all contribute to development of antibiotic resistance. Nosocomial and superinfections warrant prompt and aggressive intervention. Patients with complicating co-morbidities such as immune deficiencies, diabetes mellitus, hyperadrenocorticism, etc. will be at increased risk from these infections.

Nosocomial and resistant bacteria

Nosocomial infections should be suspected when surgical incision sites in sequential patients become infected, or when unusual resistant bacterial isolates are charted on the antibiogram.

> **Box 14.4** Common causes of failed response to antibiotic therapy.
>
> - Not a bacterial infection
> - Wrong antimicrobial drug or dose
> - *In vitro* testing does not correlate with *in vivo* effects
> - Improper drug handling
> - Inadequate duration of therapy
> - Persistent source of infection (catheters, foreign body)
> - Pocket of pus (bacteria walled off)
> - Immunoprivileged site (poor antibiotic penetration)
> - Drug misses targeted tissue site or antigen
> - Repeated (previous) antibiotic exposure
> - Superinfection – nosocomial?
> - Fast-emerging drug-resistant bacterial strain
> - Presence of ≥ 2 pathogens while treatment effective for only one
> - Immune deficiencies or immunosuppression of patient
> - Immunosuppressive comorbidities (diabetes mellitus, hyperadrenocorticism, etc.)

Environmental cultures are required to identify the source of the bacterial contamination and susceptibility patterns for antibiotic therapy. Thought must be given to areas where contact was made between the site of infection on the patient, the environment, and any equipment used. Nosocomial and resistant bacteria are typically found in common locations including clipper blades, drainage grates, cage floors, wet tables, ventilator tubing, and within disinfectant solution bottles, cold trays, scrub containers, and spray bottles.

Risk factors for hospital-acquired or resistant infections include prior treatment with antibiotics during the hospitalization; prolonged length of hospital stay; and the presence of invasive devices. Patients at high risk for resistant bacteria should initially be treated with a combination of antibiotics providing coverage for the most likely pathogens to be encountered in that specific ICU. This highlights the importance of ongoing surveillance and maintenance of an accurate hospital antibiogram. The initial treatment plan can be modified after specific culture and sensitivity results are returned.

Antibiotic deescalation

Antibiotic deescalation is a key element of responsible antimicrobial stewardship programs [31]. After culture and sensitivity results are returned (typically around day 3 of therapy), the initial empiric antibiotics protocol is stopped and the antimicrobial medications are reduced in number and/or narrowed in spectrum of activity. Deescalation is currently recommended as part of routine antimicrobial management. Benefits of deescalation include decreasing bacterial resistance pressure, cost savings, and decreased antibiotic-related adverse events. The best procedure and full scope of benefits continue to be elucidated.

Surviving Sepsis Campaign

The International Guidelines for Management of Severe Sepsis and Septic Shock have been prepared for use in the management of human patients with sepsis and septic shock [32]. Recommendations from the Surviving Sepsis Campaign for infection control that are applicable to the small animal veterinary patient and facility are provided in Table 14.11.

Table 14.11 Excerpts for infection control from the International Guidelines for Management of Severe Sepsis and Septic Shock [32].

Measure	Rationale
• Routine screening of potentially affected patients for evidence of sepsis	• Early identification of sepsis and implementation of appropriate therapy
• Hospital-based performance improvement plans	▪ Education and guideline development and implementation have demonstrated improved outcome in sepsis
• Obtain cultures prior to antimicrobial therapy (only if it will not delay therapy)	• Optimize identification of etiological agents
▪ Imaging studies should be performed promptly to confirm a source of infection	▪ Identification of a source of infection will warrant source control
• Administration of effective IV antimicrobials within the first hour of recognition of septic shock	• Each hour of delay has been associated with measurable increase in mortality in a number of (human) studies
▪ Selection and administration of empiric antibiotics likely to be effective against suspected pathogens; this may include combination therapy and should be employed for all neutropenic patients	▪ Empirical antibiotic choice is complex, with little margin for error in the septic patient. Selection of antimicrobials that cover most or all organisms is essential and should be guided by prevalence patterns and recent antibiotic exposure
• Antimicrobial regiment reassessed daily. Deescalate as soon as possible	• Narrowing the spectrum and duration of antimicrobial therapy will limit development of superinfections
▪ Empirical combination therapy should not be used for >3–5 days. Deescalate as soon as possible	▪ Combination therapy (use of two classes of antibiotics) has improved outcome but there is concern for development of resistance and additional antibiotics may not improve outcome
• Typical duration of therapy is 7–10 days	• This duration is often adequate with source control; some patients may require longer courses
▪ Antimicrobial agents should not be used in patients with severe inflammatory disease NOT associated with infection (trauma, immune disease, etc.)	▪ Limit potential development of antimicrobial resistance
• Anatomical source control should be employed within 12 hours	• Limiting specific sources of infection (septic abdomen, abscess) will increase likelihood of treatment success and decrease development of bacterial resistance
▪ Intravascular devices should be removed if believed to be a source of infection	▪ Treatment failure is likely without removal of the device
• Infection prevention measures should always be used (bandaging, gloves, hand hygiene, etc.)	• Limit development of multiresistant bacteria, horizontal transmission, and incidence of nosocomial infections

References

1. Giguère S, Prescott JF, Dowling PM. Principles of antimicrobial drug selection and use. In: Antimicrobial Therapy in Veterinary Medicine, 5th edn. Ames: John Wiley & Sons, 2013.
2. Levy MM, Dellinger RP, Townsend SR, et al. The Surviving Sepsis Campaign: results of an international guideline-based performance improvement programme targeting severe sepsis. Crit Care Med. 2010;38:367–74.
3. Kumar A, Roberts D, Wood KE, et al. Duration of hypotension before initiation of effective antimicrobial therapy is the critical determinant of survival in human septic shock. Crit Care Med. 2006;34(6):1589–96.
4. Gonçalves-Pereira J, Pereira JM, Ribeiro O, et al. Impact of infection on admission and of the process of care on mortality of patients admitted to the Intensive Care Unit: the INFAUCI study. Clin Microbiol Infect. 2014;20(12):1308–15.
5. Allison RW, Meinkoth JH. Hematology without the numbers: in-clinic blood film evaluation. Vet Clin North Am Small Anim Pract. 2007;37(2):245–66.
6. Bonczynski JJ, Ludwig LL, Barton LJ, Loar A, Peterson ME. Comparison of peritoneal fluid and peripheral blood pH, bicarbonate, glucose, and lactate concentration as a diagnostic tool for septic peritonitis in dogs and cats. Vet Surg. 2003;32(2):161–6.
7. Mouat EE, Davis GJ, Drobatz KJ, Wallace KA. Evaluation of data from 35 dogs pertaining to dehiscence following intestinal resection and anastomosis. J Am Anim Hosp Assoc. 2014;50(4):254–63.
8. Szabo SD, Jermyn K, Neel J, Mathews KG. Evaluation of postceliotomy peritoneal drain fluid volume, cytology, and blood-to-peritoneal fluid lactate and glucose differences in normal dogs. Vet Surg. 2011;40(4):444–9.
9. Huizenga NA, de Herder WW, Koper JW, et al. Decreased ligand affinity rather than glucocorticoid receptor down-regulation in patients with endogenous Cushing's syndrome. Eur J Endocrinol. 2000;142(5):472–6.
10. Studdert VP, Phillips WA, Studdert MJ. Recurrent and persistent infections in related Weimaraner dogs. Aust Vet J. 1984;61:261.
11. Couto CG, Krakowka S, Johnson G, et al. In vitro immunologic features of Weimaraner dogs with neutrophil abnormalities and recurrent infections. Vet Immunol Immunopathol. 1989;23:103.
12. Skelly BJ, Franklin RJM. Recognition and diagnosis of lysosomal storage diseases in the cat and dog. J Vet Intern Med. 2002;16:133.
13. Debenham SL, Millington A, Kijas J, et al. Canine leucocyte adhesion deficiency in Irish red and white setters. J Small Anim Pract. 2002;43:74.
14. Yang TJ. Pathobiology of canine cyclic hematopoiesis (review). In Vivo. 1987;5:297.
15. Latimer KS, Webb JL. Leukocytes. In: Duncan and Prasse's Veterinary Laboratory Medicine Clinical Pathology, 5th edn. Chichester: John Wiley & Sons, 2011.
16. Jackson ML. Leukocytes in health and disease. In: Textbook of Veterinary Internal Medicine, 7th edn. Ettinger SJ, Feldman EC, eds. St Louis: Elsevier Saunders, 2010.
17. Prieur DJ, Collier LL. Inheritance of the Chediak–Higashi syndrome in cats. J Hered. 1981;72:175.
18. Hirsch VM, Cunningham TA. Hereditary anomaly of neutrophil granulation in Birman cats. Am J Vet Res. 1984;45:2170.
19. Latimer KS, Kircher IM, Lindl PA, et al. Leukocyte function in Pelger–Huet anomaly of dogs. J Leukoc Biol. 1989;45:301.
20. Latimer KS, Rakich PM, Thompson DF. Pelger–Huet anomaly in cats. Vet Pathol. 1985;22:370.
21. Foster AP. Immunomodulation and immunodeficiency. Vet Dermatol. 2004;15(2):115–26.
22. Perryman LE. Molecular pathology of severe combined immunodeficiency in mice, horses, and dogs. Vet Pathol. 2004;41(2):95–100.
23. Felsburg PJ, Hartnett BJ, Henthorn PS, Moore PF, Krakowka S, Ochs HD. Canine X-linked severe combined immunodeficiency. Vet Immunol Immunopathol. 1999;69(2-4):127–35.
24. Boothe DM. Small Animal Clinical Pharmacology and Therapeutics, 2nd edn. St Louis: Elsevier Saunders, 2012.
25. Kohanski MA, Dwyer DJ, Hayete B, et al. A common mechanism of cellular death induced by bactericidal antibiotics. Cell 2007:130(5):797–810.
26. Blondeau JM. New concepts in antimicrobial susceptibility testing: the mutant prevention concentration and mutant selection window approach. Vet Dermatol. 2009;20(5-6):383–96.
27. Sprung CL, Annane D, Keh D, et al. Hydrocortisone therapy for patients with septic shock. N Engl J Med. 2008;358(2):111–24.
28. Dellinger RP. Steroid therapy of septic shock: the decision is in the eye of the beholder. Crit Care Med. 2008;36(6):1987–9.

29. Spivey JM. The postantibiotic effect. Clin Pharm. 1992;11(10):865–75.

30 30.Brahmi N, Blel Y, Kouraichi N, et al. Impact of ceftazidime resitriction on gram-negative bacterial resistance in an intensive care unit. Infect Chemother. 2006;12(4):190–4.

31. Masterton RG. Antibiotic de-escalation. Crit Care Clin. 2011;27(1):149–62.

32. Dellinger RP, Levy MM, Rhodes A, et al. Surviving Sepsis Campaign: International Guidelines for Management of Severe Sepsis and Septic Shock. Crit Care Med. 2013;41(2):588–95.

33. Rebar AH, MacWilliams PS, Feldman BF, et al. A Guide to Hematology in Dogs and Cats. Jackson Hole: Teton NewMedia, 2002.

34. Boothe DM. Treatment of bacterial infections. In: Small Animal Clinical Pharmacology and Therapeutics, 2nd edn. Boothe DM, ed. St Louis: Elsevier Saunders, 2012: p 286.

35. Barsanti JA. Genitourinary infections. In: Infectious Diseases of the Dog and Cat, 4th edn. Greene CE, ed. St Louis: Elsevier Saunders, 2012: p 1026.

36. Boothe DM. Treatment of bacterial infections. In: Small Animal Clinical Pharmacology and Therapeutics, 2nd edn. Boothe DM, ed. St Louis: Elsevier Saunders, 2012: p 307.

37. Center SA. Hepatobiliary Infections. In: Infectious Diseases of the Dog and Cat, 4th edn. Greene CE, ed. St Louis: Elsevier Saunders, 2012: p 985.

38. Barsanti JA. Genitourinary infections. In: Infectious Diseases of the Dog and Cat, 4th edn. Greene CE, ed. St Louis: Elsevier Saunders, 2012: p 1040.

39. Sirinarumitr K. Medical treatment of benign prostatic hypertrophy and prostatitis in dogs. In: Kirk's Current Veterinary Therapy XIV. Bonagura JD, Twedt DC, eds. St Louis: Elsevier Saunders, 2009: p 1047.

40. Kent M. Bacterial infection of the central nervous system. In: Infectious Diseases of the Dog and Cat, 4th edn. Greene CE, ed. St Louis: Elsevier Saunders, 2012: p 1046.

41. Lee-Fowler T, Reinero C. Bacterial respiratory infections. In: Infectious Diseases of the Dog and Cat, 4th edn. Greene CE, ed. St Louis: Elsevier Saunders, 2012: pp 945–6.

42. Calver CA, Thomason JD. Cardiovascular infection. In: Infectious Diseases of the Dog and Cat, 4th edn. Greene CE, ed. St Louis: Elsevier Saunders, 2012: p 914.

43. Plumb DC. Plumb's Veterinary Drug Handbook, 8th edn. Stockholm: Pharm-Vet Inc., 2015.

44. Silverstein DC, Hopper K. Small Animal Critical Care Medicine, 2nd edn. St Louis: Elsevier Saunders, 2015.

Further reading

Allison RW, Meinkoth JH. Hematology without the numbers: in-clinic blood film evaluation. Vet Clin North Am Small Anim Pract. 2007;37(2):245–66, vi.

Boothe DM. Small Animal Clinical Pharmacology and Therapeutics, 2nd edn. St Louis: Elsevier Saunders, 2012.

Giguère S, Prescott JF, Dowling PM. Principles of antimicrobial drug selection and use. In: Antimicrobial Therapy in Veterinary Medicine, 5th edn. Ames: John Wiley & Sons, 2013.

Jackson ML. Leukocytes in health and disease. In: Textbook of Veterinary Internal Medicine, 7th edn. Ettinger SJ, Feldman EC, eds. St Louis: Elsevier Saunders, 2010.

Latimer KS, Webb JL. Leukocytes. In: Duncan and Prasse's Veterinary Laboratory Medicine Clinical Pathology, 5th edn. Chichester: John Wiley & Sons, 2011.

Rebar AH. Blood film evaluation. In: Small Animal Critical Care Medicine. Silverstein D, Hopper K, eds. St Louis: Elsevier Saunders, 2009.

CHAPTER 15

Gastrointestinal system motility and integrity

Jennifer Klaus

Blue Pearl Veterinary Partners, Phoenix, Arizona

Introduction

The gastrointestinal (GI) tract is a series of hollow organs, responsible for the assimilation, digestion, and absorption of ingested nutrients and expulsion of waste material. The components of the GI tract are the mouth, pharynx, esophagus, stomach, small intestines, cecum, large intestines, and anus. Effective GI motility and an intact functioning GI mucosal barrier are essential for normal digestive activity and protection from luminal pathogens.

The GI tract and liver are considered the "shock organs" of dogs [1] and suffer major changes in their motility, ultrastructure, and function during low blood flow and hypoxemic conditions [2]. The splanchnic circulation supplies the GI tract and is particularly vulnerable to hypoxia. A reservoir of pathogens is present in the GI lumen, ready to translocate to the systemic circulation should local immunological and other defensive mechanisms fail [2]. The presence of cytokines may cause the loss of epithelial tight junction barrier function. Tumor necrosis factor has been shown to have a central role in diseases associated with intestinal barrier dysfunction, such as inflammatory bowel disease or intestinal ischemia [3]. Dogs subjected to severe GI hypoxia for one hour prior to fluid resuscitation developed gut barrier failure and bacterial translocation. Gastrointestinal bacteria and endotoxin were found in the portal and systemic circulation of these dogs and resulted in sepsis and multiple organ dysfunction syndrome (MODS) [4].

Clinical signs of GI dysfunction can run the spectrum from mild changes in appetite to severe changes with sloughing intestinal mucosa. Life-threatening complications such as third body fluid spacing, loss of proteins, fluids and electrolytes, enteric bacterial translocation, sepsis, and eventually death can be a consequence of significant GI dysfunction [2].

The GI tract can complicate any disease process and impact recovery in any ICU patient. A careful assessment of diagnostic and monitoring data can assist in early recognition of potential GI tract contributions to disease. Treatment for shock and GI hypoxia should always be aggressive, replacing lost fluids and electrolytes and providing nutrition early to aid intestinal barrier cells during their healing process.

Monitoring methods

The initial history and physical examination provide a baseline of information for finding the cause of GI clinical signs and for monitoring for trends of change in the patient. Point of care (POC) testing provides important data to guide the therapy at the cage side. Many of the consequences of GI disorders are diagnosed and the response to treatment monitored with the results of the minimum database. However, making a definitive diagnosis of the GI component of the disease can require more advanced testing, to include clinicopathological testing, radiographs, contrast studies, ultrasound, or computed tomography (CT). Treatment with intravenous fluids, oxygen, analgesics, electrolyte replacement, and possibly broad-spectrum antibiotics should not be withheld in critical patients as diagnostic testing is pursued.

History

The signalment (age, sex, breed) is important since certain dog breeds can have a predisposition to GI disorders such as gastric dilation volvulus syndrome (GDV), mesenteric volvulus, and pancreatitis. While vomiting and diarrhea are the more common presenting complaints, it is important to ask about ptyalism, prehension of food, decreased ability or discomfort with opening the mouth or swallowing, facial asymmetry, and interest in food or appetite. Pharyngeal dysphagia is suspected when there is impaired initiation of the involuntary passage of food through the oropharynx. Clients might report that the pet is gagging or coughing during or after swallowing.

The actual mechanics of vomiting as well as the described color and contents of the vomitus can assist in localizing the problem within the GI tract (Figure 15.1, Table 15.1). It is important to differentiate between vomiting and regurgitation from the history [5]. Regurgitation is the passive expulsion of food or fluid from the stomach or esophagus without abdominal contractions. Most commonly, it occurs immediately after eating but can occur several hours later. The regurgitated material often includes a clear or frothy white liquid (saliva) with or without undigested or partially digested food. Regurgitation directs diagnostic efforts to problems of the esophagus or significant gastric motility disorders (passive vomiting) (see Table 15.1).

Vomiting is a centrally coordinated oral expulsion of gastric or upper duodenal contents. There are prodromal signs including lip smacking and ptyalism as well as coordinated contraction of the upper GI organs. The abdominal wall muscles are observed to forcefully contract. Bilious (yellow-green) material in the vomitus originates from the duodenum and helps to differentiate vomiting from regurgitation when the physical action has not been observed. Nonproductive vomiting can be an early sign of GDV and warrants immediate therapeutic and diagnostic investigation.

The presence of diarrhea directs diagnostic efforts toward the small and large intestines. The reported character and consistency

Monitoring and Intervention for the Critically Ill Small Animal: The Rule of 20, First Edition. Edited by Rebecca Kirby and Andrew Linklater.

© 2017 John Wiley & Sons, Inc. Published 2017 by John Wiley & Sons, Inc.

267

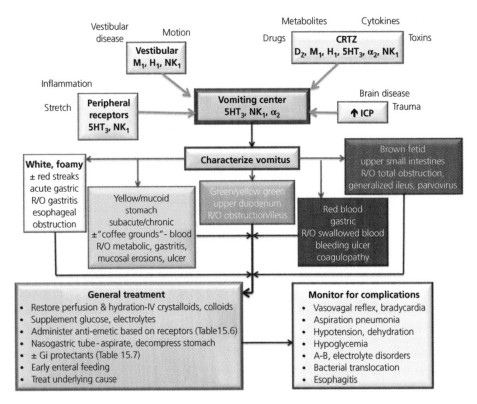

Figure 15.1 Algorithm for the general approach to a patient with vomiting. The four main mechanisms for stimulating the vomiting center with their receptor types are in light blue boxes. Some of the primary causes of stimulation of the receptors are listed surrounding each box. The final pathway for the stimulation of vomiting is through the vomiting or emetic center located in the brainstem. The character and color of the vomitus can provide an initial impression of the location within the gastrointestinal tract that is primarily affected. While many potential causes for vomiting are possible, those listed should be considered and ruled out when there is potential for life-threatening complications. General treatment guidelines are listed in the orange box, with common complications to be anticipated listed in the pink box. $5HT_3$, serotonergic receptor; α_2, adrenergic receptor; A-B, acid–base; D_2, dopaminergic receptor; GI, gastrointestinal; H_1, histaminergic receptor; M_1, cholinergic receptor; NK_1, neurokinin receptor; R/O, rule out.

Table 15.1 Common changes in force or timing of vomiting and potential pathology.

Force or timing of vomiting	Suggested pathology
Following abdominal palpation	Peripheral receptor input to vomiting
Passive effort (no outward sign)	Gastric or esophageal
Undigested food (≥6 hours post meal)	Gastric atony, pyloric obstruction
Projectile vomiting	Pyloric or upper duodenal ileus or obstruction

Table 15.2 Typical characteristics of small bowel versus large bowel diarrhea.

Small bowel	Large bowel
Projectile	"Pudding" consistency
Liquid	Mucus
Large volume	Hematochezia
Melena, steatorrhea	Few systemic alterations
Signs of systemic illness	Smaller volume
Systemic acid–base alterations	Tenesmus
Significant loss of	Increased frequency
Fluids	
Proteins	
Electrolytes	

of the diarrhea can help differentiate between these two anatomical locations (Table 15.2). Small bowel disease typically has more significant clinical consequences, with substantial fluid, electrolyte and protein loss, than does large bowel disease. Therefore, where the GI problem is located could influence the intensity of diagnostic, therapeutic, and monitoring efforts.

A report of restlessness, reluctance to lie down or any evidence of pain upon touching the abdominal region can direct diagnostic efforts to rule out potentially life-threatening problems such as GDV, mesenteric volvulus, septic peritonitis, or necrotizing pancreatitis. Exposure to medications (i.e., antibiotics, anticholinergics) or toxins (i.e., numerous plant toxins, cleaning agents, and chemicals) with GI side effects or medications that have potential GI toxicity (i.e., nonsteroidal-antiinflammatory medication and steroids)

is important historical information. A review of current prescription and over-the-counter medications might reveal recent treatment with protein pump inhibitors or gastroprotectants, as well as oral medications that can be seen on radiographs (bisthmus subsalicylate, Pepto-Bismol®).

Feeding habits should be explored, with focus on the degree of appetite and when the pet last ate normally. Information regarding the type and consistency of the food, any prescription diets, a recent change in content, brand or bags/cans, or treats and access to table scraps (human food) or trash can provide important information to guide diagnostics. Rarely, contamination of pet foods occurs in commercial diets, followed by a recall of the food. If the history warrants further investigation, there are internet resources available to alert the clinician to current and common pet food recalls (Table 15.3).

Physical examination

Physical examination findings attributable to the GI tract typically start with assessment of temperature, pulse, and respiration. Fever combined with GI signs will direct efforts toward treating infectious, inflammatory or septic conditions. Hypothermia can be a consequence of shock, with poor perfusion due to GI fluid loss. Heart and pulse rate, combined with mucous membrane color, pulse intensity and capillary refill time, provide a reflection of peripheral perfusion, often affected by substantial acute fluid and electrolyte loss into the GI tract. Chronic fluid losses can cause dehydration without impacting perfusion, resulting in tacky or dry mucous membranes with mild dehydration and prolonged skin tent or sunken eyes with more severe dehydration. Increased respiratory rate and effort can be a consequence of aspiration of vomitus, pain or acute respiratory distress syndrome secondary to sepsis associated with GI disorders.

Direct examination of the GI tract begins with the oral cavity, pharynx, and teeth [5]. Hypersalivation, discharge or malodor from the oral cavity can suggest gingivitis or systemic metabolic disease. Tooth health is evaluated as a source of infection or anorexia. Abnormalities in the integrity of the jaw and bite could reflect traumatic injury or renal secondary hyperparathyroidism, or neuromuscular disorders, such as tetanus or (masseter) muscle myositis. Oral mucous membrane, tongue or gingival discoloration, ulcers or masses are recorded. Evaluation of the sublingual area may reveal ulceration, injury, ranulas or string foreign bodies. The pharynx is then examined externally by palpation or visualized orally following sedation if disease is suspected in this area, such as pharyngeal dysphagia.

Abdominal examination should focus on the presence of discomfort, distension, organ abnormalities, and GI sounds. Abnormalities can be detected on abdominal palpation in both dogs and cats, and include cranial organomegaly (liver or spleen enlargement), a distended urinary bladder, masses, intestinal impaction with feces, GI foreign material, increased intestinal thickness, and a gravid uterus. In cats, large or small kidneys and an enlarged spleen may also be differentiated. If the abdomen is generally distended, the clinician should palpate and ballot to differentiate between fat, free abdominal fluid, abdominal muscle weakness or organ enlargement. A positive fluid wave requires a large volume of fluid (40 mL/kg) to be present [6].

Abdominal pain is a significant finding and should be differentiated from spinal pain or generalized pain or anxiety. The pain is then localized as cranial, midabdominal, caudal or generalized abdominal pain. A review of the organs located in that abdominal region can direct diagnostic efforts. This physical finding could indicate severe problems and warrants timely testing, including radiographs, ultrasound, and laboratory analysis, including abdominal fluid analysis [7].

Auscultation of the abdomen should be done at least twice daily for patients with potential GI disorders. Listening with a stethoscope directly under the abdomen is preferred in smaller patients, and a four-quadrant approach is used when listening to larger dogs. If no GI sounds are heard within two minutes, ileus is present and warrants concern for mechanical or functional obstruction. Increased GI sounds can signify hypermotility.

The rectal examination completes the examination of the caudal abdomen. The prostate in males, cervix or caudal uterus in females, urethra and aortic pulse should be palpated ventrally. Anal sacs are examined at the 4 and 8 o'clock positions and should be easily expressed. Sublumbar lymph nodes should be palpated dorsally. Masses, strictures or other pelvic canal abnormalities such as perineal hernias should be identified as well as anal tone noted. The character of the rectal mucosa and pelvic and sacral bone structure are also noted. Fecal character is evaluated to determine if constipation, obstipation or diarrhea is present. Melena and hematochezia can be indicative of significant increases in intestinal permeability or the first sign of a coagulation disorder [1,2]. Point of care testing in the ICU can guide initial stabilization and diagnostic testing.

Point of care diagnostics

Point of care diagnostics can not only provide invaluable information on the cause of GI disturbance, but may also help determine the severity of disease and direct urgent care.

Minimum database

The minimum database will provide the initial POC testing and consists of a packed cell volume (PCV), total protein (TP), blood urea nitrogen (BUN), blood glucose, electrolytes, blood gas, and coagulation profile. Hemoconcentration due to severe dehydration or third body fluid spacing can elevate the PCV and TP. A PCV ≥60% with little to no increase in protein concentration and acute onset of raspberry jam-like bloody diarrhea should prompt consideration of hemorrhagic gastroenteritis (HGE) in dogs [8]. Blood in the stool or vomitus necessitates assessment of coagulation, to include platelet estimate, prothrombin time, and activated partial thromboplastin time. Severe inflammation of the GI tract can cause albumin loss and lower the TP. Blood glucose can be decreased with sepsis, neonatal malnutrition, hypoadrenocorticism, xylitol toxicity or severe liver dysfunction [7]. Elevations in BUN with concentrated urine suggests dehydration and renal hypoperfusion, digested blood in the GI tract, a high-protein diet, or postrenal obstruction [9]. Anorexic animals with diarrhea often present with significant electrolyte changes, including sodium (Na^+), chloride (Cl^-), potassium (K^+), and magnesium (Mg^{++}) loss. Hyperkalemia with hyponatremia should prompt consideration of adrenocortical insufficiency or whipworm (*Trichuris vulpis*) infection, both of which can present with diarrhea [7]. Hypokalemia is the most common electrolyte abnormality in the vomiting patient [5].

Acid–base status trends towards metabolic acidosis due to intravascular volume deficits associated with vomiting, diarrhea or third body fluid spacing. However, metabolic alkalosis in concert with hypochloremia with or without hyponatremia and hypokalemia points to gastric outflow or high duodenum obstruction. Rarely, patients with gastrinomas or with frequent unrelenting vomiting without obstruction will also develop metabolic alkalosis [5].

Fecal examination

A fecal examination is done as a POC test for patients with diarrhea (especially in younger animals). A direct fecal exam in addition to zinc sulfate centrifugation should be performed. In dogs with diarrhea within the United Sates, 29.6% of those less than six months of age had intestinal parasites, while those greater than one year of age had a 6.1% prevalence of parasites. Whipworms, however, seem to be the only parasite detected with increased frequency in dogs over six months of age, attributable to the long prepatent period and lack of direct transmission from dams to pups [10]. Similar to dogs, the prevalence for the majority of parasites is highest in cats less than six months of age. Hookworms and tapeworms, however, are more commonly found in cats between one and five years of age [11].

Giardia and *Trichuris* can be difficult to identify, requiring multiple fecal examinations or other modalities to make the diagnosis. Enzyme-linked immunosorbent assays can be used as POC snap tests to detect canine parvovirus, *Giardia* spp., and *Cryptosporidium parvum* antigens. Repeat fecal examination is also important, since as many as 41.5% of all treated cats and dogs with a history of parasites are positive for at least one parasite on repeat fecal examination following treatment [11].

Initial clinicopathological testing

A complete blood cell count (CBC), serum biochemistry, and urinalysis are evaluated. Ideally, blood and urine are collected prior to intravenous fluid administration. Neutropenia prompts testing for parvoviral enteritis, but can also be associated with other causes of viral enteritis, sepsis or infection with *Salmonella* spp. Leukocytosis with immature neutrophils (bands) is a common finding with systemic infection or inflammation. A stress leukogram featuring leukocytosis with lymphopenia and eosinopenia is a nonspecific finding, common with gastroenteritis in any debilitated animal. A normal leukogram in a systemically ill patient should prompt an adrenal corticotropin stimulation test for adrenocortical insufficiency [7].

A complete serum biochemical profile will evaluate concurrent organ dysfunction. The BUN, creatinine, and urinalysis can indicate renal dysfunction as a cause of uremic GI ulceration. Hyperphosphatemia, when renal function is normal, can occur with massive cell necrosis, such as GI thrombosis, torsions or entrapment. Amylase and lipase blood tests provide very little insight into the etiology of GI distress. SNAP canine (or feline) pancreatic lipase testing is more sensitive and specific for pancreatitis, but false negatives and positives are common. Positive canine pancreatic lipase levels have been detected in dogs with heart disease, hyperadrenocorticism, renal disease, ehrlichiosis and obesity [12–16]. Levels of amylase, lipase, and canine-specific pancreatic lipase on abdominal fluid tests may provide additional insight in dogs suspected of having pancreatitis [17]. Elevated blood ammonia (NH_3) levels may indicate severe liver dysfunction or portosytemic shunting, which can lead to signs of hepatic encephalopathy, vomiting or diarrhea. Portovascular anomalies may lead to severe GI distress, GI ulcerations, and sepsis. Blood ammonia levels should be run immediately (or stored on ice, separated from red blood cells (RBCs)) to avoid false elevation due to production by aging RBCs, or false decrease in samples exposed to air [18–20]. Elevation of NH_3 levels should prompt additional diagnostics of liver function.

Other fecal diagnostics

Inflammatory changes on a fecal smear can provide indication for fecal culture or bacterial PCR testing. Fecal culture, however, can be insensitive, with only 10.8% of dogs with diarrhea having positive cultures for pathogens, some of which are potentially false positives [21]. Acid-fast staining can also be used to confirm *Campylobacter jejuni* on a fecal smear [7]. Real-time fecal PCR

testing is also available in dogs and cats and detects toxin genes or organisms associated with disease with increased sensitivity over fecal culture. The results can be confounding, however, as virtually all of the tested bacteria, including *Campylobacter* spp., *E. coli*, *Salmonella* spp. and *Clostridium* spp. have been isolated from clinically healthy dogs and cats [22]. Of concern, however, is the potential impact of zoonotic bacterial infections on human health. Zoonotic bacteria include *Salmonella* spp., *Campylobacter* spp., *Clostridium difficile*, *Shigella* spp., and *Yersinia enterocolitica* [7,22].

Abdominal effusions

Abdominal effusion occurs in patients as a consequence of increased capillary hydrostatic pressure, decreased capillary oncotic pressure, vascular permeability, obstruction of lymphatic drainage or a combination of these factors. When the effusion is of a large quantity, fluid can be collected by the four-quadrant abdominocentesis technique. Ultrasound-guided centesis or a diagnostic peritoneal lavage (Box 15.1) are necessary to collect fluid from specific abdominal locations or when the quantity of fluid is small [23].

Abdominal imaging should be performed prior to abdominal fluid collection techniques to avoid the iatrogenic introduction of peritoneal air during the procedure. Fluid collected should be placed in an EDTA tube for cytology, a serum tube for chemistry analysis, and a sterile tube for culture. If the sample is hemorrhagic, it should not clot. Clotting is often seen with inadvertent parenchymal organ puncture and, less commonly, peracute hemoabdomen [23]. A focused abdominal sonogram for trauma (AFAST) scan is sensitive for the diagnosis of abdominal fluid accumulations after trauma (Figure 15.2) [24].

Diagnostic peritoneal lavage (see Box 15.1) can prove helpful when diagnosing focal abdominal disease, such as septic peritonitis, which has been compartmentalized by omentum. Biochemical test results of the fluid must be interpreted in light of the dilution of the sample [23].

Fluids obtained by direct paracentesis can be classified as a transudate, modified transudate or exudate based on cell count and total protein analysis [23]. A transudate is extravascular fluid with low protein content and low cell counts. It typically results from increased capillary hydrostatic pressure or diminished capillary colloidal osmotic pressure. The few cells present are typically mononuclear cells. An exudate is an extravascular fluid with high

---

Box 15.1 Steps to perform a diagnostic peritoneal centesis and lavage.

1. The urinary bladder is emptied by ultrasound-guided cystocentesis or a urinary catheter is placed.
2. With the patient in dorsal recumbency, a skin site 2–3 cm caudal to the umbilicus is clipped and prepared with aseptic scrub. Local anesthetic is placed in the skin, subcutaneous tissue, and muscle at the site of catheter insertion.
3. A peritoneal dialysis catheter (for lavage) or a fenestrated 20 G or 18 G over-the-needle catheter (for therapeutic or diagnositic centesis) is introduced at the prepared skin site and directed towards the pelvic inlet.
4. Gentle aspiration of the catheter is performed and any fluid recovered saved for analysis.
5. If no fluid is retrieved, warmed (body temperature) 0.9% sodium chloride is infused (20–22 mL/kg) is infused. The catheter is capped off and the animal allowed to stand and move around.
6. The catheter is then aspirated with the animal standing, when possible, and the recovered fluid saved for analysis.

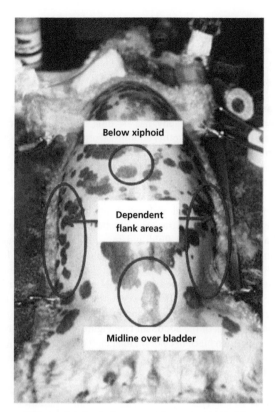

Figure 15.2 Focused abdominal sonogram for trauma (AFAST) scan. The areas outlined by the red circles provide a high yield for demonstrating free abdominal fluid. This may be performed in lateral or dorsal recumbency.

protein content and/or high cell counts; it implies vascular damage, inflammation, infection or hemorrhage.

A portion of the recovered fluid is centrifuged and a cytological preparation made of the pellet (exudates with high cell counts may be examined with a direct smear). Romanowsky-type staining (Diff-Quik® Stain Kit, Imeb, San Marcos, CA) can be used for cytological evaluation and a gram stain can be performed if bacteria are present to help direct antibiotic therapy. Cytology of the fluid may show evidence of inflammation (white blood cells (WBCs)), infection (bacteria, especially if intracellular), and GI rupture (fibers from plants, meat or other sources). Cytological evaluation alone is up to

87–100% accurate in dogs and cats in making the diagnosis of septic peritonitis [25,26]. Aspiration of bowel loop contents could lead to observation of free bacteria and create a false impression of septic peritonitis. Therefore, the presence of intracellular bacteria or other infectious agent is key to making that diagnosis [23].

Bile peritonitis can also be confirmed when cytology demonstrates phagocytosis of golden-green-blue granular pigment by inflammatory cells. However, not all patients with bile peritonitis will have these cytological abnormalities. When the total bilirubin of the abdominal fluid is twice that of serum, the diagnosis of bile peritonitis is likely [27]. However, hemolysis in either sample can elevate the bilirubin result and must be considered when interpreting results [23].

Other biochemical testing of abdominal fluid can include quantification of glucose, lactate, creatinine, and potassium. Abdominal serum amylase and lipase levels have been proposed for the diagnosis of pancreatitis, but have not been validated at this time [23]. The author recommends using the supernatant of the spun abdominal fluid sample on a dry chemistry analyzer for these tests, as POC tests calibrated for whole blood have not been validated for abdominal effusion.

A study evaluated abdominal fluid glucose concentration compared to serum concentration in companion animals. It was found that a decrease of 20 mg/dL or greater in abdominal fluid glucose to serum glucose was 100% sensitive and specific for the diagnosis of septic peritonitis in dogs. In cats, the same gradient was 86% sensitive and 100% specific in dogs [28]. In the same study, a small number of dogs had a blood-to-fluid lactate difference of −2.0 mmol/L which was also 100% sensitive and specific for a diagnosis of septic peritoneal effusion [28]. Interestingly, degenerate neutrophils and glucose and lactate levels after celiotomy seem to be unreliable predictors of septic peritonitis. A sudden increase in fluid volume, neutrophil quantity, and/or intracellular organisms may be required to diagnose septic peritonitis in postoperative patients [29]. Other patient-specific parameters of clinical deterioration may be necessary to make the diagnosis. The results from an abdominal fluid sample that provide support for surgical intervention are listed in Table 15.4.

An abdominal fluid creatinine to peripheral blood creatinine ratio greater than 2.0 in the dog and cat is a highly sensitive and specific indicator of uroperitoneum. An abdominal fluid potassium to peripheral blood potassium ratio of 1.4 in dogs and 1.9 in cats is also supportive of uroperitoneum [30,31]. Aerobic and anaerobic cultures and susceptibility of abdominal fluid should be submitted based on cytological evidence of an inflammatory process [23,25,26].

Table 15.4 Abdominal fluid sample evaluation.*

Parameter	Significant alteration	Indication of
PCV	$\geq$5% increase on repeated sampling	Ongoing hemorrhage
WBC**	>20 000, increasing with repeated sampling	Septic abdomen, severe inflammation or necrosis
Differential**	Predominant cell is neutrophil (>90%)	As above
Cytology**	Intracellular bacteria, hypersegmented and vacuolated WBC, plant or meat fibers	As above
Amylase	>200 IU activity, increasing with repeated lavage	Severe pancreatitis, pancreatic abscess or necrosis
Lipase	Greater than the lipase in the serum, increasing with repeat sampling	As above
Bilirubin	Greater in abdominal fluid than serum	Ruptured biliary tract
Creatinine	Greater in abdominal fluid (2×) than serum	Ruptured urinary tract
Potassium	Greater in abdominal fluid (1.4×) than serum	As above
Glucose	Greater in serum than abdominal fluid*	Septic abdomen

* Postoperative free abdominal fluid evaluation has not shown a high diagnostic yield in dogs [29].
** Test results also valid for abdominal lavage fluid samples.
PCV, packed cell volume; WBC, white blood cell.

Imaging

The patient must be stabilized prior to performing potentially stressful imaging procedures. Fluid resuscitation with appropriate analgesia and/or sedation in addition to oxygen supplementation are provided as indicated and continued throughout the imaging procedure [23].

Radiography and contrast procedures

Radiography is rapid and readily accessible. Images compatible with pancreatitis, generalized ileus, aerophagia, and free abdominal fluid can direct the need for specific diagnostic or therapeutic procedures. Disorders that require surgical intervention, such as GDV (compartmentalization of stomach gas), linear foreign material (small bowel plication with C-shaped small intestine gas pockets), uterine distension in nongravid animals, and rupture of hollow viscus or abdominal wall perforation (free abdominal gas) can also be quickly identified [23]. However, radiographic changes may not be diagnostic for other surgical conditions such as nonlinear (particularly textile) foreign body obstruction, intussusception, and mesenteric or other organ volvulus. Assessment of small intestinal diameter width to lumbar vertebra 5 height ratios have also been examined in several studies [32,33] but do not necessarily offer additional information. If an abnormal intestinal pattern is present, contrast studies, repeating the radiographs in 6–12 hours or alternative imaging modalities may provide further information if the patient is stable.

Gastrointestinal contrast studies may be appropriate for ruling out small bowel obstruction in selected patients. A negative contrast gastrogram (10–30 mL/kg of air inserted through a nasogastric tube) may outline a gastric foreign object. The air is suctioned out following the study, and the tube may be fixed in place for monitoring and therapeutic purposes. When there is no evidence of GI perforation, 30% barium sulfate suspension (Liquid E-Z-Paque®, E-Z-EM Canada Inc.) may be administered orally or through a nasogastric or orogastric tube at a dose of 10–12 mL/kg; confirmation of tube placement must be performed prior to administration of barium. The risk of barium aspiration pneumonia exists, and necessitates that contrast be administered cautiously in patients with impaired swallowing reflex, gastric distension or persistent vomiting [23,34]. Lateral and ventrodorsal radiographic views are taken at 0, 15, 30, 60, 90, 120, and 180 minutes after administration or until the contrast agent reaches the colon [24].

When the possibility of GI tract perforation exists, an iodinated contrast agent, such as diatrizoate sodium (Hypaque® Sodium Oral Powder, Nycomed, Princeton, NJ), is chosen instead of barium, and administered as a 30% solution at an oral dose of 2–20 mL/kg. Note, however, that an increased frequency of radiographs may be required since iodinated contrast agents hasten small intestinal transit time (normal time is 3–4 hours in dogs and 1–4 hours in cats) [23]. Ultrasound is an important alternative to consider when a GI perforation is suspected.

In patients with a history of trauma, it may be important to determine the integrity of the abdominal compartment. Diaphragmatic tears (without herniation) may not be evident on plain radiographs and a positive contrast peritoneogram may be considered. A peritoneal catheter is placed and 1 mL/lb (2.2 mL/kg) of water-soluble contrast agent is injected into the peritoneal space. Leakage of the contrast outside the normal abdominal cavity often warrants surgery, to reduce organs to their normal position and to prevent organ entrapment or ischemia. Peritoneal contents which herniate into the thorax causing stomach entrapment or evidence of GI leakage warrant immediate surgical intervention.

Thoracic radiographs should be evaluated for evidence of cardiorespiratory disease, esophageal disease or foreign body, and aspiration pneumonia. Thoracic radiographs can also screen for acute lung injury, acute respiratory distress syndrome, metastatic neoplasia, enlarged lymph nodes, and mass lesions [23].

Ultrasound

Abdominal ultrasonography has become an invaluable tool to evaluate the GI tract and other abdominal organs. Though operator dependent, ultrasound of the stomach, small intestine, and colon can aid in diagnosing obstructive lesions, inflammation, and neoplastic disease. Gas can preclude complete visualization of portions of the GI tract, so ultrasound can frequently be useful in concert with abdominal radiographs, where gas can help to delineate disease [35].Ultrasound can be used to retrieve peritoneal and retroperitoneal fluid and to aspirate or biopsy various abdominal structures. Doppler ultrasound can assess for blood flow to a particular organ or structure [23].

The abdominal focused abdominal sonogram for trauma (AFAST) is a rapid and efficient way for even inexperienced ultrasonographers to identify free abdominal fluid. The probe is placed in four positions of the abdomen (see Figure 15.2) to identify free fluid (most often black in color on image). If only a scant amount of fluid is noted, rechecking in 6–12 hours is advised as fluid may continue to accumulate and be more accessible.

CT scan

Computed tomography (CT) imaging offers superior tissue contrast. Helical CT provides multiple sections imaged simultaneously, significantly reducing scan and anesthetic time [36]. In companion animals, abdominal CT has been beneficial in defining liver, spleen, pancreatic, adrenal gland and urinary tract anomalies and parenchymal organ perfusion [37]. Acute necrotizing pancreatitis has been differentiated from nonnecrotizing pancreatitis using CT.

Endoscopy

Endoscopy enables the visualization of the mucosal surface of the pharynx, esophagus, stomach, upper duodenum, rectum, and colon. Biopsies can also be taken during this procedure when indicated. In addition, it becomes an important tool for noninvasive removal of selected esophageal or gastric foreign bodies.

Virtual endoscopy of the esophagus and stomach has been simulated using helical CT. Advantages of this included visualization of gastric surfaces from any angle, quantitative lesion measurement with three-dimensional (3D) software processing, increased speed and the differentiation of intramural and extramural lesions. Limitations of the CT virtual image include retention of fluid or solid food obscuring anatomy, inability to obtain information regarding mucosal color and texture, and an inability to obtain biopsies or retrieve gastrointestinal foreign material [38].

Exploratory laparotomy

Surgical exploration still has an important role in critical care medicine when other diagnostic methodology has not provided the necessary information or other diagnostic methods are limited or unavailable. The decision to progress to anesthesia in a critical patient must be weighed thoughtfully. Common indications for exploratory laparotomy are listed in Box 15.2. In the event that no definitive cause of the GI disorder is determined, visualization at surgery provides a direct assessment of organ structure with biopsies taken of all appropriate tissues, whether or not they are

Box 15.2 Indications for timely abdominal exploratory.

- Lack of a diagnosis in a deteriorating patient
- Free abdominal air (in closed abdominal cavity)
- Bacteria seen within WBCs in abdominal fluid
- Plant fibers seen in free abdominal fluid or DPL fluid
- Significant or continued abdominal hemorrhage
- Torsion or entrapment of abdominal organ(s)
- Evidence of organ ischemia
- Penetrating abdominal foreign bodies or wounds
- Failure to respond to medical therapy
- Rupture of a major abdominal organ
- Debridement of infected wounds, muscles, fascia
- To relieve intestinal obstruction
- Perforation of abdominal organ
- To obtain biopsies
- Postoperative acute abdominal pain
- Nonpenetrating bite wounds of the abdomen with crushing injury

DPL, diagnostic peritoneal lavage; WBC, white blood cell.

grossly abnormal. When vomiting or diarrhea is the primary clinical problem, biopsies of the stomach and small intestinal segments (duodenum, jejunum, and ileum) will provide histopathological evidence of the health of the tissues sampled. Large bowel biopsies are indicated only when disease is localized to this section of bowel [23]. Other organs from which samples may be collected include the liver, gallbladder, pancreas, kidneys, lymph nodes, and bladder wall.

Equipment-based patient monitoring

Monitoring for complications of vomiting can include electrocardiogram (ECG) for arrhythmias associated with a vasovagal reflex, blood pressure for perfusion changes associated with shifts in intravascular volume or electrolyte changes, and arterial blood gas or pulse oximetry to assess oxygenation concerns associated with possible pulmonary infiltrates, most commonly from aspiration pnuemonia. Monitoring the central venous pressure (CVP) can follow trends of change in intravascular volume. The amount of fluid and air retrieved from the nasogastric (NG) tube can provide insight into the volume of fluid lost through third body fluid spacing into the stomach as well as an indirect impression of gastric motility.

The muscosal surfaces of the GI tract have a relatively high blood flow and have been used as an indicator of tissue perfusion in shock. The measured tissue carbon dioxide (CO_2) levels and calculated tissue pH of the GI tract have been correlated with various shock parameters and have provided a means for early detection of shock in a variety of models [39,40]. Gastric tonometry, sublingual or buccal capnography, orthogonal polarization spectral imaging (OPSI), and sidestream dark field (SDF) technologies have been evaluated using a portion of the GI tract, but, at this time, have not been widely adapted for the veterinary clinical setting.

Gastric tonometry has been used as a monitoring tool in shock and sepsis. The procedure requires the insertion of a special nasogastric tube with a saline- or gas-filled balloon at the tip. The thin wall of the balloon allows the partial pressure of carbon dioxide (pCO_2) of the gastric mucosa to equilibrate with the contents of the balloon tip. The pCO_2 of the saline in the balloon tip is measured and the pH is subsequently calculated and expressed as pHi. The pHi has been correlated with tissue perfusion parameters such as lactate and cardiac index. The results are therefore assessed as a reflection of blood flow to the stomach. Although gastric tonometry

has demonstrated that a normalization of pHi is associated with therapeutic success, it has fallen out of favor in human ICUs since the results have not impacted outcome [41].

Sublingual or buccal capnometry is another attractive methodology for monitoring a portion of the GI tract in patients with shock. Tissue capnometry directly measures CO_2 levels of the sublingual or buccal mucosa. The results have been correlated with the severity of shock and have been used as a guide for resuscitation procedures in experimental animals [42–45]. The procedure has been shown to provide useful information in a variety of studies, and could become an important monitoring tool in the future.

Visual microcirculatory evaluation of superficial capillary beds continues to gain recognition as an effective technology to monitor capillary perfusion of the GI tract. OPSI and SDF technologies use various energy wavelengths to optimize visualization of hemoglobin flowing through a capillary bed. This allows the operator to observe and measure the microcirculation. Video and still images are collected. Data can then be calculated that reflects the density and heterogenicity of the capillary beds. This technology is being evaluated as a guide for resuscitation of septic patients [46–48]. OPSI is in its clinical infancy and its clinical application has yet to be defined.

Gastrointestinal disorders

The most common clinical evidence of a GI disorder is vomiting or diarrhea. The mechanism and cause of each are extensive and warrant separate consideration. Impaired GI motility and loss of the protective mucosal barrier can occur as a cause or a consequence of GI disease. When GI disease causes enlarged intraabdominal organs or dramatic abdominal fluid accumulation within the closed cavity, intraabdominal hypertension can occur. Each can cause patient deterioration and life-threatening complications, such as massive fluid, protein and electrolyte loss, bacterial translocation, blood loss, severe pain, and eventually death.

Vomiting

The vast array of underlying diseases, and the number of medications that can cause vomiting, make vomiting a possible complication in every ICU patient. Poor perfusion, dehydration, electrolyte imbalance, and acid–base disorders are critical complications to be anticipated. Esophagitis, aspiration pneumonia, and malnutrition are serious secondary problems that can severely compromise the recovery of the patient from the underlying disorder [5]. The physical act of vomiting can be exhausting to the patient, and when the vagus nerve is stimulated, bradycardia ensues. Loss of consciousness and cardiac arrest can occur secondary to this vasovagal reflex. Knowledge of the cause and suspected mechanism initiating vomiting is important for providing timely and appropriate therapy.

Vomiting evolved as a protective means to remove toxic or noxious ingesta from the GI tract. The emetic center provides the neurological initiation of the vomiting action and is composed of several nuclei located in the medulla oblongata of the brainstem. It is rich in serotonergic ($5HT_3$), adrenergic (α_2), and neurokinetic (NK_1) receptors which can be activated one of three ways: by direct stimulation, by humoral signaling secondary to blood-borne substances activating the chemoreceptor trigger zone (CRTZ) or through other neuronal pathways leading to the emetic center (see Figure 15.1). The neuronal pathways include vagal, sympathetic, vestibular, and cerebrocortical afferents or the nearby nucleus tractus solaris pathways.

Each can be activated by peripheral receptors located throughout the body [5]. Commonly, the underlying disorder will activate more than one mechanism to stimulate vomiting.

The GI tract contains the largest number of peripheral receptors (mostly $5HT_3$ and NK_1 receptors) on vagal afferent neurons, with the duodenum having the highest concentration. The presence of inflammatory or cytotoxic substances will activate release of serotonin or substance P, which then activates $5HT_3$ or NK_1 receptors, respectively [5]. Vomiting can also be triggered by peripheral receptors in the kidneys, uterus, and urinary bladder whose sympathetic nerves send afferent impulses to the emetic center. The pharynx and tonsillar fossa use the afferent fibers of the glossopharyngeal nerve to trigger vomiting.

Substances in the circulating blood directly activate the CRTZ located in the fourth ventricle of the brain; this is devoid of the blood–brain barrier. The CRTZ contains dopaminergic (D_2), cholinergic (M_1), histaminergic (H_1), $5HT_3$, α_2, and NK_1 receptors, which can trigger afferent neurons to the emetic center. Cats differ from dogs in that they have poorly developed D_2 and H_1 receptors, while α_2 receptors are more important than in the dog. This is the reason why xylazine and dexmedetomodine (α_2 agonists) can be administered to cause emesis in the cat while apomorphine and endogenous histamine are less effective in that species [5].

Vestibular pathways pass through the CRTZ en route to the emetic center. The vestibular pathway contains M_1, H_1, and NK_1 receptors which can be triggered by motion sickness, inner ear inflammation or cerebellar lesions.

The underlying causes of vomiting, therefore, include not only primary GI tract disorders (such as intestinal foreign body, gastritis) but also systemic disease and lesions of non-GI organs containing peripheral receptors for vomiting. These secondary GI problems can include metabolic disease (such as uremia, liver failure, pancreatitis, sepsis), central nervous system disease (such as elevated intracranial pressure, vestibular disease), stretch or inflammation of organ serosa or submucosa (such as acute splenic torsion, uterine torsion), and drugs or toxins that stimulate the CRTZ [5]. A list of the more common causes of vomiting in the critical ICU patient is given in Table 15.5.

The cause and suspected mechanism(s) initiating vomiting should guide the selection of the antiemetic(s) most appropriate for the patient. A list of antiemetics, their site of action, recommended dose, and potential side-effects is presented in Table 15.6.

General guidelines for treating the ICU small animal patient with vomiting are presented in an algorithm (see Figure 15.1). The treatment strategy begins with restoring and maintaining perfusion with intravenous infusion of crystalloids. The addition of hydroxyethyl starch encourages intravascular fluid retention, and should be considered in patients with significant third body fluid spacing (see Chapter 2). It is not uncommon for patients to continue to have significant continued fluid losses when reperfusion of the GI occurs. Maintenance fluid therapy with the crystalloid, sometimes in combination with colloid may require higher than anticipated fluid volumes in the vomiting patient; continued fluid therapy should include replacement, maintenance, and ongoing losses when calculated. Frequent monitoring of patient peripheral perfusion parameters, heart rate, blood pressure, CVP, and physical hydration parameters is vital for making timely adjustments to fluid infusion rates to meet the needs of the patient. Electrolyte and acid–base status are evaluated. Patients with hypochloremic metabolic alkalosis are treated with 0.9% sodium chloride as the initial crystalloid of choice. Glucose is supplemented as necessary for hypoglycemia. Antiemetics are selected based on the estimated mechanism(s) that are stimulating the vomiting center, the receptor(s) most likely being affected (see Figure 15.1), the route of administration, and duration of action and potential side-effects of the antiemetic.

Nasogastric tubes provide a simple, rapid, and inexpensive means of decompressing the stomach to minimize risk for continued emesis and aspiration pneumonia, monitor fluid losses, and allow early enteral nutrition. The NG tube should be suctioned every 2–6 hours, depending on the rate of fluid or gas accumulation. The quantities of gas and air are recorded to follow trends of accumulation and to get an impression of gastric emptying. Often a critical animal will not stop vomiting until gastric decompression has reduced peripheral receptor input. Gastric protectant drugs (Table 15.7) are used when gastric erosions or ulcers are anticipated (see Mucosal ulceration below).

Table 15.5 Common general causes of vomiting in the ICU small animal patient.

Primary GI problems	Seondary GI problems
Inflammation	Pancreatic pathology
Infection	Hepatic pathology
Foreign body	Biliary pathology
Ulceration	CNS disease
Gastric or bowel ischemia	Vestibular disease
Gastric or bowel distension	Motion sickness
Ileus	Peritonitis
Dietary indiscretions	Systemic infection
Dietary allergies	Systemic inflammation
Ingested toxins	Systemic medications
Administered medications	Renal pathology
GI parasites	Metabolic disease
GI distension	Distension of capsule or serosa of spleen or liver
Herniation\performation of GI tract	Urinary bladder, gallbladder, uterus distension
Intusussception	Heartworm disease (cats)
Gastric or mesenteric volvulus	Hypoadrenocorticism
	Hyperadrenocorticism
	Hyperthyroidism (cats)
	Toxicity

CNS, central nervous system; GI, gastrointestinal.

Table 15.6 Antiemetics commonly administered in veterinary medicine with their receptor, site of action, dose, and side-effects. Adapted from [5,8,50].

Drug	Receptor antagonists	Site of action	Dose	Side-effects
Chlorpromazine	α_2, D_2, M_1, H_1	CRTZ, emetic center	0.05–0.5 mg/kg IV, IM, SC q 8–12 h	Hypotension, sedation
Prochlorpromazine	α_2, D_2, M_1, H_1	CRTZ, emetic center	0.1–0.5 mg/kg, IM, SC q 8–12 h	Hypotension, sedation
Metoclopramide	D_2 (low dose), $5HT_3$ (high dose)	CRTZ	0.1–0.5 mg/kg IV SC, IM, PO q 8–12 h or CRI 1–2 mg/kg IV q 24 h	Gastric prokinetic, extrapyramidal effects if overdosed
Ondansetron	$5HT_3$	CRTZ, emetic center, vagal afferents	0.5–2 mg/kg IV, PO q 12–24 h	Decreases efficacy of tramadol
Dolasetron	$5HT_3$	CRTZ, emetic center, vagal afferents	0.6–1 mg/kg IV, SC, PO q 24 h	
Maropitant	NK_1	CRTZ, emetic center, vagal afferents, vestibular	1 mg/kg SC q 24 h or 2–6 mg/kg PO q 24 h	
Meclizine hydrochloride	H_1	CRTZ, vestibular	2–10 mg/kg up to 10 kg or 2–6 mg/kg over 10 kg PO q 24 h	Sedation, dry mouth

CRI, constant rate of infusion; CRTZ, chemoreceptor trigger zone.

Table 15.7 Gastroprotective medications, their mechanism of action, dose, and other notes. Adapted from [8,50].

Drug	Mechanism of action	Dose	Comments
Famotidine	Histamine$_2$-receptor antagonist	0.5–1 mg/kg q 12–24 h PO, IV, IM, SC	Reduce dose with renal impairment, possible hemolytic reaction with rapid IV infusion in cats
Calcium Carbonate	Binds with HCl to form neutral salts and water	25–50 mg/kg/day PO q 6–12 h	Short duration of action
Omeprazole	Proton pump inhibitor	0.5–1 mg/kg q 24 h PO	Must give delayed-release tablets whole Elevation in gastric pH decreases absorption of pH-dependent drugs (ketoconazole, digoxin) and may prolong elimination of drugs eliminated by CYP450 (cyclosporine, diazepam, phenytoin, warfarin, theophylline, propranolol)
Pantoprazole	Proton pump inhibitor	1 mg/kg q 24 h IV or 1 mg/kg bolus then 0.1 mg/kg/h	Lower potential for adverse drug events vs omeprazole but potential for similar drug interactions most effective acid-blocker
Sucralfate	Sucrose sulfate and aluminum hydroxide salt	0.25–1 g PO q 8 h	No adverse effects. Requires acidic environment for efficacy. Can impair absorption of other drugs so provide 2 hours in between other medication administration
Misoprostol	Prostaglandin analogue	2–5 µg/kg PO q 12 h	Less effective at decreasing intraluminal pH than famotidine; absorbed drug reaching the intestine can cause intestinal secretion, smooth muscle contraction, and subsequent diarrhea

Diagnosis and treatment of the underlying cause of vomiting are essential once the patient is stable. There is a potential for serious complications in any vomiting patient. A list of complications with recommended monitoring procedures can include vagsovagal reflex and bradycardia (ECG, heart rate), aspiration pneumonia (respiratory rate and effort, pulse oximetry), hypotension (heart rate, blood pressure, peripheral perfusion physical parameters, CVP), hypoglycemia (blood glucose), acid–base imbalances (blood gas), electrolyte imbalances (blood electrolytes), and bacterial translocation with sepsis (body temperature, mentation, blood glucose, blood pressure, white blood cell count).

Diarrhea

Diarrhea is a common problem in the critical ICU patient. Underlying disorders responsible for patient admission to the ICU (such as parvovirus enteritis, hemorrhagic gastroenteritis, heat stroke, and severe traumatic shock) can result in massive fluid loss and electrolyte alterations secondary to diarrhea. However, diarrhea can also be a consequence of hospitalization and treatment. For example, the initiation of enteral feeding with a high-fat diet, the administration of drugs that slow GI motility or irritate the bowel, and the development of stress colitis can each result in diarrhea.

Most of the digestion and absorption of nutrients occurs within the small bowel, making these segments of the GI tract eminently important to the health of the patient. Malabsorption and maldigestion are therefore typically problems of the small bowel. The large bowel is responsible for removing water and key nutrients from the waste material and transporting the unwanted material for excretion. The colon produces mucus to provide lubrication of the fecal material to aid in expulsion.

There are four mechanisms responsible for the formation of diarrhea, occurring alone or in combination:
- the presence of osmotically active particles in the intestinal lumen
- excessive solute secretion by the intestinal mucosa
- impaired absorption of water and solutes by the intestinal mucosa
- intestinal motility disorders [1,49].

Osmotic diarrhea occurs when fecal water content increases as a result of the presence of nonabsorbable solutes in the GI tract. Overeating, sudden diet changes, maldigestion or malabsorption can all contribute. Secretory diarrhea can be stimulated by enteric hormones, fatty acids, bile acids, and pathogenic bacterial endotoxins (which enhance bowel secretions). Gastrointestinal pathogens known to stimulate secretory diarrhea include *Staphylococcus aureus*, *Escherichia coli*, *Klebsiella pneumoniae*, *Salmonella typhimurium*, *Campylobacter* spp., *Yersinia enterocolitica*, and *Clostridium perfringens* [49].

Damage to the GI mucosal barrier will impair sodium and water reabsorption, potentiating the loss of water, electrolytes, and proteins into the intestinal lumen. Cells sloughed from the damaged intestinal wall can contribute an osmotic mechanism to the diarrhea, as well [49]. Hemorrhagic diarrhea represents a loss of mucosal integrity and predisposes to bacterial translocation and sepsis [2].Finally, decreased GI motility can affect intestinal transit time and result in insufficient absorption of water, proteins, nutrients, and electrolytes, causing diarrhea.

It is important to differentiate between small bowel and large bowel diarrhea when considering etiology as well as the consequences of the diarrhea to the patient (see Table 15.2). Small bowel diarrhea results in more dramatic fluid, electrolyte, protein, and acid–base alterations compared to large bowel diarrhea. The disorders that cause small bowel diarrhea are typically more severe than the more common causes of large bowel diarrhea. Large volumes of liquid diarrhea passed without urgency are signs of small intestinal diarrhea. Steatorrhea and melena can also occur from small bowel lesions. Loss of body weight and condition is expected with chronic small intestinal diarrhea due to insufficient absorption of nutrients. Hematochezia and mucus secreted around the fecal material are typical of large bowel diarrhea. Tenesmus and increased frequency of smaller quantities of stool are also signs of large bowel diarrhea [5]. Diarrhea not improving in 14 days or episodic diarrhea is considered chronic.

Parvovirus diarrhea and HGE are two of the most common causes of hemorrhagic diarrhea in dogs in the ICU. The HGE syndrome in dogs causes acute hemorrhagic small bowel diarrhea, acute dehydration, and poor perfusion. Hallmarks of the syndrome include acute onset, significant dehydration, blackberry jam consistency diarrhea, and elevated PCV with normal or low TP, likely due to enteric blood loss and splenic contraction. The cause is unknown, but *Clostridium perfringens* overgrowth may be a contributing factor in some patients. Both causes of hemorrhagic diarrhea can be fatal without aggressive supportive therapy [8].

The therapeutic goals for treating diarrhea in an ICU patient should include:
- restoration of perfusion and hydration
- correction of significant electrolyte and acid–base disorders
- treatment of the underlying cause of the diarrhea
- elimination of any factors contributing to the cause of diarrhea.

Care is taken to isolate animals with potentially contagious (such as parvovirus, feline panleukopenia) or zoonotic (such as *Campylobacter* spp. or *Salmonella* spp.) causes of diarrhea.

The intravascular administration of crystalloids will restore perfusion and interstitial fluid balance. The addition of hydroxyethyl starch as a colloid will promote intravascular retention of the crystalloid. This reduces the amount of crystalloid available to extravasate into the GI lumen and contribute to diarrhea. The choice of crystalloid will be guided by the electrolyte status. Potassium supplementation may be required once perfusion has been restored. Significant GI hemorrhage can necessitate transfusion with blood products in the most severe cases. Significant hypoproteinemia may warrant supplementation with plasma products.

Treatment of the underlying cause might involve administration of anthelmentics for intestinal parasites, glucocorticosteroids and mineralocorticoids for hypoadrenocorticism, or surgical removal of a mass or foreign body. The indication for antibiotics with diarrhea is controversial. The large numbers of normal resident anaerobic bacteria provide some protection to the gut. Anaerobic gut bacteria live in the mucous layer next to the epithelial cells and serve to prevent adherence of enteric pathogens [2].

Because of this, the use of antibiotics may not be justified as a treatment for simple diarrhea.

However, for patients with evidence of loss of intestinal mucosal barrier integrity, for instance with severe hemorrhagic diarrhea, parenteral bactericidal antibiotic therapy is warranted with the goal of eliminating enteric bacteria which have translocated into the systemic circulation. Positive blood cultures and fecal cultures can further help to tailor specific antibiotic therapy [7]. Initial antibiotic selection in these critical situations should address the potential for gram-positive and -negative aerobic and anaerobic bacterial species.

Intestinal protectants (such as bismuth subsalicylate or barium) have been used in an attempt to coat the gastric and upper duodenal mucosa and reduce diarrhea. Metronidazole has antibacterial and antiinflammatory effects and is useful in the treatment of inflammatory bowel disease in dogs and cats. The metronidazole is generally administered at 10–20 mg/kg in dogs and 5.0–7.5 mg/kg in cats twice daily. Lower doses are chosen for patients with hepatic insufficiency; patients should be monitored for neurological signs that may develop with high cumulative doses.

Colonic motility modifiers are sometimes employed to manage diarrhea, but are not a common addition to therapy in the ICU patient. It is difficult to determine whether or not motility is a component of the cause of diarrhea, calling into question their value in the ICU. The primary agents used are opioids, including diphenoxylate and loperamide [50]. Diphenoxylate hydrochloride is a meperidine derivative with μ-receptor effects on the GI wall, stimulating smooth muscle segmentation, decreasing peristalsis, and increasing fluid absorption. Systemic opiate effects can occur due to blood–brain barrier penetration, giving it the potential for abuse and a schedule V drug designation. Bitter atropine is often present in combination to decrease abuse potential and to dry salivary secretions. Doses are 0.1–0.2 mg/kg PO q 8 hours in dogs and 0.05–0.1 mg/kg PO q 12 hours in cats [50]. Loperamide hydrochloride is a butyramide derivative with μ-opioid agonist activity similar to diphenoxylate, though it does not cross the blood–brain barrier or cause systemic opioid effects. Doses are 0.08–0.2 mg/kg PO q 8–12 hours in dogs and 0.08–1.16 mg/kg PO q 12–24 hours in cats [50].

Motility disorders

The most important GI delayed motility disorders of small animals can impact the esophagus (megaesophagus), stomach (gastric distension), small intestine (ileus and mechanical obstruction) or colon (constipation) [41]. Mechanical obstruction, primary enteritis, postsurgical pseudoobstruction, hypoadrenocorticism, severe electrolyte abnormalities, nematode infection, intestinal sclerosis, and radiation enteritis have been described in dogs and cats as causes of decreased small intestinal motility. The sequelae include pain, fluid, electrolyte and acid–base disorders, and overgrowth of resident bacteria with potential for bacterial translocation.

The enteric nervous system (ENS) is part of the autonomic nervous system and controls the neural pathways for GI motility [51]. It is able to function without input from the spinal cord or the cephalic brain. Sensory neurons monitor for changes in luminal activity such as distension, chemistry (pH, osmolarity, specific nutrients), and mechanical stimulation. They stimulate interneurons that then stimulate efferent secretomotor neurons. These can stimulate a wide range of effector cells, to include smooth muscle cells, epithelial cells that secrete or absorb fluids, submucosal blood vessels, and enteric endocrine cells. Acetylcholine is the primary neurotransmitter in the ENS.

The motor activity of the GI tract performs three primary motor functions: segmental contractions (nonpropulsive "churning" movements of the luminal contents), propulsion (progressive wave of relaxation followed by contraction), and sphincter tone (coordinated activity of smooth muscle to allow hollow organs to hold luminal contents). Feeding stimulates both churning and propulsion of the small intestines. These activities are regulated largely by ENS neural and hormonal stimuli. Modulation of intestinal smooth muscle is largely a function of calcium concentration (Ca^{++}). Agonists regulate Ca^{++} through G-protein receptor-initiated release of intracellular calcium or the opening and closing of calcium channels [51]. Drugs such as calcium channel blockers or anticholinergic agents can therefore have a significant and negative effect on GI motility.

Vomiting and diarrhea are the most common clinical signs indicating a GI motility disorder. However, reduced or absent motility in the critical ICU patient can occur without causing any specific outward physical signs and still negatively impact patient recovery. The cause can be a primary lesion of the GI tract or can occur as a consequence of metabolic changes (such as calcium alterations, hypokalemia, ischemia), inflammatory mediators, dietary changes or drugs that affect the smooth muscle contraction, ENS stimulation or blood flow to the GI tissues.

Esophageal dilation and dysfunction

Megaesophagus is a condition where esophageal peristalsis is abnormal and the esophagus is enlarged. Regurgitation is the primary clinical sign. Chronically affected patients may have a thin body condition. True megaesophagus can be a congenital condition (often secondary to persistent right aortic arch), secondary to diseases such as hypothyroidism, myasthenia gravis or other inflammatory myopathies or systemic lupus, compared to esophageal dilation and dysfunction which can occur in any critically ill patient secondary to anesthesia or sedation, electrolyte abnormalities, hypoglycemia, GDV, esophagitis, or esophageal foreign bodies, lead toxicity, etc.

Megaesophagus and esophageal dilation can complicate the medical management of any critical patient due to the difficulty in providing enteral nutrition and the high possibility of aspiration pneumonia and esophagitis.

A complete neurological exam is done to identify any neurological deficits or neuromuscular dysfunction associated with causes of megaesophagus (such as myasthenia gravis, inflammatory myopathies, systemic lupus erythematosus) [5]. Cervical and thoracic radiographs are needed to evaluate for generalized esophageal dilation, esophageal foreign bodies or masses, thymoma or focal esophageal dilation (as seen with stricture or vascular ring anomaly). Radiographs also screen for aspiration pneumonia. Contrast radiography, endoscopy, and/or videofluoroscopy can be done for further esophageal assessment. Once megaesophagus has been identified, additional clinicopathological testing is performed to include complete thyroid profile, adrenocorticotropic hormone stimulation test, acetylcholine receptor antibody test, lead level assay, and antinuclear antibody titer [5].

Therapy for megaesophagus should target the underlying pathology and address secondary complications such as aspiration pneumonia (see Chapter 8) and esophagitis. Dietary modification, including feeding small frequent meals from an elevated position, can be used to reduce regurgitation. The best food consistency for each patient will vary, requiring that semisolid, solid, soft, and liquid diets are tested. Holding the patient's forelimbs upright after they have eaten, with gentle coupage, may help stimulate the movement of food down the esophagus and into the stomach. Bailey chairs may be helpful but require training.

Gastroprotectant drugs (see Table 15.7) will raise the pH of the gastric fluid and are used to reduce the occurrence of reflux esophagitis when regurgitation is occurring. Cisapride and metoclopramide (see Table 15.8) may enhance lower esophageal sphincter pressure and tone [5]. Celecoxib, a cyclooxygenase-2 (COX-2) inhibitor, has been shown to increase the lower esophageal pressure in dogs without impacting gastric emptying time [51]. Celecoxib and other COX-2 inhibitors warrant further investigation for the treatment of esophageal hypomotility [52].

Gastric distension

Gastric distension can occur from an excess of gastric contents, such as food bloat or aerophagia, or from problems causing abnormal gastric motility and emptying. Disorders of gastric emptying can arise from mechanical obstruction, poor motility or a combination of both. Clinical signs typically manifest as either vomiting or nonproductive vomiting, and, often, abdominal distension. Undigested or partially digested food vomited 6–8 hours after eating suggests gastric outflow obstruction or gastric paresis as the cause [5]. Mechanical obstruction of the pylorus can occur due to foreign bodies, malignancy, gastric torsion or volvulus, and pyloric hypertrophy.

The causes of abnormal gastric motility are more complex, occurring secondary to gastric neuronal or smooth muscle dysfunction. The end result is uncoordinated or ineffective contractions between the antrum, pylorus, and duodenum. Primary conditions causing gastric hypomotility include gastric infectious or inflammatory diseases, mucosal ulceration, and postsurgical gastroparesis [53]. Secondary conditions impacting gastric motility include metabolic disorders (uremia, hypoglycemia), electrolyte disturbances (hypokalemia, hypercalcemia), acute stress, acute abdominal or peritoneal inflammation and prescribed drugs (cholinergic antagonists, adrenergic agonists, and opioids) [53]. Dogs recovering from gastric dilation and volvulus have been shown to experience gastric neuronal and smooth muscle abnormalities causing delayed gastric emptying [54].

The presence of gastric distension can cause serious complications in the critical ICU patient. Effective peristalsis is not possible in the widely dilated stomach. In the most critical patients with GDV, compromise to gastric blood flow is prominent and will cause gastric tissue hypoxia and eventually necrosis. The enlarged stomach can prevent full expansion of the diaphragm and restrict ventilation and oxygenation. Gastric compression of the vena cava can impair venous return to the heart, reducing cardiac output. Splenic engorgement can occur as arterial blood is pumped into the spleen but venous outflow is limited due to gastric compression. The stomach will begin to serve as a third body fluid space with fluids, electrolytes, and proteins extravasating from the damaged gastric capillaries into the lumen of the stomach. Aspiration of gastric fluid or materials into the trachea should be anticipated, with aspiration pneumonia potentially becoming a life-threatening problem. Silent aspiration is possible (no outward signs of regurgitation), with vasovagal reflex a potential result.

Treatment of gastric distension will incorporate restoration of systemic perfusion, correction of electrolyte disorders, gastric decompression, treatment of underlying disorders, and medical management of gastric motility using smooth muscle prokinetic agents (Table 15.8) [53]. Gastric decompression can expose the general circulation to the locally produced cytokines and vasoactive mediators formed during tissue hypoxia, making intravascular fluid support prior to decompression crucial for an optimal result. Lidocaine infusions have been advocated for GDV patients to

Table 15.8 Mechanism, site of activity, indications, and doses of gastrointestinal motility modifying drugs [50].

Drug classification/ mechanism	Sites of activity	Indications	Dose	Other properties
Dopaminergic (D_2) antagonists				
Metoclopramide	GES, stomach, intestine, CRTZ	Vomiting, gastroesophageal reflux, delayed gastric emptying, ileus/ pseudoobstruction	0.2–0.5 mg/kg PO, IV q 8 h 0.01–0.02 mg/kg/h IV CRI	α_2-adrenergic antagonist β_2-adrenergic antagonist 5-HT_4-serotonergic agonist 5-HT_3-serotonergic antagonist
Serotonergic (5-HT_4) agonists				
Cisapride	GES, stomach, intestines, colon	Gatroesophageal reflux, delayed gastric emptying, ileus/ pseudoobstruction, constipation, chemotherapy-induced vomiting	0.1–0.5 mg/kg PO q 8 h	5-HT_3- serotonergic antagonist 5-HT_1- serotonergic antagonist 5-HT_2- serotonergic agonist
Motilin-like drugs				
Erythromycin	GES, stomach, intestines, colon	Gastroesophageal reflux, delayed gastric emptying, constipation (dogs)	0.5–1.0 mg/kg PO/IV q 8 h	5-HT_3- serotonergic antagonist
Acetylcholinesterase inhibitors				
Ranitidine	Stomach, colon	Delayed gastric emptying, constipation	1.0–2.0 mg/kg PO q 8–12 h	H_2-histaminergic antagonist
Nisatidine	Stomach, colon	Delayed gastric emptying, constipation	2.5–5.0 mg/kg PO q 8 h	H_2-histaminergic antagonist
µ-Opioid agonist				
Loperamide hydrochloride	Intestines, colon	Inhibits GI motility and prokinetic propulsion (antidiarrheal)	0.08–0.2 mg/kg PO q 8–12 h in dogs and 0.08–1.16 mg/ kg PO q 12–24 h in cats	Bloat and sedation, paralytic ileus; use in cats is controversial
Diphenoxylate	As above	As above	0.1–0.2 mg/kg PO q 8 h in dogs and 0.05–0.1 mg/kg PO q 12 h in cats	As above

BID, twice daily; CRTZ, chemoreceptor trigger zone; GES, gastroesophageal sphincter; 5-HT, 5-hydroxytryptamine; IV, intravenous; PO, per os; QID, four times daily; SID, once daily; TID, three times daily.

decrease arrhythmias, acute kidney injury, and hospitalization time [55], though some studies have not validated these properties [56]. Oxygen supplementation may be beneficial during the IV administration of crystalloids sometimes in combination with hydroxyethyl starch, which are infused to restore perfusion. The colloids will aid in minimizing extravasation of additional fluids into the stomach. Once perfusion has been restored, electrolyte disorders can be addressed. Gastric decompression can be accomplished by external gastric trocarization or placement of an orogastric or nasogastric tube.

Trocarization can be done using a short large-bore needle or over-the-needle catheter on the left or right cranial dorsolateral abdomen. The clinician should introduce the trocar in the area with the greatest tympany, after aseptic skin preparation [8]. Orogastric intubation is another means of gastric decompression used when solid material is filling the stomach. However, heavy sedation or general anesthesia is required. Endotracheal intubation is essential during this gastric decompression and lavage procedure to reduce the risk of aspiration pneumonia. The orogastric tube length is marked to the level of the last rib, lubricated, and gently passed to the premeasured mark. Esophageal, pharyngeal, and oral regions must be suctioned following orogastric lavage.

Decompression and removal of gas and fluid using a NG tube require minimal or no sedation and the tube can be secured in place and used to maintain decompression while the underlying disorder is being treated (Figure 15.3). Intermittent suctioning of the NG tube allows removal of gastric fluid and air to keep the stomach empty and minimize gastric contents available for reflux into the trachea. A low-pressure suction device, such as the Thorovac® (Andersen, Haw River, NC), can be attached to the NG tube for continuous decompression. This is an option when intermittent syringe suctioning has been inadequate to relieve gastric pressure or high volumes of gastric fluid are recovered. The NG tube will also

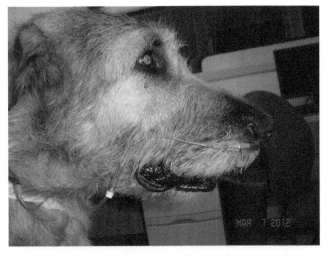

Figure 15.3 A nasogastric tube that has been secured using a suture in the nasal planum and lateral aspect of the maxilla followed by a collapsing Chinese finger trap.

facilitate direct gastric feeding, important for the return of motility, and administration of oral medications.

Ileus

Ileus, also called paralytic ileus or adynamic ileus, is the temporary absence of normal contractile movements of the intestinal walls, caused by the failure of peristalsis rather than by mechanical obstruction. It can be generalized, affecting the entirety of the small or large intestines, or segmental when only a local portion of the intestine is affected. Generalized ileus commonly occurs for 24–72 hours after abdominal surgery, particularly when the intestines have been manipulated. Ileus may also be caused by peritonitis or other abdominal inflammatory conditions. It commonly accompanies inflammatory bowel diseases such as parvovirus diarrhea or hemorrhagic gastroenteritis. Disorders outside the intestine, such as kidney failure, hypothyroidism or electrolyte disorders (such as hypokalemia or hypercalcemia), may cause ileus as well. Drugs, especially opioid analgesics and anticholinergic drugs, are a common cause.

Ileus will provide a site for significant third body fluid spacing in the critical patient. Tissue and capillary fluids, proteins, and electrolytes will extravasate into the distended, poorly contracting, and often inflamed bowel. Vascular compromise of the intestines and bacterial translocation are of immediate concern.

Treatment is initiated by stabilizing perfusion with IV fluid therapy. The addition of hydroxyethyl starch as a colloid can reduce the amount of water available to extravasate into the third body fluid space. Electrolyte disorders are corrected and analgesics used that have minimal effect on GI motility. It is important to identify and treat any cause of mechanical obstruction prior to treating with prokinetic drugs. Once mechanical obstruction has been eliminated as a problem, prokinetic drugs (see Table 15.8) are administered followed by enteral feeding early in the treatment process [53].

Constipation

Constipation refers to bowel movements that are infrequent or hard to pass and is a common cause of painful defecation. Severe constipation includes obstipation (failure to pass stools or gas) and fecal impaction. The colon is responsible for the reabsorption of water from the feces. In the ICU patient, severe dehydration and impaired patient mobility can predispose to constipation. Other causes of constipation include obstructed defecation and colonic hypomotility. This can progress to bowel obstruction and become life threatening. Causes of hypomotility include diet, hormonal disorders such as hypothyroidism, side-effects of medications, and rarely heavy metal toxicity. English Bulldogs, Boston Terriers, and Manx cats are predisposed to constipation if malformation of the sacral spinal cord is present. Perianal fistulas in German Shepherd dogs can precipitate dyschezia and constipation. Megacolon is most common in middle-aged male cats while intact male dogs may have prostatomegaly that predisposes to constipation [5].

Tenesmus and dyschezia are common signs of constipation, requiring evaluation for both intraluminal (colonic neoplasia, inflammatory polyps, foreign bodies, strictures) and extraluminal (pelvic fractures, extraluminal masses, organomegaly) causes [5]. Megacolon in cats provides a classic example of colonic hypomotility. In cats with megacolon, 96% of cases of obstipation are accounted for by idiopathic megacolon (62%), pelvic canal stenosis (23%), nerve injury (6%), or Manx sacral spinal cord deformity (5%) [57]. A smaller number of cats have megacolon as a complication of colopexy (1%) and colonic neoplasia (1%). Colonic hypo- or aganglionosis is suspected in another 2% of cases [57].

Mild episodes of constipation cause straining and abdominal discomfort. Systemic dehydration in a critical patient can trigger significant colonic water reabsorption, leaving dry and impacted fecal material. Initial management incorporates systemic rehydration and deobstipation. Moderate or recurrent episodes may require medical intervention such as dietary modification, water enemas, oral and/or suppository laxatives or osmotic agents such as lactulose and colonic prokinetic agents (see Table 15.8). Patients with intermittent or recurrent constipation should be evaluated for underlying diseases (such as renal disease or hyperthyroidism).

Disorders of mucosal integrity

The mucosal lining of the GI tract consists of the epithelial layer as well as an underlying layer of loose connective tissue known as the lamina propria. This underlying layer contains capillaries, enteric neurons, immune cells, and a thin layer of smooth muscle. The surface area of the epithelial layer is amplified by microvilli on the epithelial cell surface, evagination of the epithelial layer to form villi, and invagination to form crypts. A mucus layer overlies the entire intestinal epithelium. The majority of microorganisms in the lumen of the bowel can be found in the outer mucous layer. However, there is an inner, protected, and unstirred layer directly adjacent to the epithelial surface that is relatively sterile. The sterility is due to the high concentration of antimicrobial proteins that play a crucial role in maintaining the intestinal mucosal barrier. Bacteria are further sequestered within the mucus through secretion of immunoglobulin A (IgA). Local B-cells produce bacteria-specific IgA to trap them in the mucus or opsonize luminal bacteria that have internalized into the lamina propria [58].

The intestinal epithelial cells, however, are by far the most important part of the mucosal barrier. These cells form a continuous monolayer and include enterocytes (absorptive), goblet cells (mucus secreting), enteroendocrine cells (produce GI hormones), and Paneth cells (secretory, antimicrobial). At the apical surface of the villi, the enterocytes possess microvilli that form a brush border containing digestive enzymes and transporter receptors for metabolism and uptake of dietary antigens (incompletely digested food particles). The enterocyte must transport water and desired nutrients while maintaining an effective barrier to harmful macromolecules and microorganisms. Water, low molecular weight molecules, and small ions cross between the epithelial cells (paracellular route) while larger molecules pass through the epithelial cell (transcellular route). Tight junction complexes link the intercellular spaces between adjacent epithelial cells. The tight junctions expressed at the crypt are more permeable to larger molecules (radius up to 50 angstrom) while villous tight junctions only allow smaller molecules (<6 angstrom) to pass. The transcellular route occurs through pinocytosis or selective receptor-mediated endocytosis. Many of the molecules entering by the transcellular route are degraded by intracellular lysosomes [58].

Damage can occur from direct insult to the mucus or epithelial layer of the mucosal barrier from causes such as heat stroke, ingestion of caustic materials, infectious agents such as internal parasites, parvovirus or other enteral viral infections, overgrowth of pathogenic GI bacteria, GI neoplasia or inflammatory bowel disease. The presence of cytokines systemically or within the bowel wall can alter the interepithelial tight junctions and impair the normal intestinal selectivity. Any condition that causes an interruption of blood flow to the bowel, even when transient, can alter the intestinal epithelial barrier. Problems such as severe hypotension and shock (splanchnic vasoconstriction), mesenteric thrombosis, severe bowel distension or organ torsion are potential causes. Medications (such as glucocorticosteroids and nonsteroidal antiinflammatory drugs) and the stress of illness can also interrupt capillary flow and result in damage to the mucosa.

The GI signs of increased mucosal permeability can vary and include inappetance, vomiting with blood, diarrhea (with or without blood), abdominal distension, ileus and even the passing of mucosal strands in the diarrhea. Systemic signs that can result from alterations in the GI epithelial barrier include poor perfusion, dehydration, anemia, peripheral edema, fever, depression, abdominal pain, and abdominal distension. Disruption to any portion of the epithelial barrier can lead to poor uptake of nutrients, loss of water, proteins and electrolytes into the bowel, impaired GI motility and uptake of pathogens and endotoxins into the systemic circulation.

Treatment of disorders causing a breakdown of the mucosal barrier should incorporate the following:

- restore perfusion and hydration
- provide adequate analgesics
- restore electrolyte imbalances
- treat the inciting cause
- provide broad-spectrum bactericidal antibiotic support if bacterial translocation is likely
- maintain GI tract decompression
- promote GI motility
- start early enteral feeding to provide nutrients for the restoration of the epithelial layer [59,60].

The loss of albumin is anticipated. Resuscitation with a combination of crystalloid and hydroxyethyl starch colloid can promote fluid retention within the vasculature and reduce the amount of fluid available to extravasate into the bowel lumen through the damaged mucosal barrier.

Mucosal ulceration

An ulcer is formed when there is damage to the mucosal epithelial barrier that is focal and deep enough to cause bleeding. Critically ill humans undergoing mechanical ventilation, coagulopathy, shock, trauma or multiple organ failure have been found to have an increased risk for developing stress ulcer formation. The same risk factors are expected with dogs and cats [59]. Hemodynamic compromise predisposes to GI ulcerations and hemorrhage. Mucosal hypoperfusion in concert with decreased GI motility during shock leads to increased contact time for gastric acid and other harmful substances [59]. There is also a reduction in prostaglandin synthesis, decreasing mucous and bicarbonate secretion. Upon restoration of GI blood flow, reactive oxygen species can cause cell death [59]. Additional causes of GI ulceration in the ICU patient include nonsteroidal antiinflammatory or corticosteroid administration, severe renal and hepatic disease, infiltrative GI disease, neoplasia (especially gastrin-producing tumors), and the stress of illness and hospitalization [60].

The incidence of stress-related mucosal disease has not been established in veterinary patients, but is between 6% and 100% of critically ill human patients, typically occurring within 24 hours of hospitalization [59–63]. Stress-related ulcer disease is a spectrum from stress-related injury with superficial diffuse mucosal erosions and insignificant bleeding to stress-related ulceration with focal ulcers penetrating into the submucosa. The latter carries an increased risk of bleeding that could require blood transfusion and hemodynamic stabilization [64].

Making a diagnosis of GI hemorrhage is the first step to diagnosing ulcers. Clinical signs can be obvious, such as blood aspirated from an NG tube or the patient having hematemesis or melena. These patients must be evaluated for the presence of a coagulation disorder. The diagnosis of an ulcer is based on visualization of mucosal surfaces through endoscopic evaluation of the esophagus, stomach, and duodenum or at the time of surgical exploratory [59]. Biopsies are taken to detect an underlying cause such as neoplasia.

The key to treating GI ulceration is similar to the steps taken to prevent stress ulcer formation, and includes:

- optimizing splanchnic perfusion
- monitoring for sepsis
- establishing early enteral nutrition
- pharmacological intervention to modify intralumninal pH and support the natural mucosal defense system [60].

A gastric pH >4 is the target to prevent stress ulcers from forming, while a gastric pH >6 is targeted in patients with ulcers that have active bleeding or are at high risk for hemorrhage [62,64,65]. Therapeutic interventions such as gastric cold water lavage and surgical resection of ulcers are options to stop ongoing hemorrhage in patients with gastric ulceration. Pharmacotherapy for treatment of ulcers includes medications that reduce gastric pH, provide a protective barrier (see Table 15.7), increase prostaglandin levels, and increase motility (see Table 15.8).

Abdominal compartment syndrome

As defined in humans by the World Society on Abdominal Compartment Syndrome, abdominal compartment syndrome (ACS) is defined as a sustained intraabdominal pressure >20 mmHg (>27.2 cmH$_2$O) which is associated with new organ dysfunction or failure, with or without an abdominal perfusion pressure of <60 mmHg [66]. Abdominal compartment syndrome occurs when:

- tissue fluid within the peritoneal and retroperitoneal space (edema, retroperitoneal blood or free fluid in the abdomen) accumulates in such large volumes that the abdominal wall compliance threshold is crossed and the abdomen can no longer stretch
- there is a decrease in compartmental volume in the abdomen
- there is an increase in externally applied pressure on the abdomen.

Once the abdominal wall can no longer expand, any further fluid leaking into the abdominal tissues or cavity results in fairly rapid rises in the pressure. If the pressure continues to rise over 20 mmHg and organs begin to fail, the intraabdominal hypertension has now progressed to the end-stage of the highly fatal process termed abdominal compartment syndrome.

The syndrome is characterized by compression of the vena cava causing decreased venous return and ventricular filling, and subsequent decreased cardiac output. Excursion of the diaphragm is reduced, causing decreased functional residual capacity in the lungs. Increases in intrathoracic pressure also occur which compress the cerebral venous outflow tract. This in combination with decreased cardiac output can result in decreased cerebral perfusion pressure. As pressure in the abdomen rises, blood flow to organs decrease and urine output drops as the renal veins and urinary collecting system are directly compressed. In the GI tract, there is impaired healing and GI wall edema, while hepatic blood flow is also diminished [67].

The causes of ACS have been categorized as primary (treatment requiring surgery or interventional radiology), secondary (medical intervention), and recurrent. The underlying cause of the disease process is capillary permeability caused by the systemic inflammatory response syndrome (SIRS). In humans, common conditions causing abdominal compartment syndrome include patients receiving high volumes of IV crystalloids for resuscitation, undergoing mechanical ventilation, severe abdominal or pelvic injury, and emergency laparotomy procedure. Gastrointestinal perforation, bile peritonitis, abdominal masses, and pregnancy have also been documented as associated with abdominal compartment syndrome [67].

The World Society on Abdominal Compartment Syndrome has established an intraabdominal hypertension grading system (Table 15.9) to establish a uniform designation for the severity of intraabdominal pressure elevations [66].

In veterinary medicine, the measurement of intraabdominal pressures is in the early stages of discovery. Experimentally, normal intraabdominal pressures are 1.5–5.1 mmHg (2–7 cm H$_2$O) in dogs [58] and 3.8–6.5 mmHg (5.2–8.8 cmH$_2$O) in cats [68]. A few studies have documented intraabdominal hypertension post laparotomy in

Table 15.9 Intraabdominal hypertension grading system from the World Society on Abdominal Compartment Syndrome.

Grade of intraabdominal hypertension	Intraabdominal pressure
Grade I	12–15 mmHg (16.3–20.4 cmH$_2$O)
Grade II	16–20 mmHg (21.8–27.2 cmH$_2$O)
Grade III	21–25 mmHg (28.6–34 cmH$_2$O)
Grade IV	>25 mmHg (>34 cmH$_2$O)

Box 15.3 Steps to measure intraabdominal pressure.

1. Place a Foley urinary catheter.
2. Attach a three-way stopcock to the catheter and then to a sterile urinary collection system.
3. A water manometer is attached to the first stopcock and is leveled with the symphysis pubis.
4. The second stopcock is attached to a 250 mL bag of 0.9% NaCl with an attached 20–35 mL syringe to empty the bladder.
5. To obtain a measurement, the urinary bladder is emptied and 0.5–1 mL/kg of saline is instilled into the urinary bladder.
6. The manometer is then filled with saline.
7. The intraabdominal pressure is measured where the meniscus equilibrates, minus the zero level difference.

Optimal patient position has not been established, but must remain the same between measurements for comparison [71,72]. In cats, right lateral recumbency seems to yield a higher pressure than sternal recumbency [71,73].

dogs or with disease that resulted in a visibly distended abdomen [69]. In addition, ACS has been documented in a dog with babesiosis [70] and cats with experimental chronic obstructive pancreatitis [71]. A method for measuring intraabdominal pressure in small animals using a water manometer is similar to performing a CVP measurement and is described in Box 15.3.

The treatment for ACS involves decompression, often warranting a decompressive laparotomy with management of an open abdomen. However, prevention of ACS is preferred to emergency surgery, which can further exacerbate the inflammatory response and worsen the patient's condition [67]. If identified early, intraabdominal hypertension may be decreased before ACS occurs. Options that have been used in human medicine include gastric decompression, rectal decompression with enemas, urinary decompression, changing body position, the use of diuretics, hemodialysis and the use of sedation, analgesia or neuromuscular blockade to increase abdominal wall compliance [72].

Humans with intraabdominal hypertension who develop ACS have a 20% survival rate [73]. The survival rate in small animal patients with ACS is unknown. If a small animal patient is considered at risk for developing ACS, preventative measures such as an epidural to relax abdominal muscles, NG tube placement, enemas and a urinary catheter can each be used as noninvasive decompressive measures. Surgical decompression with open abdomen should be considered in veterinary patients when ACS is confirmed [67].

Nutrition

The majority of patients with increased mucosal permeability will benefit from early enteral feeding (see Chapter 16). Early enteral nutrition improves nitrogen balance, wound healing, and host immune function, augments cellular antioxidant systems, decreases

hypermetabolic response to tissue injury, and preserves intestinal mucosal integrity. Studies demonstrate better preservation of lymphocyte, neutrophils, and gut-associated immune function, aiding the host defense mechanism, in enterally fed humans and animals [74]. Clinically, this results in decreased length of hospital stay and a lower incidence of in-hospital infections [74]. There are selected cases that may benefit from starvation for 12–48 hours, such as those with mild secretory and osmotic diarrhea, since the absence of nutrients in the GI tract reduces secretions and osmotically active particles [7]. However, the vast majority of patients will benefit from therapeutic nutrition.

Dogs with parvovirus that received early enteral nutrition by nasoesophageal tube had a return of appetite and cessation of vomiting and diarrhea one day earlier than those animals fasted 12 hours beyond cessation of vomiting. The dogs receiving early enteral feeding also experienced significant weight gain and decreased mortality. Gut permeability testing in those dogs suggested improved gut barrier function limiting bacterial translocation [75]. Similarly, in dogs with septic peritonitis where nutrition was instituted within 24 hours postoperatively, significantly less time in the hospital (1.6 days) was required in comparison to those fasted over 24 hours postoperatively [76].

Certain dietary components may also influence GI recovery. Glutamine is considered a nonessential amino acid in health, but becomes conditionally essential in states of illness or injury. In these states of catabolism, amino acids, most importantly glutamine and arginine, are released from muscle and provide a source of fuel for intestinal enterocytes as well as leukocytes and macrophages. Glutamine is rapidly depleted from the body as it is the preferred energy source for enterocytes during stress and plasma levels can remain depleted for up to three weeks post illness or injury. Although glutamine supplementation has shown some promise in human medicine [77,78], the optimal quantities of glutamine supplementation and the indication for supplementation have yet to be determined in veterinary medicine.

Arginine is an essential amino acid and is an intermediary in the urea cycle, with a deficiency resulting in high blood NH$_3$ and hepatic encephalopathy. Cats have increased susceptibility to arginine deficiency and develop clinical signs of deficiency more rapidly than dogs [79]. Lower levels in dogs with critical illness appear to negatively impact survival [80]. In humans, arginine levels were reduced in trauma and postoperative patients but not in patients with sepsis. Supplementation of arginine in nonseptic critically ill patients appears to improve outcomes [81].

However, arginine does not appear to be decreased in patients with sepsis and supplementation is suspected to induce nitric oxide synthase (iNOS) from activated myeloid cells, promoting the production of nitric oxide. In sepsis, excess nitric oxide can potentiate hypotension and organ dysfunction. In canine sepsis, arginine administration resulted in increased plasma arginine, increased nitric oxide and worsened shock, organ dysfunction, and mortality. Therefore, the provision of arginine to patients with sepsis is not recommended [82]. The reader is referred to Chapter 16 for further information.

Feeding tubes

Nasosophageal (NE) and NG tubes offer an advantage over more invasive tubes, since they can be placed with minimal or no sedation. Nasogastric tubes can facilitate gastric decompression, enteral drug administration, and initiation of enteral feedings. Liquid medications and diets are typically required due to tube diameter size [83,84]. Recently, a study comparing dogs with various diseases fed by either

NE or NG tubes did not identify a difference in complication rate between the two methods of feeding. The study groups, however, were small and not matched for disease severity [85]. Another study demonstrated that cats with acute pancreatitis tolerated NG feeding well with minimal complications [86]. Various tubes used for enteral nutrition are discussed in Chapter 16.

References

1. Guilford WG, Center SA, Strombeck DR, Williams DA, Meyer DJ. Strombeck's Small Animal Gastroenterology. Philadelphia: Saunders, 1996: p 351.

2. Grenvik A, Ayres SM, Holbrook PR, Shoemaker WC. Textbook of Critical Care. Philadelphia: Saunders, 2000: p 1621.

3. Turner JR. Intestinal mucosal barrier function in health and disease Nature Rev Immunol. 2009;9:799–809.

4. Zhi-Yong S, Yuan-Lin D, Xiao-Hong W. Bacterial translocation and multiple system organ failure in bowel ischemia and reperfusion. J Trauma Acute Care Surg. 1992;32(2):148–53.

5. Ettinger SJ, Feldman EC, eds. Textbook of Veterinary Internal Medicine: Diseases of the Dog and the Cat, 7th edn. St Louis: Elsevier Saunders, 2010: pp 2–9, 189–209.

6. Herold LV, Devey JJ, Kirby R, Rudloff E. Clinical evaluation of hemoperitoneum in dogs. J Vet Emerg Crit Care 2008;18(1):40–53.

7. Hackett TB. Gastrointestinal complications of critical illness in small animals. Vet Clin North Am Small Anim Pract. 2011;41(4):759–66, vi.

8. Silverstein D, Hopper K. Small Animal Critical Care Medicine. Philadelphia: Elsevier Health Sciences, 2008: pp 558–62.

9. Stockham SL, Scott MA. Fundamentals of Veterinary Clinical Pathology. Ames: Iowa State Press, 2002: pp 298–96.

10. Little SE, Johnson EM, Lewis D, et al. Prevalence of intestinal parasites in pet dogs in the United States. Vet Parasitol. 2009;166(1):144–52, 289–90.

11. Gates MC, Nolan TJ. Endoparasite prevalence and recurrence across different age groups of dogs and cats. Vet Parasitol. 2009;166(1–2):153–8.

12. Han D, Choi R, Hyun C. Canine pancreatic-specific lipase concentrations in dogs with heart failure and chronic mitral valvular insufficiency. J Vet Intern Med. 2015;29(1):180–3.

13. Adrian AM, Twedt DC, Kraft SL, Marolf AJ. Computed tomographic angiography under sedation in the diagnosis of suspected canine pancreatitis: a pilot study. J Vet Intern Med. 2015;29(1):97–103.

14. Cartier MA, Hill SL, Sunico S, et al. Pancreas-specific lipase concentrations and amylase and lipase activities in the peritoneal fluid of dogs with suspected pancreatitis. Vet J. 2014;201(3):385–9.

15. Mawby DI, Whittemore JC, Fecteau KA. Canine pancreatic-specific lipase concentrations in clinically healthy dogs nad dogs with naturally occurring hyperadrenocorticism. J Vet Intern Med. 2014;28(4):1244–50.

16. Mylonakis ME, Xenoulis PG, Theodorou K, et al. Serum canine pancreatic lipase immunoreactivity in experimentally induced and naturally occurring canine monocytic ehrlichiosis (Ehrlichia canis). Vet Microbiol. 2014;169 (3–4):198–202.

17. Chartier MA, Hill SL, Sunico S, et al. Pancreas-specific lipase concentrations and amylase and lipase activities in the peritoneal fluid of dogs with suspected pancreatitis. Vet J. 2014;201(3):385–9.

18. Cote E, ed. Clinical Veterinary Advisor, 2nd edn. St Louis: Elsevier Mosby, 2011: p 1444.

19. Berent AC, Weisse C. Hepatic vascular anomalies. In: Textbook of Veterinary Internal Medicine, vol. 2, 7th edn. Ettinger SJ, Feldman EC, eds. St Louis: Elsevier Saunders, 2010: pp 1649–72.

20. Stockham SL, Scott MA. Liver function. In: Fundamentals of Veterinary Clinical Pathology. Ames: Iowa State Press, 2002: pp 480–3.

21. Cave NJ, Marks SL, Kass PH, Melli AC, Brophy MA. Evaluation of a routine diagnostic fecal panel for dogs with diarrhea. J Am Vet Med Assoc. 2002;221(1):52–9.

22. Marks SL, Rankin SC, Byrne BA, Weese JS. Enteropathogenic bacteria in dogs and cats: diagnosis, epidemiology, treatment, and control. J Vet Intern Med. 2011;25(6):1195–208.

23. Beal MW. Approach to the acute abdomen. Vet Clin North Am Small Anim Pract. 2005;35(2):375–96.

24. Lisciandro GR. Abdominal and thoracic focused assessment with sonography for trauma, triage, and monitoring in small animals. J Vet Emerg Crit Care 2011;21(2):104–22.

25. Lanz OI, Ellison GW, Weichman G, van Gilder J. Surgical treatment of septic peritonitis without abdominal drainage in 28 dogs. J Am Anim Hosp Assoc. 2001;37(1):87–92.

26. Ruthrauff CM, Smith J, Glerum L. Primary bacterial septic peritonitis in cats: 13 cases. J Am Anim Hosp Assoc. 2009;45(6):268–76.

27. Owens SD, Gossett R, McElhaney MR, Christopher MM, Shelly SM. Three cases of canine bile peritonitis with mucinous material in abdominal fluid as the prominent cytologic finding. Vet Clin Pathol. 2003;32(3):114–20.

28. Bonczynski JJ, Ludwig LL, Barton LJ, Loar A, Peterson ME. Comparison of peritoneal fluid and peripheral blood ph, bicarbonate, glucose, and lactate concentration as a diagnostic tool for septic peritonitis in dogs and cats. Vet Surg. 2003;32(2):161–6.

29. Szabo SD, Jermyn K, Neel J, Mathews KG. Evaluation of postceliotomy peritoneal drain fluid volume, cytology, and blood-to-peritoneal fluid lactate and glucose differences in normal dogs. Vet Surg. 2011;40(4):444–9.

30. Schmiedt C, Tobias KM, Otto CM. Evaluation of abdominal fluid: peripheral blood creatinine and potassium ratios for diagnosis of uroperitoneum in dogs. J Vet Emerg Crit Care 2001;11(4):275–80.

31. Aumann M, Worth LT, Drobatz KJ. Uroperitoneum in cats: 26 cases (1986–1995). J Am Anim Hosp Assoc. 1998;34(4):315–24.

32. Finck C, d'Anjou MA, Alexander K, et al. Radiographic diagnosis of mechanical obstruction in dogs based on relative small intestinal external diameters. Vet Radiol Ultrasound. 2014;55(5):472–9.

33. Ciasca TC, David FH, Lamb C. Does measurement of small intestinal diamter increase diagnostic accuracy of radiography in dogs with suspected intestinal obstruction? Vet Radiol Ultrasound 2013;54(3):207–11.

34. Moon M, Myer W. Gastrointestinal contrast radiology in small animals. Semin Vet Med Surg (Small Anim). 1986;1:121–43.

35. Larson MM, Biller DS. Ultrasound of the gastrointestinal tract. Vet Clin North Am Small Anim Pract. 2009;39(4):747–59.

36. Ohlerth S, Scharf G. Computed tomography in small animals – basic principles and state of the art applications. Vet J. 2007;173(2):254–71.

37. Bertolini G, Prokop M. Multidetector-row computed tomography: technical basics and preliminary clinical applications in small animals. Vet J. 2011;189(1):15–26.

38. Yamada K, Morimoto M, Kishimoto M, Wisner ER. Virtual endoscopy of dogs using multidetector row CT. Vet Radiol Ultrasound 2007;48(4):318–22.

39. Ruffolo DC. Gastric tonometry: early warning of tissue hypoperfusion. Crit Care Nurs Q. 1998;21(3):26–32.

40. Weil MH. Tissue pCO2 as a universal marker of tissue hypoxia. Minerva Anestesiol. 2000;66(5):33–7.

41. Palizas F, Dubin A, Regueira T, et al. Gastric tonometry versus cardiac index as resuscitation goal in septic shock: a multicenter, randomized, controlled trial. Crit Care 2009;13(2):R44.

42. Cammarata GA, Weil MH, Castillo CJ, et al. Buccal capnometry for quantitating the severity of hemorrhagic shock. Shock 2009;31(2):207–11.

43. Xu J, Ma L, Sun S, et al. Fluid resuscitation guided by sublingual partial pressure of carbon dioxide during hemorrhagic shock in a procine model. Shock 2013;39(4):361–5.

44. Povoas HP, Weil MH, Tang W, et al. Comparisons between sublingual and gastric tonometry during hemorrhagic shock. Chest 2000;118(4):1127–32.

45. Weil MH, Nakagawa Y, Tang W, et al. Sublingual capnometry: a new noninvasive measurement for diagnosis and and quantitation of severity of circulatory shock. Crit Care Med. 1999;27(7):1225–9.

46. De Backer D, Ospina-Tascon G, Salgado D, et al. Monitoring the microcirculation in the critically ill patient: current methods and future applications. Intensive Care Med. 2010;36(11);1813–25.

47. Vincent JL, DeBacker D. Microcirculatory alterations in the critically ill. Hosp Pract. 2009;37(1):107–12.

48. Nencioni A, Trzeciak S, Shapiro NI. The microcirculation as a diagnostics and therapeutic target in sepsis. Intern Emerg Med. 2009;4(5):413–18.

49. Tams TR. Handbook of Small Animal Gastroenterology. Philadelphia: Saunders, 1996: pp 246–66.

50. Boothe DM. Small Animal Clinical Pharmacology and Therapeutics. Philadelphia: Saunders, 2001.

51. Binder HJ. Organization of the gastrointestinal system. In: Medical Physiology, 2nd edn. Boron WF, Boulpaep EL, eds. Philadelphia: Elsevier, 2005: pp 883–93.

52. De La Fuente SG, McMahon RL, Clary EM, et al. Celecoxib (Celebrex) increases canine lower esophageal sphincter pressure. J Surg Res. 2002;107(1):154–8.

53. Washabau RJ. Gastrointestinal motility disorders and gastrointestinal prokinetic therapy. Vet Clin North Am Small Anim Pract. 2003;33(5):1007–28.

54. Hall JA, Solie TN, Seim HB, Twedt DC. Gastric myoelectric and motor activity in dogs with gastric dilatation-volvulus. Am J Physiol. 1993;265:G646.

55. Bruchim Y, Itay S, Shira BH, et al. Evaluation of lidocaine treatment on frequency of cardiac arrhythmias, acute kidney injury and hospitalization time in dogs with gastic dilatation and voluvulus. J Vet Emerg Crit Care 2012;22(4):419–27.

56. Buber T, Saragusty J, Ranen E, et al. Evaluation of lidocaine treatment and risk factors for death associated with gastric dilatation and volvulus in dogs: 112 cases (1997–2005). J Am Vet Med Assoc. 2007;230(9):1334–9.

57. Washabau RJ, Hasler AH. Constipation, obstipation, and megacolon. Consult Feline Int Med. 1996;3:104–13.

58. Salim SY, Soderholm JD. Importance of disrupted intestinal barrier in inflammatory bowel diseases. Inflamm Bowel Dis. 2011;7(1):362–80.

59. Monnig AA, Prittie JE. A review of stress-related mucosal disease. J Vet Emerg Crit Care. 2011;21(5):484–95.

60. Giger U. Blood typing and cross-matching. In: Kirk's Current Veterinary Therapy XIV. Bonagura JD, Twedt DC, eds. St Louis: Elsevier, 2009: pp 497–501.

61. Choung RS, Talley NJ. Epidemiology and clinical presentation of stress-related peptic damage and chronic peptic ulcer. Curr Mol Med. 2008;8(4):253–7.

62. Ali T, Harty RF. Stress-induced ulcer bleeding in critically ill patients. Gastroenterol Clin North Am. 2009;38(2):245–65.

63. Stollman N, Metz DC. Pathophysiology and prophylaxis of stress ulcer in intensive care unit patients. J Crit Care 2005;20(1):35–45.

64. Spirt MJ. Stress-related mucosal disease: risk factors and prophylactic therapy. Clin Therapeut. 2004;26(2):197–213.

65. Fennerty MB. Pathophysiology of the upper gastrointestinal tract in the critically ill patient: rationale for the therapeutic benefits of acid suppression. Crit Care Med. 2002;30(6 Suppl):S351–5.

66. Malbrain ML, Cheatham ML, Kirkpatrick A, et al. Results from the International Conference of Experts on Intra-Abdominal Hypertension and Abdominal Compartment Syndrome. I. Definitions. Intensive Care Med. 2006;32(11):1722–32.

67. Nielsen LK, Whelan M. Compartment syndrome: pathophysiology, clinical presentations, treatment, and prevention in human and veterinary medicine. J Vet Emerg Crit Care 2012;22(3):291–302.

68. Conzemius MG, Sammarco JL, Holt DE, Smith GK. Clinical determination of preoperative and postoperative intra-abdominal pressures in dogs. Vet Surg. 1995;24(3):195–201.

69. Rader RA, Johnson JA. Determination of normal intra-abdominal pressure using urinary bladder catheterization in clinically healthy cats. J Vet Emerg Crit Care 2010;20(4):386–92.

70. Joubert KE, Oglesby PA, Downie J, Serfontein T. Abdominal compartment syndrome in a dog with babesiosis. J Vet Emerg Crit Care 2007;17(2):184–90.

71. Karanjia ND, Widdison AL, Leung F, Alvarez C, Lutrin FJ, Reber HA. Compartment syndrome in experimental chronic obstructive pancreatitis: effect of decompressing the main pancreatic duct. Br J Surg. 1994;81(2):259–64.

72. An G, West MA. Abdominal compartment syndrome: a concise clinical review. Crit Care Med. 2008;36(4):1304–10.

73. Vidal MG, Ruiz Weisser J, Gonzalez F, et al. Incidence and clinical effects of intra-abdominal hypertension in critically ill patients. Crit Care Med. 2008;36(6):1823–31.

74. Marik PE, Zaloga GP. Early enteral nutrition in acutely ill patients: a systematic review. Crit Care Med. 2001;29(12):2264–70.

75. Mohr AJ, Leisewitz AL, Jacobson LS, Steiner JM, Ruaux CG, Williams DA. Effect of early enteral nutrition on intestinal permeability, intestinal protein loss, and outcome in dogs with severe parvoviral enteritis. J Vet Int Med. 2003;17(6):791–8.

76. Liu DT, Brown DC, Silverstein DC. Early nutritional support is associated with decreased length of hospitalization in dogs with septic peritonitis: a retrospective study of 45 cases (2000–2009). J Vet Emerg Crit Care 2012;22(4):453–9.

77. Wischmeyer PE. Clinical applications of l-glutamine: past, present, and future. Nutr Clin Pract. 2003;18(5):377–85.

78. Heyland D, Muscedere J, Wischmeyer PE, et al. A randomized trial of glutamine and antioxidants in critically ill patients. N Engl J Med. 2013;368(16):1489–97.

79. Kerl ME, Johnson PA. Nutritional plan: matching diet to disease. Clin Tech Small Anim Pract. 2004;19(1):9–21.

80. Chan DL, Rozanski EA, Freeman LM. Relationship among plasma amino acids, c-reactive protein, illness severity, and outcome in critically ill dogs. J Vet Intern Med. 2009;23(3):559–63.

81. LaPierre CD. Should peri-operative arginine containing nutrition therapy become routine in the surgical patient? A systematic review of the evidence and meta-analysis. International Anesthesia Research Society 2010:449.

82. Kalil AC, Sevransky JE, Myers DE, et al. Preclinical trial of l-arginine monotherapy alone or with n-acetylcysteine in septic shock. Crit Care Med. 2006;34(11):2719–28.

83. Prittie J, Barton L. Route of nutrient delivery. Clin Tech Small Anim Pract. 2004;19(1):6–8.

84. Saker KE, Remillard RL. Critical care nutrition and enteral-assisted feeding. In: Small Animal Clinical Nutrition, 5th edn. Topeka: Mark Morris Institute, 2010: pp 439–76.

85. Yu MK, Freeman LM, Heinze CR, Parker VJ, Linder DE. Comparison of complication rates in dogs with nasoesophageal versus nasogastric feeding tubes. J Vet Emerg Crit Care 2013;23(3):300–4.

86. Klaus JA, Rudloff E, Kirby R. Nasogastric tube feeding in cats with suspected acute pancreatitis: 55 cases (2001–2006). J Vet Emerg Crit Care 2009;19(4):337–46.

CHAPTER 16
Nutritional status

Caroline Tonozzi

VCA Aurora Animal Hospital, Aurora, Illinois

Introduction

Tell me what you eat, and I will tell you what you are.

(Jean Anthelme Brillat-Savarin, 18th century)

Starvation is the lack of food. "Simple starvation" occurs when a previously healthy animal has not eaten for a 72-hour period. The body will respond by decreasing the metabolic rate to conserve energy and to maintain body mass. Glucose is produced from glycogen and fat stores in this situation and used to make energy. Once the animal resumes eating, these compensatory metabolic changes are rapidly reversed, and the animal returns to normal.

Illness and injury can cause a catabolic state that results in a reduced prognosis for recovery. Anorexia, nausea, pain, discomfort or the physical inability to eat will also lead to starvation. This form is called "stressed starvation" and occurs when a patient has been either anorexic for ≥3 days due to a severe illness or malnourished at the time of presentation for an illness. Increased release of stress hormones (cortisol, glucagon, catecholamines) and inflammatory cytokines shifts energy production away from glucose and fat to lean muscle proteolysis (Figure 16.1) [1]. Marked proteolysis exceeds protein synthesis, with energy consumed during the process. Muscle wasting will occur while fat deposits are spared, causing a negative nitrogen and energy balance [2]. Delayed wound healing, altered immune function, gastrointestinal (GI) dysfunction, and weakened skeletal and respiratory muscle strength contribute to a worse overall prognosis for recovery. Many of the effects of protein-calorie malnutrition on the immune response are listed in Table 16.1.

The small bowel is a primary component of the immune system due to the abundant amount of lymphoid tissue present and the protective mucosal barrier function. The GI mucosal cells extract the majority of their nutrients from the enteral side of the bowel rather than from the capillaries. Certain nutrients, specifically glutamine, arginine, nucleotides, omega-3 fatty acids, and dietary fiber, are required for growth and normal function of the mucosal epithelial cells and lymphoid tissue [3,4]. IgA is secreted into the GI lumen to prevent adherence of microbes to the mucosa.

During states of starvation in critically ill animals, the enterocytes become malnourished and are unused, rapidly causing villus atrophy. Transit time within the bowel is increased with decreased absorptive capacity and increased bacterial proliferation within the lumen. The mucosal barrier becomes damaged, causing an increase in GI mucosal permeability. Various factors have been found to promote the translocation of luminal pathogens. These factors include luminal bacterial overgrowth, impaired host defense mechanisms, protein-calorie malnutrition, trauma, critical illness, and interruption of the luminal nutritional stream [5]. The subsequent bacteremia may contribute to the "two-hit" theory of critical illness, with the second physiological injury potentially arising from the bowel [6].

A deficiency of a specific nutrient can cause specific life-threatening problems. Thiamine deficiency in the cat can lead to dementia, seizures, and coma. Carnitine deficiency in the Boxer can cause cardiomyopathy. Taurine deficiency in the cat can cause blindness or dilated cardiomyopathy. Vitamin A deficiency can cause blindness. A list of common nutrient components, their functions, and possible consequences of deficiency is provided in Table 16.2.

When illness limits the intake of adequate nutrients, a prolonged recovery time is anticipated. Protein-calorie malnutrition will impair immune function and result in a greater risk of infection. However, providing nutritional support early in the course of hospitalization has been shown to improve outcome of both human and veterinary ICU patients [7,8]. A positive correlation has been found between the type of nutritional support provided, the amount of energy produced, and the outcome from critical illness [9,10].

The goals of nutritional support are to meet nutritional requirements, reverse metabolic consequences of malnutrition (such as muscle loss), and improve recovery time [2]. A nutritional plan is prepared for the small animal patient on the first day of hospitalization. The plan should address the following four questions:

- Is the patient ready for feeding?
- How should the patient be fed?
- What should the patient be fed?
- Is there a need for pharmaconutrition (supplementation of the prepared diet)?

Diagnosis

Information derived from diagnostic and monitoring procedures will be incorporated into the patient nutritional assessment. The data collection begins with a thorough history and physical examination, followed by cage-side point of care (POC) laboratory testing, clinicopathological testing, and diagnostic imaging. The goal is to create a nutritional plan that answers the four questions above. The World Small Animal Veterinary Association has produced a Global Nutrition Toolkit containing guidelines and forms to assist the veterinary team in creating an optimal nutritional plan for small animal patients (http://www.wsava.org/nutrition-toolkit). Monitoring procedures will assess the response to feeding, with the goal of minimizing complications and maximizing outcome.

Monitoring and Intervention for the Critically Ill Small Animal: The Rule of 20, First Edition. Edited by Rebecca Kirby and Andrew Linklater.
© 2017 John Wiley & Sons, Inc. Published 2017 by John Wiley & Sons, Inc.

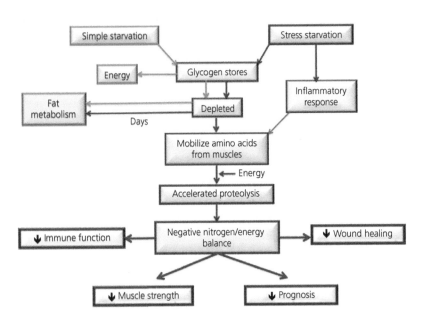

Figure 16.1 Mechanism of "stress" starvation compared to "simple" starvation. Green arrows: simple starvation. Red arrows: stress starvation.

Table 16.1 Effects of protein-calorie malnutrition on immunity.

Component	Effect
Hypoalbuminemic malnutrition associated with infection or inflammation; modulated by hormones and cytokines (IL-1, TNF-alpha)	Depletes visceral protein (albumin) stores; depressed cell-mediated immunity
Humoral immunity	Decline in production of IG, secretory antibodies, complement
Neutropenia	Capacity of neutrophils to kill phagocytosed bacteria decreased; decreased cytokine secretion
Immune components Complement, interferon production, opsonization, plasma lysosome production, acute-phase reactants	Depressed production and/or function
Thyroid, lymphoid tissues	Atrophy, decreased peripheral T-lymphocytes, impaired response of lymphocytes to mitogens; depressed response to contact sensitivity, inflammatory reactions, and vaccines
Anatomical barriers	Disrupted, atrophy of skin and GI mucosa

Adapted from: Saker KE. Nutrition and immune function. Vet Clin North Am. 2006;36;1199–224 [41].
GI, gastrointestinal; IG, immunoglobulin; IL, interleukin; TNF, tumor necrosis factor.

History and physical examination

The history begins with the species and signalment (age, sex, breed). There are different nutritional requirements for the dog compared to the cat (Table 16.3). Young growing animals, gestating or lactating females, and geriatric animals will have differing caloric and nutritional needs. Breed-related nutritional concerns such as predisposition for carnitine deficiency in Boxers, Doberman Pinschers, Great Danes, Irish Wolfhounds and other giant breeds and primary hyperlipidemia in Miniature Schnauzers and Shetland Sheepdogs can become important.

Past medical history and exposure to medications or toxins will guide the nutritional plan. Renal disease, liver disease, diabetes mellitus, pancreatitis, protein-losing disease, and hypothyroidism are but a few of the chronic or recurrent disease states that can warrant a nutritional plan that might require alterations and supplementation. The diet history is necessary and should include the type and brand of food, amount fed, frequency of feeding, and length of time fed the current diet. Cats are carnivores and require many of their nutrients from meat-based diets (see Table 16.2). Weight gain or loss and the period of time for the weight change are recorded as well as any food allergies.

Current history should include when the patient last had a normal appetite, and the progression of change in appetite and food intake through to presentation. Any signs of GI dysfunction, such as bloating, excessive borborygmus, flatulence or eructation, salivating, nausea, regurgitation, vomiting, diarrhea or constipation, should be recorded. Any problems with food prehension, chewing or swallowing could become important.

The physical examination begins with the temperature, pulse rate and intensity, respiratory rate and effort, and body and muscle condition scores. Hyperthermia suggests an increased demand for calories (increased metabolic rate). Hypothermia implies a slower metabolic rate that may be due to poor perfusion and shock, especially in the cat. Correction of the hypothermia is necessary before initiating the nutritional plan. Tachycardia (dogs), poor or absent peripheral pulses, pale mucous membrane color, and prolonged capillary refill time are physical peripheral perfusion parameters that indicate shock. Rapid or labored breathing requires active contraction of the respiratory muscles and an important expenditure of energy. Dehydration can be determined by tenting of the skin, dry mucous membranes and corneas, and eyes sunken within the orbit. Resuscitation and initial stabilization of circulatory and respiratory distress are required prior to initiating the nutritional plan (Figure 16.2).

A complete physical examination is required, with particular attention given to the body weight, body condition score (BCS) (Figure 16.3) and muscle condition score (MCS) (Figure 16.4). A BCS <4/9 is low and >5/9 is high, each potentially prompting an adjustment in total calories to be fed and percentage distribution of protein, fats, and carbohydrates. Hepatomegaly and icterus are

Table 16.2 Important nutrients to be supplemented in diets for critical small animal patients [40,42,43].

Nutrient decreased	Functions	Clinical consequences	Notes
Water (most important nutrient)	Water is necessary for cellular life, chemical and metabolic reactions, transport of nutrients and other substances, cushion joints and brain tissues, body temperature regulation, and elimination of wastes	Dehydration; poor skin turgor, dull, dry corneas, mucous membranes, oliguria, eventually death	Severe deficit causes poor perfusion
Arginine (essential amino acid for dog and cat)	Entry into urea cycle with high blood ammonia; stimulates release of GH, insulin, glucagon; substrate for nitric oxide production; promotes collagen deposition in wounds; stimulates T-cell function and growth of lymphocytes	Dementia, seizures, altered consciousness; poor wound healing, poor immune response	Cats lack intestinal pyrroline-5-carboxylate synthase to make precursor ornithine; enriched diets enhance immune function and wound healing; better results if combined with omega-3 fatty acids; energy and protein requirements must be met for good result of supplementation
Glutamine (essential amino acid in catabolic state)	Synthesis pathway attenuated in critical illness; low levels signal skeletal muscle protein catabolism; provides fuel for rapidly dividing enterocytes, endothelial cells, renal tubular cells and lymphocytes; essential nucleotide precursor	Muscle wasting, gastrointestinal signs with poor healing, immune system dysfunction infection; supplement could cause azotemia in renal failure, high ammonia in liver failure	Decreased IC concentration in critical illness; unstable in solution; immune enhancing when added to standard diets; enhances GI tolerance in shock; ideal in early management of critical surgical patients
Carnitine	Key component of lipid metabolism and energy production	Myocardial disease in some dogs; possible hepatic lipidosis cats	
Taurine	Required to synthesize bile acids to absorb dietary fats; regulates calcium flux; neurotransmission; antioxidant; stabilizes cells membranes; may have role in bioelectrical potentials, myocardium, retinas	Reproductive failure, developmental abnormalities, retinal degeneration, dilated cardiomyopathy	Cats cannot synthesize and have ongoing loss in feces and urine
Thiamine (vitamin B1)	Helps convert carbohydrates to glucose for energy production; needed to form ATP by all cells, especially brain	Deficit causes GI (vomiting, salivation), and neurological signs (ventroflexion of head and neck, vocalization, dementia, seizures, abnormal gait, stupor)	Cats very susceptible; diets deficient or thiaminase in some GI bacteria and in some raw fish common causes; water-soluble vitamin
Vitamin A	Hormone-like growth factor for epithelial and other cells; necessary for light absorption in retina; important for immune function, gene transcription and protein formation	Blindness, impaired immunity	Cats must ingest preformed vitamin A; lack dioxygenase enzymes in the intestinal mucosa to split the beta-carotene molecule to vitamin A aldehyde
Arachidonic acid (essential omega-6 fatty acid)	Maintains cells wall integrity	Poor hair coat quality, poor tissue integrity	Cats cannot produce from linoleic acid; animal source fats required for cats
Niacin (vitamin B3)	Helps convert carbohydrates to glucose for energy; helps use fats and proteins; affects nervous system, skin, eyes, hair coat	Diarrhea, flaky skin, poor response to stress	Cats cannot convert tryptophan to niacin; high meat diet required; high doses can cause "flushing"; water-soluble vitamin
Zinc	Role in protein and nucleic acid metabolism	Depressed wound healing, increased protein catabolism, depressed immune function	
Omega-3 fatty acids	Source of energy in dogs and cats; incorporated into cell membranes, maintain membrane fluidity, permeability, receptor functions; precursors to eicosanoids (omega-3 derived less metabolically active than omega-6 derived eicosanoids); antiinflammatory – inhibit production of inflammatory mediators; positive effect immune barrier of skin		Must be incorporated in cell membranes to be metabolically active; supplementation could increase vitamin E requirements

ATP, adenosine triphosphate; GH, growth hormone; GI, gastrointestinal; IC, intracellular.

signs compatible with hepatic lipidosis in the cat and warrant early nutrition as a key component of therapy.

The physical examination findings are used to select the feeding tube most appropriate for the patient. Problems within the oral cavity, altered mentation, and profound weakness are but a few of the viable reasons to initiate tube feedings. Nasogastric or naso-esophageal tubes may be an ideal choice for short-term (≤5 days) enteral feeding. An esophagostomy or gastrostomy tube might be the better choice if resolution of an oral problem is going to take ≥5 days. Evidence of gastric paresis or ileus (bloated abdomen, reduced

Table 16.3 Nutritional requirements for adult cats and dogs [40].

Nutrient	Adult cats	Adult dogs
Type (source)	Carnivore (meat)	Omnivore (meat and plant)
Essential amino acids	Arginine, histidine, isoleucine, leucine, lysine, methionine, phenylalanine, threonine, tryptophan, valine, and taurine	Arginine, methionine, histidine, phenylalanine, isoleucine, threonine, leucine, tryptophan, lysine, and valine
Protein %*	30–45%	15–30%
Fats %*	10–30%	10–20%
Carbohydrates %*	<50%	50%

* % dry matter basis.

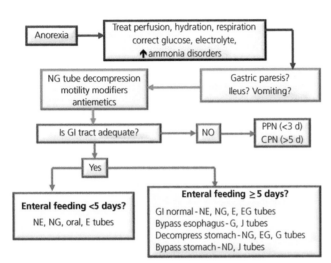

Figure 16.2 An algorithm to help determine when and how to initiate a nutritional plan.

or absent bowel sounds, regurgitation) might direct placement of a tube with the distal end within the stomach to allow gastric decompression. Should it be necessary to bypass the stomach and upper duodenum, a jejunostomy tube is selected. A list of enteral feeding tube sites with tube size, indication, advantages, and potential complication is provided in Table 16.4. The finding of nausea or retching on abdominal palpation or diarrhea found on rectal examination will become important when prescribing the method of enteral feeding (Figure 16.5). The use of antiemetics and motility modifiers may be warranted, as well.

Point of care laboratory testing

The minimum database is obtained by POC testing and consists of the packed cell volume (PCV), total protein (TP), blood glucose, blood urea nitrogen (BUN), electrolyte panel (sodium (Na^+), potassium (K^+), chloride (Cl^-), ionized calcium (Ca^{++}) and magnesium (Mg^{++})), blood gas, coagulation profile, platelet estimate, and urinalysis.

The PCV and TP are evaluated together for an indication of dehydration or acute blood loss, requiring volume support prior to initiating any form of nutritional support. Anemia warrants an assessment of the need for iron supplementation. Low TP could warrant a higher percentage of calories from protein in the diet. Hyperglycemia might merit a lower percentage of carbohydrates in the diet and the administration of insulin while hypoglycemia could justify a higher percentage of carbohydrates. Examination of the serum for lipemia can direct a lower percentage of fat in the diet calculations where icterus, especially in the cat, can direct

diagnostics for hepatic lipidosis. A high BUN can suggest renal disease, directing further testing and possibly altering the selection of diet to reduce the percentage of protein. A low BUN can bring concern for liver failure and hepatoencephalopathy, potentially warranting a lower percentage of dietary protein with an emphasis on branched chain amino acids.

Prolongation of clotting times should trigger an assessment to determine the need for calcium and vitamin K supplementation. Significant electrolyte disorders should be corrected during the initial stabilization period and prior to implementation of the nutritional plan. Acid–base disorders should be stabilized prior to feeding when possible and monitored closely since metabolic acidosis can occur during parenteral feeding. The urinalysis should provide evidence of the kidneys' ability to concentrate urine (specific gravity), proteinuria, glycosuria, and crystal formation, each a potential marker for dietary adjustments.

Clinicopathological testing

A complete blood count (CBC) and serum biochemical profile should be submitted, with blood ammonia and thyroid panel. The presence of neutropenia or lymphopenia could indicate depression of immune function and warrant supplementation of specific nutrients, vitamins or minerals (see Tables 16.1 and 16.2). Hypoalbuminemia, as a component of low TP associated with infection or inflammation, warrants support of the immune system and supplementation of protein from the diet. The baseline serum phosphorus is very important in assessing the potential for refeeding syndrome, with hypophosphatemia requiring careful monitoring and supplementation (see Nutritional disorders, later in this chapter). High blood ammonia can justify lowering the protein in the diet. Low levels of thyroid hormone or high cholesterol might support a lower percentage of fat in the diet and potential adjustment of required calories.

Diagnostic imaging

Imaging begins with plain thoracic and abdominal radiographs to assess organ size, position, and structure. An assessment of the entire length of the GI tract is important for evidence of obstruction, megaesophagus, stricture, gastric distension, ileus, fluid-filled bowel, abdominal mass or peritoneal fluid. An assessment of the size of the caudal vena cava can provide an indication of intravascular volume and direct fluid stabilization prior to nutritional support. Special attention should be given to any evidence of aspiration pneumonia, which could contribute to the decision concerning the type of feeding tube (see Table 16.4) and the need for gastric decompression and antiemetics.

A radiograph should be taken centering over the distal (internal) end of the feeding tube after placement to confirm the

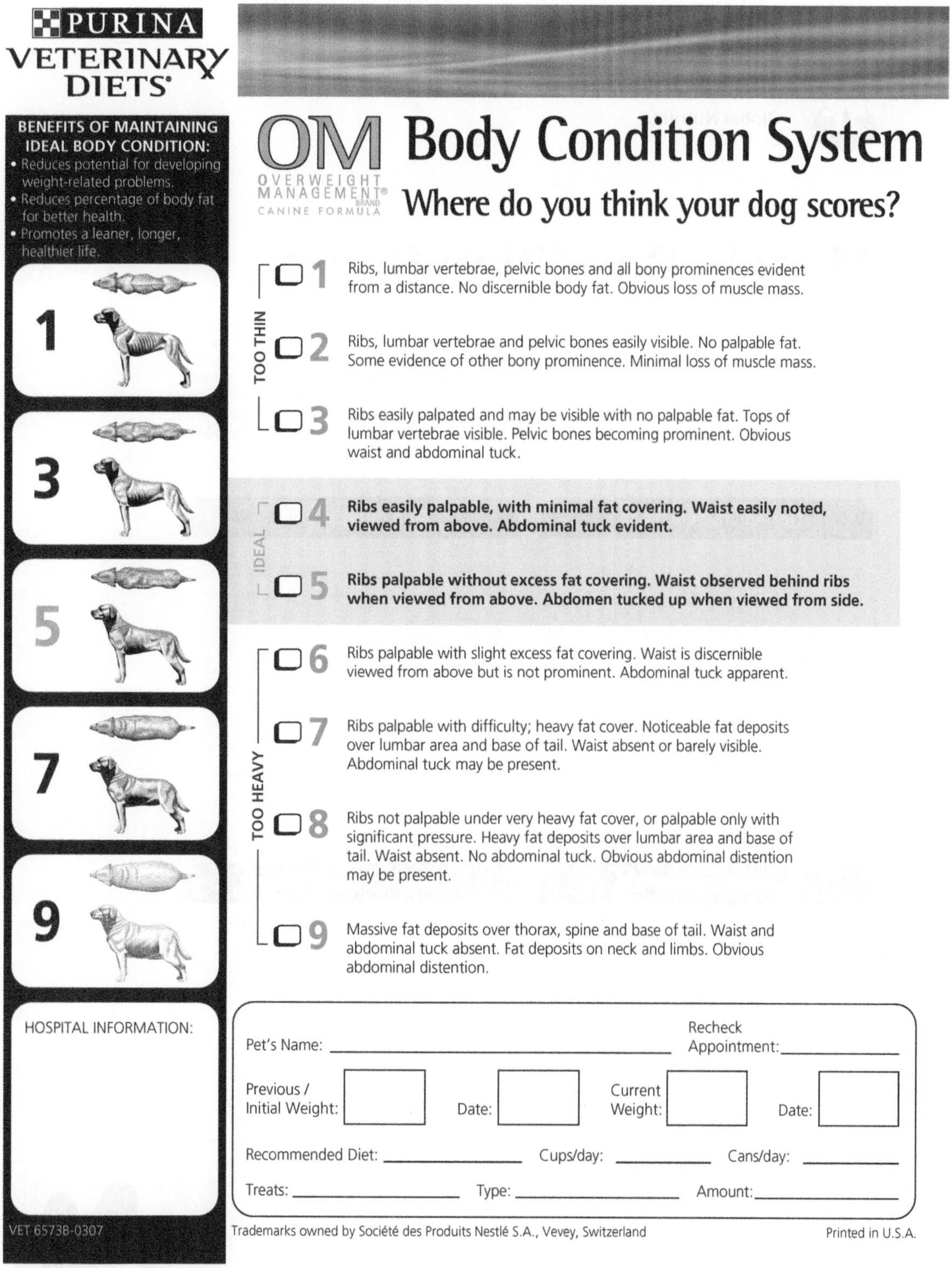

OM Body Condition System

OVERWEIGHT MANAGEMENT® BRAND CANINE FORMULA

Where do you think your dog scores?

PURINA VETERINARY DIETS®

BENEFITS OF MAINTAINING IDEAL BODY CONDITION:
- Reduces potential for developing weight-related problems.
- Reduces percentage of body fat for better health.
- Promotes a leaner, longer, healthier life.

TOO THIN

☐ **1** Ribs, lumbar vertebrae, pelvic bones and all bony prominences evident from a distance. No discernible body fat. Obvious loss of muscle mass.

☐ **2** Ribs, lumbar vertebrae and pelvic bones easily visible. No palpable fat. Some evidence of other bony prominence. Minimal loss of muscle mass.

☐ **3** Ribs easily palpated and may be visible with no palpable fat. Tops of lumbar vertebrae visible. Pelvic bones becoming prominent. Obvious waist and abdominal tuck.

IDEAL

☐ **4** Ribs easily palpable, with minimal fat covering. Waist easily noted, viewed from above. Abdominal tuck evident.

☐ **5** Ribs palpable without excess fat covering. Waist observed behind ribs when viewed from above. Abdomen tucked up when viewed from side.

TOO HEAVY

☐ **6** Ribs palpable with slight excess fat covering. Waist is discernible viewed from above but is not prominent. Abdominal tuck apparent.

☐ **7** Ribs palpable with difficulty; heavy fat cover. Noticeable fat deposits over lumbar area and base of tail. Waist absent or barely visible. Abdominal tuck may be present.

☐ **8** Ribs not palpable under very heavy fat cover, or palpable only with significant pressure. Heavy fat deposits over lumbar area and base of tail. Waist absent. No abdominal tuck. Obvious abdominal distention may be present.

☐ **9** Massive fat deposits over thorax, spine and base of tail. Waist and abdominal tuck absent. Fat deposits on neck and limbs. Obvious abdominal distention.

HOSPITAL INFORMATION:

Pet's Name: _____

Recheck Appointment: _____

Previous / Initial Weight: _____   Date: _____

Current Weight: _____   Date: _____

Recommended Diet: _____ Cups/day: _____ Cans/day: _____

Treats: _____ Type: _____ Amount: _____

VET 6573B-0307   Trademarks owned by Société des Produits Nestlé S.A., Vevey, Switzerland   Printed in U.S.A.

Figure 16.3 Body condition score for dogs. A similar system may be used for cats. Used with permission from Nestlé Purina Pet Care.

location and to discover any curling or kinking of the tube that needs correction prior to feeding. Endoscopy can be used to place gastrostomy tubes and direct placement of a feeding tube through the pylorus into the upper duodenum. Advanced imaging with ultrasound, computed tomography or nuclear magnetic resonance imaging may be necessary to diagnose the underlying problem.

Advanced testing

Indirect calorimetry is a technique that provides accurate estimates of energy expenditure from measures of carbon dioxide production and oxygen consumption during rest and steady-state exercise. There are open and closed circuit methods. The technology has advanced to fully portable, electronic equipment that provides continual and instantaneous breath-by-breath values of pulmonary gas

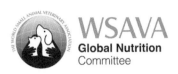

Muscle Condition Score

Muscle condition score is assessed by visualization and palpation of the spine, scapulae, skull, and wings of the ilia. Muscle loss is typically first noted in the epaxial muscles on each side of the spine; muscle loss at other sites can be more variable. Muscle condition score is graded as normal, mild loss, moderate loss, or severe loss. Note that animals can have significant muscle loss even if they are overweight (body condition score > 5/9). Conversely, animals can have a low body condition score (< 4/9) but have minimal muscle loss. Therefore, assessing both body condition score and muscle condition score on every animal at every visit is important. Palpation is especially important with mild muscle loss and in animals that are overweight. An example of each score is shown below.

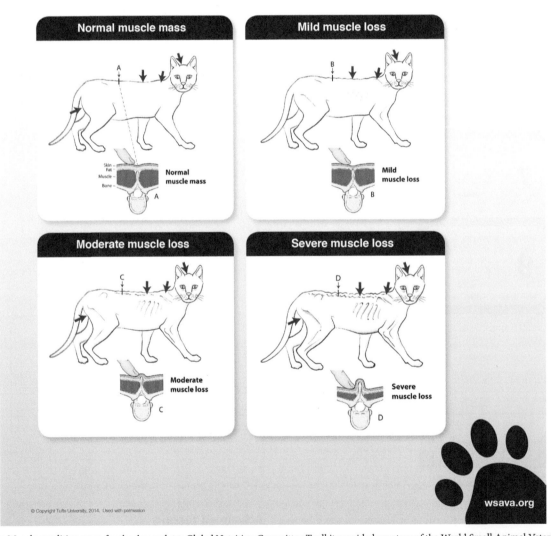

Figure 16.4 Muscle condition score for the dog and cat. Global Nutrition Committee Toolkit provided courtesy of the World Small Animal Veterinary Association. These guidelines were first published in J Small Anim Pract. 2011;52(7):385–96, published by John Wiley and Sons Ltd, and are published here with permission.

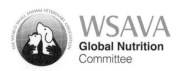

Muscle Condition Score

Muscle condition score is assessed by visualization and palpation of the spine, scapulae, skull, and wings of the ilia. Muscle loss is typically first noted in the epaxial muscles on each side of the spine; muscle loss at other sites can be more variable. Muscle condition score is graded as normal, mild loss, moderate loss, or severe loss. Note that animals can have significant muscle loss if they are overweight (body condition score > 5). Conversely, animals can have a low body condition score (< 4) but have minimal muscle loss. Therefore, assessing both body condition score and muscle condition score on every animal at every visit is important. Palpation is especially important when muscle loss is mild and in animals that are overweight. An example of each score is shown below.

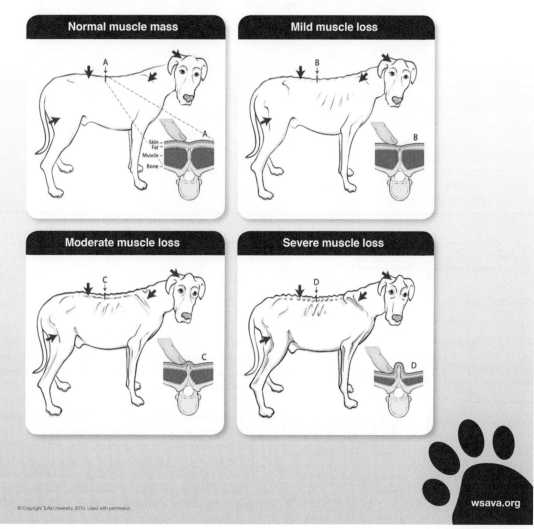

wsava.org

Figure 16.4 (*Continued*)

Table 16.4 Common small animal enteral feeding tube location, size, indication, advantages, and disadvantages.

Tube location	Indications	Advantages	Disadvantages	Notes
Nasogastric Size: 5–12 Fr	<7 days; aspiration of gastric fluid, air; deposit food in stomach	Only mild sedation required; inexpensive; no incisions; monitor gastric fluid/air; gastric decompression; easy removal	Irritation to nose (epistaxis, rhinitis); can cause irritation to gastric mucosa; dacryocystitis; can stimulate vomiting; aspiration pneumonia; small diameter tubes; liquid diet required	Ideal for early trickle-flow feeding; excellent for severely emaciated animals; radiograph confirms placement
Nasoesophageal Size: 5–12 Fr	<7 days; feeding small volumes, liquid diet	Only sedation required; inexpensive; no surgical incisions; unlikely to stimulate vomiting or irritate gastric mucosa	Irritation to nose (epistaxis, rhinitis); can cause irritation to gastric mucosa; dacryocystitis; can stimulate vomiting; aspiration pneumonia; small diameter tubes; liquid diet required; not ideal if increased intracranial pressure	Ideal for early trickle-flow feeding; excellent for severely emaciated animals
Esophagostomy Size: 12–22 Fr	≥5 days; functioning esophagus; oral and pharyngeal disease (bypasses mouth and pharynx)	Short surgical procedure; remains for weeks to months if needed; easy removal; can feed canned food mixed with water or liquid diet	Requires anesthesia w/tracheal intubation; incisions in skin and esophagus; possible infection at stoma site	Excellent for cats with hepatic lipidosis; possible placement of tube through esophagus into mediastinum
Gastrostomy Size: 18–24 Fr balloon or mushroom tipped	≥14 days; oral, pharyngeal or esophageal disorders, permanent supplemental feeding, altered level of consciousness	Remains for weeks to months if needed; leaves head and neck free; can feed canned food mixed with water or liquid diet; easy removal after 14 days	Requires surgery or endoscopy for placement; incision through gastric and abdominal body wall required; possibility of peritonitis, abscess, fasciitis; stoma must form prior to removal of tube	
Jejunostomy Size: 5–12 Fr	≥7 days; bypass mouth, esophagus, stomach and duodenum (pyloric obstruction, pancreatitis, gastric motility disorders, biliary disease)	Feed liquid diet by constant rate of infusion	Requires laparotomy for placement; stoma formation required prior to removal; possibility of peritonitis or abdominal abscess; requires liquid diet	Primarily used for in-hospital feeding of critical patients; requires monomeric diet
Nasoduodenal or nasojejunal Size: 5–12 Fr	<7 days; bypass mouth, esophagus, stomach and duodenum (pyloric obstruction, pancreatitis, gastric motility disorders, biliary disease)	Feed liquid diet by constant rate infusion; no surgery required	Requires endoscopy or fluoroscopy for placement; not ideal if increased intracranial pressure; required liquid diet	Primarily used for in-hospital feeding of critical patients; requires monomeric diet

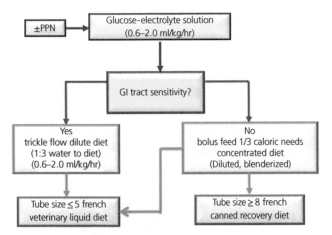

Figure 16.5 Decision-making schematic for the initiation of enteral feeding in a critically ill small animal with anorexia.

exchange. Open-flow indirect calorimetry has been described in the dog and found to provide accurate data regarding oxygen consumption, carbon dioxide production, and resting energy expenditure [11]. While the calculation for the resting energy requirement (RER) is only an estimation, the measured resting energy expenditure in dogs provides a more accurate determination [11]. Indirect calorimetry is carried out on an individual basis. Disadvantages of

indirect calorimetry include the lack of equipment availability, cost of equipment, time required for testing, and expense.

Monitoring methods

Routine assessment of parameters related to nutrition should occur at least a twice daily (Table 16.5). Physical assessment should include body weight, BCS, perfusion and hydration status, and food consumption or delivery. While the body weight may fluctuate daily based on the fluid status and the underlying disease, a gain or loss in body weight of >1 kg in a 24-hour period should be investigated. The amount of fluids given by IV or oral route is assessed to determine the impact this could have. A change in BCS during hospital stay would indicate a severe metabolic challenge and support the patient's need for nutritional intervention. Alterations in mentation or level of consciousness should prompt further investigation for glucose alterations, serious electrolyte disorders, thiamine deficiency, refeeding syndrome or hepatoencephalopathy associated with protein in the diet or swallowing and digesting blood. The catheter site used for infusion of peripheral parenteral nutrition (PPN) or central parenteral nutrition (CPN) is evaluated for heat, redness, irritation or pain.

Monitoring the gastric residual volume (GRV) can be helpful in assessing tolerance to enteral feeding. A nasogastric or gastrostomy tube is used to aspirate gastric contents (fluid and air).

Table 16.5 Parameters used to assess the impact of the nutritional plan in the critically ill dog and cat.

Monitored parameter	Impact	Notes
Body weight	Should remain constant or slightly increase after stabilization	Is a function of fluid input (IV and oral fluids), third body fluid spacing, fluid losses (urine, vomit, diarrhea, gastric aspiration, evaporation from panting)
BCS, MCS	Should only improve over time	A decline suggests an inadequate nutritional plan
Physical perfusion parameters (heart rate, body temperature, mucous membrane color, pulse intensity, capillary refill time)	Poor perfusion implies an intravascular volume deficit if cardiac function is adequate	Will have significant effect on fluid balance and body weight
Physical hydration parameters (skin turgor, mucous membrane and corneal moisture, eye position in bony socket)	Dehydration implies inadequate fluid balance; peripheral edema, chemosis or rapid, labored breathing can indicate overhydration	Both can affect body weight. An abnormality in hydration requires immediate adjustment of quantities of IV and oral fluids administered
Feeding tube productivity	Air and fluid aspirated should be quantified	Can serve as an estimate of GRV, guiding enteral diet volume and concentration
Neurological exam	Onset of dementia, depressed mentation, stupor, coma or seizures warrants rapid assessment of the nutritional plan	Glucose, electrolyte, and thiamine concentrations are assessed and stabilized. Concern for HE in a patient with liver disease warrants treatment with lactulose by enema and orally. An alteration in the dietary protein may be required
Catheter sites for CPN, PPN	Examined for heat, redness, swelling, pain, exudate	Any evidence of inflammation warrants removal of catheter and replacement in a different location
Blood glucose (2× daily)	Alterations warrant evaluation of carbohydrate source and quantity in diet and assessment for glucose disorders	
Serum electrolytes (2× daily)	Na^+, K^+, Ca^{++}, Mg^{++}, and PO_4^- are evaluated for alterations	Total body deficits can be present in spite of normal serum levels. Abnormalities could suggest refeeding syndrome and require stabilization

BCS, body condition score; CPN, central parenteral nutrition; GRV, gastric residual volume; HE, hepatic encephalopathy; MCS, muscle condition score; PPN, peripheral parenteral nutrition.

Gastric residual volume is the volume of fluid aspirated from the stomach after a given period of time and before a new feeding [12,13]. High GRV has been correlated with a higher incidence of vomiting or regurgitation, leading to aspiration pneumonia and cessation of feeding in humans [14]. However, an increased GRV in the canine patient had no significant correlation with the occurrence of vomiting or aspiration pneumonia [15]. A high GRV can be an indication of enteral feeding intolerance (see Nutritional disorders, later in this chapter), requiring an adjustment in the amount, concentration or frequency of feeding.

Formulating the nutritional plan

Every patient in the ICU deserves a nutritional plan formulated to meet his or her individual needs. Evaluating the history, physical examination, laboratory results, and diagnostic imaging results provides the initial nutritional assessment of the patient. Specific factors considered include current body weight, recent change in body weight, BCS, MCS, activity level, level of consciousness, condition of GI tract, blood glucose, presence of lipemia, and, of course, the underlying disease process.

Patient preparation
Oxygenation, ventilation, perfusion, bleeding, and hydration are key patient parameters requiring rapid stabilization prior to initiating any type of feeding regimen. Oxygen supplementation and intravenous fluid therapy (see Chapter 2) are common therapeutic interventions incorporated into the initial resuscitation plan. Serious electrolyte abnormalities, including disorders of Na^+, K^+,

Ca^{++}, and PO_4^-, must be addressed (see Chapter 6). Hypoglycemia ≤ 60 mg/dL (3.33 mmol/L) is treated with IV dextrose (0.5 g/kg) and high blood ammonia reduced with oral lactulose or lactulose enemas prior to feeding. Hyperglycemia due to a diabetic crisis must be managed (see Chapter 5) prior to complicating glucose management with enteral or parenteral feeding.

Evaluation of the GI tract will determine the need for gastric decompression or antiemetic, GI protectants, and motility modifying drugs. Common GI drugs used in the ICU, their mechanism of action, and dose are listed in Tables 15.6, 15.7, and 15.8, in Chapter 15. Short-term intravenous amino acid solutions and trickle-flow gastric feeding of glucose-electrolyte oral solutions may provide a method of support and testing of gastric tolerance while determining the ability of the GI tract to tolerate feeding.

Feeding methods
There are only two routes for providing nutrition in the critically ill patient: enteral and parenteral. Providing nutrition through a functional digestive system is the preferred route of feeding. Maintenance of normal gut flora depends on normal GI motility and nourishment of the enterocytes. This form of feeding is less expensive, stimulates the immune system, decreases hospitalization days, and minimizes the metabolic consequences of refeeding [16–20].

Enteral feeding methods
Oral voluntary feeding is ideal but rarely results in consistent intake of adequate quantities of the desired nutrients in critically ill small animals. Oral forced feeding is not recommended and can lead to food aversion, excessive salivation, and stress to the animal.

Appetite stimulants, such as cyproheptadine (cats only: 0.1–0.5 mg/kg PO q 8–12 h) and mirtazapine (3.75 mg/cat PO q 3 days; 0.55 mg/kg PO q 24 h, maximum dose 30 mg per day), can be given but do not result in consistent intake of nutrition, making them unreliable for critical patients.

Tube feeding provides a convenient and consistent method for delivering a desired quantity and concentration of diet to the GI tract. Choosing the ideal feeding tube depends on the desired diameter and length of the tube, ease of placement, comfort level to the patient, cost of placement, and the estimated length of time the tube will be in place. Table 16.4 lists common sizes, indications, advantages, and disadvantages for nasogastric (NG), nasoesophageal (NE), esophagostomy (E), gastrostomy (G), jejunostomy (J), nasoduodenal (ND), and nasojejunal (NJ) tubes. Feeding tube placement should be confirmed by radiography, endoscopy or at the time of surgery. Complications include tube dislodgment, misplacement, inadvertent tube removal by patient, local infection or inflammation, or clogged tubes from medications or food. For surgically placed G or J tubes, early dislodgment may cause further complications such as peritonitis or fasciitis. Should the patient vomit a tube, there is a possibility that the animal can bite and swallow the tube segment, creating a gastric foreign body. When the tube is no longer needed, it is removed and confirmation that the entire tube has been removed is made (measure removed tube length against identical unused tube). Any stoma present is cleaned and allowed to heal by second intention.

Nasal and J tubes must be small in diameter to pass through the nose or into the bowel, limiting the diet to liquid formulations. Diluted blended canned diets can be placed through the larger diameter E and G tubes.

Enteral tube feeding can occur by one of two methods: bolus feeding (liquid or blended diets) and trickle-flow feeding (liquid). Figure 16.5 provides a schematic for determining which methods might be most appropriate for the individual patient. Bolus feeding is chosen when the GI tract is assessed as having normal motility and function. Bloat, poor motility, vomiting or frequent bouts of diarrhea are signs of GI sensitivity justifying the selection of trickle-flow feeding methods. Box 16.1 outlines the method for bolus feeding a patient an enteral diet. Box 16.2 outlines the method for trickle-flow (continuous rate of infusion) feeding. Nursing care for feeding tubes is found in Table 20.6.

Parenteral feeding methods

Parenteral feeding is used in patients that cannot tolerate enteral feeding. Severe GI sensitivity and neurological disease when the animal does not have a protected airway are two of the more common indications. Two different types of parenteral nutrition are available: central parenteral nutrition (CPN) and peripheral parenteral nutrition (PPN). CPN has been called total parenteral nutrition, but the "total" nutritional requirements are seldom delivered. The diet is more complete in CPN than PPN, providing glucose, lipids, amino acids, vitamins, and minerals. This results in a hyperosmolar solution that must be delivered through a central vein. PPN may only provide a portion of the total calories most commonly through carbohydrates and amino acids. PPN should be reserved for patients that need nutritional maintenance not nourishment, do not have severe disease, need short-term maintenance or are also receiving enteral nutrition. Any type of parenteral administration is intended to be a short-term supplement only, and is not intended for long-term feeding.

Central parenteral nutrition solutions are administered through a central venous catheter, requiring strict sterility of the catheter and administration sets to be maintained. The catheter insertion

---

Box 16.1 Bolus enteral feeding through tubes.

- Confirm accurate placement of the feeding tube (flushing with saline, radiograph, visualize at surgery or endoscopy).
- Wait 24 hours after placement of gastrostomy and jejunostomy tubes before use.
- Liquid concentration diets can be used for any size of feeding tube.
- Diluted blenderized diets can be used if >8 Fr feeding tube.

Bolus feedings

- Warm the food to body temperature.
- Day 1: one-third of the calculated RER is divided into 4–6 small feedings of 5–20 mL.
- Flush the tube with 3–5 mL of water before feeding to clear debris.
- Inject food through tube over several minutes; slow the rate if retching, drooling or swallowing observed.
- Flush the tube with 3–5 mL of water after each feeding and cap off the feeding tube.
- Day 2+: increase the volume of the diet by one-third/day depending upon patient tolerance of the caloric intake.
- Aspirate nasogastric or gastrostomy tubes prior to each feeding to ensure gastric emptying; if more than half of the previous meal persists, skip the next feeding and consider adding a motility modifier.
- Unblock a tube blockage by flushing a cola product or enzymatic solution into the tube overnight; replace the tube if still blocked.
- Increase the volume and decrease the frequency of feedings once stable on RER.
- Clean the wounds and change bandages every two to three days as necessary for esophagostomy, gastrostomy, and jejunostomy tubes.
- Place Elizabethan collars to prevent inadvertent removal of tubes.

RER, resting energy requirement.

Box 16.2 Trickle-flow tube feeding (continuous rate of infusion) of liquid diet.

- Flush the tube with 3–5 mL of water before starting infusion to clear debris.
- Day 1: place water or glucose-electrolyte solution sufficient for 4–8 hours into infusion bag to test GI tolerance of infusion.
- Place IV infusion line into bag and through pump. Consider adding blue food coloring to identify the water or glucose electrolyte solution.
- Infuse glucose-electrolyte/water solution at 0.6–2 mL/kg/h.
- Aspirate nasogastric or gastrotomy tubes every 2–4 hours to ensure gastric emptying; if more than half of the infused volume persists, consider adding motility modifier (such as metoclopramide, cisapride, ranitidine).
- Begin feeding liquid diet once patient is tolerating water or glucose-electrolyte solution.
- Place one-third of calculated RER in infusion bag, dilute with or water to desired daily volume (typically 1:3 dilution).
- Warm diet to room temperature.
- Begin CRI of diluted liquid diet at 0.6–2.0 mL/kg/h; slow the rate if retching, drooling or swallowing observed.
- Flush and aspirate tube periodically to ensure patency and evaluate residual volumes.
- Gradually increase concentration of diet by 25–33% every 12–24 hours until full strength.
- Gradually increase volume q 12–24 h to reach calculated RER.

CRI, constant rate infusion; RER, resting energy requirement.

site should undergo a surgical preparation and scrub and the catheter set-up must be handled aseptically. Surgical draping is recommended during catheter placement. Single- or multilumen central catheters can be used. Administration of the CPN solution is through a 1.2 μm in-line filter. If a single-lumen catheter is used, it should be dedicated to the infusion of CPN and not used for blood draws or the administration of medications. Multilumen catheter can have multiple uses, as long as the CPN infusion port is dedicated.

Peripheral parenteral nutrition solutions have a lower osmolality (≤550 mOsm/L) and may be safely given through a peripheral vein. Phlebitis, while uncommon, can still be a complication of PPN administration. Other IV fluids can be administered through this same catheter.

Depending on the route of administration, the volume of fluid administered through the diet should be factored into the daily maintenance fluid requirements for the patient. Catheter insertion sites and stoma sites should be kept clean and dry, with periodic examination for evidence of inflammation or infection.

Diet selection

The RER (also called resting energy expenditure) is an approximation of the calories (kilocalories (kcal)) the patient requires to maintain homeostasis at rest. It can be measured by indirect calorimetry or estimated by the calculations shown in Box 16.3. For ease, Table 16.6 provides the estimated RER according to kilogram and pound weight for most adult dogs and Table 16.7 provides the estimated RER for most weights of cats [9].

To avoid overfeeding of obese patients, an estimated lean body weight is used for the estimation of RER. Illness factors were advocated in the past, but the addition of an illness factor has not been shown to counter protein catabolism or improve outcome in small animal patients. Administration of the patient's 100% RER has not been shown to have a greater benefit than feeding approximately 65% of RER in critically ill human patients [21].

Enteral diets

An initial evaluation of the GI tract tolerance of enteral feeding can be made by trickle-flow infusion (0.6–2.0 mL/kg/h) of a glucose-electrolyte oral solution (such as Rebound OES®, Virbac Animal Health, Fort Worth, TX). It may be helpful to add a small amount of (blue) food coloring to identify this fluid when aspirating the feeding tube to estimate GRV. Delayed gastric emptying will cause accumulation of the infused electrolyte solution and can warrant the addition of a motility modifier drug and decreasing the trickle-flow rate of infusion.

Veterinary polymeric diets are available for enteral feeding of the dog and cat. Liquid veterinary critical care diets for dogs and cats, the calories per milliliter, the distribution of calories, and protein supplementation are listed in Table 16.8. Concentrated polymeric

veterinary diets for dogs and cats are most commonly called "recovery diets" and are listed with their calorie and protein content in Table 16.9. Polymeric diets contain intact protein, polysaccharides, and long-chain triglycerides that are well tolerated by veterinary patients [21,22].

Table 16.6 Calorie needs for an average healthy adult dog in ideal body condition.

Weight (kg)	Weight (lb)	Kilocalories/ day	Weight (kg)	Weight (lb)	Kilocalories/ day
2	4.4	140	26	57.2	970
3	6.6	190	27	59.4	1000
4	8.8	240	28	61.6	1020
5	11	280	29	63.8	1050
6	13.2	320	30	66	1080
7	15.4	360	31	68.2	1100
8	17.6	400	32	70.4	1130
9	19.8	440	33	72.6	1160
10	22	470	34	74.8	1180
11	24.2	510	35	77	1210
12	26.4	540	36	79.2	1240
13	28.6	580	37	81.4	1260
14	30.8	610	38	83.6	1290
15	33	640	39	85.8	1310
16	35.2	670	40	88	1340
17	37.4	700	41	90.2	1360
18	39.6	730	42	92.4	1390
19	41.8	760	43	94.6	1410
20	44	790	44	96.8	1440
21	46.2	820	45	99	1460
22	48.4	850	46	101.2	1480
23	50.6	880	47	103.4	1510
24	52.8	910	48	105.6	1530
25	55	940	49	107.8	1560

Note: these recommendations are for guidance only. Dogs are individuals and some may have higher or lower calorie requirements in order to maintain an ideal trim body condition.
These guidelines were first published in J Sm Anim Pract. 2011;52(7): 385–96. Used with permission of Wiley.

Table 16.7 Calorie needs for an average healthy adult cat in ideal body condition.

Weight (kg)	Weight (lb)	Kilocalories/day
1.0	2.2	100
1.5	3.3	130
2.0	4.4	160
2.5	5.5	180
3.0	6.6	210
3.5	7.7	230
4.0	8.8	250
4.5	9.9	270
5.0	11.0	290
5.5	12.1	310
6.0	13.2	330
6.5	14.3	350
7.0	15.4	370

Note: these recommendations are for guidance only. Cats are individuals and some may have higher or lower requirements in order to maintain an ideal trim body condition.
These guidelines were first published in J Sm Anim Pract. 2011;52(7):385–96. Used with permission of Wiley.

Box 16.3 Formulas for estimating RER in dogs and cats.

2–45 kg body weight:

$$RER(kcal/day) = (30 \times body\ weight\ in\ kg) + 70$$

<2 and >45 kg body weight:

$$RER(kcal/day) = 70(body\ weight\ in\ kg)^{0.75}$$

Table 16.8 Critical care liquid diets commercially available for small animal ICU patients.

Liquid diet	Calories per mL*	Distribution of nutrients (dry matter basis)	Protein supplementation
CliniCare Canine/Feline Liquid Diet® Abbott Animal Health, Abbott Park, IL	1 kcal/mL	Protein – 35.65% Fat – 22.17% CHO – 29.48% Fiber – 0.43% Ash – 7.395%	Arginine Glutamine Carnitine Taurine
CliniCare RF Feline® Abbott Animal Health, Abbott Park, IL	1 kcal/mL	Protein – 27.94% Fat – 29.77% CHO – 27.57% Fiber – 0.46% Ash – 6.87%	Arginine Glutamine Carnitine Taurine
Formula V EnteralCare KC Canine® (PetAg Inc., Hampshire, IL)	0.78 kcal/mL	Protein – 32.3% Fat – 16.6% Fiber – 0%	Taurine Arginine DL-methionine Carnitine
Formula V EnteralCare KC Feline® (PetAg Inc., Hampshire, IL)	0.69 kcal/mL	Protein – 41.6% Fat – 21.3% Fiber – 0%	Taurine Arginine DL-methionine Carnitine
Rebound® Liquid Diet Lactose free (VirbacVet, Fort Worth, TX)	0.73 kcal/mL	Protein – 34% Fat – 34.6% CHO – 17.3% Fiber – 1% Ash – 0.6%	Arginine Taurine
Emeraid® Critical Care HDN™ Critical care for canines (Emeraid, Cornell, IL)	2.0 kcal/mL	Protein – 34.87% Fat – 19.51% CHO – 41.16% Fiber – 4.46%	Taurine L-tryptophan L-lysine Cysteine L-threonine DL-methionine Glutamine Arginine Branched chain amino acids
Emeraid® Critical Care HDN™ Critical care for felines (Emeraid, Cornell, IL)	1.90 kcal/mL	Protein – 40.1% Fat – 28.2% Fiber – 3.82% CHO – 27.88%	L-tryptophan Glutamine Arginine Branched chain amino acids Taurine DL-methionine L-threonine cysteine

* Values are approximate.
CHO, carbohydrate.

After determining the RER, the protein, fat, and carbohydrate requirements desired are calculated (see Table 16.3) and the most appropriate diet selected based upon calorie and distribution of nutrients. Typically, the liquid diets are diluted with water or oral electrolyte solution and administered by bolus or trickle-flow feeding techniques (see Boxes 16.1 and 16.2). The concentration is increased over the first 24–48 hours of feeding, and then the volume, working to reach the total RER within 3–5 days, if tolerated.

Monomeric or elemental diets are liquid diets containing nutrients that require little or no digestion. The composition is usually amino acids, glucose, and oligosaccharides, with some fatty acids. There are no veterinary monomeric liquid diets available for the dog and cat. Products for human use include Peptamen® (Baxter Health Care, Deerfield, IL), Vivonex HN® (Norwich-Eaton Pharmaceuticals, Norwich, NY), and Vital HN® (Ross Products Division, Abbot Laboratories, Abbot Park, IL) [23]. Administration of these diets would be by trickle-flow feeding using the guidelines in Box 16.2.

These diets might be indicated for treatment of severe GI diseases such as pancreatitis or short bowel syndrome or demonstrated intolerance of a polymeric diet [24]. However, these diets lack essential nutrients for the dog and cat and should be used only on a short-term basis or should be supplemented to meet nutritional needs.

Vomiting, diarrhea, and regurgitation may occur if the patient is overfed, fed too quickly, or the osmolarity of the food is too high. Lowering the volume of food administered or increasing the timing of food infusion can address these problems. The diet should be at room temperature and may require further dilution with water to lower the osmolarity.

Parenteral diets

Commercial formulations for CPN have not been adequately evaluated in veterinary patients. Most often, the CPN diet is a composition of protein from a commercial 8.5% amino acid solution, lipids from a commercial 20% lipid solution, and carbohydrates

Table 16.9 Critical care concentrated diets commercially available for small animal ICU patients.

Diet	Calories	Analysis	Comments
Maximum Calorie® (Iams Co, Dayton, OH)	333 kcal/can	Protein – 41% Fat – 35% CHO – 12.7% Fiber – 2.9% Ash – 8.2%	DL-methionine Taurine
Urgent Care a/d® (Hill's Pet Nutrition, Topeka, KS)	180 kcal/can	Protein – 44.2% Fat – 30.4% CHO – 15.4% Fiber – 1.3%	Glutamine Taurine Branched chain amino acids
Recovery RS® (Royal Canin, St Charles, MO)	184 kcal/can	g/1000 kcal: Protein – 98.9 Fat – 64.8 Fiber – 14.4	Taurine
CN Critical Nutrition® (Nestlé Purina Pet Care, St Louis, MO)	208 kcal/can	Protein – min 9.5% Fat – min 7.5% Fiber – max 1.5% Moisture 75%	DL-methionine Taurine

CHO, carbohydrate.

Table 16.10 Guidelines for calculating central (total) parenteral nutrition formulation from 8.5% amino acid solution, 20% lipid solution, and 50% dextrose solution.

Central (total) parenteral nutrition calculations	Sums
Nutrient goals (grams/100 kcal) *Protein dogs (cats)* 15–25% of RER calories 4–6 g/100 kcal (6 g/100 kcal) Hepatic/renal failure 2–3 g/100 kcal (3–4 g/100 kcal) Protein-losing disease 6 g/100 kcal (6 g/100 kcal)	
Lipids 30–50% of remaining RER	
Carbohydrates 30–50% of remaining RER	
Protein 8.5% amino acid solution = 0.085 g protein/mL RER kcal × (g protein desired/100 kcal) = #g protein desired/day g protein desired/day × 0.085 g/mL = # mL of amino acid solution/day (A) 4 kcal/g protein × g protein desired/day = kcal from protein RER kcal – kcal from protein = kcal from fats and CHO (1/2 from each)	A
Lipids 20% lipid solution = 2 kcal/mL remaining kcal ÷ 2 = kcal from lipids (same # kcal for CHO) kcal from lipids ÷ 2 kcal/mL = # mL of lipid solution/day (B)	+ B
Carbohydrates 50% dextrose = 1.7 kcal/mL kcal from CHO ÷ 1.7 kcal/mL = # mL of dextrose solution/day (C)	+ C
Add nutrient volumes together	=
Total volume of nutrient solution/day	Total volume (mL)

Adapted from: Chan D, Freeman L. Nutrition in critical illness. Vet Clin North Am Small Anim Pract. 2006;36:1225–41.[1].
CHO, carbohydrate; RER, resting energy requirement.

from a 50% dextrose solution. The procedure for calculating the amount of each nutrient to combine to make the CPN diet specific for the patient is outlined in Table 16.10. The diets are created for the individual patient, noting that animals with hypertriglyceridemia may not require lipid supplementation. The compounding of these solutions should occur within a laminar flow hood to avoid bacterial contamination. Some human hospitals and compounding pharmacies can mix the solution based on a prescription providing the volume and final concentration of each component [25].

Similar to enteral nutrition, CPN is initiated at 25% of RER and gradually increased to full RER over 48–72 hours. The bag of admixture lasts 24 hours, with any remaining solution being discarded after that period of time. The patient should not be disconnected from the solution at any time while receiving CPN to avoid bacterial contamination of the diet or catheter. The volume delivered daily depends on patient status with fluid therapy infusion adjusted to include the CPN volume to avoid fluid overload. Discontinuation of CPN should occur when enteral feeding has been initiated through voluntary or tube feeding.

Peripheral (or partial) parenteral nutrition can play a role in the early transition period onto an enteral feeding regime. This solution is not meant to meet RER calories, but instead can supplement essential amino acids and carbohydrates sufficient to minimize or eliminate the proteolysis of critical illness. Table 16.11 provides a procedure for compounding PPN using the same protein, lipid, and carbohydrate sources as CPN but calculated for lower concentrations in the admixture. A commercial solution (Procalamine®, B. Braun Medical,Bethlehem, PA) containing a lower percentage of branched chain amino acids (3%) and a carbohydrate source (3% glycerin) diluted in a maintenance electrolyte solution (Na+ 35 mEq/L; K+ 24.5 mEq/L) can be administered with or without additional maintenance crystalloids or colloids through a peripheral vein. This can provide a lower level of nutritional support while testing the GI tract for tolerance of enteral feeding.

Complications of CPN and PPN can be mechanical, caused by disconnection, line breakage, or occlusion of the administration apparatus. Sepsis and thrombosis or phlebitis at the catheter site may result from administration of the hyperosmolar solution or bacterial contamination from exogenous or hematogenous sources. High-dose lipid emulsion may cause immunosuppression via granulocyte and reticuloendothelial cell dysfunction. Monitoring of physical perfusion parameters, fluid balance, body weight, electrolytes (including phosphorus), glucose, and creatinine is a daily necessity.

An assessment of dogs and cats receiving PPN found the most common metabolic complication was hyperglycemia, followed by lipemia and hyperbilirubinemia. Most complications were mild and did not require discontinuation of PPN. Septic complications were rare, with all affected animals eventually being discharged from the hospital. The presence, type, and number of complications of PPN did not impact the duration of hospitalization or outcome. However, animals that received supplemental enteral nutrition survived more often than those receiving PPN exclusively [26].

A review of dogs and cats receiving more than their calculated RER by PN found that hyperglycemia was also the most common metabolic complication. A high creatinine in dogs was the only complication associated with mortality. Chronic kidney disease in

Table 16.11 Guidelines for calculating peripheral (partial) parenteral nutrition formulation from 8.5% amino acid solution, 20% lipid solution, and 50% dextrose solution.

Peripheral (partial) parenteral nutrition calculations	Sums
Partial ER (PER) = RER × 0.70	
Calorie calculations and distribution	
Small dogs and cats (3–10 kg)	
0.20–0.25 × PER for both protein and CHO	
0.60 × PER for lipids	
Medium dogs (11–30 kg)	
0.33 × PER for each (protein, CHO, and lipids)	
Large dogs (>30 kg)	
0.50 × PER for CHO	
0.25 × PER for both protein and lipid	
Protein	
8.5% amino acid solution = 0.085 g protein/ mL = 0.34 kcal/mL	A
PER kcal desired ÷ 0.34 kcal/mL = mL amino acid solution/day (A)	
Lipids	+
20% lipid solution = 2 kcal/mL	B
PER kcal ÷ 2 = kcal from lipids = # mL of lipid solution/ day (B)	
Carbohydrates	+
50% dextrose = 1.7 kcal/mL	C
PER from CHO ÷ 1.7 kcal/mL = # mL of dextrose solution/ day (C)	
Add nutrient volumes together	=
Total volume of nutrient solution/day	Total volume (mL)

Adapted from: Chan D, Freeman L. Nutrition in critical illness. Vet Clin North Am Small Anim Pract. 2006;36:1225–41.[1].
CHO, carbohydrate; RER, resting energy requirement.

Box 16.4 Nutrition and drug interactions [25,39].

Drugs compatible with CPN solutions

Aminophylline
Ampicillin
Cefazolin
Chloramphenicol
Cimetidine
Clindamycin
Digoxin
Diphenhydramine
Dopamine
Erythromycin
Furosemide
Gentamicin
Heparin
Insulin (regular)
Lidocaine
Metoclopramide
Penicillin G
Phytonadione
Ranitidine
Ticarcillin

dogs, hepatic lipidosis in cats, and longer duration of inadequate caloric intake before PN in both species were negatively associated with survival. Factors positively associated with survival included longer duration of PN administration in both species, enteral feeding in cats with any disease, and enteral feeding in dogs with respiratory disease [27].

Dietary additives

The pharmaconutrition concept considers nutrients as drugs, ideally provided separately from standard enteral or parenteral nutrition regimens in supraphysiological doses [28]. Current evidence suggests that low trace element and vitamin levels are associated with higher risk of death, systemic inflammatory response syndrome (SIRS), and higher oxidative stress, particularly in the most seriously ill human patients [29]. Most plasma micronutrient concentrations (except for vitamin E and copper) decrease with increasing severity of SIRS. Capillary leakage is associated with redistribution of micronutrients from the circulation. In addition, fluid loss, hemodilution, dehydration, and the standard enteral or parenteral nutrition regimens may compound low plasma levels of micronutrients in SIRS.

Oxidative stress overcomes the endogenous antioxidant defenses of the host in critical illness. The most up-to-date evidence in human medicine is supported by animal models and reinforces the concept that pharmaconutrition with high-dose micronutrient

supplements such as selenium, zinc, and antioxidant vitamins (C, E) is able to reduce oxidative stress, decrease infections, and reduce mortality. Enteral glutamine, arginine, and nucleotide supplementation have been found to augment the nonspecific host response to infection and support the health of the GI tract [30]. The optimal composition, dose, timing, and duration of therapy are key factors that still need to be established in humans and in veterinary small animal patients.

Vitamin B complex consists of folic acid, thiamine, riboflavin, niacin, pantothenic acid, pyridoxine, and cobalamin, essential for metabolism of glucose, fat, and protein by the liver. These water-soluble vitamins act as co-enzymes for the tricarboxylic acid cycle, energy production, and red blood cell metabolism [25]. All critical patients on fluid therapy should have 1 mL B vitamin complex (B-Vitamin Complex, Henry Schein Animal Health, Dublin, OH) per 100 kcal of RER/day added to the IV fluids or diet.

The addition of probiotics to the veterinary nutritional menu provides an option for balancing the GI flora with "good" bacteria. Products such as Fortiflora® (Purina Veterinary Diets, Nestlé, St Louis, MO) or Prostora® (Iams Company, Dayton, OH) provide bacteria such as *Enterococcus faecium* as well as vitamin C, vitamin E, beta-carotene, zinc, manganese, iron, copper, and sodium selenite. The goal of supplementing these nutrients is to promote GI health and boost the immune response.

The addition of IV drugs to the PN solution must be done with extreme caution. Common drugs used in the ICU that can be incorporated into the amino acid, glucose, and lipid mixture are listed in Box 16.4.

Nutritional disorders

There are several diseases or disorders seen in the dog and cat that are caused by an excess or deficiency of a single nutrient or group of nutrients (such as proteins, carbohydrates or fats). Table 16.12 provides a list of common nutritional problems, the mechanism of the

Table 16.12 Common medical problems associated with excess or deficiency of nutrients in the dog and cat.

Problem	Mechanism	Signs	Treatment
Hepatoencephalopathy	Imbalance of aromatic amino acids (phenylalanine, tryptophan and tyrosine) to branched chain amino acids (leucine, isoleucine, and valine) proposed leading to generation of false neurotransmitters	Mental depression, seizures, dementia, altered consciousness, coma, death	Treat liver disease; administration of branches chain amino acids not proven to be beneficial treatment in humans
Thiamine deficiency (primarily cats)	Thiaminase in raw fish; thiamine-deficient diets; prolonged, severe anorexia	Ventroflexion of neck, dementia, vocalization, seizures, coma	Administer 50-100 mg/kg thiamine IV or IM; B vitamin complex supplementation
Copper toxicity (hepatopathy) (West Highland White Terrier, Doberman Pinscher, Bedlington Terrier, Skye Terrier; rare in cats)	Lack of hepatic enzymes for biliary excretion; copper accumulation; breed predisposition	Chronic hepatitis, cirrhosis or failure	Symptomatic for liver failure, low protein, low copper diets, penicillamine (10–15 mg/kg PO q 12 h dogs) to chelate copper; zinc 100 mg to decrease copper GI absorption
Zinc toxicity	Usually from ingestions of nuts, bolts, pennies, toys, jewelry, some lotions; red blood cell hemolysis (mechanism not described)	Anemia, vomiting, diarrhea, hemoglobinuria, icterus, kidney failure possible; diagnosis by radiographs to find object, blood zinc levels; gastritis	Remove object providing zinc; red blood cell or whole-blood transfusion; fluid diuresis; GI protectants
Increased dietary protein in kidney disease	Acute and chronic increase in dietary protein affects renal blood flow and GFR; can induce renal hypertrophy and increased GFR and glomerular pressure in animals	Signs of kidney disease or failure: polyuria, polydipsia, hypertension, proteinuria, azotemia, uremia	High protein an issue only if renal injury or disease is present; use renal diets with protein, phosphorus, sodium restriction; supplementation with omega 3-fatty acids; protein restriction not preventative of kidney disease
Obesity	Excess of calories from any source; increased health risks; diabetes mellitus, cardiovascular disease, arthritis, lipidosis; early mortality in dogs and cats; fat produces hormones and cytokines, stimulates chronic inflammation	Clinical signs of chronic disease, arthritis	Dietary and behavioral modification. Higher protein and lower caloric intake; increase exercise
Feline hepatic lipidosis	Fasting or anorexia in cats; obesity predisposing factor; hepatic fat intake exceeds output; fat accumulation in hepatic cells; impaired liver function, can progress to liver failure; can be secondary to diabetes mellitus, hyperthyroidism	Icterus, vomiting, diarrhea, drooling, enlarged liver	Correct fluid balance, glucose and electrolyte alterations; key treatment is enteral feeding (E and G tubes ideal); vitamin K may be required for coagulation, lactulose for HE and dextrose for hypoglycemia may also be required
Carnitine deficiency (Boxer, Doberman Pinscher, Great Dane, Irish Wolfhound, other large breeds)	Carnitine must be transported to cardiac and skeletal muscle; inadequate fat usage for energy production	Dilated cardiomyopathy, heart disorders	Treat heart disease; dietary source milk and meat; l-carnitine supplementation (50–100 mg/kg/day PO q 8 h dogs, q 2–4 h cats); may or may not show improvement of heart disease
Taurine deficiency	Maintains function of retinal photoreceptor cells; affects K^+ efflux from cardiac cells	Dilated cardiomyopathy; blindness (cats especially)	Treat heart disease; taurine supplementation (20–25 mg/kg PO q 12 h dogs; 250–500 mg/cat q 12–24 h)
Nutritional secondary hyperparathyroidism	Meat-rich diets; too much PO_4^- compared to Ca^{++}	Bone fractures, bone resorption	Calcium supplementation; change diet to meet normal 2.5:1 Ca^{++}: PO_4^- ratio; treat fractures – slow healing
Hypervitaminosis A	Liver-rich diets; oversupplementation (cats most likely); inhibits intramembranous and endochondral ossification, results in dystrophic calcification	Excessive bone formation; bone deformities	
Vitamin D toxicity	Intestinal absorption of calcium; bone resorption; usually due to oversupplementation	Chronic kidney failure, arrhythmias	Blood work shows low phosphorus and high calcium
Skin disease	Deficiencies in omega-6 polyunsaturated fatty acids, zinc, vitamin A, B vitamins	Scaly or flaky skin, pruritus, seborrhea, alopecia	Fatty acid supplementation; elimination diet for allergens, B vitamin supplementation

GFR, glomerular filtration rate; GI, gastrointestinal; HE, hepatic encephalopathy.

resulting disorder, clinical signs of the problem, and general treatment recommendations.

There are also specific disorders that can result from the administration of nutritional support in the ICU. Enteral feed intolerance, refeeding syndrome, and drug–food interactions are potential complications that require early recognition, appropriate intervention, and careful monitoring to optimize patient recovery.

Enteral feeding intolerance

Feeding intolerance can manifest with one or more of the following clinical features: large GRV, GI symptoms, which can include vomiting, diarrhea, abdominal distension, and inadequate delivery of enteral nutrition. A precise range of volume has not been described to define a large GRV for the dog and cat. However, there is no reported difference in GRV in dogs fed by continuous compared to intermittent bolus enteral feeding. In addition, there was no correlation between the GRV in the dog and the occurrence of vomiting or regurgitation with enteral feeding [14].

The prevalence of enteral feeding intolerance in critical human patients is close to 30% [31]. While the incidence in small animal ICU patients is unknown, GI signs warranting adjustment in feeding procedures or the use of a motility modifier are not uncommon. The clinical signs most typically result from impaired gastroduodenal motility and absorption, but other GI abnormalities such as impaired barrier function may also contribute.

The response to enteral GI intolerance can incorporate one or more of the following:
- add an antiemetic if vomiting is occurring
- add a motility modifier if vomiting or GRV observed to match diet volume input
- dilute the diet
- reduce the volume of infusion
- adjust the content of the diet
- discontinue enteral feeding for 12–24 h.

While erythromycin has a stronger effect on gastric motility, metoclopramide has been reported as the most frequently prescribed agent for stimulating GI motility in response to feeding intolerance in humans [31].

Refeeding syndrome

The refeeding syndrome can be defined as the potentially fatal fluid and electrolyte shifts that may occur in malnourished patients receiving either enteral or parenteral feeding [32]. These shifts result from hormonal and metabolic changes and may cause serious complications. The hallmark biochemical feature of refeeding syndrome is hypophosphatemia. However, the syndrome is complex and may also feature abnormal sodium and fluid balance, changes in glucose, protein and fat metabolism, thiamine deficiency, hypokalemia, and hypomagnesemia [33]. Malnutrition is the strongest risk factor in humans. When parenteral feeding solutions contain phosphorus, the incidence declines from 100% to 18%.

With prolonged fasting, there is protein and muscle breakdown, with muscle and other tissues reducing their use of ketone bodies and instead using fatty acids as their main energy source [34]. There is a decrease in intracellular minerals, such as phosphorus, with a reduction in renal excretion of these minerals.

During refeeding of carbohydrates, there is an increase in insulin release and a decrease in the secretion of glucagon. Insulin promotes glycogen, fat and protein synthesis, which requires the presence of phosphorus, magnesium, and thiamine. Insulin also stimulates the movement of potassium into the cells. Phosphorus and magnesium also move to the intracellular space, with water following by osmosis. This lowers even further the serum concentrations of phosphorus, magnesium, and potassium.

In the refeeding syndrome, the insulin surge causes an increased uptake and use of phosphate in the cells, resulting in both intracellular and extracellular phosphate deficits. This affects almost every metabolic system of the body (energy production and storage, acid–base balance, hemoglobin affinity for oxygen, cell membrane integrity).

While serum concentrations may remain normal, there is a whole-body deficit of K^+. This affects the electromechanical membrane potential and can lead to arrhythmias and even death. Magnesium deficits cause a decrease in oxidative phosphorylation and ATP production, abnormalities in DNA, RNA, and ribosome structural integrity, and impaired membrane potential. Cardiac and neuromuscular signs (such as seizures, tetany, tremors) can be a consequence.

Glucose intake after starvation suppresses gluconeogenesis due to endogenous insulin release (see Chapter 5). Excessive administration can lead to hyperglycemia with glycosuria and the dehydration, metabolic acidosis and ketoacidosis that can follow. Lipogenesis follows which can cause hepatic lipidosis, hypercapnia, and eventually respiratory failure. Thiamine, an essential co-factor for carbohydrate metabolism, is deficient and can initiate serious neurological problems (such as dementia, seizures, coma).

The introduction of carbohydrate to the diet leads to a rapid decline in renal excretion of Na^+ and water [35]. The administration of fluids to maintain normal urine output can lead to volume overload with pulmonary edema, heart failure, and arrhythmias as potential consequences.

Patients that have been without food for >5 days are considered at risk in human ICUs [34]. Thorough assessment should identify the small animal patient that is susceptible through diet history, electrolyte levels (to include phosphorus), and blood glucose results. To avoid refeeding syndrome, the patient is fed ≤50% of the estimated RER. The guidelines in Boxes 16.1 and 16.2 recommend feeding one-third of the RER, which should provide a safe approach for the patient. Thiamine supplementation (50–100 mg/day IM or IV) is warranted in all patients during feeding in the ICU. Careful attention to fluid balance helps to avoid overhydration and electrolyte levels are monitored and corrected as indicated (see Chapter 6).

Treatment of the refeeding syndrome requires the temporary cessation of feeding and immediate stabilization of airway, breathing (see Chapter 8), and circulation (see Chapter 2). Cardiac and neurological function should be assessed and treatment initiated as indicated. Patient warming may be required with immediate attention given to the correction of critical electrolyte (Na^+, K^+, Mg^{++}, phosphorus) abnormalities. Thiamine should be administered by injection. Careful monitoring is required as the patient is reintroduced to feeding.

Drug–food interactions

The clinical significance of drug–food interactions can be variable in humans and has not been clearly defined for the dog and cat. Generally, the effect of food on drugs can result in a reduction in the drug's bioavailability and potentially alter drug clearance. Numerous drugs display clinically important differences in pharmacokinetics when administered with food relative to when administered under fasted conditions. A multitude of mechanisms could be responsible for food effects, including delayed gastric emptying, drug solubility due to the presence of food and digestive fluids, the formation of drug–food complexes, alterations in hepatic blood flow and modulation of drug-metabolizing enzymes by constituents of food [36].

The type, amount, and timing of foods consumed can influence drug dissolution, absorption, distribution, metabolism, and excretion [37]. High-fat meals may enhance the absorption of some oral medications (such as griseofulvin). The calcium in milk-based enteral diets could inhibit the oral absorption of doxycycline or tetracycline.

The fat, protein, and carbohydrate components of the diet can also affect drug pharmacokinetics and dynamics. High-fat meals will increase plasma concentrations of free fatty acids, which could displace a drug from binding sites on plasma albumin. High-protein diets increase the activity of the hepatic cytochrome p450 oxidative system and enhance the metabolism of numerous drugs. High electrolyte intake could diminish the action of diuretic agents. In addition, drugs could inhibit the concentration of important nutrients. Some laxatives will decrease lipid digestion and absorption, thereby affecting the absorption of the fat-soluble vitamins. Tetracycline and doxycycline will bind iron and decrease its absorption. Coumadins inhibit the function of vitamin K. Long-term treatment with phenobarbital and other anticonvulsants has been found to cause excessive metabolism and deficiency of vitamin D in humans.

A poor nutritional status could affect the drug detoxification system, making it more inefficient [38]. Nutritional factors (including proteins, carbohydrates, fats, vitamins, and minerals) could affect the efficiency of the hepatic cytochrome p450 oxidative system. Diets restricted in calories, protein, or essential fatty acids, as well as those having low-quality protein or high sugar content, can affect the component enzymes, cytochrome p450, and cytochrome p450 reductase. In addition, deficiencies of specific vitamins (riboflavin, ascorbic acid, vitamins A and E) and minerals (iron, copper, zinc, magnesium) could affect the cytochrome p450 system.

The full impact of diet and nutrition on drug therapy in the dog and cat is unknown at this time. It is important to review the list of pharmaceuticals given to the critical patient, including herbal and over-the-counter medications, in light of their nutritional status and nutritional support. Adjustment may be required in drug or diet composition, dose, timing or route of administration to avoid negative drug–food interactions.

References

1. Chan D, Freeman L. Nutrition in critical illness. Vet Clin North Am Small Anim Pract. 2006;36:1225–41.
2. Caesar MP, Langouche L, Coudyzer W, et al. Impact of early parenteral nutrition on muscle and adipose tissue components during critical illness. Crit Care Med. 2013;41(10):2298–309.
3. Shikora SA. Special nutrients for gut feeding. In: Nutrition Support. Theory and Therapeutics. New York: Chapman and Hall, 1997: pp 285–301.
4. McCwen KC, Bistrain BR. Immunonutrition: problematic or problem solving? Am J Clin Nutr. 2003;77:764–70.
5. Rombeau JL. Enteral nutrition and critical illness. In: Enteral Nutrition. New York: Chapman and Hall, 1994: pp 25–36.
6. Johnson V, Gaynor A, Chan DL, Rozanski E. Multiple organ dysfunction syndrome in humans and dogs. J Vet Emerg Crit Care 2004;14(3):158–66.
7. Zaloga GP. Early enteral nutritional support improves outcome. Hypothesis or fact? Crit Care Med. 1999;27:259–61.
8. Brunetto MA, Gomes MOS, Andre MR, et al. Effects of nutritional support on hospitalized outcome in dogs and cats. J Vet Emerg Crit Care 2010;20(2):224–31.
9. World Small Animal Veterinary Association Global Nutrition Committee. Nutrition Toolkit. Available at: www.wsava.org/nutrition-toolkit (accessed 1 June 2016).
10. O'Toole EL, McDonell WN, Wilson BA, Mathews KA, Miller CW, Sears WC. Evaluation of accuracy and reliability of indirect calorimetry for the measurement of resting energy expenditure in healthy dogs. Am J Vet Res. 2001;62(11):1761–7.
11. O'Toole EL, Miller CW, Wilson BA, Mathews KA, Davis C, Sears W. Comparison of the standard predictive equation for calculation of resting energy expenditure with indirect calorimetry in hospitalized and healthy dogs. J Am Vet Med Assoc. 2004;225(1):58–64.
12. Edwards S, Metheny N. Measurement of gastric residual volume: state of the science. Med Surg Nurs. 2000;9:125–8.
13. Horn D, Chaboyer W, Schluter P. Gastric residual volumes in critically ill pediatric patients: a comparison of feeding regimens. Aust Crit Care 2004;17:98–103.
14. Holahan M, Abood S, Hauptman J, et al. Intermittent and continuous enteral nutrition in critically ill dogs: a prospective randomized trial. J Vet Intern Med. 2010;24:520–6.
15. Dhaliwa R, Heyland DK. Nutrition and infection in the intensive care unit: what does the evidence show? Curr Opini Crit Care 2005;11(5):461–7.
16. Gramlich L, Kichian K, Pinkilla J, et al. Does enteral nutrition compared to parenteral nutrition result in better outcomes in critically ill adult patients? A systematic review of the literature. Nutrition 2004;20(10):843–8.
17. Atkinson S, Sieffert E, Bihari D. A prospective, randomized, double-blind, controlled clinically trial of enteral immunonutrition in the critically ill. Crit Care Med. 1998;26(7):1164–72.
18. Radriazzani D, Bertolini G, Facchini R, et al. Early enteral immunonutrition vs. parenteral nutrition in critically ill patients without severe sepsis: a randomized clinical trial. Intensive Care Med. 2006;32(8):1991–8.
19. Mazak T, Ebisawa K. Enteral vs parenteral nutrition after gastrointestinal surgery: a systematic review and meta-analysis of randomized controlled trials in the English literature. J Gastrointest Surg. 2008;4:739–55.
20. Krishman JA, Parce PB, Martinez A, et al. Caloric intake in medical ICU patients. Chest 2003;124(1):297–305.
21. Souba,WW. Nutritional support. N Engl J Med. 1997;338:41–8.
22. Proulx J. Nutrition in critically ill animals. In: The Veterinary ICU Book. Jackson Hole: Teton NewMedia, 2002: pp 202–17.
23. Hopkins B. Enteral nutrition products. In: Nutrition in Critical Care. St Louis: Mosby, 1994: pp 439–49.
24. Michel KE. Interventional nutrition for the critical care patient: optimal diets. Clin Tech Small Anim Pract. 1998;13(4):204–10.
25. Remillard RL. Nutritional support in critical care patients. Vet Clin North Am Small Anim. 2002;32:1145–64.
26. Chan DL, Freeman LM, Labato MA, Rush JE. Retrospective evaluation of partial parenteral nutrition in dogs and cats. J Vet Intern Med. 2002;16(4):440–5.
27. Queau Y, Larsen JA, Kass PH, Glucksman GS, Fascetti AJ. Factors associated with adverse outcomes during parenteral nutrition administration in dogs and cats. J Vet Intern Med. 2011;25(3):446–52.
28. Manzanaresa W, Langloisb PL, Hardyc G. Update on antioxidant micronutrients in the critically ill. Curr Opin Clin Nutr Metab Care 2013;16(6):719–25.
29. Berger MM, Shenkin A. Update on clinical micronutrient supplementation studies in the critically ill. Curr Opin Clin Nutr Metab Care 2006;9(6):711–16.
30. Santora R, Kozar RA. Molecular mechanisms of pharmaconutrients. J Surg Res. 2010;161(2):288–94.
31. Gungabissoon U, Hacquoil K, Bains C, et al. Prevalence, risk factors, clinical consequences and treatment of enteral feed intolerance during critical illness. J Enteral Parenteral Nutrit. 2015;39(4):441–8.
32. Solomon SM, Kirby DF. The refeeding syndrome: a review. J Parenter Enteral Nutr. 1990;14:90–7.
33. Perrault MM, Ostrop NJ, Tierney MG. Efficacy and safety of intravenous phosphate replacement in critically ill patients. Ann Pharmacother. 1997;31:683–8.
34. Hisham M, Mehanna J, Moledina, Travis J. Refeeding syndrome: what it is and how to prevent and treat it. Br Med J. 2008;336:1495–8.
35. Veverbrants E, Arky RA. Effects of fasting and refeeding: studies on sodium, potassium and water excretion on a constant electrolyte and fluid intake. J Clin Endocrinol Metab. 1969;29:55–62.
36. Harris RZ, Jang GR, Tsunoda S, et al. Dietary effects on drug metabolism and transport. Clin Pharmacokinet. 2003;42(13):1071–88.
37. Hathcock JN. Metabolic mechanisms of drug–nutrient interactions. Fed Proc. 1985;44(1):124–9.
38. Bidlack WR, Brown RC, Mohan C. Nutritional parameters that alter hepatic drug metabolism, conjugation, and toxicity. Fed Proc. 1986;45(2):142–8.
39. Trissel LA. Handbook on Injectable Drugs, 9th edn. Bethesda: American Society of Hospital Pharmacists, 1996.
40. Kerl ME, Johnson PA. Nutritional plan: matching diet to disease. Clin Tech Small Anim Pract. 2004;19(1):9–21.
41. Saker KE. Nutrition and immune function. Vet Clin North Am. 2006;36:1199–224.
42. Michel KE. Interventional nutrition for the critical care patient: optimal diets. Clin Tech Small Anim Pract. 1998;13(4):204–10.
43. Souba WW, Kimberg VS, Plumley D, et al. The role of glutamine in maintaining a healthy gut and supporting the metabolic response to injury and infection. J Surg Res. 1990;48:383–91.

CHAPTER 17

Temperature

Conni Wehausen

Animal Emergency and Referral Center of Minnesota, St Paul, Minnesota

Introduction

Alterations of body temperature are common in the critical small animal patient, providing insight into systemic and environmental conditions affecting the animal. In general, heat will increase and cold will decrease the metabolic rate. When all parts of the heat-regulating mechanism operate smoothly, body temperature stays near the normal temperature or "set-point" temperature of the body. However, there are times when body temperature can go awry.

Significant changes in the body temperature can be a consequence of one or more problems, such as:

- an altered metabolic rate
- impaired perfusion
- drug administration
- circulating toxins or mediators
- exposure to harmful environmental temperature extremes.

Measuring body temperature is a vital component of every physical examination, with temperature reported in either degrees Fahrenheit (°F) or degrees Celsius (°C). The formulae to convert between °F and °C are given in Box 17.1.

Homeostatic mechanisms maintain a normal temperature *range* rather than a fixed value, with the body temperature oscillating around the desired normal set-point temperature of the body. Normal rectal body temperature in the dog and cat varies throughout the day between 99.5 °F and 102.5 °F (37.5–39.2 °C) in the dog and 100–103.1 °F (37.8–39.5 °C) in the cat [1]. The set-point may vary with changing environments or differing activity levels and is controlled by thermoregulation.

Thermoregulation is the process of maintaining body temperature by balancing heat production and heat loss. Body heat is a product of heat-generating metabolism as well as absorption of environmental heat. The basal metabolism of the truncal organs, brain, and skeletal muscle produces body heat, with accelerated metabolism resulting in accelerated heat production [1,2]. Increased muscle (shivering), hormone (thyroxine, growth hormone), catecholamine (epinephrine, norepinephrine), and sympathetic activity can all contribute to increased metabolism and heat production [2]. The skin and subcutaneous fat act to insulate the body and retain heat.

To maintain normothermia, heat loss must match heat input and production (Figure 17.1). Heat is transferred from the body core to the skin through a dynamic vasculature system, allowing the skin temperature to fluctuate [2]. Four mechanisms allow heat loss from the skin to the surroundings. *Conduction* is the transfer of heat from the body directly to an object it comes into contact with (such as a metal table or kennel surface). *Convection* is the transfer of heat from the body to the air that surrounds it. *Radiation* is the transfer of heat through electromagnetic waves to surrounding objects that do not come into direct contact with the body. *Evaporation* is heat loss that occurs when water is turned into vapor (seen with panting and sweating) [1–3].

The process of thermoregulation is controlled by the hypothalamus (Figure 17.2). The anterior hypothalamus contains warm-sensitive, cool-sensitive, and temperature-insensitive neurons that determine the desired set-point of the body. The preoptic nuclei in the anterior hypothalamus act as central temperature sensors, sensing both heat and cold in the blood circulating through the hypothalamus. Temperature receptors in the skin sense peripheral temperatures while core receptors sense the temperature in the abdominal viscera, spinal cord, and great vessels. Information is then transferred to the posterior hypothalamus where the signals are integrated to control thermoregulation [1,2] through stimulation of the autonomic nervous system. During hyperthermia (temperatures above the set-point), the hypothalamus initiates mechanisms to decrease temperature by causing vasodilation of blood vessels in the skin, inhibiting chemical thermogenesis (decrease heat production), and causing the animal to pant and, in some species, to sweat. During hypothermia (temperatures below the set-point), the hypothalamus initiates mechanisms to increase temperature by causing vasocontriction of the skin vasculature to minimize heat loss, stimulating piloerection to trap insulating air close to the body, and increasing heat production through shivering, sympathetic excitation, and increased thyroxine secretion. Hypothermia can stimulate behavioral changes causing the animal to seek warmth and curl up to conserve heat [2].

Following the trends of change in body temprature can provided insight into the metabolic demands on the ICU patient. While measuring the body temperature can be a simple procedure, determining the underlying cause of a temperature change and the possible consequences provides a stimulating challenge.

Initial diagnostics and monitoring methods

Careful assessment of the results of diagnostic and monitoring procedures is necessary to identify a potential source of a critical temperature change. Important information can be derived from the history, physical examination, clinicopathological testing, diagnostic imaging, and monitoring procedures.

Monitoring and Intervention for the Critically Ill Small Animal: The Rule of 20, First Edition. Edited by Rebecca Kirby and Andrew Linklater.
© 2017 John Wiley & Sons, Inc. Published 2017 by John Wiley & Sons, Inc.

Initial history and physical examination

The history begins with the signalment (age, sex, breed) and can reveal variables potentially contributing to changes in body temperature, such as a breed predisposition to altered heat regulatory mechanisms (such as brachycephalic breeds), dysregulation of temperature in geriatric dogs and cats, poor heat generation in toy breeds or very young animals or a genetic predisposition to malignant hyperthermia. Exposure to elevated or cold environmental temperatures, vigorous exercise, inadequate access to water or shelter, and important past medical problems (such as collapsing trachea, laryngeal paralysis, hypothyroidism) are factors that could affect thermoregulation identified through

history. A list of prescribed drugs (human and veterinary), exposure to possible toxins or recreational stimulants and any over-the-counter medications administered could reveal a potential source of temperature change. Table 17.1 lists drugs known to affect thermoregulation.

Physical examination begins with temperature, pulse rate and intensity, and respiratory rate and effort. Core body temperature will provide a true reflection of the internal body temperature and can be measured using a pulmonary artery catheter, esophageal probe or urinary bladder thermistor. These techniques are invasive, require heavy sedation or anesthesia for placement and precise positioning to obtain reliable measurements [4,5]. More commonly, minimally to noninvasive methods are utilized to measure temperature in veterinary patients and include rectal, auricular, and axillary thermometry. The methods available to measure body temperature are listed in Table 17.2 with recognized advantages and disadvantages of each technique [4,6–8]. The rectal temperature remains the "gold standard" for the noninvasive estimation of the core temperature by a peripheral method.

Box 17.1 Temperature conversion formulas.

$°F = (°C \times 1.8) + 32$ or $°F = (°C \times 9/5) + 32$

$°C = (°F - 32) \times 0.556$ or $°C = (°F - 32) \times 5/9$

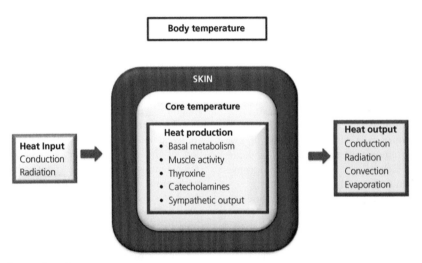

Figure 17.1 Maintenance of normothermia.

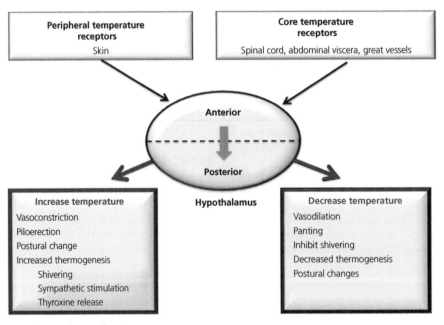

Figure 17.2 Hypothalamic regulation of normothermia.

Table 17.1 Drugs which affect body temperature.

Temperature elevation	Temperature reduction
Methylxanthine derivatives	Muscle relaxants
Caffeine, theobromine, chocolate	Sedatives
Illicit/recreational drugs	Narcotics
Marijuana, cocaine, amphetamines, cocaine	Anesthetics
Belladonna alkaloids	Nonsteroidal antiinflammatory drugs
Atropine, scopolamine	Glucocorticosteroids
Antibioitics	Antipsychotic drugs
Tetracyclines, beta-lactams, sulfonamides	
Sympathomimetics (allergy/ADHD/diet drugs)	
Amphetamines, ephedrine, pseudoephedrine, phenylpropanolamine	
Inhaled anesthetics (malignant hyperthermia)	
Allergy drugs	
Loratadine, promethazine	
Mental illness drugs	
Thioridazine, chlorpromazine, prochlorperazine	
Major tranquilizers	
Phenothiazines, butyrophenones, thioxanthenes	
Blood pressure drugs	
Mecamylamine, beta-blockers	
Migraine drugs (triptanes)	
Opioids	

ADHD, attention deficit hyperactivity disorder.

Table 17.2 Methods of temperature measurement.

Thermometry site	Advantages	Disadvantages	Comment
Rectal Mercury in glass Digital	Easy, inexpensive, widely available Requires 3 minutes contact time Equilibration type requires 1 minute contact time; predictive requires 10–15 seconds, calculates final result	Fecal material can affect contact with rectal mucosa. Patient discomfort, increased stress response [7]. Could spread infectious disease [9,10]. Avoid if anal area trauma, wounds or masses Potential for leakage of mercury – not recommended.	Rectal thermometry is the "gold standard" for peripheral estimate of core temperature [4,6,11]. Requires contact with rectal mucosa. Two types of rectal thermometers, which have similar reported results [12,13]
Pulmonary artery	Accurate core body temperature	Invasive and costly. Requires placement of pulmonary artery catheter	The ideal method for measuring core body temperature
Esophageal	Highly accurate reflection of core temperature	Considered invasive, used primarily during anesthesia. Requires specialized equipment	Placement of sensor is in the lower 1/3 of esophagus close to heart and aorta [14]
Urinary bladder	Highly accurate reflection of core temperature	Considered invasive, used during anesthesia or ICUs. Requires specialized equipment. Results affected by urine flow and volume.	Urine temperature is a reflection of temperature of renal blood flow (20% of cardiac output) [15]
Auricular	Reasonably priced. Veterinary brands available. Generally nonstressful to patient. Can use device in axillary region, as well	Temperatures reported as variable, poorly correlating with rectal and pulmonary arterial temperatures. Under estimates core temperature, especially if hyperthermia.[6,8,16–18] Affected by ceruminous debris or fluid behind tympanic membrane.	Uses infrared thermometry to measure heat from tympanic membrane and ear canal [8,12]. Tympanic membranes share blood supply with hypothalamus for good indication of core temperature [4,19,20]
Axillary	Found to be less stressful in dogs [7]	Wide variation in correlation with rectal temperatures.[18,21–23] Found less accurate if higher body condition scores.[21]	Can use digital rectal or auricular thermometer. Place at the midpoint of the axilla as far anterior as possible against the thorax [21]
Toe web	Large difference with rectal temperature suggests poor peripheral perfusion. Can use to assess response to treatment for perfusion abnormalities	Not an accurate method without comparison to rectal temperature.	Can use rectal thermometer or thermistor probe. Place between toes of rear paw and compare to rectal temperature. Toe web normally 2–9 °F (1–4 °C) lower than rectal temperature

Table 17.3 Common clinical signs associated with altered body temperature.

Body system	Hypothermia	Hyperthermia
Cardiovascular	Hypotension, dysrhythmias: pulse deficit (bradyarrhythmias), decreased cardiac output (shock); ECG: prolonged PR interval, wide QRS, J waves, Afib, Vtach, Vfib	Early (dogs: tachycardia, hyperemia, CRT <1 sec, bounding pulses Later (dogs,cats): bradycardia, weak pulses, CRT >2 sec, pale membranes, dysrhythmias: pulse deficit
Respiratory	Initially increased RR, then decreased respiratory depth and rate; finally apnea	Rapid RR (panting), loud upper airway noises, cyanosis if airway obstruction; increased respiratory rate and effort with crackles if lung edema or hemorrhage
CNS/neuromuscular	Altered mentation, shivering (dogs), stiff movements and hyporeflexia	Altered mentation, obtunded stupor, comatose, seizures, tremors
Renal	Polyuria (cold diuresis)	Dehydration, oliguria, anuria, hematuria, pigmenturia
Gastrointestinal	Decreased bowel sounds, ileus	Vomiting, diarrhea, blood, and mucosa from rectum, decreased bowel sounds, ileus
Coagulation	Bleeding from venipuncture sites, petechiation, ecchymosis	Bleeding from venipuncture sites, petechiation, ecchymosis
Skin/subcutaneous tissues	Cold to touch, vasoconstriction, piloerection, necrosis if frostbite	Vasodilation, hyperemia, skin tenting with dehydration, blistering, burns

Afib, atrial fibrillation; CNS, central nervous system; CRT, capillary refill time; RR, respiratory rate; Vfib, ventricular fibrillation; Vtach, ventricular tachycardia.

Heart rate, pulse intensity, capillary refill time, and mucous membrane color constitute the physical peripheral perfusion parameters used to assess tissue perfusion. Both high and low extremes in body temperature can cause hypovolemia and inadequate perfusion. Hydration is often affected, with dehydration reflected by dry mucous membranes, dull corneas, poor skin turgor, and sunken eye position.

Other clinical signs resulting from a body temperature change can be either focal and specific to the temperature change (such as burns with heat or frostbite with cold) or signs that are nonspecific to body temperature (such as shock, dehydration, panting). Any area of pain, heat or swelling is investigated as a site of infection or inflammation. A careful examination of the joints and deep palpation of bones may reveal a hidden site of inflammation. A list of organ systems and the clinical signs commonly associated with hyper- and hypothermia is provided in Table 17.3. Point of care (POC) testing (minimum database), clinicopathological testing, and diagnostic imaging are used to further define the cause and expose the consequences of a temperature abnormality.

Point of care testing

The POC minimum database should consist of packed cell volume (PCV), total proteins (TP), glucose, blood urea nitrogen (BUN), electrolytes, blood gas analysis, and coagulation profile (including platelet number estimate and buccal mucosal bleeding time). The PCV can reveal hemoconcentration due to dehydration or anemia due to blood loss or red blood cell lysis with either temperature extreme. Thrombocytopenia is common with both temperature disorders. Azotemia can also occur due to dehydration, hypovolemia or direct cytotoxic injury to the cells of the kidney. Hyperglycemia can be seen associated with an initial stress response, followed by hypoglycemia associated with glucose consumption with either hyper- or hypothermia.

Electrolyte results are assessed to identify hypernatremia since temperature alterations can stimulate the loss of free water. Potassium concentrations can be elevated with muscle necrosis or lowered through diuresis, each a potential serious consequence of an extreme alteration in body temperature. Blood gases often show metabolic acidosis with high blood lactate in patients with hyperthermia. Hypothermic patients often have respiratory acidosis.

Coagulopathies are common, with the prothrombin time (PT) and activated partial thromboplastin time (aPTT) frequently prolonged as a result of coagulation factor consumption surpassing production.

Alterations in coagulation parameters (PT, aPTT) should be interpreted cautiously in hypothermic patients since the tests are run at a controlled (normal body) temperature and do not necessarily reflect *in vivo* coagulation [24]. Platelet function can be abnormal, demonstrated by a prolongation of the buccal mucosal bleeding time.

Clinicopathological testing

A thorough evaluation of a patient for the consequences or causes of an unexplained change in temperature can be quite extensive. A complete blood count (CBC), serum biochemical profile, and urinalysis will provide an initial screen for problems associated with alterations in body temperature. The white blood count may be high with active inflammation or infection or low due to consumption and margination seen during sepsis. Nucleated red blood cells are seen in up to 90% of dogs with heat stroke [25]. Animals with a fever may show evidence of anemia with spherocytosis, nucleated red cells and reticulocytosis from immune-mediated diseases or nonregenerative anemia associated with chronic infectious or inflammatory diseases.

There are many chemistry abnormalities seen in patients with abnormal body temperature, with specific changes dependent upon the cause and the organs impacted by disease. Heat stroke often results in elevated liver enzymes and total bilirubin due to hepatocellular hypoxia. Urinalysis may reveal pigmenturia (myoglobin or hemoglobin), hematuria, proteinuria, renal tubular casts or isosthenuria due to urinary tract injury from temperature extremes. Urinary tract infections may be the primary indicator of systemic infection that is causing fever. Special testing may be requested, such as fluid analysis, culture and susceptibility testing, serology for infectious diseases, aspiration and cytology of mass lesions, immune panels, toxicology screening, and drug levels.

Diagnostic imaging

Diagnostic imaging begins with plain thoracic and abdominal radiographs. Thoracic radiographs are evaluated for pulmonary, cardiac or pleural space abnormalities. Pulmonary infiltrates can be found with pneumonia, cardiogenic, and noncardiogenic causes of edema, pulmonary hemorrhage, neoplasia, and acute lung injury or acute respiratory distress syndrome. Abdominal radiographs provide an initial assessment of bone density and structure, peritoneal fluid or air and organ size, shape, and position.

Ultrasound may provide a more detailed evaluation of organs for evidence of cysts, fluid, infiltrates, hemorrhage, cardiac disease or anatomical abnormalities. Free abdominal or pleural fluid or mass lesions can be aspirated and evaluated by culture, cytology, and biochemistry as indicated. Advanced imaging with computed tomography or nuclear magnetic resonance may be used to better define the extent and nature of a suspected or confirmed abnormality.

Monitoring techniques

Physical patient parameters provide the basis for continuous monitoring of the ICU patient with an abnormal body temperature. Frequent assessment of the physical peripheral perfusion parameters, hydration status, mentation, and respiratory rate and rhythm will aid in the early detection of consequences of extreme alterations in temperature (such as poor perfusion, dehydration, depressed mentation, seizures, labored breathing, panting). Indirect blood pressure monitoring provides additional information regarding peripheral perfusion, with trends of change monitored during and after resuscitation. The body temperature can be continuously monitored by inserting an indwelling rectal thermistor that provides data to a digital monitor, often found as part of the electrocardiogram (ECG) or other multiparameter monitoring equipment. The ECG can detect cardiac rate and rhythm abnormalities frequently noted with temperature abnormalities and allow timely intervention. Pulse oximetry and end-tidal CO_2 monitoring may be indicated for patients with respiratory changes.

Disorders of body temperature

Investigation of the physiological responses to hyperthermia and hypothermia provides insight into possible causes and potential complications. Fever, heat stroke, and malignant hyperthermia represent common hyperthermia syndromes encountered in the ICU patient. The systemic inflammatory response syndrome (SIRS) is anticipated in these patients. Hypothermia can be a consequence of critical problems in the ICU patient such as excessive heat loss (sedation, anesthesia or surgery), impaired circulation, and severe metabolic disease. Regardless of the cause, the effects of hyperthermia and hypothermia on patient perfusion and metabolism can be significant.

Hyperthermia

Hyperthermia is defined as an elevation in body temperature; this occurs when internal heat production or external heat input is greater than heat loss. It has been characterized as either pyrogenic (due to endogenous or exogenous pyrogens) or nonpyrogenic (due to environmental or metabolism-related heat sources) [25]. Pyrogenic hyperthermia is referred to as "fever."

A pyrogen is a heat-inducing substance that causes the thermoregulatory set-point in the anterior hypothalamus to rise or "reset" [26]. This higher temperature is now the new "normal" temperature for the animal. Exogenous pyrogens come from an external source and include substances such as bacterial endotoxins and other microbial products, viruses, incompatible blood products, and drugs. These exogenous pyrogens stimulate the body to produce additional pyrogens. These are called endogenous pyrogens and are low molecular weight proteins produced by phagocytic leukocytes and released into the circulation. Factors causing pyrogenic hyperthermia (fever) in small animals are listed in Table 17.4.

Nonpyrogenic hyperthermia occurs when heat from the environment or heat generated from exercise and metabolism exceeds heat dissipation mechanisms. This causes the body temperature to rise above the thermoregulatory set-point of the hypothalamus [25]. Factors causing nonpyrogenic hyperthermia in small animals are listed in Table 17.5.

Elevated body temperature can have severe deleterious effects on patients and cause prominent clinical signs (see Table 17.3). When body temperature rises, heat receptors stimulate the thermoregulatory center, immediately triggering cooling mechanisms (vasodilation, decreased metabolic rate, panting). Over time, the body begins to acclimate to a warmer body temperature by enhancing cardiovascular performance, stimulating the renin-angiotensin-aldosterone axis resulting in salt conservation by the kidneys, increasing glomerular filtration rate, expanding plasma volume, and increasing the ability to resist exertional rhabdomyolysis [27]. Heat stress activates the acute-phase response, resulting in production of both proinflammatory and antiinflammatory cytokines. Finally, heat shock proteins are formed to protect cells from injury by decreasing denaturation of protein and regulating the baroreceptor response to prevent hypotension [28].

The ICU patient may present with an elevated body temperature or develop the problem during hospitalization. The causes of fever or pyrogenic hyperthermia (infection, inflammation, immune disorder, neoplasia) are vastly different from the causes of nonpyrogenic hyperthermia (heat stroke, malignant hyperthermia, drug reaction), with temperature extremes (>106 °F (41.1 °C)) more likely with the nonpyrogenic causes.

Fever

The onset of fever in an ICU patient triggers an investigation for both infectious and noninfectious etiologies. The source of the inciting exogenous pyrogens can include infection (bacterial, viral, rickettsial, protozoal, parasitic, fungal), inflammation (ischemia, internal hemorrhage, necrosis), neoplasia or immune-mediated disease [26]. In humans, fevers have noninfectious origins in 25–50% of cases and the incidence in veterinary patients is thought to be similar [29–31]. Treatments commonly administered in the ICU can also act as exogenous pyrogens and cause fever. Blood transfusion, drug administration, and invasive medical procedures (such as indwelling catheter placement) can result in transfusion reaction, drug reaction, and catheter-related phlebitis respectively. Drugs have been found to cause increased body temperature in at least five ways: altered thermoregulatory mechanisms, drug administration-related fever, fever from the pharmacological action of the drug, idiosyncratic reactions, and hypersensitivity reactions [32]. The more common causes of infectious and noninfectious fever are listed in Table 17.4.

The body response to exogenous pyrogens is initiated by production of endogenous pyrogens that reset the hypothalamic thermoregulatory set-point [26]. Studies on the peripheral and central action of cytokines demonstrated that peripheral cytokines can communicate with the brain in several ways, including stimulation of afferent neuronal pathways and induction of the synthesis of a noncytokine pyrogen (prostaglandin E2) in endothelial cells in the periphery and in the brain. Cytokines synthesized in the periphery may cross the blood–brain barrier and act directly through neuronal cytokine receptors [33]. Following a rise in the set-point, the animal will increase heat production and decrease heat loss. Patients with true fever (reset set-point) are not likely to show signs of heat dissipation (such as panting) and may be curling up or shivering to generate heat and reduce heat loss.

Fever rarely leads to body temperatures high enough to result in host tissue damage. In fact, fever is thought to be an adaptation that has evolved to protect the body from invading pathogens. Fever has been shown to strengthen immune function by enhancing neutrophil and lymphocyte function, improving the antimicrobial activity of antibiotics and decreasing the availability of iron needed by bacteria to replicate [29,30]. Increased survival has been seen in both humans and animals with elevated body temperature in the face of infection [34,35].

Table 17.4 Common causes of fever.

Body system	Infectious etiology	Noninfectious etiology
Cardiovascular	Catheter infection Endocarditis	Vasculitis Thrombophlebitis Thromboemboli
Endocrine		Hypoadrenocorticism
Gastrointestinal	Infectious diarrhea Cholangiohepatitis Peritonitis	Pancreatitis Hepatitis Bowel infarct
Immune		IMHA IMTP
Integument/muscle	Wound infection Abscess	Surgical wounds Trauma Burns
Nervous	Meningitis	Steroid-responsive meningitis Intracranial hemorrhage
Reproductive	Pyometra Prostatitis	
Respiratory	Pneumonia Pyothorax Upper respiratory infection Bacterial Viral	Aspiration pneumonitis Atelectasis ARDS Pulmonary thromboembolism
Systemic	Rickettsial Fungal Protozoal Parasitic	Neoplasia Paraneoplastic syndrome SIRS Transfusion reaction
Urinary	UTI Pyelonephritis	
Other		Hemorrhage into confined spaces Drugs

ARDS, acute respiratory distress syndrome; IMHA, immune-mediated hemolytic anemia; IMTP, immune-mediated thrombocytopenia; SIRS, systemic inflammatory response syndrome; UTI, urinary tract infection.

Table 17.5 Common factors predisposing to nonpyrogenic hyperthermia.

Decreased heat dissipation
Abnormal upper airway
Tracheal collapse
Brachycephalic airway syndrome
Laryngeal paralysis
Obesity

Exposure to high environmental temperatures
Lack of water and shade
Enclosed environment
Inadequate ventilation
Heat cramps
Heat exhaustion
Heat stroke

Increased muscle activity
Exercise (exertional)
Seizures
Tremors, twitching

Hypothalamic disorders

Drugs (see Table 17.1)
Malignant hyperthermia
Vasoconstrictive drugs

Increased metabolic rate
Hyperthyroidism
Pheochromocytoma

Despite the many benefits of fever, there are deleterious effects associated with the amount and duration of temperature rise. Elevated body temperature increases metabolic demand and oxygen consumption. This has been found to lead to secondary neurological insult in human patients with ischemic stroke, traumatic brain injury, and myocardial injury [34]. Fever can result in patient discomfort, reducing activity and appetite and leading to longer hospital stays. The intensified microbial killing may also damage host tissue due to increased immune response [36].

Determining and treating the underlying cause of the fever is crucial to halting pyrogen production and establishing a body temperature within the normal range. The initial diagnostic testing often provides clues to identifying the source. However, when it does not, or when fever develops in an otherwise stable ICU patient, a search for the hidden source of pyrogens causing the "fever of unknown origin" is begun.

Diagnosis of fever of unknown origin

The basic components of the diagnostic approach to a patient with fever of unknown origin are listed in Table 17.6. Underlying problems such as infection, immune-mediated diseases, neoplasia, inflammation, and ischemia are common inciting causes. The history is reviewed and refined with emphasis on past medical problems and potential exposure to drugs or toxins. Current medications administered in the ICU are reviewed to identify any potential drug

Table 17.6 Diagnostic testing for causes of fever of unknown origin in critically ill dogs and cats.

Thorough history
Thorough physical examination
   Orthopedic (deep bone palpation, joints)
   Neurological
   Ophthalmic
   Rectal
Complete blood count
Serum chemistry profile
Evaluation of thyroid function
Infectious panels (canine, feline)
Urinalysis and urine culture, susceptibility
Imaging
   Radiography: abdominal, thoracic, orthopedic
   Ultrasonography: abdominal, musculoskeletal, retrobulbar
   Echocardiography: evaluate heart valves for endocarditis
   Computed tomography or magnetic resonance imaging of affected areas
Specific clinicopathological tests (as indicated)
   Bone marrow evaluation
   Arthrocentesis
   Cerebral spinal fluid analysis
   Fungal antigen or antibody testing
   Blood cultures
   Wound culture
   Serology, PCR or other evaluation for specific infectious diseases
   Serology for immune-mediated diseases
   Aspirates of affected regions with cytology and culture, susceptibility

offenders. Environmental sources of heat such as heating blankets, hot water bottles, excessive bedding, and poor ventilation (such as enclosed oxygen hoods or cages, or cages that are too small) are identified. The physical examination is repeated and compared to admission findings, with any areas of pain, swelling or inflammation becoming a focus. Catheter and any other skin penetration sites are examined for inflammation and infection. Wounds are uncovered and examined, with bandages checked for evidence of purulent exudate. Nosocomial infections have been reported to occur in up to 30% of hospitalized humans and provide a similar concern for hospitalized animals [26].

The initial clinicopathological data is compared with more current test results. Occult infections may be found within the reproductive tract, urinary tract, pulmonary tree, central nervous system or peritoneum. Additional clinicopathological testing is often required to identify these sources, submitting samples such as blood, urine or body fluid for culture and susceptibility (Table 14.1), blood for serology for infectious agents, blood for immune panels and cytology of aspirated masses, organs or fluid. A search of the major organs for ischemia, necrosis, thrombosis, infiltrative neoplasia or abscessation is made, often through imaging, or exploratory surgery when other options have failed to reveal the source.

Treatment of fever

Mild-to-moderate temperature elevations (102.9–105 °F (39.4–40.6 °C)) are typical and often beneficial to the body in the defense against the causative pathogen. More often, cooling procedures afford little or no benefit to these patients. While cooling the body may transiently reduce the body temperature, the reset set-point will direct the body to increase the body temperature again. This will raise the metabolic rate and oxygen, water, and electrolyte consumption. However, rare extremes in body temperature (>106 °F

(>41.1 °C)) warrant immediate cooling measures to bring the temperature down to 103 °F (39.4 °C) (Table 17.7).

Fluid balance is a major component of patient support during treatment of the underlying problem. Hypovolemia causing perfusion deficits must be restored. A combination of crystalloid (10–30 mL/kg IV dogs; 10-15 mL/kg cats) and colloid (hydroxyethyl starch: 10–20 mL/kg IV dogs; 5 mL/kg IV cats) is optimal to restore intravascular volume and promote vascular fluid retention. High normal resuscitation end-points are chosen for these patients unless there is concern for internal hemorrhage, lung or brain edema or oliguric renal failure (see Chapter 2). Additional colloid (5 mL/kg IV dogs, cats), and crystalloids (5–10 mL/kg dogs, cats) volume increments can be infused to titrate the intravascular volume and pressure to the desired end-points. Rehydration should occur over 4–12 hours unless there is concern for fluid overload.

Fever indicates an elevation in metabolic rate and water consumption and loss through heat dissipation. Therefore, maintenance fluid requirements will be higher (~2–10 mL/kg/h higher) than normal in the animal with a fever. The patient may benefit from a constant rate infusion of hydroxyethyl starch (0.6–1.0 mL/kg/h) with the crystalloid maintenance fluids to promote vascular retention of infused fluids. Patients with fever are often anorexic, making enteral or parenteral nutrition part of the treatment plan as early as possible.

Antibiotic therapy should be reserved for patients with a known or strongly suspected bacterial infection to avoid drug resistance. Antibiotic selection will be based upon the susceptibility of the most likely pathogen at the infection site(s), the drug pharmacodynamics and pharmacokinetics, patient factors (such as known allergies, concurrent drug administration, perfusion, hydration), and drug availability (see Chapter 18).

The addition of antipyretic therapy to the treatment plan can be considered for patients with temperatures >106 °F (41.1 °C) or with fevers >104 °F (40 °C) for more than 2–3 days while definitive treatment is in progress. Medication options typically include nonsteroidal anti-inflammatory drugs (NSAIDs) and acetaminophen (or paracetamol, dogs only). The NSAIDs block cyclooxygenase (COX) enzymes and prostaglandin synthesis, allowing the hypothalamic set-point to reset at a lower temperature. However, potential side-effects of most NSAIDs include gastrointestinal irritation and ulceration, renal injury, and inhibition of platelet function. Their use is to be avoided in patients with poor perfusion, gastrointestinal (GI) compromise, preexisting renal disease, or impending surgery. Acetaminophen (or paracetamol) appears to also inhibit the COX enzyme (possibly COX-3) system and the production of PGE2 in the brain but has little effect on peripheral COX enzymes. This reduces the amount of the systemic side-effects reported with other NSAIDS [37]. However, acetaminophen toxicity has been widely reported in the dog and cat, preventing the routine use of this drug in these species [38,39]. The NSAID dipyrone has been reported to lead to bone marrow suppression and should also be avoided [40]. A recent human study found that the use of NSAIDs and acetaminophen in febrile patients increased mortality in septic patients but not in those without infection [41].

Glucocorticoids (0.25–1 mg/kg/day) can block both fever and the acute-phase response. Steroid use should be reserved for patients with known noninfectious causes of fever in which blocking these adaptive responses will not be detrimental. Glucocorticoids are often required in immune-mediated causes of fever, and higher doses are used for immunosuppression. Phenothiazines can also decrease body temperature by causing peripheral vasodilation and depressing thermoregulation. These drugs can cause significant hypotension and sedation and should be used with caution in critical patients.

Table 17.7 Methods of cooling.

Method of cooling*	Advantages	Disadvantages
At-home methods		
Using a fan to increase convective losses	Simple	None
Hose with cool water	Simple, fast, effective	Make sure to run water for 30 seconds to remove hot water from hose. Cool water only
Applying cool, damp towels to the body	Simple	Hypothermia if prolonged, wetting fur may exacerbate hypothermia
Submersion in cold water	Rapid conductive losses	Discomfort, risk of exacerbating hypothermia, peripheral vasoconstriction decreasing heat loss, cumbersome
Alcohol to paw pads	Simple	May not have enough cooling effect, skin irritation
Ice packs in inguinal/axillary region	Simple	Peripheral vasoconstrction, discomfort for patient
In-hospital methods		
All at-home cooling methods applicable		
Room temperature IV fluids	Require IV fluids for hypovolemia	May not cool large animal rapidly enough; need to place IV catheter
Fans (with or without cool water on skin)	Heat dissipation through convection and evaporation, inexpensive, readily available	Possible patient discomfort
Cold water GI lavage (gastric or colonic)	Gastric lavage may decrease bleeding from gastric ulcers	Other methods are as effective. Cumbersome, risk of aspiration pneumonia, expense, patient cleanliness is compromised, time-consuming to implement
Peritoneal or bladder cool water lavage	Can rapidly cool core temperature	Other methods are as effective and faster. Expense, patient discomfort, need to maintain sterility, time-consuming to implement

*Stop cooling at 103°F or 39.5°C; avoid ice cold water - causes peripheral vasoconstriction, trapping heat.
GI, gastrointestinal.

The Rule of 20 becomes an important component of the treatment and monitoring plans for the ICU patient with fever. Many critically ill animals have a SIRS disease process with an associated increase in vascular permeability, hypoalbuminemia, and impaired perfusion. There can be devastating consequences from extreme or prolonged temperature elevations. A careful and methodical review of the organ systems at least twice daily is warranted during the febrile episode.

Heat stroke

Three syndromes are described as part of the heat illness syndrome of nonpyrogenic hyperthermia: heat cramps, heat exhaustion, and heat stroke. Heat cramps are muscle spasms caused by loss of sodium, chloride, potassium, and water due to heat exposure. Heat exhaustion is seen when water and electrolyte loss results in clinical signs of fatigue, diarrhea, and vomiting. Heat stroke has been defined as "a form of hyperthermia associated with a systemic inflammatory response leading to a syndrome of multiorgan dysfunction in which encephalopathy predominates" [27].

Classic heat stroke results from exposure to high environmental temperature while exertional heat stroke occurs following strenuous exercise [27]. Environmental temperatures rise rapidly in closed environments with poor ventilation. The temperature in a closed car can reach 120 °F (48 °C) in 20 minutes when it is only 75 °F (24 °C) outside [26]. In animals, 70% of heat loss occurs through radiation and convection through the skin. As the environmental temperature approaches body temperature, the primary mechanism of heat loss is by evaporation through panting [28,42]. Animals that are brachycephalic, obese or have altered respiratory systems (such as tracheal collapse and laryngeal paralysis) are at greater risk of hyperthermia. In the ICU, confinement of animals in

small, poorly ventilated spaces (such as small oxygen cages or poorly ventilated oxygen collars) can result in an ineffective respiratory rate and effort for dissipating the additional heat.

In heat stroke, there is failure of the thermoregulatory system, an exaggerated acute-phase inflammatory response and failures in the protective heat shock cellular responses. Direct endothelial damage from heat and activation of the coagulation cascade begin to contribute to decompensation [26,28]. Endotoxin is released from the intestines and absorbed systemically due to increased intestinal and vascular permeability. The animal with heat stroke has systemic inflammation (SIRS) with anticipated vasodilation, increased vascular permeability, and inadequate cardiac output. Evaporative water loss, third body fluid spacing due to increased vascular permeability, fluid loss through vomiting and diarrhea, inadequate fluid intake, and vasodilation result in severe hypovolemia and dehydration. Multiple organ dysfunction is a hallmark of heat stroke and can include disseminated intravascular coagulation (DIC), cardiac arrhythmias, acute kidney injury, hepatic dysfunction, gastrointestinal hemorrhage and necrosis, seizures, coma, and eventually death [26,43,44].

The clinical signs at presentation will depend upon the duration and severity of the heat exposure, with higher temperatures causing more severe signs. The body temperature of the dog or cat with heat stroke can vary at presentation, depending on the type of cooling measures initiated prior to transport and the perfusion status of the animal. Most dogs display signs of a hyperdynamic cardiovascular response (red mucous membranes, rapid capillary refill time, and tachycardia). Up to 25% of patients with heat stroke develop ventricular arrhythmias [45] and pulse deficits. Gastrointestinal signs such as vomiting or diarrhea are anticipated. Blood and strips of intestinal mucosa may leak from the rectum due to third body fluid spacing, GI ulceration, and necrosis of intestinal epithelium. Petechiae and ecchymoses seen in the skin and mucous membranes are due to thrombocytopenia associated with endothelial damage and eventually DIC. Harsh lung sounds or crackles may be auscultated with lung abnormalities as a consequence of aspiration, acute lung injury or acute respiratory distress syndrome or pulmonary hemorrhage secondary to DIC. The mental status will vary from depressed mentation to obtunded to comatose. Up to 35% of canine heat stroke patients may have seizures [45]. Oliguria is likely present due to severe dehydration and acute kidney injury associated with poor renal perfusion and rhabdomyolysis causing myoglobinuria and pigment nephropathy. Brown or red urine is common due to myoglobinuria or hematuria, respectively.

Mortality rate for dogs with heat stroke is reported to be as high as 50% and 64% [44,46]. Hypoglycemia, DIC, acute renal failure, seizures, delayed admission, and obesity have been found to be associated with an increased risk of death [42]. A novel scoring system for heat stroke in dogs has been reported and is based on the evaluation of 13 parameters that include clinical signs, complications, and clinicopathological data observed during the first 24 hours. Higher scores corresponded with lower probability of survival. The proposed scoring system is presented in Table 17.8 [47] and can be adapted as additional data is accumulated. Edema, hyperemia, congestion, and necrosis have been reported in multiple organs of dogs with fatal heat stroke on histopathology. A study described cerebral edema, hemorrhage, hyperemia, and neuronal necrosis in the brain of canine heat stroke victims [48]. The severity of the consequences of heat stroke necessitate timely and aggressive therapy to minimize complications and improve patient survival.

Treatment of heat stroke
The faster cooling measures are initiated, the better the chance for patient survival from heat stroke. In humans, lowering the temperature to 102 °F (38.9 °C) within an hour of presentation lowered the mortality rate from 33% to 15% [49]. Rapid cooling is believed to provide similar survival benefits in veterinary patients.

Cooling measures should be started by the pet owner prior to and continued during transport, but must not delay transit time. Options for cooling at home and in hospital are presented in Table 17.7 with the major advantages and disadvantages listed for each method. Owners can wet the fur using a hose (making sure hose water is cool) or towels presoaked with cool water. Submersion in iced cold water is avoided due to the resultant peripheral vasoconstriction, which limits heat dissipation and could result in drowning if the patient is neurologically impaired [45]. Active cooling is stopped when the body temperature lowers to 103.1 °F (39.5 °C) to prevent hypothermia.

Cold water gastric, bladder or peritoneal lavage and cold water enemas have been recommended as rapid core cooling methods but have been found to be associated with adverse outcomes (such as aspiration, increased GI permeability) [45]. The other noninvasive topical evaporative and convective cooling methods have been shown to be as fast or faster than these more invasive methods [50–52].

Every organ of the body is affected in heat stroke, requiring an organized and disciplined approach to patient stabilization and ICU care. The Rule of 20 provides an important checklist of life-altering factors that should be evaluated and treated in the heat stroke patient. At presentation, intravenous access is obtained immediately using one or two short, large-bore catheters and flow-by oxygen supplemented to ensure adequate blood oxygen concentrations during resuscitation. Fluid therapy is initiated and life-threatening problems such as airway obstruction (intubate and ventilate with oxygen), seizures (provide IV anticonvulsants), hypoglycemia (administer IV dextrose), and ongoing significant hemorrhage (attempt hemostasis) are rapidly addressed.

The patient will have SIRS and requires aggressive intravascular volume support. A combination of balanced isotonic crystalloid (10–20 mL/kg IV dogs; 10–15 mL/kg cats) and colloid (hydroxyethyl starch, 10–20 mL/kg IV dogs; 5 mL/kg cats) is optimal to initially restore intravascular volume and promote vascular fluid retention. High normal resuscitation end-points are chosen for these patients unless there is concern for internal hemorrhage, lung or brain edema or oliguric renal failure (see Chapter 2). Additional colloid

Table 17.8 Proposed severity scoring system for dogs presenting with heat stroke using a model with weighted values (first 24 hours). Scores higher than 36 were associated with decreased probability of survival.

Variable	Mild	Score	Moderate	Score	Severe	Score	Catastrophic	Score
Heart rate (bpm)	<108	1	109–172	2.8			>172	6.2
Glucose mg/dL	>66	1	47–66	3.6	31–46	5.5	<31	8
(mmol/L)	(3.66)		(2.6–3.67)		(1.72–2.59)		(<1.71)	
PT	<12.2	1	≥12.2	5.1				
aPTT	<17.5	1	17.5–31.9	3.2	32–50	6.9	>50	13.1
Body condition score (of 9)	<6	1	6	4.2				
Acute collapse	Absent	1	Present	3.6				
Perfusion	No shock	1	Shock	2.3				
Seizures	Absent	1	Present	2.8				
Mental status	Normal	1	Obtunded	2.7				
Petechiae, ecchymosis	Absent	1	Present	2.7				
AKI	Absent	1	Present	5.4				
DIC	Absent	1	Present	6.9				
Respiratory involvement	Absent	1	Present	5.9				

AKI, acute kidney injury; aPTT, activated partial thromboplastin time; bpm, beats per minute; DIC, disseminated intravascular coagulation; PT, prothrombin time.

Source: Adapted from Segev G, Itamar A, Savoray M, et al. A novel severity scoring system for dogs with heatstroke. J Vet Emerg Crit Care; 25(2) 2015:240–7.

(5 mL/kg IV dogs, cats), and crystalloids (5–10 mL/kg dogs, cats) boluses may be infused and titrated to the desired end-points. It is important to assess for a colloid induced coagulopathy if large volumes of hydroxyethyl starch are required to maintain resuscitation end-points. Rehydration should occur over several hours unless there is concern for fluid overload. Hypertonic saline administration is avoided in heat stroke patients due to the possibility of disorders in serum sodium, increased vascular permeability, and tenuous fluid balance with large third body fluid spaces.

Due to alterations in vascular permeability and colloidal oncotic pressure (hypoalbuminemia), maintenance fluid rates will be higher (~10–20 mL/kg/h) than normal initially. The patient can benefit from a constant rate infusion of colloid (0.6–1.0 mL/kg/h) with the crystalloid maintenance fluids to promote vascular retention of infused fluids. The damage to the GI tract creates a third body fluid space, anorexia, vomiting and watery diarrhea, each compounding fluid loss and necessitating increased volumes to maintain adequate fluid balance. Enteral nutrition should be part of the treatment plan as early as possible.

Dextrose (0.5 g/kg IV as 25% solution) is given if the blood glucose is <60 mg/dL (3.33 mmol/L) at presentation. Blood glucose is closely monitored and the patient supplemented with dextrose orally or through intravenous maintenance fluids if hypoglycemia persists.

Anticonvulsants (diazepam 0.5–2.0 mg/kg IV or PR, midazolam 0.07–0.22 mg/kg IV or IM or levetiracetam 10–60 mg/kg IV or IM) should be administered to patients with seizures (see Figure 12.2 and Table 12.8). Protocols for cerebral edema and increased intracranial pressure are instituted for heat stroke patients with seizures or altered level of consciousness (see Figure 12.3 and Table 12.9). Maintenance anticonvulsants (phenobarbital 2–4 mg/kg IV or IM to maximum of 24 mg/kg) may be needed if seizure activity or twitching persists. Repeated neurological examinations are essential to detect any decline in brain or spinal cord function from heat damage.

Analgesia and sedation are provided after the initial life-threatening complications have been addressed. It is important to provide adequate pain relief with drugs that will not have a detrimental effect on vasomotor tone or cardiac output. A combination of a benzodiazepine and opioid given IV is effective and can be reversed if there are unwanted side-effects (see Chapter 19).

Monitoring and controlling the body temperature is essential after the initiation of cooling. To avoid hypothermia and the resultant vasoconstriction and shivering, cooling procedures are stopped when the rectal temperature drops to 103.1 °F (39.5 °C). While mild hypothermia is acceptable, rectal temperatures <99 °F (37.2 °C) warrant mild warming procedures to optimize peripheral blood flow. This would be an ideal patient for continuous monitoring of the rectal temperature.

The breakdown in the GI mucosal barrier predisposes to the absorption of endotoxins, bacteria, and other toxic products. A combination of intravenous antibiotics effective against gram-positive and gram-negative aerobic bacteria and against anaerobic bacteria is necessary during the period of hospitalization (see Chapters 14 and 18). GI protectants such as famotidine (0.5–1 mg/kg q 12–24h PO, IV, IM, SC) and sucralfate (0.25–1 g PO q 8h) are provided to reduce the impact of GI compromise (see Chapter 15). The placement of a nasogastric tube early in the treatment plan allows decompression of the stomach to minimize vomiting and aspiration pneumonia, the oral administration of glucose and medications and early enteral feeding of the damaged GI tract. Promotility agents (such as metoclopramide 0.1–0.5 mg/kg IV SC, IM, PO q 8–12h or CRI 1–2 mg/kg IV q 24h, erythromycin 0.5–1 mg/kg q 8h or cisapride

(0.1–0.5 mg/kg PO TID) help manage ileus and can decrease peripheral receptor input to the vomiting center.

It should be assumed that the animal suffering heat stroke has a coagulation disorder. Initial findings can vary from mild thrombocytopenia to fulminant DIC, with frequent reevaluation of coagulation necessary. Blood product administration may become part of the fluid therapy plan, as deemed necessary. Whole blood is given (after type and cross-matching as time and patient condition permit) when anemia, hypoproteinemia, and coagulation problems are identified. Fresh frozen plasma (10 mL/kg) can be administered to provide coagulation factors, antithrombin, and albumin if DIC is suspected. While improving capillary blood flow is the mainstay of therapy for DIC, the use of heparin can be considered along with blood component therapy (see Chapter 9).

An ECG will identify any important arrhythmias, with anti-arrhythmic drugs administered when the arrhythmia is deemed to be contributing to perfusion deficits or prefibrillatory arrhythmia (see Chapter 11). Repeated auscultation of the lungs and monitoring of the respiratory rate, effort, and pulse oximetry can detect pulmonary disorders, such as edema, hemorrhage or infection, resulting from the heat stroke, SIRS or fluid therapy. Acute kidney injury contributes to the mortality rate of patients with heat stroke and warrants close observation of urine output, fluid balance, blood pressure and blood creatinine and BUN. Periodic evaluation of the urine for glycosuria with normal blood glucose or renal tubular cell casts can provide an early indication of renal tubular damage.

Malignant hyperthermia

Malignant hyperthermia, also known as canine stress syndrome in dogs, is a rare life-threatening condition seen in dogs (Greyhounds, Labrador Retrievers) and cats, as well as humans, swine, and horses. Malignant hyperthermia is consistently triggered in susceptible animals by excitement, apprehension, exercise, or environmental stress. Giving certain anesthetics or specific drugs that affect the neurological and muscular systems also consistently triggers malignant hyperthermia in susceptible animals. These drugs can induce a drastic and uncontrolled increase in skeletal muscle oxidative metabolism, which overwhelms the body's capacity to supply oxygen, remove carbon dioxide, and regulate body temperature.

This syndrome is characterized by abnormally high body temperature, muscle rigidity, very rapid and irregular heartbeat, increased respiratory rate, unstable blood pressure, pulmonary edema, impaired blood coagulation, kidney failure, and death.

There is no simple test to diagnose the condition, but genetic testing is available to identify dogs that have the autosomal dominant gene responsible for the syndrome in dogs [53]. Diagnosis during an episode is based on the development of clinical signs. Signs can develop slowly or rapidly, but once observed, body temperature increases rapidly and can reach 113 °F (45 °C).

Rapid recognition of malignant hyperthermia is essential for success in treatment. Any inciting cause (inhaled anesthetics) should be discontinued. Dantrolene sodium is the treatment and is given at 1 mg/kg rapidly IV and repeated until symptoms subside or a maximum cumulative dose of 10 mg/kg has been reached. Should signs recur, the administration can be repeated. Dantrolene is a postsynaptic muscle relaxant that uncouples excitation-contraction in skeletal muscle cells. It achieves this by inhibiting calcium ions release from sarcoplasmic reticulum stores. Supportive care as outlined for heat stroke above is provided. The mortality rate is high with malignant hyperthermia, and aggressive treatment is warranted [54].

Hypothermia

Hypothermia occurs when the body loses heat faster than it can be produced due to increased heat loss, decreased heat production or alterations in thermoregulation. Reducing the core temperature by just a few degrees can alter the physiology of almost every system and organ. Hypothermia causes a linear reduction in both heart rate and cardiac output in line with metabolic rate, with these changes considered physiological rather than pathological [55]. However, as temperature drops, reduced metabolism leads to a decrease in CO_2 production, with the resultant fall in pCO_2 exerting a negative effect on cerebral blood flow. The resultant alkalosis has been reported to increase the risk of seizure activity [55]. Simultaneously, there are risks of impaired immunity, abnormal hemostasis, and altered glucose metabolism. In addition, the metabolism and clearance of a large number of regularly administered drugs are slowed during hypothermia [56]. The effect of inotropic therapies potentially required to support cardiac output can be blunted when the core temperature is low [56].

Hypothermia is diagnosed when the body temperature is <99°F (37°C) in the dog and cat and can be classified as primary or secondary [1]. Primary hypothermia (also called accidental or environmental hypothermia) is caused by exposure to low environmental temperatures with normal body heat production. Primary hypothermia (cold exposure) is classified as mild with body temperatures 90–99°F (32–37°C), moderate at 82–90°F (28–32°C), severe at 68–82°F (20–28°C) and profound at <80°F (<20°C). Animals appear to tolerate a lower core body temperature due to exogenous or environmental factors compared to endogenous causes.

Secondary hypothermia occurs when heat production within the body and thermoregulation are altered by endogenous factors. Because the clinical signs are more pronounced at higher temperatures from secondary hypothermia, the classification of severity is different than that proposed for environmental exposure. Secondary hypothermia can be classified in the dog and cat as mild at body temperatures of 98–99.9°F (36.7–37.7°C), moderate at 96–98°F (35.5–36.7°C), severe at 92–96°F (33–35.5°C) and critical at temperatures <92°F (<33°C) [57].

Hypothermia in the ICU small animal patient is more frequently secondary in origin, resulting from or compounded by conditions such as poor perfusion, trauma, severe sepsis, drugs, hypoglycemia, hypothyroidism, sedatives, anesthesia, organ dysfunction, and surgery [57]. Hypothermia is common in sedated or anesthetized patients, requiring close monitoring and heat support to prevent the consequences of low body temperature. Severe injury and shock are frequently associated with abnormalities in patient body temperature. Substantial increases in mortality have been associated with severe hypothermia in humans experiencing trauma when their body temperatures are below 95°F (35°C). Although shock severity is an important predictor of outcome in these patients, hypothermia independently contributes to the substantial mortality associated with trauma [58].

The specific effect the lower body temperature has on the patient varies with the degree of hypothermia and the species, with dogs and cats appearing to differ somewhat in their response. Clinical signs associated with secondary hypothermia in dogs and cats are listed in Table 17.3. Dogs with mild secondary hypothermia initially have tachycardia, peripheral vasoconstriction, and tachypnea associated with increased catecholamine release [1]. Cats will typically have a normal or slower heart rate. Mild and moderate secondary hypothermia causes canine patients to shiver if not anesthetized, but this rarely occurs in the cat.

As the body temperature continues to decline (from mild to moderate secondary hypothermia), the dog will develop bradycardia due to decreased spontaneous depolarization of pacemaker cells, and the patient becomes refractory to atropine [24]. Both dogs and cats become mentally dull due to a decline in cerebral metabolic rate [1]. Cold diuresis can occur in either species when the body senses an increased blood volume due to peripheral vasoconstriction and decreases antidiuretic hormone production and increases glomerular filtration rate [1] Urine output can subsequently increase and lead to dehydration.

Moderate to severe secondary hypothermia causes a progressive drop in the metabolic rate. Patients will have an altered mentation: obtunded or comatose. Decreased hepatic metabolism can lead to slower anesthetic recovery. Bradycardia persists but the myocardium becomes irritable with atrial dysrhythmias occurring earlier in hypothermia. Hypothermia can also result in decreased platelet function and number, decreased coagulation factor (enzyme) activity, and decreased tissue factor-factor VIIa complex activity [59]. There can be exacerbation of hemorrhage, contributing to morbidity and mortality in trauma patients and animals undergoing surgery (see Chapter 9).

As the core temperature falls to critical levels, ventricular arrhythmias are often noted, with occasional premature ventricular contractions progressing to ventricular tachycardia and eventually ventricular fibrillation [24]. Hypotension occurs as the vessels lose their affinity for norepinephrine and become vasodilated [1]. Respiratory rate and depth decrease as decreased cellular metabolism results in lower CO_2 production [1]. There is a shift to the left of the oxygen-hemoglobin dissociation curve contributing to tissue hypoxia. Patients develop acute tubular necrosis and acute kidney injury as renal blood flow declines.

In the final stages of hypothermia, the patient is unconscious and nonresponsive with dilated pupils and severely depressed respiratory rates. Ventricular fibrillation is common but will not respond to electrical defibrillation until the patient is warmed [60]. Occasionally, seizures may occur towards the end, and death may occur from apnea [1].

Hypothermia typically causes an elevation in PCV due to decreased plasma volume. Thrombocytopenia is often seen due to platelet sequestration in the spleen or consumption. Hyperglycemia is often found initially due to increased catecholamine and cortisol release and a decreased metabolic rate. However, the glucose concentration soon declines due to glycogen depletion and impaired gluconeogenesis [57]. Potassium is decreased in mild hypothermia due to intracellular redistribution and elevated in severe cases due to impairment of the sodium-potassium-ATPase pump [57].

The cat has a very distinct physiological response to shock, manifesting with hypotension, bradycardia, and hypothermia. It appears that the norepinephrine (NE) released during the early phase of shock may contribute to a centrally mediated hypothermia in the cat [61]. In the cat, moderate hypothermia may then reduce the release of NE centrally and locally in the heart, each contributing to hypotension and bradycardia [62]. Finally, an increase in parasympathetic outflow through a vasovagal type reflex in hypothermic cats may perpetuate a relative or true bradycardia. Management of the hypothermia plays a key role in successful resuscitation from hypovolemic shock in the cat.

A careful assessment of the patient history, physical examination, minimum database, and initial clinicopathological tests will aid in the identification of any underlying health problems causing the hypothermia. Particular attention is given to the perfusion parameters (blood pressure, heart rate, pulse intensity, capillary refill time) since poor perfusion can cause hypothermia or result from the temperature disorder. Diseases such as renal failure, liver failure, hypothyroidism, and ingestion of certain drugs or toxins (see Table 17.1) can lead to hypothermia and will require therapy specific for the cause. The more life-threatening complications of hypothermia such as coagulopathy, hypoglycemia, cardiac arrhythmias, depressed ventilation, and altered level of consciousness are pursued and stabilized when found abnormal.

Treatment of hypothermia

Controlled rewarming and intravascular volume resuscitation are the two most critical components of patient resuscitation from hypothermia of any cause. There are three types of rewarming strategies: passive surface, active external, and active core rewarming techniques (Table 17.9) [57]. The most effective method of rewarming patients in veterinary medicine is not known.

Passive rewarming is used for mild hypothermia when the patient has adequate intravascular volume. The patient is wrapped in dry blankets to prevent further heat loss and heat production occurs by shivering. However, shivering is rare in the cat, and will lead to increased oxygen consumption in the patient.

Moderate hypothermia requires active external rewarming. Forced air blankets, warm water bottles, and circulating water blankets can be applied to the thorax and abdomen to increase body temperature. Hot air from hair dryers blowing directly on the animal can produce extreme temperatures and should not be used as a substitute for forced air blankets. If the patient is wet, the fur should be vigorously towel dried to prevent continued dissipation of heat. Electric blankets and warming packs such as heated rice bags should not be used due to possible burns to the skin, particularly when the patient is not able to move away from the heat source. Warm water bottles must be monitored closely as they cool, which can then remove heat from patients.

There are several potential complications with active external rewarming. As the skin and peripheral tissues warm, peripheral vessels vasodilate, allowing improved flow through the cold tissues. The cold blood from these regions circulating to central organs can result in an initial drop of core body temperature known as "afterdrop" [60]. Rewarming shock occurs when severe peripheral vasodilation in hypovolemic patients causes redistribution of blood flow to the periphery, worsening hypovolemia and perfusion [24,57]. Intravascular volume should be supplemented as active external rewarming procedures are initiated. Heat sources are not placed into direct contact with the skin of the hypothermic patient since the skin vasculature is unable to dissipate the heat and burns to the skin can occur.

Active core rewarming techniques are used when the patient has severe or critical hypothermia, which might benefit from rapidly rewarming the core temperature while avoiding peripheral vasodilation. This can be done using heated, humidified air by mask or endotracheal tube, intravenous fluids heated to 104–106.8 °F (40–42 °C), warm water bladder lavage, warm water enemas, and warm water peritoneal or pleural lavage. Studies in human patients undergoing coronary bypass surgery show that the warming of intravenous fluids can prevent decreases in systemic temperatures during surgery [63].

Many of the invasive active core rewarming methods carry potential risks. Bladder lavage may have limited efficacy due to the small surface area. Enemas and peritoneal or pleural lavage have an increased risk of electrolyte abnormalities and infection [24]. Gastric lavage is not commonly employed due to the risk of aspiration pneumonia. Often an approach using a combination of rewarming techniques is used for moderate to severe hypothermia or when there is poor response to the initial rewarming procedures. Active rewarming should be discontinued when the body temperature reaches 99 °F (37.2 °C). Passive rewarming can be continued to allow the temperature to slowly return to normal. Monitoring of temperature, blood pressure, urine output, ECG, PCV, blood glucose, electrolytes, and coagulation parameters should be performed during rewarming. Patients having open abdominal or thoracic surgery can benefit from pleural or peritoneal lavage with appropriately warmed fluids.

Hypovolemia is anticipated due to cold diuresis, inadequate fluid intake, and excessive heat expenditure as the body attempts to warm. An intravenous catheter is placed and flow-by oxygen administered to ensure adequate blood oxygen concentrations. Fluid therapy is initiated and life-threatening problems such as airway obstruction (intubate and ventilate with oxygen), seizures (provide IV anticonvulsants), hypoglycemia (administer IV dextrose), and ongoing significant hemorrhage (attempt hemostasis) are rapidly addressed. Fluid resuscitation will consist of an isotonic crystalloid solution

Table 17.9 Warming methods.*

Method of warming	Advantages	Disadvantages/comment
Passive external Wrap in dry blankets, decrease exposure to cool surfaces	Inexpensive, easy	May be ineffective and relies on generation of internal heat; shivering may increase oxygen consumption
Active external Forced air blanket Warm water bottles Circulating water blanket Hair dryer Electric blanket Warming packs (e.g. rice bags)	Required for moderate hypothermia, very effective methods	May cause peripheral vasodilation exacerbating hypovolemia, "afterdrop" phenomenon, burns (particularly with electric blankets, warming packs, and hair dryers – these are not recommended)
Active internal Heated/humidified air Heated IV fluids Warm water lavage (gastric, bladder, rectal, cavitary)	Effective in increasing core temperatures or preventing open cavitary heat losses	Cumbersome, more expensive to initiate and keep patient clean, risk of aspiration, bladder lavage less effective

* Warming should be discontinued when body temperature reaches 99 °F (37.2 °C).

(10–15 mL/kg IV) administered in conjunction with rewarming. The administration of colloid (hydroxyethyl starch, 5 mL/kg IV) can facilitate intravascular retention of administered fluids during resuscitation [57]. Lactated Ringer's is avoided due to concern regarding the capability of the liver to metabolize the lactate [24,60]. Low normal resuscitation end-points are selected for hypothermic patients since overzealous fluid administration can lead to interstitial edema and pulmonary edema. Additional colloid (5 mL/kg increments IV) is infused if needed to titrate to the desired resuscitation end-points. Additional crystalloids (5–10 mL/kg) can be given as well, to support hydration if severe dehydration is still present. In the cat, fluid resuscitation is halted when the indirect arterial systolic blood pressure is above 60 mmHg, and active external rewarming initiated to bring the rectal temperature ≥98 °F. Additional crystalloids and colloids can then be infused, if needed, to reach the desired end-points.

Maintenance fluids will have to be adjusted to meet metabolic needs while avoiding volume overload. Intravenous infusion of maintenance crystalloids can begin at 2–4 mL/kg/h IV with the goal to match fluid loss through metabolism, urine, and any third body fluid spaces. The patient can benefit from a constant rate infusion of colloid (0.6–1.0 mL/kg/h) with the crystalloid maintenance fluids to promote vascular retention of infused fluids. Potassium supplementation may be required in the maintenance fluids if hypokalemia is a component of the patient's problems.

The Rule of 20 should be used, at least twice daily during the critical stabilization period, to assess the status of the patient suffering from protracted moderate to severe or critical hypothermia. Oxygen therapy is continued in patients experiencing hypotension, hypoventilation or pulmonary edema. Dextrose (0.5 g/kg IV of 25% solution) supplementation is provided if blood glucose is ≤60 mg/dL (3.33 mmol/L). The serum potassium may be high from muscle necrosis (requiring diuresis) or low from cold diuresis (requiring potassium supplementation). An ECG is done to assess for arrhythmias as a consequence of hypothermia or hyperkalemia and specific treatment provided when the arrhythmia is affecting perfusion or is prefibrillatory. A coagulopathy is to be anticipated. Fresh frozen plasma (10 mL/kg IV) can be administered to provide coagulation factors, antithrombin, and albumin. Thromboembolic disease can be a result of cold-induced vascular damage and can require specific intervention (see Chapter 9). The neurological examination is repeated frequently since cerebral edema can be a result of prolonged hypothermia. Treatment for increased intracranial pressure is provided if the level of consciousness has failed to improve (see Chapter 12). Promotility drugs and GI protectants are warranted to minimize ileus and protect the GI mucosa during the recovery period.

The prognosis is difficult to predict in the dog and cat. The duration and degree of hypothermia, the inciting cause, and the timely initiation of careful resuscitative procedures are each likely to contribute to patient morbidity and mortality. In humans presenting with environmental hypothermia, indicators of a poor prognosis include prehospital cardiac arrest, severe hypotension, azotemia, need for endotracheal intubation, hyperkalemia, and thromboembolism [24]. Patients with mild hypothermia or that have a rapid response to therapy have a good prognosis. Hypothermia has been reported associated with serious complications or a poor prognosis in dogs with pancreatitis [64], spontaneous hemoperitoneum in cats [65], and female dogs with pyometra (marker of peritonitis, prolonged hospitalization) [66].

Preventing hypothermia in the ICU

Heavy sedation, anesthesia, post surgery, post cardiac arrest, serious metabolic illness, hypotension, and multiple drug therapies are but a few of the common causes of hypothermia in the ICU. Very young animals, toy breeds, and geriatric patients are at greater risk of developing hypothermia than the general small animal ICU population. Blankets, warm IV fluids, warm circulating air blowers, hot water bottles, warmed lavage fluids, and circulating warm water blankets are all methods that can be employed to minimize the development of hypothermia. Preoperative and intraoperative warming, followed by postoperative warming during recovery have been found to reduce hypothermia in humans and should be considered the standard of care in the small animal ICU patient [67,68].

Therapeutic hypothermia

Induced hypothermia as a treatment for cardiac arrest and traumatic brain injury began in the 1940s, with many studies reporting benefits compared to "expected outcome" or historical controls [69]. But significant problems in patient management and variable outcomes through the years have prevented its routine use in human prehospital or hospital settings. Through the years, a better understanding of mechanisms involved, better management of the side-effects of hypothermia and better methods of inducing and maintaining hypothermia have prompted ongoing research into this therapeutic tool.

The processes termed postresuscitation disease, reperfusion injury, and secondary brain injury may continue for hours to days after the initial injury and can be retriggered by new episodes of ischemia [70]. All of these processes have been found to be temperature dependent, stimulated by fever and can be mitigated or blocked by mild to moderate hypothermia. Hypothermia has been shown to be protective to the brain of experimental animals (including dogs) and humans undergoing oxidative stress [71]. Inducing hypothermia is recommended in newborns with hypoxic ischemic encephalopathy [72] and in adults following cardiac arrest [73].

Therapeutic hypothermia in humans has been classified as mild (93–95 °F, 34–35 °C), moderate (90–93 °F, 32–33.9 °C), moderate-deep (86–89.4 °F, 30–31.9 °C), and deep (<86 °F, <30 °C) [74]. Studies on mechanisms underlying the protective effects of hypothermia point to four key factors determining success or failure of cooling treatments [69]:

- speed of induction of hypothermia, with rapid initiation after injury
- duration of cooling, which depends on the severity of the initial injury and the time to reaching target temperature
- speed of rewarming, which should be slow to avoid reinitiation of the original destructive process
- proper management and prevention of side-effects.

Experiments in dogs undergoing ice-cold saline flush (containing oxygen and glucose) to induce profound hypothermia (<50 °F, <10 °C) allowed for satisfactory neurological recovery after three hours of exsanguination cardiac arrest [75]. Toy breed dogs have been successfully maintained with surface-induced hypothermia (68–75 °F, 19.8–23.8 °C) and low-flow cardiopulmonary bypass during open heart surgery for selected congenital deformities [76], and therapeutic hypothermia (91.4–95 °F, 33–35 °C) has been reported in a dog to control severe seizures associated with traumatic brain injury [77]. Reports describing the clinical or experimental use of therapeutic hypothermia in the cat are lacking. General guidelines have not been established at this time in veterinary medicine.

References

1. Todd J, Powell LL. Hypothermia. In: Small Animal Critical Care Medicine. Silverstein D, Hopper K, eds. St Louis: Elsevier Saunders, 2009: pp 720–2.
2. Guyton AC, Hall JE. Body temperature, temperature regulation and fever, In: Textbook of Medical Physiology, 11th edn. Philadelphia: Elsevier Saunders, 2006: pp 889–901.
3. Hemmelgarn C, Gannon K. Heatstroke: thermoregulation, pathophysiology and predisposing factors. Comp Cont Educ Samll Anim Pract. 2013:35(7):E1–6.
4. Southward ES, Mann FA, Dodam J, et al. A comparison of auricular, rectal and pulmonary artery thermometry in dogs with anesthesia induced hypothermia. J Vet Emerg Crit Care 2006;16(3):172–5.
5. Moran DS, Mendal L. Core temperature measurement, methods and current insights. Sports Med. 2002;32(14):879–85.
6. Greer RJ, Cohn LA, Dodam J, et al. Comparison of three methods of temperature measurement in hypothermic, euthermic, and hyperthermic dogs. J Am Vet Med Assoc. 2007;230:1841–8.
7. Gomart SB, Allerton FJW, Gommeren K. Accuracy of different temperature reading techniques and associated stress response in hospitalized dogs. J Vet Emerg Crit Care 2014;24(3):279–85.
8. Kunkle GA, Nicklin CF, Tamboe DL. Comparison of body temperature in cats using a veterinary infrared thermometer and a digital rectal thermometer. J Am Anim Hosp Assoc. 2004;140:42–6.
9. Livornese LL, Dias S, Samel C, et al. Hospital-acquired infection with vancomycin-resistant Enterococcus faecium transmitted by electronic thermometers. Ann Intern Med. 1992;117(2):112–16.
10. Brooks SE, Veal RO, Kramer M, et al. Reduction in the incidence of Clostridium difficile-associated diarrhea in an acute care hospital and a skilled nursing facility following replacement of electronic thermometers with single use disposables. Infect Control Hosp Epidemiol. 1992:13(2):98–103.
11. Fulbrook P. Core temperature measurement: a comparison of rectal, axillary and pulmonary artery blood temperature. Intensive Crit Care Nurs. 1993;9:217–25.
12. Jensen BN, Jensen FS, Madsen S, et al. Accuracy of digital tympanic, oral, axillary and rectal thermometers compared with standard rectal mercury thermometers. Eur J Surg. 2000;166(11)848–51.
13. Nuckton TJ, Goldreich D, Wendt F, et al. A comparison of 2 methods of measuring rectal temperature with digital thermometers. Am J Crit Care 2001;10(3):146–50.
14. Bloch EC, Ginsber B, Binner RA Jr. The esophageal temperature gradient in anesthetized children. J Clin Monit. 1993;9(2):73–7.
15. Fallis WM. Monitoring urinary bladder temperature in the intensive care unit: state of the science. Am J Crit Care 2002;11:38–45.
16. Craig JV, Lancaster GA, Taylor S, et al. Infrared ear thermometry compared with rectal thermometry in children: a systematic review. Lancet 2002;360(9333):603–9.
17. Huggins R, Glaviano N, Negishi N, et al. Comparison of rectal and aural core body temperature thermometry in hyperthermic, exercising individuals: a meta-analysis. J Athl Train. 2012;47(3):329–38.
18. Lamb V, McBrearty AR. Comparison of rectal, tympanic membrane and axillary temperature measurement methods in dogs. Vet Rec. 2013;173:524–8.
19. Rexroat J, Benish, K, Fraden J. Clinical accuracy of Vet-Temp instant ear thermometer: comparative study with dogs and cats. San Diego: Advanced Monitors Corporation, 1999. Available at: www.admon.com/wp-content/uploads/2010/09/Humane-Society-White-Paper.pdf (accessed 2 June 2016).
20. Gonzalez AM, Mann FA, Preziosi S, et al. Measurement of body temperature by use of auricular thermometers versus rectal thermometers in dogs with otitis externa. J Am Vet Med Assoc. 2002;221:378–80.
21. Goic JB, Reineke EL, Drobatz KJ. Comparison of rectal and axillary temperatures in dogs and cats. J Am Vet Med Assoc. 2014;244(10):1170–5.
22. Craig JV, Lancaster GA, Williamson P, et al. Temperature measured at the axilla compared with rectum in children and young people: systematic review. Br Med J. 2000;320:1174–8.
23. Fulbrook P. Core body temperature measurement: a comparison of axilla, tympanic membrane and pulmonary artery blood temperature. Intensive Crit Care Nurs. 1997;13:266–72.
24. Winfield WE. Accidental hypothermia, In: The Veterinary ICU Book. Jackson Hole: Teton NewMedia, 2002: pp 1116–29.
25. Walters JM. Hyperthermia, In: The Veterinary ICU Book. Jackson Hole: Teton NewMedia, 2002: pp 1130–6.
26. Miller JB. Hyperthermia and fever. In: Small Animal Critical Care Medicine. St Louis: Elsevier Saunders, 2009: pp 21–6.
27. Bouchama A, Knochel JP. Heat stroke. N Engl J Med. 2002;346:1978–88.
28. Drobatz KJ. Heat stroke. In: Small Animal Critical Care Medicine. St Louis: Elsevier Saunders, 2009: pp 723–6.
29. Lagutchik MS. Fever in the ICU patient. In: The Veterinary ICU Book. Jackson Hole: Teton NewMedia, 2002: pp 671–84.
30. Öncü S. A clinical outline to fever in intensive care patients. Minerva Anestesiol. 2013;79(4):408–18.
31. Rehman T, de Boisblanc BP. Persistent fever in the ICU. Chest 2014;145(1):158–65.
32. Cuddy ML. The effects of drugs on thermoregulation. AACN Clin Issues 2004;15(2):238–53.
33. Conti B, Tabarean I, Andrei C, et al. Cytokines and fever. Front Biosci. 2004;9:1433–49.
34. Launey Y, Nesseler N, Malledant Y, et al. Clinical review: fever in septic ICU patients – friend or foe? Crit Care 2011;15(3)222–9.
35. Jiang Q, Cross AS, Singh I, et al. Febrile core temperatures is essential for optimal host defense in bacterial peritonitis. Infect Immun. 2000;68(3):1265–70.
36. Rice P, Martin E, He J, et al. Febrile-range hyperthermia augments neutrophil accumulation and enhances lung injury in experimental gram-negative bacterial pneumonia. J Immunol. 2005;174:3676–85.
37. Greco A, Ajmone-Cat MA, Nicolini A, et al. Paracetamol effectively reduces prostaglandin E2 synthesis in brain macrophages by inhibiting enzymatic activity of cyclooxygenase but not phospholipase and prostaglandin E synthase. J Neurosci Res. 2003;71(6):844–52.
38. Court MH, Greenblatt DJ. Molecular basis for deficient acetaminophen glucuronidation in cats. An interspecies comparison of enzyme kinetics in liver microsomes. Biochem Pharmacol. 1997;53(7):1041–7.
39. McConkey SE, Grant DM, Cribb AE. The role of para-aminophenol in acetaminophen-induced methemoglobinemia in dogs and cats. J Vet Pharmacol Ther. 2009;32(6):585–95.
40. Kramer M. Chronic toxicity of pyrazolones: the problem of nitrosation. Br J Clin Pharmacol. 1980;10(Suppl 2):313S–317S.
41. Lee BH, Inui D, Suh G, et al. Association of body temperature and antipyretic treatments with mortality of critically ill patients with and without sepsis: multi-centered prospective observational study. Crit Care 2012;16(1):R33.
42. Bruchim Y, Klement E, Saragusty J, et al. Heat stroke in dogs: a retrospective study of 54 cases (1999–2004) and analysis of risk factors for death. J Vet Intern Med. 2006;20:38–46.
43. Johnson SI, McMichael M, White G. Heatstroke in small animal medicine: a clinical practice review. J Vet Emerg Crit Care 2006;16(2):112–19.
44. Bruchim Y, Klement E, Saragusty J, et al. Heat stroke in dogs: a retrospective study of 54 cases (1999–2004) and analysis of risk factors of death. J Vet Intern Med. 2006;20:38–46.
45. Hemmelgarn C, Gannon K. Heatstroke: clinical signs, diagnosis, treatment and prognosis. Comp Cont Educ Samll Anim Pract. 2013;35(7):E1–7.
46. Drobatz KJ, Macintire DK. Heat-induced illness in dogs: 42 cases (1976–1993). J Am Vet Med Assoc. 1996; 209(11):1984–99.
47. Segev G, Aroch I, Savoray M, et al. A novel severity scoring system for dogs with heatstroke. J Vet Emerg Crit Care 2015;25(2):240–7.
48. Bruchim Y, Loeb E, Saragusty J. Pathological findings in dogs with fatal heatstroke. J Comp Pathol. 2009;140(2–3):97–104.
49. Vicario SJ, Okabajue R, Haltom T. Rapid cooling in classic heatstroke: effect on mortality rates. Am J Emerg Med. 1986;4(5):394–8.
50. White JD, Riccobene E, Nucci R, et al. Evaporation versus iced gastric lavage treatment of heatstroke: comparative efficacy in a canine model. Crit Care Med. 1987;15(8):748–50.
51. Syverud SA, Barker WJ, Amsterdam J, et al. Iced gastric lavage for treatment of heatstroke: efficacy in a canine model. Ann Emerg Med. 1985;14(5):424–32.
52. White JD, Kamath R, et al. Evaporation versus iced gastric lavage treatment of heatstroke: comparative efficacy in a canine model. Am J Emerg Med. 1993;11(1):1–3.
53. Roberts MC, Mickelson JR, Patterson E, et al. Autosomal dominant canine malignant hyperthermia is caused by a mutation in the gene encoding the skeletal muscle calcium release channel (RYR1). Anesthesiology 2001;95(3):716–25.
54. O'Brien PJ, Cribb PH, White R, et al. Canine malignant hyperthermia: diagnosis of susceptibility in a breeding colony. Can Vet J. 1983;24(6):172–7.
55. Wood T, Thoresen M. Physiological responses to hypothermia. Semin Fetal Neonatal Med. 2015;20(2):87–96.
56. Zhou J, Poloyac SM. The effect of therapeutic hypothermia on drug metabolism and response: cellular mechanisms to organ function. Expert Opin Drug Metab Toxicol. 2011;7(7):803–16.
57. Oncken AK, Kirby R, Rudloff E. Hypothermia in critically ill dogs and cats. Comp Cont Educ Small Anim Pract. 2001;23(6):506–21.
58. Martin RS, Kilgo PD, Miller P, et al. Injury-associated hypothermia: an analysis of the 2004 National Trauma Data Bank. Shock 2005;24(2):114–18.
59. Van Poucke S, Stevens K, Marcus A, Lance M. Hypothermia: effects on platelet function and hemostasis. Thromb J. 2014;12(1):31.
60. Haldane S, McCullough S, Raffe M. Hypothermia. Standards Care. 2003;5(5):6–10.
61. Myers RD, Beleslin DB, Rezevani AH. Hypothermia: role of alpha 1- and alpha 2-noradrenrgic receptors in the hypothalamus of the cat. Pharmacol Biochem Behav. 1987;26(2):373–9.

62. Kitagawa H, Akiyama T, Yamazaki T. Effects of moderate hypothermia on in situ cardiac sympathetic nerve endings. Neurochem Int. 2002;40(3):235–42.

63. Jensen KO, Jensen JM, Sprengel K. Practicability of avoiding hypothermia in resuscitation room phase in severely injured patients. J Med Eng Technol. 2015;39(4):223–5.

64. Pápa K, Máthé A, Abonyi-Toth Z, et al. Occurrence, clinical features and outcome of canine pancreatitis (80 cases). Acta Vet Hung. 2011;59(1):37–52.

65. Culp WT, Weisse C, Kellogg M, et al. Spontaneous hemoperitoneum in cats: 65 cases (1994–2006). J Am Vet Med Assoc. 2010;236(9):978–82.

66. Jitpean S, Ström-Holst B, Emanuelson U, et al. Outcome of pyometra in female dogs and predictors of peritonitis and prolonged postoperative hospitalization in surgically treated cases. BMC Vet Res. 2014;10:6.

67. Munday J, Hines S, Wallace K, et al. A systemic review of the effectiveness of warming interventions for women undergoing cesarean section. Worldviews Evid Based Nurs. 2014;11(6):383–93.

68. Roberson MC, Dieckmann LS, Rodriguez R, et al. A review of the evidence for active preoperative warming of adults undergoing general anesthesia. Am Assoc Nurse Anesth J. 2013;81(3):351–6.

69. Polderman KH. Mechanisms of action, physiological effects, and complications of hypothermia. Crit Care Med. 2009;37(7 Suppl):S186–202.

70. Polderman KH. Induced hypothermia and fever control for prevention and treatment of neurological injuries. Lancet 2008;371(9628):1955–69.

71. Antonic A, Dottori M, Leung J, et al. Hypothermia protects human neurons. Int J Stroke 2014;9(5):544–52.

72. Jacobs SE, Berg M, Hunt R, et al. Cooling for newborns with hypoxic ischaemic encephalopathy. Cochrane Database Syst Rev. 2013;1:CD003311.

73. Arrich J, Holzer M, et al. Hypothermia for neuroprotection in adults after cardiopulmonary resuscitation. Cochrane Database Syst Rev. 2012;9:CD004128.

74. Polderman KH, Herold I. Therapeutic hypothermia and controlled normothermia in the intensive care unit: practical considerations, side-effects, and cooling methods. Crit Care Med. 2009;37(3):1101–20.

75. Wu X, Drabek T, Tisherman S, et al. Emergency preservation and resuscitation with profound hypothermia, oxygen, and glucose allows reliable neurological recovery after 3h of cardiac arrest from rapid exsanguination in dogs. J Cereb Blood Flow Metab. 2008;28(2):302–11.

76. Kanemoto I, Taguchi D, Yokoyama S, et al. Open heart surgery with deep hypothermia and cardiopulmonary bypass in small and toy dogs. Vet Surg. 2010;39(6):674–9.

77. Hayes GM. Severe seizures associated with traumatic brain injury managed by controlled hypothermia, pharmacologic coma, and mechanical ventilation in a dog. J Vet Emerg Crit Care 2009;19(6):629–34.

Further reading

Hemmelgarn C, Gannon K. Heatstroke: thermoregulation, pathophysiology and predisposing factors. Comp Cont Educ Small Anim Pract. 2013;35(7):E4. An excellent review of the thermoregulation and pathophysiology of heat stroke.

Hemmelgarn C, Gannon K. Heatstroke: clinical signs, diagnosis, treatment and prognosis. Comp Cont Educ Small Anim Pract. 2013;35(7):E3. An easy-to-follow article highlighting the clinically important aspects of heatstroke.

Oncken AK, Kirby R, Rudloff E. Hypothermia in critically ill dogs and cats. Comp Cont Educ Small Anim Pract. 2001;23(6):506–21. A comprehensive review of hypothermia in small animal patients.

Öncü S. A clinical outline to fever in intensive care patients. Minerva Anestesiol. 2013;79(4):408–18. A well-written overview of causes of fever in a human ICU and recommended treatment.

CHAPTER 18
Drug selection and dosing regimens

Dawn Merton Boothe

College of Veterinary Medicine, Auburn University, Auburn, Alabama

Introduction

The goal of drug therapy is to induce in the patient a desired pharmacological response for an adequate period of time while avoiding adverse drug events. Reaching this goal requires the administration of the right drug (drug selection), in the right amount (dosing regimen), at the right time (dosing interval). The magnitude of response to any drug is determined by the concentration of the drug and the affinity of the drug for the targeted receptors. The desired response could be due to the original drug that was administered, the metabolites of the administered drug or a combination of effects. This includes "prodrugs" which are drugs that must be activated prior to eliciting the intended response.

Dosing regimens are composed of a route, dose (such as mg/kg) and interval (such as every eight hours: q 8h). The goal is to achieve and maintain the desired response throughout the dosing interval. The route of administration of a drug is mandated by the drug preparation and by patient needs. Therefore, it is the drug dose and interval that are most often manipulated to achieve the goals of drug therapy. The therapeutic range of a particular drug is characterized by a plasma drug concentration (PDC). The C_{min} is the minimum PDC below which therapeutic failure is likely to occur. The C_{max} is the maximum PDC above which side-effects, adverse events or toxicities are more likely to occur.

When deciding to initiate drug therapy, 10 basic questions should be considered (Box 18.1). The selection of the right drug for a critical patient requires knowledge of the effect that factors specific to the patient (Table 18.1) can have on drug **a**bsorption, **d**istribution, **m**etabolism, and **e**xcretion (ADME). To achieve the optimal drug response with minimal negative side-effects, it is necessary to carefully select the drug(s) and give special consideration to drug dose and interval of administration for each drug prescribed.

Drug selection

Benefit versus risk should be the most important determinant of drug selection. The objective is to assess whether the drug is necessary and beneficial and determine if the effects are measurable and safe. Unfortunately, the most effective drug can also be associated with the greatest risk of adverse effects.

The individual characteristics of a drug should be evaluated during the drug selection process. The pharmacodynamics of a drug describes the concentration and subsequent pharmacological effects of that drug. Drug pharmacokinetics describes the properties responsible for maintaining effective drug concentrations, to include bioavailability, absorption, distribution, metabolism, volume of distribution (Vd), half-life, and elimination.

The ideal drug should incorporate one or more of the following pharmacological traits:

- a wide therapeutic index (a much higher dose is needed to reach toxicity than for the desired effect; such as antimicrobials)
- the drug effects can be reversed (such as opioids)
- the drug has selectivity at specific receptors (such as beta- or alpha-adrenergic selective drugs; cyclooxygenase 2 selective nonsteroidal antiinflammatory drugs).

While receptor specific drugs are generally associated with fewer adversities, the "selectivity" may be lost with overdosing. Similar changes in magnitude and direction should occur between the drug concentrations in the plasma and drug concentrations at the targeted tissue or receptor. This is determined by appropriate drug dosing and by drug absorption and distribution.

Selection of antimicrobials justifies special consideration. The initial drug is typically chosen empirically, based on common etiological agents and drug qualities. Little information exists to support empirical selection of antimicrobials in the critically ill small animal patient, yet these patients can be the most vulnerable to therapeutic failure. Unfortunately, the advent of antimicrobial resistance is limiting efficacy of many commonly prescribed antimicrobial drugs. It is critical that the antibiotic choice is made with knowledge of the most current antibiograms that have been prepared specifically for the veterinary hospital or geographical region. An estimation of the likelihood for resistance can be determined. The procedures for hospital antibiotic surveillance and compilation of an antibiogram can be found in Chapter 14. Many commercial veterinary laboratories can provide a current antibiogram for the geographical region or for the specific veterinary hospital.

Drug disposition

Both patient factors and drug factors (ADME) will have an important impact on drug disposition or behavior. Patient factors (see Table 18.1) will include normal physiological differences as well as pathological factors caused by the disease. Drug factors include a wide variety of drug–drug (and potentially drug–diet) interactions that may alter the response of the individual patient. Significant interactions have been reported between drugs and some dietary supplements in human patients. A review of all current medications and supplements becomes important to determine any potential of negative drug interactions and to ascertain whether any new clinical signs could be the result of one or more of the drugs.

The drug concentration at the site of action generally parallels PDC, and is determined by four simultaneously occurring drug activities: absorption, distribution, metabolism, and excretion.

Monitoring and Intervention for the Critically Ill Small Animal: The Rule of 20, First Edition. Edited by Rebecca Kirby and Andrew Linklater.
© 2017 John Wiley & Sons, Inc. Published 2017 by John Wiley & Sons, Inc.

Figure 18.1 provides a schematic demonstrating the general pathways for drug ADME.

The most common method of drug movement is by passive diffusion and as such, the single most important determinant of how much drug moves is the concentration of diffusible drug. Water-soluble drugs primarily distribute to the extracellular fluid (ECF) while lipid-soluble drugs tend to penetrate cell membranes. The extent of drug movement depends on the size of the body compartments to which the drug is being distributed. The apparent volume of tissue distribution (Vd) is the volume of tissue which dilutes the drug and is calculated by Vd = dose/PDC.

Small, lipid-soluble and unionized drug molecules are more likely to move beyond cell membranes or other barriers. A drug that is ionized will be trapped at the site. In general, the closer the bodily fluid or tissue pH is to the pKa of the drug (equal parts ionized versus unionized), the more diffusible the drug. Although passive drug movement predominates, the importance of active transport through efflux or influx proteins is being recognized. These transport pumps generally move weak acids, weak bases or organic (nonionizable) drugs against a concentration gradient. Their role in renal and biliary excretion is well recognized. These pumps can

markedly impact drug absorption and prevent effective drug penetration at isolated sites, such as the brain, cerebral spinal fluid, eye, prostate, and testicles,

Absorption can be described by the rate and extent of the drug being absorbed and the systemic bioavailability of the drug. The bioavailability is the percent or fraction (F) of a drug dose that reaches systemic circulation. By definition, a drug given intravenously is 100% bioavailable (F = 1). The difference between an IV dose and a non-IV dose is represented by the formula: Dose non-IV = dose IV/F. Intravenous administration is common in the critically ill patient. Although the risk of an exaggerated response might be increased, an advantage to IV administration is the removal of the effect of disease, diet or other drugs on drug absorption.

Many factors influence oral drug absorption. Because of the large surface area in the small intestines, most oral drugs are absorbed from that location. The rate and extent of oral drug absorption are influenced primarily by environmental pH (generally acidic but becoming more alkaline distally), motility, epithelial permeability, surface area, blood flow, and bile salt production. Transport proteins (P-glycoprotein in particular) and drug-metabolizing enzymes in intestinal epithelial cells can markedly contribute to differential drug absorption.

Even drugs that are well absorbed after oral administration may not have a high systemic bioavailability. First-pass metabolism occurs when much of the absorbed drug is extracted by the portal circulation. For these first-pass drugs, the oral dose is generally much higher than the parenteral dose. Alternate routes, including transmucosal or rectal administration, might be considered for such drugs. Further, systemic bioavailability of these drugs is markedly influenced by changes in portal blood flow.

Parenteral (subcutaneous, intramuscular) absorption is influenced primarily by surface area and regional blood flow. Many drugs are modified to prolong parenteral absorption by the addition of salts or esters that will release the drug. The parenteral and oral administration of drugs should be avoided in critical patients until regional perfusion is restored.

Transdermal administration deserves special consideration. The stratum corneum is a major barrier to absorption of all except the most lipophilic of drugs. FDA-approved special delivery systems such as transdermal patches or liquids may effectively deliver drug by increasing epithelial permeability by altering temperature or hydration. However, caution is recommended when using compounded complex delivery systems since there may be limited data to support the safety, efficacy or quality of such preparations.

Distribution is one of two drug movements that eliminates drug from plasma. Distribution includes movements of the drug from plasma into tissues and back again, with elimination from the body the final movement. Factors that determine distribution include regional blood flow, tissue-drug binding, and transport proteins. Protein binding, principally to albumin, causes a lipid-soluble drug to be sufficiently water soluble, allowing the drug to move through the body. However, while protein bound, the drug is inactive.

The amount of tissue to which an IV administered drug is distributed is the main determinant of PDC. The Vd simplistically is the volume of tissue which dilutes the drug and can be calculated by Vd = dose/PDC. As such, if a target PDC and the Vd of a drug are known, the dose needed to achieve the desired PDC (and thus the desired response) can be calculated by Dose (mg/kg) = PDC (mg/L) × Vd (L/kg). Since dose is directly proportional to Vd, an

Table 18.1 Patient factors affecting drug pharmacodynamics and pharmacokinetics.

Factor	Effect	Examples of drugs affected	Adjustment
Fluid balance Increased fluid balance: IV fluid administration, fluid retention (except for third body compartments)	↓ Plasma and tissue drug concentrations; Half-life (this may be offset by ↑ clearance of renally eliminated drugs)	Water-soluble antibiotics: aminoglycosides, beta-lactams	Increase dose to enhance efficacy; Longer dosing interval to avoid adverse effects
Poor peripheral tissue perfusion: dehydration, hypovolemia, vasoconstrictive drugs	↓ Absorption SC, IM (primarily rate); ↑ PDC due to smaller volume of distribution; ↑ Distribution to brain and heart; ↓ Decreased renal clearance until volume replacement occurs) (prolonged)	Any drug, but the risk is greater with water-soluble drugs. Care with cardioactive and CNS active drugs in particular	Anticipate longer onset to response; Decrease dose particularly for CNS or cardioactive drug until volume replaced (this may also shorten half-life); Prolong interval in anticipation of longer duration of effect, particularly in patients with altered renal function
Compartmentalized third body fluid space: ascites, pleural effusion	↑↓ or no change in half-life; Impact depends on distribution of drug: decreased volume of distribution if a water-soluble drug. If lipid soluble, dose on total body weight. Binding to effluxed proteins		Half-life may not change even if profound changes in distribution or clearance; Dose based on lean body weight or BSA
Hypoalbuminemia	↑ Renal clearance if organ function normal (shorter half-life); ↑ Free drug available at receptor (longer half-life)	Antimicrobials: cefovecin, doxycyline; Imidazole antifungals; All nonsteroidal antinflammatories	Decrease dose if abnormal clearance; prolong interval, particularly if abnormal clearance
↑ Inflammatory proteins/acute-phase proteins	↑ binding by basic drugs; will facilitate clearance of flow-limited drugs	Lidocaine, opioids	May need to alter dose
Renal disease Uremic toxins	Altered tissue receptors; ↓ Competition for drug binding sites; change conformation/affinity for binding protein	NSAIDS, selected penicillins, furosemide, anticonvulsants	
Abnormal proximal tubular secretion	↓ Excretion; abnormal transport of drugs and organic acids	Penicillins, cephalosporins, NSAIDs, sulfonamides, several diuretics	Reduce dose using creatinine clearance; Adjust dosing interval for drugs that accumulate; adjust either interval or dose for drugs that do not accumulate
↓ Renal blood flow	↓ Excretion; abnormal transport of drugs and bases; ↓ Renal extraction	Cimetidine, procainamide, morphine derivatives; Penicillins, sulfates, glucuronide conjugates	Adjust dosing interval for drugs that accumulate; adjust either interval or dose for drugs that do not accumulate
Liver disease Hepatoportal/intrahepatic shunting Chronic liver disease	↓ Flow-dependent metabolism; ↓↓ Phase I and II drug metabolism/clearance	Propranolol, verapamil, prazosin, morphine derivatives; Diazepam, prednisolone, phenylbutazone, phenytoin, theophylline, cimetidine, antipyrine	Reduce dose; Addition of liver protective drugs may be beneficial: N-acetylcysteine, sAME, milk thistle
Cholestasis	↓ Activity/amount p450; ↓ drug elimination in bile	Doxycycline, clindamycin, digitoxin, naproxin	Reduce dose

(Continued)

Table 18.1 (Continued)

Factor	Effect	Examples of drugs affected	Adjustment
Sepsis			
Increased capillary permeability	↑ Vd	Aminoglycoside	Increase dose
Hyperperfusion	↑ Renal and hepatic clearance of flow-dependent drugs		Increase dose
	↑ Rate **of** hepatic metabolism; ↓ PDC		
Brain trauma	↑ Rate of hepatic metabolism		May need to alter dose
Biliary tract disease	Bilirubinemia competes for albumin binding site		May need to alter dose
Electrolyte, acid–base disorders	Altered receptor sensitivity to drugs	Hyperkalemia effect on digitalis, quinidine, procainamide	Delay drug administration until correction or consider altered dose
Δ pH	Δ drug distribution		
Gastrointestinal disorders	Poor absorption of oral drugs; drug binding to effluxed proteins		Use parenteral routes of administration
Abnormal mucosal transport, motility, blood flow, efflux of proteins			
Nutritional status			
Obesity	↑ Fat distribution of lipophilic drugs		
Poor enteral feeding; enterocyte atrophy w/in 3 days	Poor absorption; abnormal hepatic drug metabolism		
Oral feeding	Diet impacts on absorption of oral drugs		
Fever	Poor oral absorption	Amoxicillin	Avoid oral drugs
Cardiovascular disease			
Na+, H₂O retention	Δ Vd/drug distribution	Lidocaine, digoxin	
Hypertension/vasoconstriction	↓ Hepatic clearance		
↓ Cardiac output	Redistribute blood flow; ↑ drug to brain & heart; ↓ absorption SC, IM, oral; ↓ clearance of flow-dependent drugs		
Species			
Feline	Deficiency of some glucuronyl transferases in Phase II metabolism; deficient in many phase I metabolism enzymes; different responses to some drugs	Opioids, dopamine, fluoroquinolones	Avoid drugs that form toxic metabolites; closely adhere to drug recommendation for the species

BSA, body surface area; CNS, central nervous system; NSAID, nonsteroidal antiinflammatory drug; PDC, plasma drug concentration; sAME, S-adenosyl methionine; Vd, volume of distribution.

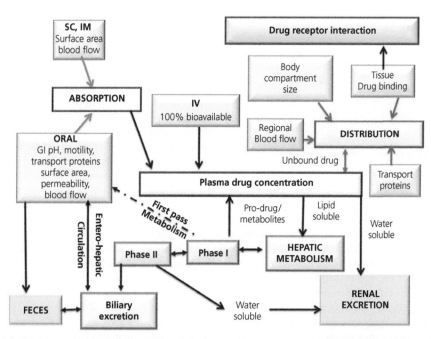

Figure 18.1 Schematic of drug movements from absorption through elimination. Response to a drug reflects the extend of drug–receptor interaction and thus concentration of drug at the tissue. Tissue drug concentrations generally parallel plasma concentrations, which in turn reflect four simultaneous drug movements. Drug absorption depends on the route of administration, with intravenous (IV) providing 100% drug bioavailability. Oral absorption is impacted primarily by gastrointestinal pH, motility, surface area, and epithelial permeability. First-pass metabolism by the liver decreases oral bioavailability. Factors that affect drug distribution include protein binding, regional blood flow, transport proteins, tissue-drug binding, and body compartment size. Elimination of the plasma drug concentration can be through hepatic metabolism for lipid-soluble drugs, which undergo Phase I and possibly Phase II metabolism, or renal excretion of water-soluble drugs. Lipid-soluble drugs also may be excreted in the bile, some of which will undergo enterohepatic circulation. Each of the drug movements is impacted by the concentration of diffusible drug and thus drug lipophilicity, molecular weight, and drug pKa. GI, gastrointestinal; IM, intramuscular; SC, subcutaneous.

increase in the Vd necessitates that the dose is also increased to maintain the same PDC. Likewise, if the Vd decreases (such as dehydration), the PDC will increase, possibly resulting in toxicity. When the drug is given by a nonintravenous route, then the dose must be further modified by F (Dose non-IV = dose IV/F).

All drugs initially distribute to plasma (about 0.05% of body weight). Drugs that are tightly and significantly (>80%) bound to plasma proteins generally remain in the plasma and have a Vd ≤0.1 L/kg. The fraction of unbound drug can be easily influenced by changes in protein concentration and by competition with other drugs or compounds; however, this unbound fraction may be more rapidly cleared, decreasing the risk of adverse reaction.

Drug solubility affects the distribution of the drug. Water-soluble drugs primarily distribute to the ECF (20–30% of body weight,) resulting in a Vd generally between 0.2 and 0.3 L/kg. Lipid-soluble drugs tend to penetrate cell membranes, being distributed to total body water (60% or more of body weight) with a Vd ≥0.6 L/kg. Drugs that are ion trapped, bound to tissue proteins or accumulate for other reasons are removed from plasma and are characterized by higher PDC. This often results in Vd >1 L/kg. Because distribution of a drug can remove it from the organs of clearance, the half-life of these drugs tends to be long, and the time to steady state, the point at which both safety and efficacy can be assessed, will also be prolonged. Once an equilibrium is reached between drug distribution and elimination, the decline in PDC reflects only drug elimination from the body.

Metabolism is the means by which the body converts a lipid-soluble drug, which will be passively reabsorbed as urine is concentrated in the renal tubule, into a water-soluble drug, which will not be passively reabsorbed and will subsequently be excreted. Most drug metabolism occurs in the liver. Hepatic clearance of a drug is affected by hepatic blood flow and the intrinsic metabolism and protein binding of the drug. The influence of each of these varies with the drug, and determines whether the drug metabolism is "flow-limited" or "capacity-limited." For "flow-limited" drugs (such as lidocaine, most beta-adrenergic drugs, most opioids, benzodiazepines), clearance is dependent only on the rate of delivery to the liver and thus changes directly and proportionately with changes in hepatic blood flow. Orally administered drugs enter the portal circulation and undergo "first-pass metabolism." These drugs are characterized by a high hepatic extraction (>70% with each passage) and are not impacted by protein binding. Clearance of "capacity-limited" drugs (most nonsteroidal antiinflammatories, diazepam, prednisolone, phenylbutazone, phenytoin, theophylline, cimetidine, and antipyrine) is limited by the intrinsic metabolic capacity of the liver. Protein binding can prevent the clearance of capacity-limited drugs.

Hepatic drug metabolism is generally accomplished in two phases. Phase I metabolism enzymes (primarily cytochrome p450; CYP450) most often inactivate a drug. However, drugs may also be converted to an active metabolite with equal or less activity. Prodrugs must be converted to an active metabolite (such as enrofloxacin converted to ciprofloxacin; prednisone converted to prednisolone). Phase I metabolism also can metabolize a drug to a toxic metabolite, with such drugs increasing the risk of hepatotoxicity. Toxic metabolites are also common sources of haptens, molecules that associate with tissues and cause an allergic response.

Phase I metabolism is often, but not always, a prelude to Phase II

Box 18.2 Formulas to modify drug dose or interval with renal disease.

New dose = old dose × normal Cr/pt Cr
New interval = old interval × pt Cr/normal Cr
Using creatinine clearance:
New dose = old dose × pt CrCl/normal CrCl
New interval = old interval × normal CrCl/pt CrCl
CrCl = [U_{cr} (mg/dL) × Uvolume (mL/min) ÷ S_{cr} (mg/dL)] ÷ BW (kg)

Cr, creatinine; Crcl, creatinine clearance; pt, patient; S_{cr}, serum creatinine; U_{cr}, urine creatinine.

---

metabolism. Phase II hepatic metabolism results in the addition of a large water-soluble molecule to the drug, generally rendering the drug inactive (or nontoxic), and facilitating its renal excretion (or, less commonly, biliary excretion). As such, Phase II metabolism is often protective in nature. Common conjugates include glucuronide (some deficiencies in the cat) and glutathione, the latter being particularly effective in scavenging toxic drug metabolites. However, the liver's protective Phase II metabolic capacity is both dose and duration dependent. Acetylation often produces active metabolites and is a reaction in which the dog is deficient.

The metabolic pathway of each drug varies markedly with the chemistry of the drug and the species of the patient. Over 20 superfamilies of CYP450 have been identified. Species differences are marked, with many drugs able to induce or inhibit many of these enzymes.

Excretion is the drug movement that clears drug or its metabolites from the body. The kidney is the most important organ of excretion. All drugs undergo glomerular filtration; however, the extent of excretion of that drug in urine depends on how much is passively resorbed, which in turn depends on lipid solubility, ionization, and molecular weight. In addition to glomerular filtration, which is a passive process, many drugs are actively secreted into the urine in the proximal tubules by way of transport proteins.

All drug movements in the kidney are influenced by renal blood flow. Therefore, any disease or drug that affects renal blood flow will have an impact on renal drug clearance. The extent of renal clearance of a drug can be predicted based on creatinine clearance or serum creatinine, which can be used to modify dosing regimens (Box 18.2). However, urine pH can have a profound effect on the extent of renal excretion of a drug. In contrast to renal clearance, biliary clearance is slow. Generally, very large drugs are excreted in the bile (such as macrolides, cyclosporine).

Drug dosing interval

Drug metabolism and excretion are responsible for drug elimination from the body. The drug elimination half-life is the basis of the dosing interval. At one half-life, 50% is eliminated; with the next half-life, 50% of the remaining drug is eliminated (25%) for a total of 75%; at three half-lives, a total of 87.5% is eliminated, which is generally sufficient for resolution of clinical response. Half-life also determines the time to reach steady-state equilibrium. This occurs when the amount of drug leaving the body is equal to the amount reaching the systemic circulation during a dosing interval. Steady state is reached after 3–5 drug half-lives have lapsed once a new dosing regimen has started. Steady state is relevant only for a drug that is given as multiple dosing (including constant rate infusion (CRI)) rather than single dosing. In addition, only drugs that

accumulate with multiple dosing will reach steady state. This occurs only when a drug is given at a dosing interval that is shorter than or not much longer than its half-life. If the dosing interval is substantially longer than the half-life, most of each dose is eliminated before the next dose; accumulation is minimal and steady state is not reached. However, if the dosing interval is substantially shorter than the half-life, much of the previous dose remains in the body when the next dose is given. The drug begins to accumulate, with the magnitude dependent on how much shorter the interval is compared to the half-life. For such drugs, the amount of fluctuation during an interval is very small. A drug given at an interval equal to its half-life will accumulate two-fold at steady state. The time to steady state (and thus the maximum effect) is solely dependent on elimination half-life, requiring 3–5 half-lives of the same preparation at the same dosing regimen.

If the time to reach steady state will take too long (such as with anticonvulsants in a dog with status epilepticus), a loading dose can be given which is calculated based on Vd and target PDC. It is for this reason that a loading dose is also given prior to initiating a CRI for some drugs. It is important to note that after administration of a loading dose, the patient is not at steady state; rather, predicted steady-state concentrations have been achieved. The maintenance dose is designed to maintain what is achieved with the loading dose. If it does not, then PDC will either decline or increase until steady state is reached after 3–5 half-lives of maintenance dosing. For example, if the half-life of fentanyl is three hours, then steady state may not occur until nine hours after a CRI is begun. A loading dose may be appropriate since maximum drug efficacy may not occur for nine hours. Likewise, safety cannot be accurately assessed until nine hours have passed. Consideration should be given to the half-lives of drugs that are mixed together in a CRI so that all drugs reach steady state simultaneously for maximum effect. Otherwise, the efficacy and safety of each drug must be assessed at the appropriate steady state.

The patient, the disease, and drug factors influence the drug elimination half-life. For example, if Vd of a drug decreases (such as in a dehydrated patient), PDC increases and more drug is in each volume that is cleared by the liver or kidney. Elimination increases (half-life is shorter) even if clearance does not change. However, if clearance were also to decrease (such as occurs with decreased glomerular filtration rate (GFR)), less volume would be going through the kidney and thus elimination and half-life might not change, despite profound differences in drug disposition. If fluids replace the volume, as Vd normalizes, then half-life will finally become prolonged due to decreased clearance.

Diagnostic and monitoring procedures

The critically ill small animal patient is likely to have at least two or more drugs prescribed in their treatment plan in addition to IV fluids and nutritional supplementation. The polypharmaceutical approach, while potentially life saving, can also result in drug-induced adverse reactions. Important information can be gained from the history, physical examination, cage-side point of care (POC) laboratory testing, and clinicopathological testing that can assist in drug selection and the prescribing of drug dose and intervals. Monitoring procedures must then be initiated to assess the therapeutic benefits and to assist in the early detection of any adverse reactions attributable to the drug therapy.

The history and physical examination

The history and physical examination are critical to the process of drug selection and determining the appropriate dose and interval for the patient. The signalment will provide the age, sex, and breed, which can affect drug pharmacokinetics and pharmacodynamics (see Patient factors below, and Table 18.1). Breed dispositions (including Collie, Old English Sheepdog, Long-haired Whippets, Australian Shepherds) for the ABDC delta1 gene mutation that affects drug ADME must be recognized. A complete list of prescribed and over-the-counter medications and supplementations is necessary to anticipate potential drug interactions. The diet may be important since drug–food interactions are possible. A complete list of clinical signs present will assist in identifying new signs that could be attributable to drug therapy or progression of disease. A past history of renal or liver disease may warrant consideration when making drug selections and dosing regimens.

The initial physical examination can aid in identifying alterations in Vd, such as poor perfusion, dehydration, pleural or abdominal effusions or peripheral edema. A complete physical and neurological examination should be performed, prior to the administration of medications. The physical examination is repeated a minimum of twice daily to monitor for toxic effects of the drug(s) administered. Since toxic side-effects of drugs can affect a multitude of organ systems, each drug dose and route of administration is examined for drug–drug interactions, adverse reactions attributable to one or more drug, and any therapeutic benefits of the drug.

In addition, nursing notes should record any alert for potential adverse reactions that may occur with drug administration, and the staff made aware of tolerable limits (such as heart rate or blood pressure changes). Any signs that should prompt intervention or reassessment of a drug regimen should be highlighted. Any adverse drug reaction experienced in the past or during the present hospitalization should be permanently noted in the medical record to avoid future adverse effects.

Point of care and clinicopathological testing

The minimum laboratory database (POC testing) should include packed cell volume (PCV), total protein (TP), blood urea nitrogen (BUN), blood glucose, electrolyte panel, blood gas analysis, coagulation profile, and urinalysis. The PCV and TP are assessed together and provide the earliest indication of anemia, erythrocytosis, hypoproteinemia or dehydration. A low TP brings concern for low albumin, and its effects on drug binding and transport. A high BUN brings concern for dehydration or impaired GFR, potentially affecting the Vd, drug clearance, and, together, drug elimination. A low BUN warrants further investigation for hepatic disease with drug metabolism a possible concern. Increased serum bile acids may indicate problems with either metabolism or biliary excretion. Certain drugs have undesirable side-effects if there are electrolyte disorders (such as digoxin with hypokalemia). The presence of acidemia or alkalemia could alter drug distribution and metabolism or the affinity of a receptor for the drug. The urine specific gravity in concert with BUN and serum creatinine provides an indication of kidney drug excretion. Assessment of urine sediment and urine protein for tubular cell casts or proteinuria can provide an early indication of nephrotoxicity from drug therapy, although these indicators are not sensitive.

A complete blood count and serum biochemical profile are necessary to establish a baseline indication of albumin concentration and renal and hepatic function. Tests are then repeated, as indicated, to assess the impact of drug therapy on the monitored parameter. Measuring specific drug levels may be warranted to assess efficacy and minimize adverse reactions.

Therapeutic drug monitoring (TDM) is particularly indicated for drugs with a narrow therapeutic window or for situations when therapeutic failure is life threatening. Because of the impact of patient and drug factors, TDM may be particularly useful in the critical care patient. In general, TDM can detect whether or not a patient is in the therapeutic range established for the general population of that species. However, it is important to understand that just because a patient PDC is "in the therapeutic range" and it has not responded does not mean the patient has failed that therapy. Some patients respond well below and others only at the highest end of the therapeutic range (and some beyond that). As such, the therapeutic range must be considered in the context of individual patient needs and monitoring should be implemented to determine the patient's therapeutic range.

Monitoring drug response

Monitoring is important to determine whether or not there is an appropriate response to a drug and if adverse reactions are occurring. In addition to TDM, physical examination parameters, monitoring physical parameters, laboratory testing, and equipment-based procedures may be valuable. The presence of perfusion deficits, dehydration, overhydration, edema, and third body fluid spacing can affect the Vd and drug efficacy at the prescribed dose and interval. Measuring, fluid input, and urine output along with pre- and posttreatment body weight, PCV, and TP or albumin can be surrogate markers of response to diuretic and fluid therapy. Prerenal azotemia, physical signs of dehydration, and tachycardia may be indicative of overzealous diuretic therapy. Serum electrolytes should be monitored when the patient is treated with drugs (such as diuretics) that have the ability to alter electrolytes. Response to drugs that alter hemostasis might be monitored with bleeding times or coagulation profiles (see Chapter 9).

Central venous pressure can provide an indication of central volume deficits or overload resulting from therapy or that will affect new drug therapy (see Chapter 2). Arterial blood pressure and heart rate should be monitored when using drugs that impact afterload (such as vasopressors and vasodilators, see Chapter 3). Development of tachycardia may provide an indication of overzealous afterload reduction or significant intravascular volume deficit. Beta-blockers in particular are associated with bradycardia. Antiarrhythmics can have proarrhythmic effects requiring monitoring of the electrocardiogram before and after treatment.

Monitoring clinical laboratory changes in renal function or liver leakage enzymes may be warranted for drugs that pose a risk for nephro- or hepatotoxicity. For renal function, urinalysis may indicate changes compatible with proximal tubular damage such as glucosuria in the presence of normoglycemia and cast formation. Caution is recommended when relying solely on urine parameters since they may have inadequate sensitivity.

Drug-induced changes in renal or hepatic function must be distinguished from pathological insults from other causes such as hypoxia and sepsis. In addition, it is difficult to detect an adversity to drugs if there is no defined clinical indicator of toxicity. Monitoring the impact of antimicrobials is particularly difficult. Although fever or clinical signs of inflammation may be an indicator of therapeutic failure, this is not consistently true. Because most antimicrobials are safe, erring on the side of overdosing is recommended to minimize the risk of resistance. This is true even for aminoglycosides whose toxicity is related to trough rather than peak concentrations. For more information on selection of antimicrobial agents, see Chapter 14.

Factors affecting drug therapy

Prescribing an effective and safe dosing regimen is a challenge that must be met when treating the critically ill dog and cat. A combination of drug and patient factors (see Table 18.1) must be considered when selecting a drug regimen.

Drug factors

Dysfunction of the kidneys and liver can contribute to adverse drug reactions. The effects of cardiac disease might also be profound due to the impact of poor perfusion on drug distribution and the organs of clearance. Less significant effects occur with gastrointestinal, pulmonary, endocrine, and metabolic disorders.

The impact of disease on drug metabolism and clearance can vary with the solubility (water or lipid) of the drug. Water-soluble drugs generally undergo renal excretion. Lipophilic drugs generally are metabolized by the liver prior to renal and, less commonly, biliary excretion. As such, renal disease should minimally influence these drugs.

In general, renal clearance of drugs, whether by glomerular filtration or active tubular secretion, will change proportionately with renal blood flow and can be estimated by changes in creatinine clearance or increased serum creatinine (see Box 18.2). The effects of changes in renal blood flow (usually decreased) on drug excretion are most profound if renal extraction of the drug is high (such as with penicillins, sulfates, glucuronide conjugates) but are less significant for drugs that are slowly extracted (such as aminoglycosides, diuretics, digoxin). The drug half-life will proportionately change with clearance unless offset by changes in Vd. Dosing intervals should be proportionally modified for drugs that do not accumulate. For drugs that do accumulate, either the dose or interval can be modified. An exception is the aminoglycosides that are dosed once daily so that further prolongation in dosing interval may not be necessary unless renal disease is moderate to severe.

However, any negative effect of changes in drug metabolism and clearance could be balanced or cancelled by an equal change in Vd (such as the impact of peripheral edema in the face of decreased renal clearance). Alternatively, an increase in clearance can occur during a hyperdynamic state (such as seen in early hypovolemic or septic shock) and potentially be balanced by decreased renal function. In these situations, the dosing interval of a drug may not need to be modified in the presence of disease-induced changes in clearance.

Renal clearance of lipophilic drugs may increase with aggressive fluid therapy or use of drugs which increase renal blood flow (including angiotensin converting enzyme (ACE) inhibitors in the face of renal vasoconstriction). For highly protein-bound drugs, renal clearance will increase as the drug becomes unbound. In addition to changes in drug clearance, renal disease can also alter drug disposition because of changes in electrolyte, acid–base, and fluid balance. Changes in electrolytes and acid–base balance may also be important in altering receptor sensitivity to drugs. Uremia-induced alterations in tissue receptors may also result in an altered receptor sensitivity and drug toxicity.

In general, liver disease that has impacted serum albumin, BUN, and bile acids should be assumed to have also caused a moderate to severe decrease in hepatic drug metabolism and clearance. The impact of liver disease on Phase II activity is less clear and less

profound than on Phase I. In general, decreased conjugation should be anticipated. For flow-limited drugs, anticipate that the change in hepatic clearance parallels the amount of portal blood that bypasses the liver, whether due to congenital or acquired shunting. Half-life will be prolonged, and oral bioavailability will be increased.

Diseases of the biliary tract alter the disposition of drugs eliminated through the bile. Cholestasis decreases the content or activity of cytochrome p450 drug metabolizing enzymes and thus can affect the elimination of drugs that are not secreted in bile. In general, doses of drugs eliminated principally in the bile should be reduced, particularly if the drug is characterized by a narrow therapeutic window. Because Phase II is important to organ protection, the liver and other organs are predisposed to drug-induced toxicity.

In patients for which hepatic or renal clearance is reduced, highly protein-bound drugs should not be given with one another if either is potentially toxic. In addition, highly protein-bound drugs should not be administered in the presence of endogenous protein-bound toxins which might accompany renal or liver failure.

Patient factors

Critical patient parameters such as fluid balance, third body fluid spacing, inflammation, hypoalbuminemia, and sepsis can change drug ADME (see Table 18.1). Alterations in blood flow, fluid balance, renal function or hepatic function can have an immediate and profound effect on drug pharmacokinetics. Poor perfusion from any cause results in shunting blood from the peripheral to central core circulation. When drug is not distributed to peripheral sites, normal drug ADME is altered. The PDC is preferentially shunted to the core circulation (the heart and brain), predisposing these organs to toxicity. Further, organ health is negatively impacted by hypoxia and insufficient energy substrate associated with poor perfusion. Decreased perfusion in the face of high metabolic requirements results in a mismatch that places organs at a greater risk of toxicity and decreases drug absorption (gastrointestinal tract or peripheral tissues) and clearance (kidney or liver).

These fluid shifts can have a profound influence on drug distribution, although the impact varies with the body compartment that is altered and the chemistry (water or lipid solubility) of the drug. Fluid therapy (crystalloids and colloids) and increased capillary permeability associated with SIRS diseases will alter the size of the body compartments. The impact of hyperdynamic perfusion should increase drug delivery to most tissues, also resulting in lower plasma drug concentrations. The impact of ascites is less clear, with water-soluble drugs probably not distributing to this compartment. Dosing on a mg/kg basis may markedly increase drug concentrations when there is fluid extravasation into third spaces (such as ascites). Thus, the dosing of potentially toxic drugs should be based on lean body weight or body surface area (BSA) when third spacing is present. Dehydration will have an opposite effect, generally increasing PDC until volume replacement has occurred. Volume repletion rather than dose modification should be implemented in the dehydrated patient. It should be noted, however, that aggressive fluid therapy can return the patient to a normal or even exaggerated fluid balance. Inflammatory proteins can bind free drug, making it less available, while the displacement of protein-bound drugs (such as with hypoalbuminemia) will increase the concentration of free, active drug, as well as increasing the Vd.

In addition to the impact of disease on drug response, a number of normal physiological factors can also contribute to response variability. Age extremes often are characterized by decreased function in organs of clearance, although increasingly, pediatrics demonstrate enhanced rather than decreased clearance. Gender differences in animals have not been well characterized, but differences in body composition and drug metabolizing proteins are among those impacting adverse drug reactions in humans.

Species differences (dog compared to cat) are well understood to contribute to differences in response to drugs, but less well understood is exactly what these differences are. The cat has long been recognized to be deficient in some – but not all – glucuronyl transferases associated with Phase II metabolism. However, the cat also is deficient in many Phase I enzymes (at least compared to the dog). As such, drugs that are flow-limited in some species may not be in the cat. Further, the cat appears to be rapidly depleted of its glutathione scavenging. The cat also provides an example of species differences in response to drugs. Feline hemoglobin is more susceptible to oxidation; dopamine receptors are either lacking or respond differently to dopaminergic drugs compared to dogs. Opioids are associated with increased dopamine release, causing abnormal behaviors. Cats lack efflux pumps responsible for removing fluoroquinolones from the retina. Subsequent conversion to oxygen radicals upon exposure of the accumulated drug can result in retinal degeneration.

Mutations are now a recognized cause of adverse reactions to drugs. A host of working breeds (such as Collies, Old English Sheepdogs, Long-haired Whippets, Australian Shepherds) are characterized by mutations in the ABCB delta 1 (or MDR1) gene encoding for P-glycoprotein. P-glycoprotein is an adenosine triphosphate (ATP)-driven efflux pump that restricts drug penetration into the brain, is involved in active drug elimination by the liver and kidney, and limits drug absorption in the gut. The dysfunctional proteins result in the accumulation of drugs in the central nervous system (CNS) with subsequent toxicity. Avermectins are known drugs to be avoided in these breeds, but members of the opioids (such as butorphanol, loperamide), anticancer drugs (such as vinblastine, vincristine, doxorubicin), selected antibiotics, and a plethora of other drugs (such as acepromazine) might serve as substrates for this mutated protein [1]. Dogs can be tested for the gene mutation. Drug selection, route of application, and dose modifications are necessary in affected dogs for drugs that bind to P-glycoprotein

Drug interactions

The critically ill patient is particularly predisposed to drug interactions and their negative consequences. Drug interactions can occur at the pharmaceutical, pharmacokinetic or pharmacodynamic stage of drug administration.

Pharmaceutical drug interactions occur prior to the administration or absorption of a drug. Interactions can occur as one or more of the following:
- between two drugs
- between a drug and a carrier (solvent or vehicle)
- between the drug and receptacle (including IV tubing)
- between a drug and the environment in which it is administered (gastric environment).

Any of these interactions are likely to occur in the critical care environment where IV administration and multiple drug administration are common. Drug incompatibilities can change the chemical or physical nature of a drug; several formularies, package inserts, and websites list common drug incompatibilities. Incompatible reactions can result in drug degradation due to changes in pH or

temperature, exposure to ultraviolet radiation or binding by drugs with different charges or other molecular interactions.

Unstable drugs generally have a short shelf-life when in solution. Therefore, reconstituted parenteral solutions should always be labeled with the new expiration date as well as the final concentration of diluted drug. The product label instructions should be strictly followed after reconstitution. If directed by the label, refrigeration or freezing can prolong the shelf-life. It should not be assumed that cold storage will prolong the shelf-life of the drug unless efficacy has been documented. Freezing can increase the degradation (such as ampicillin), crystallization (such as heparin, dobutamine, furosemide), and precipitation (such as insulin) of drugs. Storage at room temperature or refrigeration may result in crystayllization of some medications (mannitol). Refreezing of a previously frozen and defrosted solution increases the risk of altered efficacy.

The proper reconstituting fluid should be used to avoid inactivation of drugs. Changing the pH of a solution by improperly diluting it or mixing it with another drug can be risky. The release of some insulin is pH dependent and diluting insulin with a solution other than that provided by the manufacturer could change the pH and thus the rate of insulin release.

The pH of a solution may be necessary to keep the active drug dissolved or stable; changing the pH may result in precipitation or loss of stability. For example, acid-labile drugs (such as penicillins) can be destroyed in low pH solutions. Drugs prepared as an acid salt (such as lidocaine hydrogen chloride) or in acidic solutions (such as sodium heparin) should not be combined with alkaline solutions (sodium bicarbonate).

Often, a pharmaceutical drug interaction involving IV solutions can be detected by a visual change in the appearance of the drugs. Discoloration, cloudiness, and formation of precipitate are indications of an interaction and use of the drug should be reconsidered. If the drug has simply recrystallized, gently warming the solution may result in redissolution without loss of efficacy. However, not all interactions will result in a physical change of the appearance. Likewise, the change in physical appearance of a drug combination does not necessarily indicate that the activity of the drug has been changed. For example, diazepam has been mixed with other drugs with no observable (reported) change in drug efficacy, despite a cloudy discoloration. A pink discoloration of dopamine indicates inactivation. Discoloration of dobutamine does not preclude efficacy if the drug is used within 24 hours. Slight yellow discoloration of procainamide is acceptable; dark discoloration indicates a loss of efficacy. Any change in the physical character of a drug is a reason not to use the drug in a critically ill patient.

Drugs can bind to one another and become inactivated. Calcium solutions will cause precipitation if combined with solutions containing carbonates (such as sodium bicarbonate). Heparin is incompatible with many drugs and should not be mixed with other drugs. Saline, rather than heparin, might be used to maintain patency of catheters through which drugs will be administered. Penicillins (weak acids) will bind to and inactivate aminoglycosides (weak bases) and fluorinated quinolones, if present in sufficiently high concentrations.

Several drugs can bind to receptacles. For example, lipid-soluble drugs (such as diazepam) can bind to plastic containers; insulin binds to selected glasses and many plastics, including polyethylene and polyvinyl; aminoglycosides bind to glass. Binding to IV lines can be minimized by flushing each new system with a sufficient volume of drug-containing solution (50 mL) prior to drug administration. Drugs packaged in brown bottles (such as diazepam and furosemide) are protected from UV lighting and protection should be continued if transferred to another vial or syringe or diluted in IV fluids for CRI.

Dosing errors are one of the most adverse events that occur in human hospitals and similar errors are likely to occur in veterinary hospitals as well. Refer to Chapter 20 for a discussion on how to avoid drug errors [2].

Pharmacokinetic drug interactions occur when one drug alters the disposition of another simultaneously administered drug. These interactions can be profound and life threatening. Pharmacokinetic interactions can occur during each of the four drug movements, ADME. The most notable interactions that are likely to occur in the critically ill patient are those associated with drug transport or drug metabolizing proteins. Both classes of proteins bind with a variety of compounds, including endogenously produced substances and dietary supplements. Anything that induces the production of these proteins can increase drug clearance, increase the formation of a prodrug or the formation of a toxic metabolite. Clinically relevant drugs that act as inducers include barbiturates, anticonvulsants, and rifampin. Drugs that inhibit production of these proteins generally decrease clearance of a drug. Fungal imidazoles, chloramphenicol, and cimetidine are examples of drugs that have been demonstrated to inhibit at least one or more drugs metabolized by the canine or feline liver. Ketoconazole has been used therapeutically to prolong the half-life of cyclosporine through this mechanism. Because it also competes with cyclosporine for P-glycoprotein, absorption of cyclosporine can also be enhanced. Fluoroquinolones have a limited ability to inhibit some drugs, including methylxanthines such as theophylline.

Macrolide antibiotics also are inhibitors of some enzymes and will also inhibit P-glycoproteins. The oral bioavailability of an anticancer drug (doxetaxol), which is a substrate of P-glycoprotein, increased 17-fold in dogs treated with an inhibitor of P-glycoprotein. When this competitive approach is used for enhanced drug therapy, it is important to monitor drug levels since the impact can vary markedly with the individual patient.

Drugs that inhibit or increase gastric motility can affect drug absorption and PDC. Antisecretory drugs may alter absorption of drugs by virtue of changes in their ionization.

Pharmacodynamic interactions occur whenever the response to one drug is antagonized by another drug, generally due to competition at the receptor site. Such interactions may be synergistic or antagonistic. Some interactions are therapeutically beneficial (such as reversal of opioid sedation with either naloxone or butorphanol); other interactions may be detrimental. Pharmacodynamic interactions occur primarily at the tissue site of action.

Adjusting drug dosage or interval

The IV route should be used for administration of drugs to the critical patient when available due to potential problems with drug absorption from oral or peripheral routes. Drugs that are potentially toxic (particularly to the brain and heart) should not be rapidly administered intravenously, but instead, administered over 10–30 minutes. Because a lipid-soluble drug will distribute throughout all body tissues, doses of lipid-soluble drugs generally should be based on total body weight. Drugs with a high potential for toxicity should be dosed based on body mass. However, distribution of water-soluble drugs will be limited to extracellular fluid, and as such, doses (particularly for toxic drugs) should be based on lean body weight. Changes in either the Vd or clearance of a drug

should result in changes in the dosing regimen. Whether the dose or interval is changed depends on the drug, its Vd, and its half-life compared to the dosing interval.

Changes in Vd should result in changes in the dose and interval, particularly for drugs that accumulate with multiple dosing. It is important to remember that Vd does not indicate where a drug distributes, only that it has moved out of plasma. The larger the Vd of a given drug, the higher the dose necessary to achieve the same PDC and the longer the drug half-life. Thus a higher dose at a longer interval might be appropriate until the Vd is corrected. However, dosing on an accurate mg/kg body weight will generally accommodate changes in body compartment sizes.

A change in drug clearance results in a change in drug elimination half-life. As such, the dosing interval is most appropriately changed. However, for single dosing, no change is indicated if the Vd of the drug has not changed. For multiple dosed drugs, either the interval or the dose might change depending on whether or not the drug accumulates and how narrow the therapeutic window is for that drug.

Therapeutic failure is a concern when the efficacy of a drug is based on a continued drug presence (such as anticonvulsants) but the drug has a short half-life compared to the dosing interval. For drugs with short half-lives, lengthening the interval results in wider swings in PDCs during a single dosing interval. Thus, to avoid toxicity, decreasing the dose (rather than lengthening the interval) of drugs that depend on maintenance of a minimum drug concentration within a specified therapeutic range (such as antimicrobial, anticonvulsant or cardiac drugs) may be more appropriate. For drugs with a long elimination half-life or for drugs whose effects persist in the absence of detectable drug (such as selected antibiotics, glucocorticoids, nonsteroidal antiinflammatory drugs), it may be more appropriate to prolong the interval. However, the dose might also need to be changed.

Decreases in the renal clearance of a drug tend to parallel increases in serum creatinine; lengthening the dosing interval or decreasing the dose are optional dose adjustments. This is based on changes in patient serum creatinine or patient creatinine clearance (see Box 18.2). Alternatively, allometric scaling (based on body surface area) of doses is particularly useful for predicting species differences in renal excretion. Conversions between body weight and BSA are available in Table 18.2 (dogs) and Table 18.3 (cats). Note that dose modifications should be made only for that portion of the drug undergoing renal excretion. For example, digoxin is only 50% cleared by the kidneys; a twofold increase in creatinine should result in a prolongation of the dosing interval by 50%.

Therapeutic failure with antimicrobials may reflect inappropriate dosing regimens or may be the result of a nonresponsive infection. Among the approaches to enhancing antimicrobial efficacy is assuring that the dose achieves targeted pharmacokinetic and pharmacodynamic indices. As such, minimum inhibitory concentrations (MIC) of the target drug and microbe must be known. Dosing regimens for concentration-dependent drugs (aminoglycosides, fluoroquinolones) should be designed to achieve a C_{min} to MIC ratio of 10 or more. Dosing regimens for time-dependent drugs (bacteriostatic drugs, sulfonamides, including those with potentiators) and most cell wall inhibitors (beta-lactams, including carbapenems, glycopeptides, fosfomycin) should be designed to assure that drug concentrations remain above the MIC for a significant portion of the dosing interval.

Table 18.2 Body weight (BW) to body surface area (BSA) conversion for dogs. Body surface area in square meters can be converted from mass with the following formula: BSA (m^2) = 10 × (BW in $g^{2/3}$) × 10^{-4} [3].

BW (kg)	BSA (m^2)	BW(kg)	BSA (m^2)	BW (kg)	BSA (m^2)
0.5	0.064	17	0.668	38	1.142
1.0	0.101	18	0.694	39	1.162
1.5	0.132	19	0.719	40	1.181
2.0	0.160	20	0.744	41	1.201
2.5	0.186	21	0.769	42	1.220
3.0	0.210	22	0.793	43	1.259
3.5	0.233	23	0.817	44	1.278
4.0	0.255	24	0.840	45	1.297
4.5	0.275	25	0.864	46	1.395
5.0	0.295	26	0.886	47	1.315
6.0	0.333	27	0.909	48	1.334
7.0	0.370	28	0.931	49	1.352
8.0	0.404	29	0.953	50	1.371
9.0	0.437	30	0.975	51	1.389
10.0	0.469	31	0.997	52	1.407
11	0.500	32	1.018	53	1.425
12	0.529	33	1.039	54	1.443
13	0.558	34	1.060	55	1.461
14	0.587	35	1.081	60	1.589
15	0.614	36	1.101	65	1.677
16	0.641	37	1.121	70	1.762

Table 18.3 Body weight (BW) to body surface area (BSA) conversion for cats. Body surface area in square meters can be converted from mass with the following formula: BSA (m^2) = 10.1 × (BW in $g^{2/3}$) × 10^{-4} [3].

BW (kg)	BSA (m^2)	BW (kg)	BSA (m^2)	BW (kg)	BSA (m^2)
0.1	0.022	2.2	0.169	5.2	0.300
0.2	0.034	2.4	0.179	5.4	0.307
0.3	0.045	2.6	0.189	5.6	0.315
0.4	0.054	2.8	0.199	5.8	0.323
0.5	0.063	3.0	0.208	6.0	0.330
0.6	0.071	3.2	0.217	6.2	0.337
0.7	0.079	3.4	0.226	6.4	0.345
0.8	0.086	3.6	0.235	6.6	0.352
0.9	0.093	3.8	0.244	6.8	0.360
1.0	0.100	4.0	0.252	7.0	0.366
1.2	0.113	4.2	0.260	7.2	0.373
1.4	0.125	4.4	0.269	7.4	0.380
1.6	0.137	4.6	0.277	7.6	0.387
1.8	0.148	4.8	0.285	7.8	0.393
2.0	0.159	5.0	09.292	8.0	0.400

Adverse drug reactions

Adverse reactions by definition imply harm to the patient and should be differentiated from side-effects that may be undesirable but are not likely to require corrective therapeutic intervention. Recognizing whether or not an adverse reaction has occurred in a critical patient is difficult. Therapeutic failure due to an inappropriate dosing regimen may simply be interpreted as nonresponsive disease. Toxicity may be misinterpreted as clinical manifestations of new medical problems. The criteria for adequate and inappropriate response must be established. As such, intimate familiarity with the drug(s) being used and the patient being treated is critical to anticipate the potential of adverse reactions.

The critically ill patient is particularly predisposed to problems related to either too low or too high a PDC (called type A drug reactions). Disease can impact the disposition and response of one or more of the prescribed drugs. A list of common patient factors of critically ill dogs and cats is provided in Table 18.1. It is important to remember that type A reactions might reflect an exaggerated intended response (such as tachycardia in response to dopamine) or a secondary but undesirable effect (such as peripheral vasoconstriction due to dopamine-induced norepinephrine release). Type B drug reactions are idiosyncratic, making them more difficult to avoid since they do not reflect PDC and are not predictable. Regardless of the type of adverse reaction, clinical signs, laboratory tests or other indicators of adverse response must be identified, and appropriate instrumentation available to measure the response prior to drug administration.

Therapeutic intervention may be warranted to reduce the intensity of toxicity, reduce the quantity of the offending drug or to block the effect of the drug. For most drug-induced adverse events, symptomatic treatment is appropriate. The administration of a competitive inhibitor may be an option to reduce the effect of the drug. The role of IV lipids is being defined in veterinary medicine to bind lipophilic toxic drugs and prevent their distribution into tissues. Peritoneal dialysis, hemodialysis, and hemoperfusion provide other options for enhancing the excretion or removing the drugs that have become toxic (see Chapter 13). Changing the urinary pH so that a toxic metabolite of a drug becomes ionized can prevent reabsorption and facilitate excretion of toxic metabolites, particularly if coupled with diuresis. Urinary acidification (to trap a weak base) is relatively easy to accomplish short term but alkalinzing the urine to facilitate excretion of weak acids is more difficult.

If organ damage occurs due to the generation of toxic metabolites, the administration of drugs that scavenge oxygen radicals is indicated. For example, if drug-induced hepatotoxicity is suspected (or anticipated), hepatoprotectants such as S-adenyosyl methionine or silymarin should be initiated. Acute hepatopathy can be treated intravenously with N-acetylcysteine. Administration of sodium-containing fluids is indicated to minimize drug-induced nephrotoxicity.

For some drugs, specific recommendations for drug administration have been developed to minimize the risk of toxicity. For example, once-daily administration of appropriately high doses of aminoglycosides in a well-hydrated patient can minimize aminoglycoside toxicity. Administration of the aminoglycoside in the morning has been associated with decreased toxicity in humans, and a similar approach might be taken for dogs (or treatment at night for cats). Amphotericin B is an example of a drug for which "cocktails" have been designed for drug infusion to minimize adversity. In addition, multiple dosing regimens have been recommended to decrease nephrotoxicity and the administration of sodium-containing fluids prevents marked renal vasoconstriction. If nonsteroidal antiinflammatory drugs must be used in the critically ill patient, the concurrent use of antisecretory drugs should be considered. Omeprazole consistently performs better in both dogs and cats, although an H_2-receptor blocker such as famotidine might be used while the efficacy of omeprazole is being achieved. Because these drugs decrease gastric pH, they may alter the oral absorption of weakly acidic drugs. Sucralfate is also indicated to protect the gastric mucosa but the drug can negatively affect the oral absorption of other drugs.

Constant rate infusions

The CRI drug must be added to a delivery solution in an appropriate concentration to deliver the correct dose over the desired period of time (usually µg/kg/min). Formulas for calculating CRI delivery solutions are provided in Box 18.3 and Box 20.4. Various websites provide CRI calculators for rapid and easy use.

A CRI can enhance drug safety and efficacy by minimizing an undesirable fluctuation between C_{min} and C_{max}. At steady state, by definition, the amount of drug going into the patient should equal the amount of drug irreversibly leaving the patient. Although therapeutic concentrations may occur before steady state is reached, the maximum effect will not occur until that point. Therefore, at steady state, the CRI drug at maximum concentration is equal to the drug at minimum concentration as long as the drug is being administered at the same rate during the infusion and 3–5 elimination half-lives have passed.

The rate of infusion necessary to achieve a targeted steady-state plasma drug concentration depends solely on the clearance of the drug. As with any dosing regimen, the time to reach steady-state concentration by CRI infusion is dependent on the drug being present for 3–5 half-lives.

Many critical patients may be at risk while waiting for maximum therapeutic response to a medication. A loading dose can be given in this situation, regardless of the route of administration. Note, however, that the loading dose is designed to immediately achieve steady-state drug concentrations and is calculated based on the targeted concentration and Vd. However, the patient is *not* at steady state and will not be until the same dose is administered for 3–5 half-lives. Thus, a loading dose is always accompanied by a maintenance dose to maintain drug levels while steady state is being reached. The difference between the loading and maintenance doses depends upon the drug half-life: the longer the half-life, the longer to steady state and the greater the drug accumulation.

Other considerations regarding CRI include the following.

- Distribution, not clearance, affects the concentration achieved with a loading dose. Thus, modification of a loading dose should be based on patient Vd and the concentration at steady state. Examples include obesity (reduce dose of water-soluble drug), overhydration (increase dose of water-soluble drug), dehydration (rehydrate, but if necessary approach as with altered circulation), altered circulation (decrease dose of drugs whose side-effects are manifested in the heart and brain). In general, the loading dose of highly protein-bound drugs does not need to be altered unless drug clearance is impacted by patient health.
- Administration of a drug by CRI *does not* allow rapid manipulation of PDC.
- Distribution and clearance impact the maintenance dose.
- Any time the dose is changed, 3–5 half-lives are required to reach a new steady state. Thus, the duration to response may be rapid (catecholamine vasopressors, half-lives two minutes, time to steady state (or drug elimination) six minutes) or longer (fentanyl, half-life 2–6 hours, time to maximum effect including drug elimination is 6–30 hours).
- If the drug is characterized by active or toxic metabolites, the half-life of the metabolites is often longer than the parent compound. Thus, the time to steady state, and the maximum effect achieved at steady state, must also take into account active (toxic) metabolites.

Box 18.3 Formulas for calculating constant rate infusion drug administration.

Desired mL to be delivered over 1 hour × #drops/mL (drip set dependent) divided by 3600 (60 minutes × 60 seconds)

$$M = \frac{(D)(W)(V)}{(R)(16.67)}$$

or

$$R = \frac{(D)(W)(V)}{(M)(16.67)}$$

Where:

M = number of mg of drug to add to base solution
D = dosage of drug in µg/kg/min
W = body weight in kg
V = volume in mL of base solution
R = rate of delivery in mL/h
16.67 = conversion factor

Fast formula:

Drug dosage (µg/kg/min) × BW (kg) = # mg to add to 250 mL of base solution at a rate of 15 mL/h

To calculate the desired volume to be delivered over a set time period: Volume (to be infused) × drip set rate
Divide by length of time in minutes
Equals drops per minute

Microdrip sets*: 60 drops per mL

Standard drip sets (macrodrip*): 15 drops per mL

Flashball drip sets*: 10 drops per mL

*Drops/mL will vary depending on manufacturer and are noted on individual packaging.

Adapted from: Macintire DK, Tefend M. Constant-rate infusions: practical use. Clinician's Brief 2004; 25-8. Available at: www.cliniciansbrief.com/sites/default/files/sites/cliniciansbrief.com/files/0404_procedurepro.pdf (accessed 3 June 2016).

Limitations of drug selection

The critical care patient is particularly predisposed to drug-related complications, not only because of the impact of their disease but because of the practice of polypharmacy necessary to support these patients. Dosing regimens for drugs used in critically ill small animals warrant special consideration. The package inserts accompanying drugs approved in the target species provide valuable information. The evidence of efficacy and particularly safety should be reviewed. However, the data is determined generally in healthy individuals, making the relevance to the critically ill patient potentially limited. Many drugs used in the veterinary ICU are human-approved drugs, often with even less information available to support their use in animals. When pharmacokinetic information is available, it is almost without exception based on studies in healthy animals or animal models of disease, again limiting relevance to critical care patients.

Therapeutic concentrations upon which dosing regimens are recommended may not be the same among the various species. For example, the gastrointestinal tract of animals is markedly different from that of humans, causing concern when prescribing orally administered human drugs. The bioequivalence characterizing generic drugs in humans may not translate to animals. Special consideration must also be given to drug–drug (or drug–diet) interactions, which can be lethal in any patient. Few drug or diet interactions have been reported in animals and most are extrapolated from data in humans. Yet, increasingly, differences in drug metabolizing enzymes or drug transport proteins are being demonstrated among the species, limiting such extrapolations.

Choosing the most effective drug for treatment of critically ill animals is limited by the lack of high-level evidence based information. Few clinical trials have been appropriately designed to detect a significant difference and investigators often conclude a lack of treatment effect with underpowered studies, thereby removing that potential treatment as an option. However, knowledge of the absorption, distribution, metabolism and elimination (or drug disposition) of each drug being prescribed can provide insight into the potential for therapeutic success and possibility of adverse effects or toxicity.

References

1. Geyer J, Janko C. Treatment of *MDR1* mutant dogs with macrocyclic lactones. Curr Pharm Biotechnol. 2012;13(6):969–86.
2. Grissinger M. The five rights: A destination without a map. Institute for Safe Medication Practices Medication Safety Alert. Pharm Therapeut. 2010;35(10):542.
3. Crump KT. Cancer and chemotherapy. Available at: www.vspn.org/Library/Misc/VSPN_M02045.htm (accessed 3 June 2016).

Further reading

Boothe DM, ed. Small Animal Clinical Pharmacology and Therapeutics, 2nd edn. St Louis: Elsevier Saunders, 2012.

Brundage RC, Mann HJ. General principles of pharmacokinetics and pharmacodynamics. In: Textbook of Critical Care, 6th edn. Vincent JL, Abraham E, Moore FA, et al., eds. Philadelphia: Elsevier Sanders, 2011: pp 1253–64.

Riviere JV, Papich MG, eds. Veterinary Pharmacology and Therapeutics, 9th edn. Ames: Wiley-Blackwell, 2009.

CHAPTER 19

Pain management

Armi Pigott

Lakeshore Veterinary Specialists, Milwaukee, Wisconsin

Introduction

Pain has been defined as an unpleasant sensory and emotional experience associated with actual or potential tissue damage [1]. This unpleasant feeling is conveyed to the brain by sensory neurons, giving information on the location, intensity, and, potentially, the nature of the pain. A variety of systemic alterations occur as a consequence of pain and, when left unchecked, can increase morbidity and mortality in the small animal ICU patient [1–4]. Neurohormonal changes occur in response to pain, with increased sympathetic tone, increased myocardial work and oxygen consumption, increased skeletal muscle flow, and decreased blood flow to the gastrointestinal (GI) and urinary tracts. Circulating adrenocorticotropic hormone (ACTH), cortisol, and norepinephrine are increased while circulating insulin is decreased. These changes contribute to a catabolic state that may decrease or prolong healing. Many painful patients are reluctant or unable to eat or move, contributing further to patient morbidity.

There are five neurophysiological phases involved in the sensation of pain: transduction, transmission, modulation, projection, and perception (Figure 19.1). An understanding of these steps is important since certain analgesic and anesthetic drugs can be administered to target a specific step (Box 19.1).

The *transduction* (phase 1) of a chemical, mechanical or thermal noxious stimulus is mediated by the pain receptors at the peripheral ends of the pain fibers, called nociceptors. These receptors are located in skin, mucosa, deep fascia, and connective tissue of visceral organs, ligaments, muscles, tendons, joint capsules, periosteum, and arterial vessel walls [3,5,6]. Their function is to detect and transmit the location, quality, and duration of a stimulus [3,5–7]. There are many types of nociceptors, each detecting a specific stimulus (such as heat, stretch, vibration, pressure). In the viscera, nociceptors are more sensitive to distension, twisting, and ischemic injury as noxious stimuli. The minimal stimulus required for a nociceptor to generate an electrical signal (an action potential) is called the nociceptor threshold [8]. A variety of chemical substances are responsible for the transduction of a pain signal and can include globulin and protein kinases, arachidonic acid, histamine, nerve growth factor, substance P, calcitonin gene-related peptide, potassium, serotonin, lactic acid, vasopressin, glucocorticoids, oxytocin, catecholamines, angiotensin, and endorphins/enkephalins [9,10]. The degree and duration of the stimulus determine the number of action potentials per unit of time and the duration of production of these action potentials.

Once the stimulus has been converted to an action potential, *transmission* of the signal occurs (phase 2); the electrical signal is conducted up the afferent sensory nerve fibers to the spinal cord, and depolarizes the presynaptic terminal. The presynaptic terminal interfaces with a network of interneurons and second-order neurons in the dorsal horn of the spinal cord. Interneurons can either facilitate or inhibit transmission to second-order neurons.

There are two main types of nociceptor fibers which transmit action potentials to the spinal cord. A-delta fibers (Aδ) are moderate-speed (20 m/sec), thinly myelinated fibers which are associated with initial, sharp or pricking, well-localized pain. C fibers are slower (2 m/sec), thin, unmyelinated fibers which are associated with a dull, aching, throbbing, diffuse pain. A third type of fiber, A-beta (Aß), is a fast, large-diameter, myelinated fiber that carries action potentials from mechanoreceptors. Aß fibers are believed to modulate C and Aδ activity within the dorsal horn. There is a good deal of sensory overlap between these receptors, allowing a continuum of sensation [8].

The presynaptic terminals of Aδ and C fibres release a variety of pronociceptive substances into the synaptic cleft. C fiber presynaptic terminals are known to release glutamate which activates postsynaptic alpha-amino-3-hydroxy-5-methyl-4-isoxazole propionic acid (AMPA) receptors; substance P (SP), which activates postsynaptic NK1 receptors; and calcitonin gene-related peptide (CGRP), which activates postsynaptic CGRP receptors.

In the spinal cord, the signal is either amplified or suppressed (*modulation*, phase 3) by excitatory or inhibitory interneurons that are continually bombarded with nociceptive input. Neurotransmitters of importance at this level include peptides (substance P, CGRP), amino acids (glutamate and aspartate), gamma-aminobutyric acid (GABA), nitric oxide, prostaglandins (e.g. PGE2), adenosine triphosphate (ATP), endogenous opioids, monoamines (serotonin, norepinephrine), protons, neurokinin A, and others (see Figure 19.1) [9]. Modulation is an important component of maladaptive pain (described below).

Projection (phase 4) of the signals continues their travel toward the brain through the spinal tracts. There is some controversy over which tracts are involved, but the spinothalamic, spinoreticular, spinomesencephalic, and spinohypothalamic tracts appear to be prominently involved [8,11].

Perception (phase 5) is the integration and processing of nociceptive information by the brain to recognize a stimulus as painful, and then to produce a response. The areas of the brain involved in perception are the periaqueductal gray area, reticular activating system, and thalamus. Behavioral changes may result and signals can be initiated that travel down the descending spinal tracts. These descending signals may be sent to a motor unit to evoke movement. Alternatively, the signals may synapse on inhibitory neurons in the

Monitoring and Intervention for the Critically Ill Small Animal: The Rule of 20, First Edition. Edited by Rebecca Kirby and Andrew Linklater.
© 2017 John Wiley & Sons, Inc. Published 2017 by John Wiley & Sons, Inc.

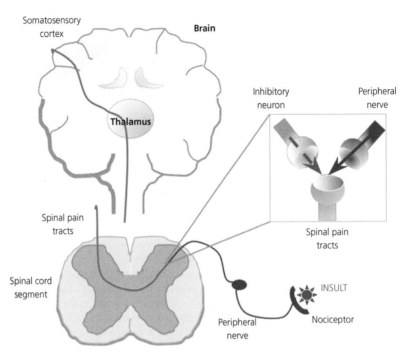

Figure 19.1 Schematic of neurological pathways for pain perception. Inflammatory mediators (such as histamine, tumor necrosis factor, interleukins, hydrogen ions) bind to one or more of the specific receptors on the nociceptor. The pain perception impulse is transmitted to the spinal cord segment through the primary afferent nerve fibers of the peripheral nerve (*burgundy line*) and synapses with spinal cord neurons in the dorsal horn of the spinal cord. Projection neurons (*blue lines*) from the dorsal horn transmit information to the somatosensory cortex through connections in the thalamus. This relays information regarding the intensity and location of the pain. Other areas of the brain are stimulated and provide descending information that regulates output from the spinal cord and the reaction to pain. In the dorsal horn of the spinal cord (*box*), the nociceptor afferent (*burgundy solid line*) releases a variety of neurotransmitters (such as ATP, glutamate, CGRP, substance P) that interact with specific receptors on the spinal pain tract neurons. This facilitates the transmission of pain messages to the brain. The tonically active inhibitory neuron (*brown dashed arrow*) receives impulses from the brain that act to inhibit the stimulation of the spinal tract pain nerves to slow or terminate the pain cycle through the release of inhibitory neurotransmitters (such as glycine, GABA). The activity of this inhibitory neuron is lessened or lost (disinhibition) during central sensitization.

dorsal horn of the spinal cord, decreasing or abolishing the noxious signals ascending to the brain. Loss or removal of this descending inhibitory signal is called disinhibition and can increase pain through decreased endogenous opioid release.

The older pain classification of acute and chronic pain has been replaced by the classification of pain as either adaptive or maladaptive [4]. *Adaptive pain* (acute) is the normal pain response to tissue injury. It can be classified as inflammatory or nociceptive, with either being a normal response to tissue damage. Nociceptive pain is a transient response to a noxious stimulus [12]. These are typically small aches and pains that are relatively innocuous and that protect the body from the environment [4]. Inflammatory pain is spontaneous pain and can include hypersensitivity to pain [12]. It occurs in response to tissue damage and the resultant inflammation caused by tissue trauma, injury, and surgery. Inflammatory pain causes suffering, and it responds to treatment [12].

Maladaptive pain is more chronic in nature and occurs when adaptive pain is untreated or poorly managed. This type of pain is classified as neuropathic, functional, or central pain. Neuropathic pain is spontaneous pain or hypersensitivity to pain resulting from damage to or a lesion of the nervous system [12]. Functional pain is a hypersensitivity to pain resulting from abnormal processing of normal input [4,12]. Central pain is pain initiated or caused by a primary lesion or dysfunction in the central nervous system (CNS) [4,12]. The thalamus typically serves as a relay station for nerve impulses from the periphery to the cortex of the brain. If adaptive pain goes untreated, the thalamus can spontaneously generate a pain signal.

Tissue damage leads to persistent and noxious stimulation of pain receptors. Damaged cells release inflammatory mediators (leukotrienes, prostaglandins, cytokines, protons) that attract inflammatory cells and the release of more chemical mediators. These mediators cause an increased sensitivity of the peripheral nociceptors by lowering their threshold for stimulation. Centrally, neurons in the dorsal horn become hyperexcitable and more sensitive to low-intensity stimuli. This phenomenon leads to pain hypersensitivity. The result is one or more of the following: a typically nonpainful stimulus is now being perceived as painful (called allodynia); a perceived increase in pain intensity from the same stimulus is now occurring over time (called wind-up pain); or there is an exaggerated response to a painful stimulus (called hyperalgesia).

Preparing an effective pain management plan is a crucial component of the treatment of the small animal ICU patient. The choice of drug(s), route of administration, and anticipated response to therapy are based on the underlying disease process that is responsible for causing the pain and the anticipation of pain hypersensitivity. The experience of pain is unique among individuals, and analgesia that is adequate for one individual might not be adequate for another. The information from the patient history, physical, orthopedic and neurological examinations, and laboratory and imaging results will be important. The best analgesic should be chosen and administered by the most effective route. Close patient monitoring is required to determine the success of analgesic therapy and for early detection of any deleterious side-effects of the drugs.

Box 19.1 Drugs that inhibit specific phases of pain.

Phase 1 – Transduction

Nonsteroidal antiinflammatory drugs
Opioids
Local anesthetics
Corticosteroids

Phase 2 - Transmission

Local anesthetics
Alpha-2-agonists

Phase 3 - Modulation

Local anesthetics
Opioids
Alpha-2-agonists
Nonsteroidal antiinflammatory drugs
N-methyl-D-aspartate (NMDA) receptor antagonists
Tricyclic antidepressants
Anticonvulsants

Phase 4 – Projection

Epidural-administered medications

Phase 5 - Perception

Inhalant anesthetic agents
Opioids
Alpha-2-agonists
Benzodiazepines
Phenothiazines
Acetaminophen

Diagnostic procedures

Pain scales have been developed that illustrate and describe the psychological and behavioral activity and response to palpation, demonstrated at varying levels of pain intensity in the cat (Figure 19.2) and dog (Figure 19.3). The World Small Animal Veterinary Medical Association Global Pain Council has developed a set of guidelines to aid the veterinary team in the recognition, assessment, and treatment of pain in the dog and cat [13]. However, there is no specific behavior that is pathognomonic for pain, and behaviors at home may differ significantly from behavior in other environments. Severely injured or ill animals may not be able to express the typical behavioral pain responses due to their underlying condition. Therefore, the diagnostic information gathered must be used to identify any underlying problems that are likely to be causing pain and to recognize any signs attributable to pain exhibited by the patient.

History

The history begins with the signalment (age, sex, breed). Age-related problems such as arthritis or severe periodontal disease are a potential cause of pain in older dogs and cats. There might be a breed disposition to potentially painful problems such as disk disease (Dachshund, Poodle, Basset Hound), orthopedic abnormalities (Rottweiler, Labrador Retriever, German Shepherd) or gastric distension (large breed dogs). Past medical problems can reveal conditions that might be associated with intermittent or low-grade continuous pain, such as neuromuscular disease, orthopedic problems, severe skin disease, chronic wounds, chronic recurrent GI

disease, or prostatitis. A list of prescribed and over-the-counter medications might reveal glucocorticosteroid or nonsteroidal antiinflammatory drugs (NSAIDs) that might be causing GI ulceration and pain.

The presenting complaint may warrant immediate concern for the animal experiencing pain (such as trauma, lameness, swelling). However, it is frequently the description of the change in behavior of the animal that provides an alert to the presence of pain. Both dogs and cats may demonstrate hiding, lack of interactions or curiosity, anxiety, submission or guarding as a response to pain. Loss of appetite may be reported or the owner may complain about the pet showing aggression, attempts to escape confinement or restraint, or unusual grooming behavior (including self-mutilation). Some animals become submissive or mentally depressed. Cats will often be lethargic and inappetent when painful.

Loss of house training is not uncommon, with cats failing to use the litter box and dogs urinating or defecating in the house or cage. In extreme situations, patients will urinate or defecate where they are lying. Vocalizing is a nonspecific behavior, with pain as the first consideration, but other causes should be investigated (such as a full urinary bladder, the need to defecate, dysphoria from medications).

Changes in body posture can include flatted ears, tail flicks, a stiff posture or gait, or guarding behavior in the cat. Dogs may lower their head and eyes, move their ears back or turn away. Altered facial expressions may also be associated with pain. In an animal that is reluctant to move due to pain, slight movement is often accompanied by other behavioral cues such as an abnormal gait, aggression, or vocalizing.

Moderate to severe abdominal or thoracic pain is often demonstrated by a reluctance to lie down. They may stand in awkward positions (such as prayer position) for prolonged periods or may constantly reposition (stand-sit-lie down-turn circles). Some animals will fall asleep in the stilted or sitting position, then begin to slump with the movement causing pain and abruptly waking to resume the original position.

Physical examination

The physical examination begins during the recording of the history, when a distant exam is performed: the posture, behavior, and gait of the patient are observed for signs of painful behavior. The physical perfusion parameters (temperature, pulse rate and intensity, heart rate and rhythm, capillary refill time (CRT), and respiratory rate and effort) are then assessed. Tachycardia, tachypnea, hyperemic mucous membranes, rapid CRT, and bounding pulses could be due to either the compensatory stage of shock or to pain, each capable of eliciting a systemic sympathetic response. Physical evidence of poor peripheral perfusion seen in the later stages of shock (prolonged CRT, tachycardia (dogs), weak peripheral pulses, and pale mucous membranes) can mask the sympathetic response from pain. Therefore, analgesics become a vital component early in the shock resuscitation plan to reduce the contributions of pain to the sympathetic response (see Chapter 2).

A careful head-to-tail examination is done, leaving manipulation of any potentially painful body regions to the latter portion of the exam. Adequate restraint is required and a muzzle or e-collar is placed (when necessary) prior to manipulation of painful areas. The head is examined for symmetry and the cranial nerves are evaluated. Ptyalism can be a sign of pain in the cat and dog, especially with severe dental or other GI disease. Mydriasis may also be a sign of the sympathetic pain response.

Your clinic name here

Date ——————————

Time ——————————

Feline Acute Pain Scale

| Rescore when awake | ☐ **Animal is sleeping, but can be aroused - Not evaluated for pain**
 ☐ **Animal can't be aroused, check vital signs, assess therapy** |

Pain Score	Example	Psychological & Behavioral	Response to Palpation	Body Tension
0	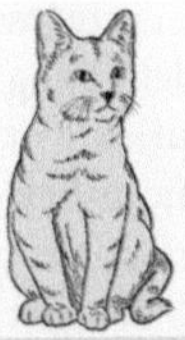	☐ **Content and quiet** when unattended ☐ **Comfortable** when resting ☐ Interested in or **curious** about surroundings	☐ **Not bothered** by palpation of wound or surgery site, or to palpation elsewhere	Minimal
1	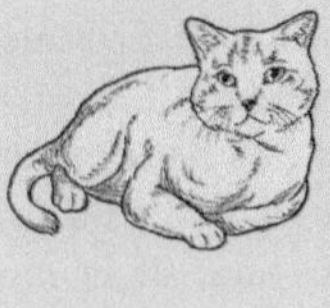	☐ **Signs are often subtle and not easily detected in the hospital setting**; more likely to be detected by the owner(s) at home ☐ Earliest signs at home may be **withdrawal from surroundings or change in normal routine** ☐ In the hospital, may be content or slightly unsettled ☐ **Less interested** in surroundings but will look around to see what is going on	☐ May or may not react to palpation of wound or surgery site	Mild
2	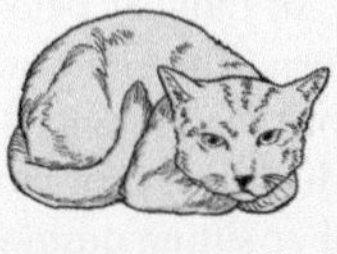	☐ Decreased responsiveness, **seeks solitude** ☐ **Quiet,** loss of brightness in eyes ☐ **Lays curled up or sits tucked up** (all four feet under body, shoulders hunched, head held slightly lower than shoulders, tail curled tightly around body) with eyes partially or mostly closed ☐ **Hair coat appears rough** or fluffed up ☐ May intensively groom an area that is painful or irritating ☐ Decreased appetite, **not interested in food**	☐ **Responds aggressively or tries to escape** if painful area is palpated or approached ☐ Tolerates attention, may even perk up when petted as long as painful area is avoided	Mild to Moderate **Reassess analgesic plan**
3	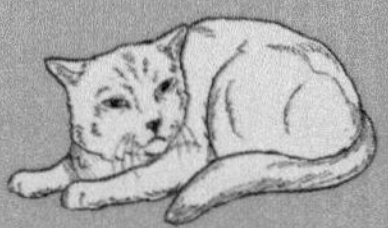	☐ Constantly **yowling, growling, or hissing** when unattended ☐ May bite or chew at wound, but **unlikely to move** if left alone	☐ **Growls or hisses at non-painful palpation** (may be experiencing allodynia, wind-up, or fearful that pain could be made worse) ☐ **Reacts aggressively** to palpation, **adamantly pulls away** to avoid any contact	Moderate **Reassess analgesic plan**
4	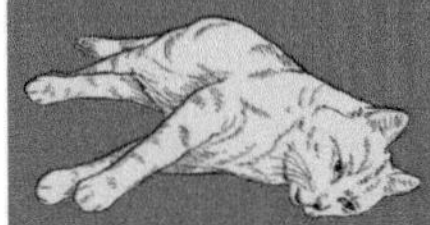	☐ Prostrate ☐ Potentially **unresponsive** to or unaware of surroundings, difficult to distract from pain ☐ Receptive to care (even aggressive or feral cats will be more tolerant of contact)	☐ **May not respond** to palpation ☐ **May be rigid** to avoid painful movement	Moderate to Severe **May be rigid to avoid painful movement** **Reassess analgesic plan**

○ Tender to palpation
✗ Warm
■ Tense

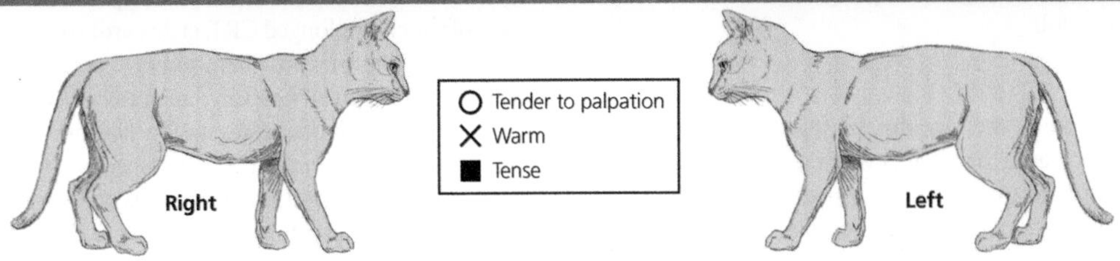

Right   **Left**

Comments _____

Colorado State University
VETERINARY TEACHING HOSPITAL

Figure 19.2 Colorado State University Feline Acute Pain Scale. Used with permission from Dr PW Hellyer, Colorado State University.

**Your clinic
name here**

Date _____

Time _____

Canine Acute Pain Scale

| Rescore when awake | ☐ **Animal is sleeping, but can be aroused - Not evaluated for pain** |
| | ☐ **Animal can't be aroused, check vital signs, assess therapy** |

Pain Score	Example	Psychological & Behavioral	Response to Palpation	Body Tension
0	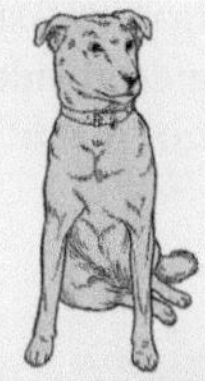	☐ **Comfortable** when resting ☐ **Happy, content** ☐ Not bothering wound or surgery site ☐ Interested in or curious about surroundings	☐ **Nontender** to palpation of wound or surgery site, or to palpation elsewhere	Minimal
1	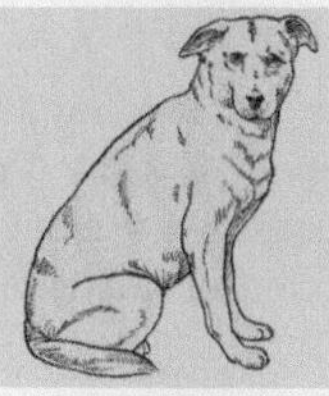	☐ **Content to slightly unsettled** or restless ☐ **Distracted easily** by surroundings	☐ **Reacts to palpation** of wound, surgery site, or other body part by **looking around, flinching, or whimpering**	Mild
2	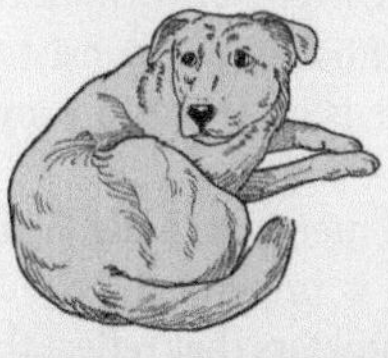	☐ Looks **uncomfortable** when resting ☐ May **whimper** or cry and may **lick or rub wound** or surgery site when unattended ☐ Droopy ears, **worried facial expression** (arched eye brows, darting eyes) ☐ **Reluctant to respond** when beckoned ☐ **Not eager to interact** with people or surroundings but will look around to see what is going on	☐ Flinches, whimpers cries, or guards/pulls away	Mild to Moderate **Reassess analgesic plan**
3	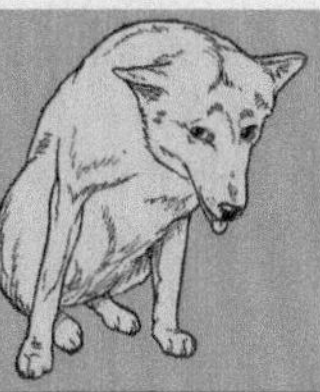	☐ **Unsettled, crying, groaning, biting or chewing** wound when unattended ☐ **Guards or protects** wound or surgery site by altering weight distribution (i.e., limping, shifting body position) ☐ **May be unwilling to move** all or part of body	☐ May be **subtle** (shifting eyes or increased respiratory rate) if dog is too painful to move or is stoic ☐ May be **dramatic**, such as a sharp cry, growl, bite or bite threat, and/or pulling away	Moderate **Reassess analgesic plan**
4	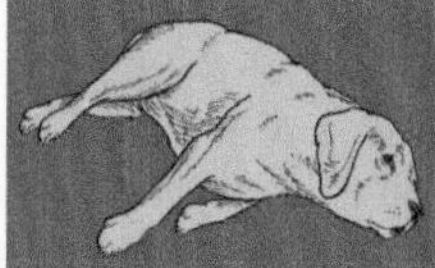	☐ **Constantly groaning or screaming** when unattended ☐ May bite or chew at wound, but unlikely to move ☐ **Potentially unresponsive** to surroundings ☐ **Difficult to distract** from pain	☐ **Cries at non-painful palpation** (may be experiencing allodynia, wind-up, or fearful that pain could be made worse) ☐ May react aggressively to palpation	Moderate to Severe **May be rigid to avoid painful movement** **Reassess analgesic plan**

○ Tender to palpation
✗ Warm
■ Tense

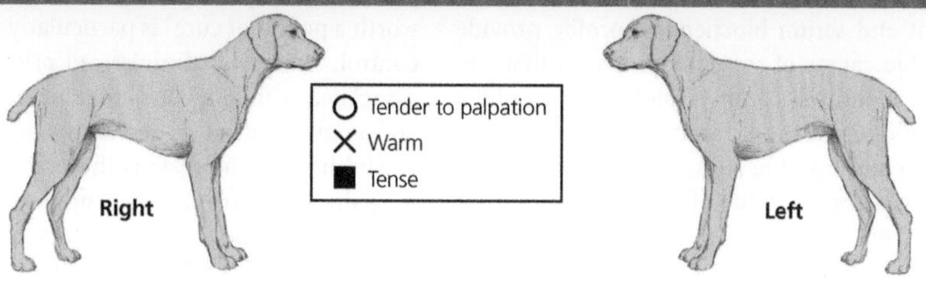

Right   **Left**

Comments _____

Figure 19.3 Colorado State University Canine Acute Pain Score. Used with permission from Dr PW Hellyer, Colorado State University.

The hands are passed along all aspects of the body, feeling for any lumps, swelling, heat, sores or wounds that could be painful. Mild pressure is applied along the vertebral column, ribcage and down the limbs to assess for discomfort or other abnormalities. Abdominal palpation may induce splinting of the abdominal muscles, suggestive of generalized abdominal pain. Analgesics may be required to allow deep palpation of abdominal structures. Urinary bladder obstruction, peritonitis, pancreatitis, acute renal toxicity, abdominal hemorrhage, bowel ischemia, gastric or splenic torsion, gastric dilation, gallbladder inflammation or outflow obstruction, abdominal trauma, and mesenteric volvulus are causes of acute abdominal pain that warrant strong analgesic support for the patient.

Neurological and orthopedic examination follows with careful manipulation of the head and neck, limbs, and joints. When testing the limb reflexes, it is important to differentiate reflex withdrawal (a reflex response) from withdrawal induced by pain (evidence of conscious recognition of pain). For example, in a nonambulatory dog with an L2–3 spinal lesion, the dog simply pulling his foot away when pinched does not indicate conscious awareness of a painful stimulus. He must also turn and look, cry out, growl, or in some way show he is aware of the painful stimulus. In equivocal cases, gently pinching an unaffected area (in the above example a digit on the thoracic limb would work well) and then comparing that response to a stimulus in the affected area can help to identify a stoic dog versus one that cannot sense the stimulus.

Careful patient evaluation can fail to demonstrate a pain response in very stoic animals. When the patient has a condition expected to cause pain (such as trauma or surgery), treatment for the expected level of pain is very appropriate.

Point of care (POC) testing

A minimum database is provided through POC in-hospital testing and should include the packed cell volume (PCV), total protein (TP), blood glucose, blood urea nitrogen (BUN), electrolyte panel, blood lactate, blood gas, coagulation profile, and urinalysis. Severe anemia, hypoglycemia, marked hyperglycemia, hypokalemia, significant azotemia, and severe acidosis can all cause weakness and mental depression, each capable of masking the physical signs of pain in the patient. Electrolyte disorders affecting sodium (Na), potassium (K), magnesium (Mg) or calcium (Ca) could impact nerve conduction and the neuromuscular response to pain. A high blood lactate suggests anaerobic metabolism, poor tissue oxygenation, and impaired perfusion. Analgesics are given and the blood lactate is monitored during fluid resuscitation for a declining trend as evidence of return of blood flow. Assessment of renal and GI function is necessary prior to administration of NSAIDs (see below).

Clinicopathological testing

A complete blood count and serum biochemical profile provide data pertaining to possible causes of systemic problems that can cause pain. A high white blood cell count, a marked neutrophilic left shift, or a low white blood cell count can indicate severe tissue inflammation. The biochemical profile is assessed to evaluate for underlying disease and to assess the ability of the liver and kidneys to metabolize and excrete the prescribed analgesic drugs. Unfortunately, at this time no systematic relationship has been demonstrated between changes in plasma enzyme activities and established assessments of pain.

The quantitation of catecholamines, cortisol, and ACTH has been used as a biochemical marker of pain in experimental animal models. However, the systolic, diastolic, and mean arterial blood pressure and heart rate have been suggested to be more sensitive than plasma ACTH or cortisol concentrations as indices of low-grade pain [14].

Imaging

Imaging provides a method for identifying a cause of recognized pain. Survey thoracic and abdominal radiographs provide the initial diagnostic imaging data once the patient has been stabilized and has received appropriate analgesics. The skeletal structures are closely examined for evidence of fracture, luxation, dislocation, inflammation, lysis or proliferative lesions that might be causing pain. Thoracic radiographs can demonstrate evidence of a mass lesion(s), pleural fluid or air, and rib or vertebral changes that might be associated with an observed pain response. Abdominal radiographs could show evidence of peritoneal fluid or air and provide an initial assessment of abdominal organ size, shape, and position.

Abdominal and thoracic ultrasound provides a more in-depth assessment of organ structure and can identify fluid pockets not seen on plain radiographs.

Monitoring procedures

The physical examination is the primary monitoring tool for assessing the presence and degree of pain. Pain scales (see Figures 19.2 and 19.3) are used to quantify the intensity of the pain and to follow the progress of pain control and patient comfort over time. These assessments rely on some objective observations but are still subject to interpretation, even between individuals. Use of the pain-scoring system in a uniform and consistent manner by each patient care team member is essential to providing optimal pain control.

Continued observation of the mental attitude, behavior, posture, and vocalization of the patient is imperative. The heart rate and blood pressure are physical parameters that reflect the demands on the sympathetic nervous system. Tachycardia and hypertension developing in an otherwise stable patient can be an early sign that the pain control is insufficient. At this time, the pain scale score is reassessed along with the analgesic drug selection, dose, and frequency of administration.

Pain management

The two key components to pain control in the acute setting are preemptive analgesia and multimodal therapy. Addressing these two components can reduce or prevent the conversion from adaptive pain to maladaptive pain. The old adage "an ounce of prevention is worth a pound of cure" is particularly applicable to preemptive pain control. Analgesia administered prior to inducing tissue trauma is associated with less wind-up, a reduced overall need for analgesia, and a reduced need for rescue analgesia [4,15–18].

Multimodal analgesia is the practice of using multiple drugs in the pain control plan. Each drug should have a different mechanism of action and be complementary or synergistic. This technique allows use of lower doses of individual drugs to achieve pain control, reducing the incidence and severity of side-effects of any one drug. Multiple drugs and routes of administration are available for use in critically ill patients. Common analgesic drugs used in the dog and cat are listed in Table 19.1 with dose, mechanism of action, and potential side-effects. Analgesic drugs frequently combined for

Table 19.1 Selected analgesic drugs and doses for dogs and cats.

Drug (duration)	Route	Dose for dog	Dose for cat	Notes
Pure mu-agonist opioids				
Fentanyl	IV CRI	2–5 µg/kg/h	2-5 µg/kg/h	May cause urine retention; can be increased or decreased based on needs. Increase dose during painful procedures
Fentanyl (15–20 min)	IV	2–5 µg/kg	1–3 µg/kg	
Fentanyl transdermal solution (Recuvyra) (3–4 d)	Proprietary intradermal injector	2.7 mg/kg	N/A	Special handling of drug and patient is required; refer to package insert
Hydromorphone	IV CRI	0.015–0.03 mg/kg/h	0.015–0.03 mg/kg/h	
Hydromorphone (2–6 h)	SC, IM, IV	0.05–0.2 mg/kg	0.05–0.1 mg/kg	
Methadone (2–6 h)	SC, IM, IV	0.2–1 mg/kg	0.1–0.5 mg/kg	Also NMDA receptor antagonist
Morphine	IV CRI	0.1–0.3 mg/kg/h	0.1–0.2 mg/kg/h	
Morphine (2–4 h)	SC, IM, slow IV	0.5–1 mg/kg	0.2–0.5 mg/kg	May cause histamine release if given fast IV
Oxymorphone (2–4 h)	SC, IM, IV	0.05–0.4 mg/kg	0.02–0.1 mg/kg	

Common side-effects of pure mu-agonist opioids include panting, nausea, sedation, mydriasis, hypothermia, hyperthermia, hyperexcitability, whining, defecation, constipation, bradycardia, respiratory depression; urinary retention has been reported with fentanyl.

Drug (duration)	Route	Dose for dog	Dose for cat	Notes
Partial mu-agonist opioids				
Buprenorphine (6–12 h)	SC, IM, IV	5–20 µg/kg	5–20 µg/kg	Sedative effects apparent in about 15 minutes but requires 30–45 minutes for analgesia to occur
Buprenorphine (Simbadol) (24 h)	SC	N/A	0.24 mg/kg	
Buprenorphine (6–8 h)	OTM	N/A	10–20 µg/kg	OTM bioavailability in dogs is only about 5% and *not* recommended

Partial mu-agonists will antagonize the pure mu-agonists. IM may be more painful than other agents. Common side-effects include respiratory depression (rare and typically at high doses). Dogs may show hypersalivation, bradycardia, hypothermia, agitation, dehydration, and miosis. Tachycardia, vomiting, and hypertension have rarely been reported. In cats mydriasis and behavioral effects (e.g. excessive purring, pacing, rolling, etc.) have been reported. Vomiting and hypothermia are rare.

Drug (duration)	Route	Dose for dog	Dose for cat	Notes
Agonist-antagonist opioids				
Butorphanol (1–4 h)	SC, IM, IV	0.1–0.4 mg/kg	0.1–0.4 mg/kg	
Butorphanol	IV CRI	0.03–0.4 mg/kg/h	0.03–0.4 mg/kg/h	Loading dose 0.1 mg/kg IV

Much better sedative than analgesic. Dogs with MDR1 mutation may have more pronounced sedation, and sedation may persist longer in these dogs. Use with caution in animals with head trauma, increased cerebrospinal fluid pressure. Adverse effects reported include sedation, excitement, respiratory depression, ataxia, anorexia, diarrhea (rare).

Drug (duration)	Route	Dose for dog	Dose for cat	Notes
Alpha-2-adrenergic agonists				
Dexmedetomidine	IM, IV	125–250 µg/m²	150–300 µg/m²	
Dexmedetomidine	IV CRI	0.5–2 µg/kg/h	1–2 µg/kg/h	

Do not use in pregnant animals, cardiovascular disease, respiratory disorders, liver or kidney disease, patients in shock, patients with severe debilitation, or severe stress due to extreme heat, cold, or fatigue. The UK label states not for use in puppies <6 months or kittens <5 months of age. Most adverse effects are extension of pharmacological action: bradycardia, vasoconstriction, muscle tremors, transient hypertension, reduced tear production, occasional atrioventricular block, decreased respiration, hypothermia, urination, vomiting, hyperglycemia. Rarely see prolonged sedation, paradoxical excitation, hypersensitivity, pulmonary edema, apnea, and death from circulatory failure. Adverse effects are generally reversed by administration of reversal agent (atipamezole), which also reverses analgesic effects. Concurrent use of atropine with bradycardia is not recommended.

Drug (duration)	Route	Dose for dog	Dose for cat	Notes
Local anesthetics				
Bupivacaine	Local infiltration, nerve blocks, IA	Up to 2 mg/kg total dose	Up to 1 mg/kg total dose	
Lidocaine	Local infiltration, nerve blocks, IA	Up to 12 mg/kg total dose	Up to 6 mg/kg total dose	
Lidocaine	IV CRI	30–80 µg/kg/min (1.8–5 mg/kg/h)	Not recommended	1–2 mg/kg IV loading dose; do *not* use the product containing epinephrine IV
Lidocaine	Transdermal patch	Apply to affected area over intact skin		

Cats are more sensitive to the cardiodepressant and CNS effects of lidocaine so use with caution in cats. Most common adverse effects are dose related and mild. CNS signs (drowsiness, depression, ataxia, muscle tremors), nausea and vomiting (usually transient). At high doses adverse cardiac effects and seizures can occur. Use with caution in patients with liver disease, congestive heart failure, shock, hypovolemia, severe respiratory depression, marked hypoxia, bradycardia, or incomplete heart block.

(Continued)

Table 19.1 (*Continued*)

Drug (duration)	Route	Dose for dog	Dose for cat	Notes
NMDA receptor antagonists				
Ketamine	Intermittent IV	0.5 mg/kg	0.5 mg/kg	NMDA receptor antagonism
Ketamine	IV CRI	0.6 mg/kg/h during surgery 0.12 mg/kg/h for next 24 h	0.6 mg/kg/h during surgery 0.12 mg/kg/h for next 24 h	NMDA receptor antagonism

Contraindicated in patients with significant hypertension, heart failure, dogs with liver failure, cats with kidney failure. Does *not* provide muscle relaxation. Increases CSF pressure at anesthetic doses (unlikely at analgesic doses). Common adverse effects include hypertension, hypersalivation, respiratory depression, hyperthermia, vomiting, vocalization, and prolonged and erratic recovery, dyspnea, seizures, muscle tremors, opisthotonus. These effects are extremely rare at analgesic doses listed above.

Drug (duration)	Route	Dose for dog	Dose for cat	Notes
Miscellaneous oral medications				
Amantadine	PO	2–5 mg/kg q 24 h	2–5 mg/kg q 24 h	NMDA receptor antagonism
Amitriptyline	PO	1–2 mg/kg q 12–24 h	0.5–1 mg/kg q 12 h	SSRI; may be useful for chronic neuropathic pain
Dextromethorphan	PO	0.5–2 mg/kg q 24 h		NMDA Receptor antagonism
Gabapentin	PO	3–10 mg/kg q 12–24 h	1.25–5 mg/kg q 24 h	Decrease dose slowly to avoid seizures; some liquid formulations contain xylitol (toxic to dogs)
Tramadol	PO	2–10 mg/kg q 8–24 h	1–5 mg/kg q 12–24 h	Useful for low-grade pain. Efficacy is questionable in cats

Amantadine has a narrow therapeutic window, and both dogs and cats are quite sensitive to overdose. May need to be compounded to provide safe appropriate dose. Adverse effects in dogs include behavioral changes, flatulence, and loose stools, especially early in therapy; limited experience/data in cats. **Amitriptyline** may reduce the seizure threshold in dogs and cats. Sedation and anticholinergic effects are the most common adverse effects. Taper slowly when discontinuing this medication. Severe adverse effects seen with severe overdose include cardiorespiratory collapse and cardiac arrhythmias. Common milder adverse effects (usually associated with overdose) include drowsiness, dry mouth, constipation, abnormal bleeding, seizures, tachycardia, fever. **Gabapentin** use with caution in animals with kidney failure; some human liquid formulations contain xylitol – do *not* use these formulations in dogs. Sedation and ataxia are most common adverse effects. **Tramadol** most common adverse effects are excessive sedation, agitation, anxiety, tremors, inappetance, vomiting, constipation, or diarrhea.

Drug (duration)	Route	Dose for dog	Dose for cat	Notes
NSAIDs				
Acetaminophen	PO	10–15 mg/kg PO q 8 h; consider q 12 h dosing if using longer than 5 days	DO NOT USE IN CATS	Hepatotoxicity and methemoglobinemia in cats; liver and renal function should be assessed beforehand
Carprofen	SC, PO	2–4 mg/kg (max dose 4.4 mg/kg/day)	(UK label; extralabel in USA) 4 mg/kg SC or IM once	Mild GI effects; rarely severe hepatic failure
Deracoxib	PO	1–2 mg/kg q 24 h		Also labeled 3–4 mg/kg PO q 24 h for postop pain
Etodolac	PO, SC	5–15 mg/kg q 24 h		
Meloxicam	IV, SC, PO, OTM	0.1–0.2 mg/kg	0.1–0.2 mg/kg injection (Metacam) ONCE	
Robenacoxib	PO, SC		1 mg/kg PO 2 mg/kg SC	Maximum 3 days
Tepoxalin	PO	10 mg/kg q 24 h		

Do *not* mix NSAIDs with steroid drugs or exceed dose – GI perforation is highly likely. Vomiting is the most common sign associated with NSAID-associated GI perforation. Most common adverse effects include vomiting, diarrhea, kidney injury, impaired platelet activity, and CNS depression. Liver and kidney function should be assessed prior to initiating therapy, and regularly with prolonged (>7–10 days) therapy. For all NSAIDs, use the minimum effective dose for long-term therapy.

Drug (duration)	Route	Dose for dog	Dose for cat	Notes
Reversal agents				
Naloxone	IM, IV, SC	0.002–0.1 mg/kg	0.002–0.1 mg/kg	Reversal for opioid drugs
Atipamezole	IM, SC (IV in emergency only)	0.05–0.2 mg/kg	0.05–0.2 mg/kg	Reverses alpha-adrenergic agonist drugs

CNS, central nervous system; CRI, constant rate infusion; CSF, cerebrospinal fluid; GI, gastrointestinal; IA, intraarticular; IM, intramuscular; IV, intravenous; NSAID, nonsteroidal antiinflammatory drug; OTM, oral transmucosal; PO, per os; SC, subcutaneous; SSRI, selective serotonin reuptake inhibitor.

Table 19.2 Opioid-lidocaine-ketamine constant rate influsion for dogs and cats with moderate pain. Choose ONE of the opioid drugs, and combine with lidocaine and ketamine. Dexmedetomidine can be added for severely painful or anxious patients if cardiovascularly stable. Use the lowest rate that produces satisfactory analgesia to reduce adverse effects. Rate can be safely tripled for patients with severe pain.

Drug	Dogs	Cats	Loading dose
Fentanyl -OR-	3 μg/kg/h	3 μg/kg/h	5 μg/kg
Hydromorphone -OR-	0.13 mg/kg/h	0.006 mg/kg/h	0.05 mg/kg
Morphine	0.1 mg/kg/h	0.1 mg/kg/h	0.3 mg/kg
Lidocaine	1.8 mg/kg/h	Not recommended	2 mg/kg (dogs only)
Ketamine	0.6 mg/kg/h	0.6 mg/kg/h	1 mg/kg
Dexmedetomidine	1 μg/kg/h	1 μg/kg/h	100 μg/m^2

multimodal analgesia in the small animal ICU patient are listed in Table 19.2 along with dose and recommended route of administration. Severe adverse drug reactions (such as hypotension, dysphoria) can warrant altering the drug(s), dose, or mode of analgesia administered.

Analgesic drugs

Analgesic drugs with different modes of action are used to target pain at different points along the pain pathway. Drug classifications that affect the peripheral nerves include NSAIDs, local anesthetics, and opioids. Drugs that work within the CNS (spinal cord and brain) include opioids, antidepressants, anticonvulsants, paracetamol (acetaminophen), and local anesthetics.

Opioids

Opioids are generally considered as an important class of analgesics for small animal patients experiencing moderate to severe pain. Endogenous opioids (such as endorphins, enkephalins) are produced by the CNS and pituitary gland and released to inhibit the transmission of pain signals. There are naturally occurring G protein-coupled opioid receptors (delta, kappa, mu, and nociception) located within both the central and peripheral nervous system and the GI tract. In the brain, stimulation of these receptors prevents the perception of pain. In the spinal cord, stimulation of opioid receptors prevents central sensitization, inhibits pain signal transmission, and inhibits neurotransmitter release. The efficacy of opioids in the peripheral tissues depends on the presence of inflammation, peripheral sensitization, and the presence or absence of hyperalgesia.

Opioid drugs are classified by their selectivity and activity at the endogenous opioid receptors. There are three pharmacological classes of opioids: pure mu-agonists, partial mu-agonists, and the kappa-agonist/mu-antagonist.

Pure mu-agonists should be selected when treating moderate to severe pain. Morphine, hydromorphone, oxymorphone, fentanyl, and methadone are the pure mu-agonists most commonly used in the dog and cat. These drugs provide superior analgesia at lower doses than the partial mu-agonists (such as buprenorphine), and the kappa-agonist/mu-antagonists (such as butorphanol) at their higher doses. Naloxone is the reversal agent for the mu-agonists.

Buprenorphine is the most widely used partial mu-agonist. It binds to the mu-opioid receptor slowly (slow onset) but with a high affinity (long duration of action). Due to its partial activity, buprenorphine provides only moderate analgesia and variable sedation, with

few adverse effects. When administered in cats, oral buprenorphine is absorbed transmucosally and provides good analgesia when dosed every six hours [19].

Butorphanol exhibits kappa-agonist/mu-antagonist activity at the opioid receptors. Receptor stimulation causes closing of influx membrane Ca channels and opening of membrane K channels, resulting in hyperpolarization of the cell membrane and suppression of transmission of action potentials in ascending pain pathways. At analgesic doses, butorphanol increases pulmonary arterial pressure and cardiac work. It also has antitussive effects. Sedation, nausea, and vomiting are possible side-effects of butorphanol administration.

Opioids often have a short half-life in dogs and cats, and therefore require frequent administration. The occurrence of undesirable side-effects after opioid administration can prompt the selection of a different opioid, addition of a sedative or switching to an analgesic with a different pharmacological action. An excitatory response to mu-agonist administration is more common in the cat and relatively uncommon in the dog. The administration of a sedative, such as acepromazine, a benzodiazepine or dexmedetomidine, in combination with the opioid, can lessen the excitatory effects. This combination can result in the synergistic effect of neuroleptanalgesia (altered awareness and analgesia) and additional sedation.

Alternatively, if the side-effects of a mu-agonist opioid are intolerable, the administration of a partial mu-agonist or kappa-agonist/mu-antagonist (such as buprenorphine or butorphanol) can be used to partially reverse the effects of the original mu-agonist drug. Naloxone can be given to fully reverse a pure mu-agonist. However, naloxone will also eliminate any analgesic effects of the mu-agonist opioid, requiring an alternate analgesic agent to be administered; the half-life of naloxone is often shorter than that of the medication being reversed, so multiple doses may be required.

Nonsteroidal antiinflammatory drugs (NSAIDS)

Nonsteroidal antiinflammatory drugs are used as antiinflammatory, analgesic, and antipyretic agents. The pharmacological action is to block the arachidonic acid cascade by inhibiting the cyclooxygenase (COX) enzymes. This reduces the production of prostaglandins, an end-product of the cascade and an inflammatory mediator that can cause an increase in the sensitivity of the peripheral nociceptors. There are three isoforms of COX enzymes: COX-1, COX-2, and COX-3. Specific NSAIDs have been developed that selectively inhibit COX-2 enzymes, with the intention of preserving the desired end-product of COX-1 activity, prostacyclin.

Nonsteroidal antiinflammatory drugs can provide excellent analgesic and antipyretic effects in the ICU patient if the source of pain is inflammation. However, careful patient selection is mandatory. The animals must have normal tissue perfusion and hydration, and adequate renal function to receive an NSAID. Box 19.2 provides guidelines for minimizing the risk factors for adverse NSAID events.

Nonsteroidal antiinflammatory drugs are highly protein bound and persist in tissue longer than in the bloodstream [20]. The response to a NSAID can improve for up to 12 weeks, partly because of binding in tissue and time needed to decrease nervous system sensitization [21]. The analgesic response can vary between individuals and switching to an alternate NSAID may be helpful when response has been inadequate.

As a class, the most common adverse effects manifest in the GI tract, renal system, and liver. Prostaglandins play an important role in the regulation of renal glomerular and gastric mucosal blood flow. Blocking prostaglandin production with NSAIDs can impair blood flow to these organs. Gastrointestinal events can range from minor decrease in appetite to severe GI bleeding or perforation. Vomiting is

Box 19.2 Guidelines for the use of nonsteroidal antiinflammatory drugs (NSAIDS).

In-hospital use
- Use proper, accurate dosing.
- Administer the minimal effective dose.
- Do not administer more than one NSAID.
- Provide a "washout period" if changing NSAID.
- Do not administer NSAIDS with corticosteroids (oral or injectable).
- Conduct appropriate patient chemistry/urine profiling.
- Conduct routine monitoring for adverse events.
- Refrain from using aspirin for pain control purposes.
- Use gastrointestinal protectants in high-risk patients.
- Minimize or avoid use in puppies and pregnant animals.
- Ensure adequate hydration and normal perfusion.
- Consider drug interactions with other medications.

At-home use
- Provide owners with verbal and written instructions.
- Dispense in approved packaging and owner information sheets.
- Conduct routine exams and blood test when on chronic NSAIDs.
- Do not refill NSAID presciptions without patient exam.
- Caution pet owner not to supplement with over-the-counter NSAIDs.

Adapted from Fox SM. Nonsteroidal anti-inflammatory drugs. In: Small Animal Anesthesia and Analgesia. Carroll GL, ed. Ames: Blackwell, 2008.

the most common sign associated with NSAID-related GI ulceration or perforation [22]. Risk factors for NSAID-associated GI perforation include inappropriate use, overdosing, simultaneous use of multiple types of NSAIDs or the use of a NSAID and a corticosteroid at the same time [22]. Renal events can include azotemia and renal failure.

Acetaminophen (paracetamol)

The mechanism of action of paracetamol (also called acetaminophen) is believed to be inhibition of the COX-3 enzyme, found in abundance in the cerebral cortex, with a weak effect on COX-1 [23]. Acetominophen will cross the blood–brain barrier, giving it potent central analgesic properties.

This drug should never be used in cats. Cats are deficient in hepatic metabolism of this drug (specifically, glucuronidation and sulfation) and are therefore more susceptible to acetaminophen toxicosis than dogs. Cats have been shown to produce signs of acetaminophen toxicosis at a dose as low as 10–mg/kg [24].

The recommended dose for dogs is 10–15 mg/kg PO q 8h. Nonrepairable liver damage has been reported at high doses in the dog. The use of acetaminophen in pregnant dogs is classified as a "potential risk" at this time.

Local anesthetics

Local anesthetics have the unique ability to produce complete blockade of sensory nerve fibers and prevent or preempt the development of secondary (central) sensitization to pain. For this reason, they are often used with opioids, alpha-2-receptor agonists, dissociative, and antiinflammatory drugs as part of a multimodal strategy to manage pain [25]. They can be administered by topical, mucosal or dermal application, by injection or infiltration into a regional site of injury or by intravenous injection for central nerve block techniques. Lidocaine can also be applied through lidocaine-impregnated dermal patches or lidocaine ointments or gels. An intravenous continuous infusion of local anesthetics can be part of a multimodal pain control protocol (see Table 19.2).

Lidocaine and bupivacaine are the local anesthetics commonly used in the dog and cat. Lidocaine alters signal conduction in neurons by blocking the fast voltage-gated Na channels in the neuronal cell membrane responsible for signal propagation [26]. With sufficient blockage, the membrane of the postsynaptic neuron will not depolarize and will thus fail to transmit an action potential. Lidocaine administered locally into the tissues has a rapid onset (1–5 minutes) and a short duration of action (60–120 minutes).

When given intravenously, lidocaine blocks Na channels in the conduction system and muscle cells of the heart. This raises the depolarization threshold, making the heart less likely to initiate or conduct early action potentials that may cause an arrhythmia [26]. Systemic exposure to excessive quantities of lidocaine mainly results in CNS signs (such as agitation, seizures) and cardiovascular effects (such as bradycardia, hypotension, arrhythmias). Drug administration should be stopped and intravenous anticonvulsant drugs may be required. Treatment with intravenous lipid emulsions (used for parenteral feeding) to reverse the effects of local anesthetic toxicity has been recommended [27].

Bupivacaine binds to the intracellular portion of voltage-gated Na channels and blocks Na influx into nerve cells, preventing depolarization. Without depolarization, no initiation or conduction of a pain signal can occur. Bupivacaine injected locally has a slower time to onset (15–30 minutes) and lasts significantly longer (3–8 hours). Bupivicaine should *not* be given intravenously. Adverse reactions typically encountered are related to the CNS and cardiovascular systems. These adverse experiences are generally dose related and due to high plasma levels from overdosage, rapid absorption from the injection site, diminished tolerance, or from unintentional intravascular injection. Excitation, tremors, depression, and seizures are possible CNS signs. Myocardial depression, decreased cardiac output, heart block, bradycardia, ventricular fibrillation, and cardiac arrest are important cardiovascular signs. Intravenous intralipid administration has been recommended to reverse the effects of bupivacaine.

Patient selection is critical for successful pain control with local anesthetics. Cats are more susceptible to the toxic effects of these two drugs and they are administered at a reduced dose in the cat, with careful monitoring. Bupivacaine should not be given to animals with cardiac arrhythmias. These agents can produce a stinging or burning sensation when applied to skin or tissues or to the pleural or peritoneal membranes. Their intracavitary use has been reported, but may have effects on cardiac output [28].

Alpha-2-agonists

The mechanisms of the analgesic actions of alpha-2-agonists have not been fully elucidated. The inhibitory neuronal actions of alpha-2-adrenoceptor agonists is through the activation of G protein-gated K channels, resulting in membrane hyperpolarization and a decreased firing rate of excitable cells in the CNS [29]. In addition, the alpha-2-adrenoceptor agonists reduce Ca conductance into nerve cells by regulating the voltage-gated Ca channels, thus inhibiting neurotransmitter release. The result is that the nerve is prevented from firing or propagating its signal to adjacent neurons.

In general, presynaptic activation of the alpha-2-adrenoceptor inhibits the release of norepinephrine, terminating the propagation of pain signals. Postsynaptic activation of alpha-2-adrenoceptors in the CNS inhibits sympathetic activity and thus can decrease blood pressure and heart rate. Combined, these effects can produce analgesia, sedation, and anxiolysis. Dexmedetomidine combines all these effects [30].

Dexmedetomidine is the alpha-2-agonist most commonly used in small animal medicine. It is a noncontrolled parenteral agent that provides good visceral analgesia and moderate sedation, with a duration of action of approximately 30–60 minutes. It can be used as a sole injectable agent for short procedures, or it can be used at very low doses administered as a constant rate infusion (CRI) as part of a multimodal pain control plan or to relieve anxiety and dysphoria.

Dexmedetomidine should *not* be used in patients with hemodynamic instability or with underlying cardiac disease. While dexmedetomidine does not appear to have any direct effects on the heart, a biphasic cardiovascular effect occurs, incorporating a transient increase of the blood pressure and a reflex decrease in heart rate [31]. This can be explained by the peripheral alpha-2B-adrenoceptor stimulation of vascular smooth muscle. Since the baroceptor reflex is well preserved, the reflex bradycardia occurring in response to a pressor stimulus is augmented [32]. The cardiovascular response to the drug can include bradycardia and hypotension. Patient selection is critical and monitoring the blood pressure and heart rate is required. Volume infusion and vasoactive drug can be given, when needed. There is argument, however, that dexmedetomidine may be beneficial in cats with hypertrophic cardiomyopathy with dynamic left ventricular outflow tract obstruction. It has been proposed that the increase in systemic vascular resistance and decrease in heart rate produced by alpha-2-agonists has the potential to temporarily eliminate the left ventricular outflow tract obstruction [33,34].

The package insert states that dexmedetomidine is also contraindicated in patients suffering from respiratory disorders, liver disease, kidney disease, shock, severe debilitation, or stress caused by extreme heat, cold, or fatigue. The medication can produce vomiting in dogs and cats following IM administration, so it should not be used when vomiting could affect increased intraocular pressure, increased intracranial pressure or increased intragastric pressure. Because alpha-2-agonists reduce uterine blood flow and may affect intrauterine pressure, dexmedetomidine is not recommended for use in pregnant animals. In addition, significant hypoventilation can occur, causing hypoxia, when alpha-2-agonists are administered with other drugs (such as opioids, ketamine, propofol). Oxygen supplementation is recommended but will not prevent respiratory acidosis.

Atipamezole (Antisedan®, Zoetis, Florham Park, NJ) is an alpha-2-antagonist that can reverse the effects of the alpha-2-agonists. Dosage recommendations for the dog are 3750 μg/m² IM (if reversing intravenous dexmedetomidine) and 5000 μg/m² IM (if reversing IM administered dexmedetomidine). A study in cats found that the IM administration of atipamezole at 2–4 times the preceding dose of the alpha-2-agonist was effective with negligible side-effects [35].

The IV administration of atipamezole is usually contraindicated, and can result in rapid relaxation of vascular tone. This coupled with bradycardia from dexmedetomidine could result in severe hypotension. The atipamezole preservative, methylparaben, can cause histamine release leading to hypotension, as well. It has been recommended that atipamezole and anticholinergics should not be used together to avoid significant increases in heart rate [36].

The routine use of anticholinergics concurrently or after treatment with dexmedetomidine is not recommended and can increase the risk of dysrhythmias. Should bradycardia result in life-threatening hypotension after dexmedetomidine injection, atipamezole should be given. Treatment with anticholinergics before administration of dexmedetomidine will prevent bradycardia, but cardiac output can still be decreased by over 50% [31].

NMDA receptor antagonists

Ketamine, dextromethorphan, and amantadine are N-methyl-D-aspartate (NMDA) receptor antagonists, with ketamine used most commonly in the dog and cat. This drug induces dissociative anesthesia, incorporating hypnosis (sedation and unconsciousness at higher doses), antinociception (intense analgesia), increased sympathetic activity, and maintenance of airway tone and respiration. The hypnotic effects appear to be largely mediated by blockade of NMDA and HCN1 (K/Na hyperpolarization-activated cyclic nucleotide-gated channel 1) receptors. The NMDA receptors play an important role in CNS sensitization to pain. In addition, cholinergic, aminergic, and opioid systems appear to play a modulatory role in both the sedation and analgesic actions of ketamine. The drug effects in chronic pain, and as an antidepressant, far outlast the actual drug levels, and are probably mediated by a neuronal response to a ketamine-induced hyperglutamatergic state [37]. Various dose recommendations (see Table 19.1) are based on the desired effects of the ketamine and the route of administration. Ketamine can be administered as an IV bolus, IM, IV by CRI, or absorbed through oral mucous membranes.

Ketamine can cause tachycardia, hypertension, respiratory problems, muscle tremors, spastic movements, vocalization, and erratic recovery when used alone at anesthetic doses. The drug should be combined with other anesthetic or analgesic agents to reduce the dose and avoid deleterious side-effects. When ketamine is used at the lower doses, behavioral or cardiovascular side-effects are uncommon. Patients with heart disease, kidney disease, seizures, head injury or eye injuries should not be given ketamine at anesthetic dose. Ketamine can interact with certain medications such as thyroid medications, narcotics, halothane, diazepam, or chloramphenicol.

Tricyclic antidepressants

Tricyclic antidepressant drugs are used in dogs and cats for their analgesic effect for chronic pain, and include amitriptyline, imipramine, fluoxetine, and clomipramine (see Table 19.1). These drugs have antihistamine, antiinflammatory, analgesic, and antidepressant effects. Amitriptyline increases synaptic activity of serotonin and norepinephrine, has significant central and peripheral anticholinergic activity, and stimulates beta-adrenergic receptors in smooth muscle. Serotonin syndrome can occur when using tricyclic antidepressants with other drugs that inhibit serotonin uptake, resulting in tachycardia, hyperresponsive reflexes, tremors, seizures, hypertension, hyperthermia, and in severe cases death.

Gabapentin

Gabapentin (see Table 19.1) is an anticonvulsant that is useful in the management of chronic neurogenic or neuropathic pain resulting from inflammation or injury to the CNS. Neuropathic pain is often not responsive to opioids. The mechanism of action appears to be through voltage-dependent Ca channel blockade, as well as increasing central inhibition or reducing the synthesis of glutamate and halting the release of excitatory neurotransmitters. However, it does not appear to interact directly with NMDA receptors. Dogs show some liver metabolism of gabapentin, but the drug is excreted mainly through the kidneys. Adverse effects are usually mild and self-limiting (drowsiness, fatigue, and weight gain) with chronic administration. Gabapentin has been used in combination with opioids and NSAIDs [38,39].

Tramadol

Tramadol (see Table 19.1) has gained wide popularity in veterinary medicine. The mechanism of action is complex, with tramadol eliciting effects as a serotonin and norepinephrine reuptake inhibitor and as a weak mu-receptor agonist. Oral bioavailability is 93% in cats but only 65% in dogs. Tramadol is metabolized to an active metabolite in cats, but not dogs. Dogs eliminate and clear tramadol more rapidly than cats. Tramadol has been shown to reduce minimum alveolar concentration of sevoflurane in cats and is reported to have an analgesic effect similar to that of morphine in dogs; however, other evidence suggests its analgesic properties may be minimal [40]. Tramadol may be used alone to treat mild pain and adjunctively in a multimodal plan to treat moderate to severe pain.

Serotonin syndrome can occur if tramadol is combined with other serotonin reuptake inhibitors. Other adverse effects of tramadol are typically mild and can include sedation, vomiting, excitation, agitation, and dysphoria. Tramadol may lower the seizure threshold in animals prone to seizures or may decrease the effectiveness of anticonvulsants.

Tramadol has the advantage of being widely available and relatively inexpensive. In 2014, tramadol became a Schedule IV drug, making DEA licensure necessary for veterinarians to prescribe the medication in the United States.

Method of drug administration

Various drug delivery methods are available for the administration of analgesics to the small animal ICU patient. Oral administration is often not a reliable means due to patient vomiting, abnormal GI function, abnormal mental status, inability to swallow, or need for nil per os (NPO).

Intermittent dosing by injection (subcutaneous, IM, IV) can be effective and requires no special equipment. This delivery method can be associated with peaks and troughs of drug concentration, which could translate to periods of excessive analgesia and sedation followed by periods of lesser and potentially inadequate analgesia. Adequate personnel over a 24-hour period are needed to prevent lapses in drug administration.

Buprenorphine (Simbadol®, Zoetis, Florham Park, NJ) and fentanyl (Recuvyra®, Elanco, Indianapolis, IN) are available in long-acting injectable preparations. The buprenorphine formulation is labeled specifically for single injection in cats with 24-hour duration, and the fentanyl product for dogs with a 72-hour duration. These preparations are less useful in the critical care patient since frequent dose adjustments may be necessary. In addition, drug interactions, protein binding, and drug elimination must be considered carefully throughout the duration of the drug effect.

Most of the opioid drugs (except methadone and buprenorphine), ketamine, lidocaine, and dexmedetomidine can be delivered by intravenous CRI. This mode of drug delivery allows easy adjustment of drug dose and avoids the peak and trough effects common with intermittent bolus therapy. A loading dose is frequently required to reach the desired plasma drug concentration prior to initiating the CRI infusion (see Chapter 18). A syringe pump or volumetric fluid infusion pump is needed to ensure appropriate delivery of the prescribed volume of drug. It is important to carefully review any recommendations for carrier solution (such as normal saline, 5% dextrose in water) when dilution of the medication is required. Monitoring is essential to ensure that the calculated dose, rate, and volume of delivery are accurate to meet the needs of the patient. The drug delivery lines and equipment are checked to confirm the patency and performance.

The infiltration of tissues or infiltration around specific nerves with local anesthetics (such as lidocaine, bupivacaine) will provide analgesia to focal areas. It is ideal when performing short, painful procedures such as laceration repairs, bone marrow aspirates, or centesis. Intracavitary infusion of local anesthetics has been used for local pain control due to peritonitis, pleuritis or postthoracostomy procedures. The localized pain from traumatic injuries such as rib fracture and skin wounds can be initially managed with local infiltration during the resuscitation phase of therapy.

Wound soaker catheters (diffusion catheter/soft tissue incision catheter, Mila International, Erlanger, KY) can be placed in large wounds at the time of repair (Figure 19.4). These catheters allow constant and focal infusion of local anesthetics to the wound. The procedure, drug dose, and catheter options are listed in Box 19.3.

Transmucosal and transdermal administration of analgesics provides a noninvasive means of drug administration. Buprenorphine and ketamine can be absorbed through the oral mucous membranes. This allows oral administration in a fractious animal when an injection is too stressful or not possible. Lidocaine is available as a transdermal patch and can be applied adjacent to wounds or incisions to increase comfort. These patches should *not* be applied directly over a wound or incision.

Fentanyl is available in a transdermal patch that can be applied to the shaved skin, providing 3–5 days of continuous analgesia. While convenient, there is a 12–24-hour lag time from the time of application until a therapeutic blood level of the drug is attained. Intravenous administration of a pure mu-agonist opioid is required during that time period. The patches are available in a variety of sizes, with patch dose recommendation base on body weight provided in Table 19.3. Unfortunately, many dogs are either slightly under or over the weight for the patch dose, necessitating additional analgesic therapy or removal of the patch to eliminate undesirable side-effects. The skin temperature and blood flow to the skin need to be constant for consistent drug delivery and this is a cause for concern in the critically ill animal. Application of a bandage over the patch to hold it in place can alter the function of the patch. Buprenorphine in a transdermal patch has not been shown to achieve therapeutic concentrations in dogs and cats.

Epidural administration of analgesics is a powerful tool for providing analgesia. Preoperative epidural injection of local anesthetics and opioids provides excellent preemptive, multimodal intraoperative analgesia, extending into the recovery period [41]. In addition, continuous epidural anesthesia can be provided by placing epidural catheters. Access to the epidural space is a technical skill that can be acquired with practice and requires little specialized equipment (spinal needles and syringes) (Figure 19.5). The procedure for performing an epidural injection is described in Box 19.4. Analgesic drugs and doses that are commonly administered as an epidural injection are listed in Table 19.4. Epidural anesthetic injections should not be administered to patients with increased intracranial pressure, clotting disorders (possibility of epidural hematoma), uncorrected hypovolemia, degenerative central or peripheral axonal diseases, anatomical abnormalities that make location of landmarks difficult, or skin infection at the site of needle penetration.

The coccygeal epidural technique provides anesthesia to the perineum, penis/vulva, urethra, colon, and anus by blocking the pudendal, pelvic, and caudal nerves without loss of motor function in the hindlimbs [42,43]. This is particularly useful for relieving

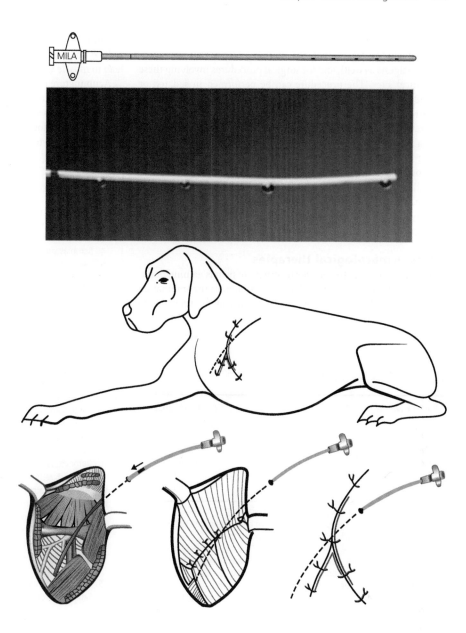

Figure 19.4 Wound diffusion catheter, Mila International. Used with permission.

Box 19.3 Steps to place a wound soaker catheter for analgesia.

1. Choose a soaker catheter. Length = long axis of wound.
2. Place the catheter in the deepest layer of the wound.
3. Injection port exits dorsally. Ensure all fenestrations in catheter remain within the wound.
4. Close the wound over the catheter.
5. Fasten catheter to skin where exits wound. Use finger trap suture or butterfly waterproof tape. Do not occlude the soft catheter when suturing.
6. Inject priming dose of bupivacaine. Ensure adequate/ease of delivery before recovery from anesthesia.
7. Continue local anesthetic infusion into wound. Continuous infusion of lidocaine (dogs only). Intermittent slow injection of bupivicaine (dogs or cats).
8. Adjust drug volume to size of wound and satisfactory pain control.
9. Continue administration of local anesthetic into wound for up to three days.
10. To discontinue, monitor for recurrence of pain for six hours after discontinuing lidocaine continuous infusion, or eight hours after last dose of bupivacaine.
11. If pain control adequate after monitoring period, remove sutures and gently pull catheter through skin to remove.
    - Mark wound catheter hub, syringes, pumps, and lines to avoid accidental IV injection of local anesthetic.
    - Sources of catheters: Mila International, Erlanger, KY and ReCathCo, Allison Park, PA.

Adapted from Abelson AL, McCob EC, Shaw S, et al. Use of wound soaker catheters for the administration of local anesthetics for postoperative analgesia: 56 cases. Vet Anesth Analg. 2009;36(6):597–602.

urethral obstruction, providing analgesia for urethral catheterization, reducing rectal, vaginal, and uterine prolapse (requires additional analgesia as well), and for surgical procedures involving these anatomical sites. The procedure can be performed in sedated or obtunded animals. Strict aseptic technique is required. Steps for performing a coccygeal epidural injection are outlined in Box 19.5. Contraindications for epidurals of any type include sepsis, pyoderma at the injection site, coagulation disorders, severe hypovolemia or hypotension, and anatomical abnormalities.

Knowledge of the pathways of nociception continues to expand, providing new targets for new analgesics in the critical small animal patient. Frequent review of the veterinary literature is required to identify these new effective drugs as they are being approved for the management of acute and chronic pain.

Nonpharmacological therapies

Nonpharmacological therapy for treatment of pain is gaining popularity in veterinary medicine and can be used alone or in combination with analgesic drugs. Areas of inflammation may be amenable to simple techniques such as intermittent application of cold packs, warm compresses, and focal hydrotherapy. Minimizing movement

of painful areas (such as bandaging or splinting a fracture) can also reduce noxious stimulation and pain in the acute setting, but can lead to muscle wasting and contracture if used long term.

Acupuncture (traditional, electroacupuncture, and percutaneous acupoint electrical stimulation) is an effective treatment for many types of pain, well tolerated by animals, and has a minimal likelihood of serious adverse effects. The mechanisms of acupuncture analgesia involve direct and indirect neurohumoral effects that

Table 19.3 Fentanyl patch dosing and application.

Patient weight	Patch dose
Cats, dogs <5 kg	12.5 µg patch
Dogs 5–10 kg	25 µg patch
Dogs 10–20 kg	50 µg patch
Dogs 20–30 kg	75 µg patch
Dogs >30 kg	100 µg patch

Practically, estimate 3 mg/kg to choose patch size.
To apply the patch, shave fur from application area. Clean skin with isopropyl alcohol and allow to air-dry. Apply patch to skin.
Because the patches are developed for human use, drug delivery in dogs and cats is inconsistent. Some animals may need adjunctive/additional drugs while others may appear severely overdosed when using the patch. Removal of the patch generally resolves signs of overdose within several hours. Severely affected animals may need naloxone for several hours following patch removal.

Box 19.4 Steps for performing an epidural injection.

1. Place in sternal or lateral recumbency.
2. Pull pelvic limbs cranially.
3. Clip 4 × 4 cm area dorsal midline: center on L7.
4. Scrub as surgical prep and drape.
5. Use strict aseptic technique.
6. Palpate landmarks:
   left and right cranial, dorsal iliac wings
   spinous process L7
   median sacral crest.
7. Locate needle insertion site, midline of lumbosacral space caudal to the dorsal spinous process of L7.
8. Insert needle slowly with bevel pointed cranial and perpendicular to the skin. Advance through skin first, then advance through:
   subcutaneous tissue
   supraspinous ligament
   interspinous ligament
   ligamentum flavum.
9. Feel a "pop" or loss of resistance as the needle enters the epidural space.
10. Remove stylet and observe hub of needle for blood or CSF; if observed, remove needle and try again.
11. Gently aspirate, if no blood or fluid accumulates in needle.
12. Slowly inject a small quantity of saline if no blood or air aspirated. There should be no resistance. Alternatively, hanging drop technique may be used.
13. Confirm correct placement of the needle.
14. Inject analgesic very slowly. Rapid injection can cause hypotension and/or ineffective epidural analgesia.
15. Remove the needle and proceed with patient care.
See Table 19.4 for epidural drugs and doses.

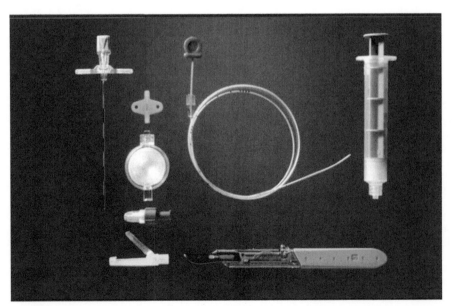

Figure 19.5 Epidural catheter kit, Mila International. Used with permission.

Table 19.4 Epidural drugs and doses for dogs and cats.

Drug	Dose for dog	Dose for cat (mg/kg)
Buprenorphine	5 µg/kg	
Butorphanol	0.25 mg/kg	0.25 mg/kg
Fentanyl	6 µg/kg	4 µg/kg
Hydromorphone	0.2 mg/kg	0.1 mg/kg
Morphine	0.1 mg/kg	0.1 mg/kg
Bupivacaine 0.5%	1 mL/4.5 kg	1 mL/7 kg
Lidocaine 20%	1 mL/3.4 kg (block to T5)	1 mL/4.5 kg (block to T5)
	1 mL/4.5 kg (block to L2)	

Adapted from: Carroll GL, ed. Small Animal Anesthesia and Analgesia. Ames: Blackwell publishing. 2008.

Box 19.5 Procedure for performing coccygeal epidural anesthesia.

1. Place in sternal recumbency.
2. Palpate the space between the sacrum and first coccygeal vertebra or the first and second coccygeal vertebrae.
3. Clip a 4×4 cm piece of skin over the area.
4. Aseptically prepare the skin.
5. Use sterile gloves and sterile procedure.
6. Reestablish the location of the most mobile joint caudal to the sacrum.
7. Penetrate skin with a 25 gauge 1 inch needle on the midline. Use index finger near the injection site as a guide for the needle.
8. Direct the needle at a 30–45° angle. Advance through the interarcuate ligament/ligamentum flavum. A palpable "pop" is possible when the ligament is penetrated.
9. Advance the needle, feeling for a little resistance as the needle enters epidural space. If bone is encountered, determine if the needle is superficial to the spinal canal or has advanced through to the floor of the vertebral canal. If superficial, keep the needle underneath the skin, redirect angle slightly cranial or caudal.
10. Inject 0.1–0.2 mL/kg of 2% lidocaine when confident that the needle is in the epidural space.

Adapted from O'Hearn AK, Wright BD. Coccygeal epidural with local anesthetic for catheterization and pain management in the treatment of feline urethral obstruction. J Vet Emerg Crit Care 2011;21(1):50–2.

block pain perception, reduce the pain response, relieve muscle spams, and reduce inflammation [44]. A review of the mechanisms and techniques utilized for treating pain in animals by acupuncture is available in literature cited in the Further reading list.

Transcutaneous electrical nerve stimulation (TENS) is a therapeutic method that electrically stimulates dermatomes to modulate pain. TENS activates nonnociceptor A-β fibers. The proposed mechanism of pain modulation occurs when more A-β fibers are activated than C fibers and A-δ fibers, resulting in diminished pain sensation [2]. TENS is also suspected to stimulate production and release of endogenous opioids [2].

Low-level laser therapy has been used to reduce pain, swelling, tissue necrosis, and inflammation in critically ill patients [45]. This laser light therapy works predominantly on a protein in mitochondria (cytochrome c oxidase) to increase ATP and reduce oxidative stress. A cascade of mitochondrial and intracellular downstream effects leads to improved tissue repair and reduced inflammation. Higher power density (>300 mW/cm²) reduces ATP production in

C fibers and A-δ fibers, resulting in an immediate neural blockade lasting up to approximately 24 hours [46]. It is reported to support soft tissue and muscle healing after trauma [47] and has been used in a variety of ICU patients including those with painful and inflammatory diseases, neurological injury [48], and organ dysfunction [49].

Massage is underutilized in veterinary medicine and likely has a role in pain management in the ICU. In the human medical community, it is recognized for success in treating muscle, nerve, and fascial disorders. It is also recognized for having a role in treating disorders of GI motility, and prevention or treatment of peripheral edema [50]. Medical massage is now taught in many veterinary physical therapy programs and medical schools. Hydrotherapy can provide significant postsurgical pain relief in some patients. Mobility exercises including assisted and nonassisted standing, walking, passive range of motion, and stretching exercises can be incorporated into the care of almost every cardiovascularly stable ICU patient [51]. This may be particularly important for patient with chronic conditions (such as osteoarthritis) who are suffering from an acute problem.

Pulse wave therapy uses high-energy sound waves, called pulses or shock waves, to stimulate and speed the healing process within the body. These sound waves release higher energy and result in deeper penetration than an ultrasound or laser. The waves travel through soft tissue at different depths to a specific treatment area. The high-energy sound waves stimulate cells and release healing growth factors in the body that reduce inflammation and swelling, increase blood flow, help bones to form and heal, and enhance wound healing.

References

1. Gaynor JS. Definitions of terms describing pain. In: Handbook of Veterinary Pain Management, 2nd edn. Gaynor JS, Muir WW, eds. St Louis: Mosby, 2009: pp 57–9.
2. Lerche P, Muir WW. Analgesia. In: Small Animal Anesthesia and Analgesia. Carroll GL, ed. Ames: Blackwell, 2008: pp 123–42.
3. Gaynor JS. The physiology of pain and principles for its treatment. In: Mechanisms of Disease in Small Animal Surgery, 3rd edn. Bojrab MJ, Monnet E, eds. Jackson: Teton New Media, 2010: pp 36–45.
4. Hellyer P, Rodan I, Brunt J, Downing R, Hagerdorn J, Robertson S. AAHA/AAFP Pain management guidelines for dogs and cats. J Am Anim Hosp Assoc. 2007;43(5):235–48.
5. Almedia T, Roizenblatt S, Tufik S. Afferent pain pathways: a neuroanatomical review. Brain Res. 2004;1000(1–2):40–56.
6. Milan M. Descending control of pain. Progr Neurobiol. 2001;66(6):355–474.
7. Dubin AE, Patapuotain A. Nociceptors: the sensors of the pain pathway. J Clin Invest. 2010;120(11):3760–72.
8. Gaynor J, Mama K. Local and regional anesthetic techniques for alleviation of perioperative pain. In: Handbook of Veterinary Pain Management, 2nd edn. Gaynor JS, Muir WW, eds. St Louis: Mosby, 2009: pp 301–33.
9. Boothe DM. Control of pain in small animals. In: Small Animal Clinical Pharmacology and Therapeutics. St Louis: Elsevier, 2012: pp 995.
10. Okuse K. Pain signalling pathways: from cytokines to ion channels. Int J Biochem Cell Biol. 2007;39(3):490–6.
11. Polgar E, Al-Khater KM, Shehab S, Watanabe M, Todd AJ. Large projection neurons in lamina I of the rat spinal cord that lack neurokinin 1 receptor are densely innervated by VGLUT-2-containing axons and possess GluR4-containing AMPA receptors. J Neurosci. 2008;28(49):13150–60.
12. Woolf CJ. Pain: moving from symptom control to mechanism-specific pharmacologic management. Ann Intern Med. 2004;140(6):441–51.
13. Mathews K, Kronen PW, Lascelles D, et al. Guidelines for recognition, assessment and treatment of pain. J Sm Anim Pract. 2014;55(5):E10–E68.
14. Peers A, Mellor DJ, Wintour EM, Dodic M. Blood pressure, heart rate, hormonal, and other acute responses to rubber-ring castration and tail docking of lambs. NZ Vet J. 2002;50(2):56–62.

15. Frerichs JA, Janis LR. Preemptive analgesia in foot and ankle surgery. Clin Podiatr Med Surg. 2003;20(2):237–56.

16. Singh H, Kundra S, Singh R, et al. Preemptive analgesia with ketamine for laparoscopic cholecystectomy. J Anesthesiol Clin Pharmacol. 2013;29(4):478–84.

17. Beilin B, Bessler H, Mayburd E, et al. Effects of preemptive analgesia on pain and cytokine production in the postoperative period. Anesthesiology 2003;98:151–5.

18. Kissin I. Preemptive analgesia. Anesthesiology 2000;93:1138–43.

19. Robertson SA, Taylor PM, Sear JW. Systemic uptake of buprenorphine by cats after oral mucosal administration. Vet Rec. 2003;152:675–8.

20. Monteiro-Steagall BP, Steagall PV, Lascelles BD. Systematic review of nonsteroidal antiinflammatory drug-induced adverse effects in dogs. J Vet Intern Med. 2013;27:1011–19.

21. Schweitzer A, Hasler-Nguyen N, Zijlstra J. Preferential uptake of the nonsteroid antiinflammatory drug diclofenac into inflamed tissues after a single oral dose in rats. BMC Pharmacol. 2009;16(9):5.

22. Lascelles BDX, Blikslager AT, Fox SM, et al. Gastrointestinal tract perforations in dogs treated with selective cyclooxygenase-2 inhibitor: 29 cases (2002–2003). J Am Vet Med Assoc. 2005;227(7):1112–17.

23. Romero-Sandoval EA, Mazario J, Howat D, et al. NCX-701 (nitroparacetamol) is an effective antinociceptive agent in rat withdrawal reflexes and wind-up. Br J Pharmacol. 2002;135:1556–62.

24. Richardson JA. Management of acetaminophen and ibuprofen toxicosis in dogs and cats. J Vet Emerg Crit Care 2000;10(4):285–91.

25. Lemke KA, Creighton CM. Paravertebral blockade of the brachial plexus in dogs. Vet Clin North Am. 2008;38(6):1231–41.

26. Sheu SS, Lederer WJ. Lidocaine's negative inotropic and antiarrhythmic actions. Dependence on shortening of action potential duration and reduction of intracellular sodium activity. Circ Res. 1985;57(4):578–90.

27. Picard J, Ward SC, Zumpe R, et al. Guidelines and the adoption of 'lipid rescue' therapy for local anaesthetic toxicity. Anaesthesia 2009;64(2):122–5.

28. Bernard F, Kudnig ST, Monnet E. Hemodynamic effects of interpleural lidocaine and bupivacaine in anesthetized dogs with and without an open pericardium. Vet Surg. 2006;25(3):252–8.

29. Birnbaumer L, Abramowitz J, Brown AM. Receptor-effector coupling by G proteins. Biochim Biophys Acta. 1990;1031:163–224.

30. Gertler R, Brown HC, Mitchell DH, Silvius EN. Dexmedetomidine: a novel sedative-analgesic agent. Proc Bayl Univ Med Cent. 2001;14(1):13–21.

31. Lemke KA. Anticholinergics and sedatives. In: Lumb and Jones' Veterinary Anesthesia and Analgesia, 4th edn. Tranquilli WJ, Thurmon JC, Grimm KA, eds. Ames: Blackwell, 2007: pp 203–39.

32. Kallio A, Scheinin M, Koulu M, et al. Effects of dexmedetomidine, a selective alpha 2-adrenoceptor agonist, on hemodynamic control mechanisms. Clin Pharmacol Ther. 1989;46:33–42.

33. Pypendop B, Verstegen J. Hemodynamic effects of medetomidine in the dog: a dose titration study. Vet Surg. 1998;27(6):612–22.

34. Kennedy MJ, Johnson, RA. Dexmedetomidine and atipamezole. Clin Brief 2015;13(8):65–7.

35. VaHa-VaHe AT. Clinical effectiveness of atipamezole as a medetomidine antagonist in cats. J Sm Anim Pract. 1990;31(4):193–7.

36. Lemke KA. Anticholinergics and sedatives. In: Lumb and Jones' Veterinary Anesthesia and Analgesia, 4th edn. Tranquilli WJ, Thurmon JC, Grimm KA, eds. Ames: Blackwell, 2007: pp 203–39.

37. Sleigh J, Harvey M, Voss L, Denny B. Ketamine – more mechanisms of action than just NMDA blockade. Trends Anesth Crit Care 2014;4(2–3):76–81.

38. Steagall PV, Monteiro-Steagall BP. Multimodel analgesia for perioperative pain in three cats. J Feline Med Surg. 2013;15(8):737–43.

39. Aghighi SA, Tipold A, Peichotta M, et al. Assessment of the effects of adjunctive gabapentin postoperative pain after intervertebral disc surgery in dogs. Vet Anesth Analg. 2012;39(6):636–46.

40. Kogel B, Terlinden R, Schneider J. Characterisation of tramadol, morphine and tapentadol in dogs in an acute pain model and Beagle dogs. Vet Anesth Analg. 2014;41(3):297–304.

41. Valverde A. Epidural analgesia and anesthesia in dogs and cats. Vet Clin North Am Small Anim Pract. 2008;38(6):37–53.

42. O'Hearn AK, Wright BD. Coccygeal epidural with local anesthetic for catheterization and pain management in the treatment of feline urethral obstruction. J Vet Emerg Crit Care 2011;21(1):50–2.

43. Skarda RT, Tranquilli WJ. Local and regional anesthetic and analgesic techniques: horses. In: Lumb and Jones' Veterinary Anesthesia and Analgesia, 4th edn. Tranquilli WJ, Thurmon JC, Grimm KA, eds. Ames: Blackwell, 2007: pp 620–2.

44. Kenney JD. Acupuncture for the treatment of pain. Am J Trad Chinese Vet Med. 2010;5(2):37–53.

45. Nadur-Andrade N, Blikslaer AT, Fox SM, et al. Effects of photobiostimulation on edema and hemorrhage induced by Bothrops moojeni venom. Lasers Med Sci. 2012;27(1):65–70.

46. Chow R, Armati P, Laakso EL, Bjordal JM, Baxter GD. Inhibitory effects of laser irradiation on peripheral mammalian nerves and relevance to analgesic effects: a systemic review. Photomed Laser Surg. 2011;29(6):365–81.

47. Fernandez KP, Alves AN, Nunes GD, et al. Effect of photobiomodulation on expression of IL-1B in skeletal muscle following injury. Lasers Med Sci. 2013;28(3):1043–6.

48. Hashimi JT, Huang YY, Osmani BZ, et al. Role of low-level laser therapy in neuro-rehabilitation. Phys Med Rehab. 2010;2(12 Suppl 2):S292–S305.

49. Hentschke VS, Janisch RB, Schmieg LA, et al. Low-level laser therapy improves the inflammatory profile of rats with heart failure. Lasers Med Sci. 2013;28(3):1007–16.

50. Millis DL. Physical therapy and rehabilitation in dogs. In: Handbook of Veterinary Pain Management, 3rd edn. Gaynor JS, ed. St Louis: Mosby, 2015: pp 383–421.

51. Gaynor JS. Energy modalities: therapeutic lasers and pulsed electromagnetic field therapy. In: Handbook of Veterinary Pain Management, 3rd edn. Gaynor JS, ed. St Louis: Mosby, 2015: pp 356–64.

Further reading

Epstein M, Rodan I, Griffenhagen G, et al. AAHA/AAFP pain management guidelines for dogs and cats. J Am Anim Hosp Assoc. 2015;52(2):67–84.

Fox F, Millis D, eds. Multimodal Management of Canine Osteoarthritis. London: Manson Publishing, 2010.

Hellyer P, Rodan I, Brunt J, Downing R, Hagerdorn J, Robertson S. AAHA/AAFP pain management guidelines for dogs and cats. J Am Anim Hosp Assoc. 2007;43(5): 235–48.

Mathews K, ed. Update on pain management. Vet Clin North Am Sm Anim Pract. 2008;38(6):1173–490.

Mathews K, Kronen PW, Lascelles D, Nolen A, Robertson S, et al. Guidelines for recognition, assessment and treatment of pain. J Sm Anim Pract. 2014;55(5):E10–E68.

Millis DL, Levine D, Taylor RA. Canine Rehabilitation and Physical Therapy. St Louis: Saunders, 2004.

Silverstein D, Hopper K, eds. Small Animal Critical Care Medicine, 2nd edn. St Louis: Elsevier Saunders, 2015.

WSAVA Global Pain Council Guidelines. Available at: www.wsava.org/guidelines/global-pain-council-guidelines (accessed 3 June 2016).

CHAPTER 20

Veterinary nursing care

Heather Darbo and Cheryl Page
Lakeshore Veterinary Specialists, Glendale, Wisconsin

Introduction

Critical thinking is the intellectually disciplined process of skillfully conceptualizing, analyzing, synthesizing, and applying information that is generated by observation, experience, reflection, reasoning, and communication. An understanding of physiology, a basic knowledge of drug action, and a keen sense of observation combine to create the critical thinking skills required for critical care nursing. The responsibility of the critical care veterinary nurse (also termed technician or nurse technician) is to work as part of a cohesive healthcare team for the benefit of the patient. A systematic approach is essential and the Rule of 20 provides an organized framework for evaluating the patient, anticipating potential complications and recognizing important changes in clinical signs.

The veterinary nursing staff also serve as advocates for the animals in the ICU. Veterinary medicine is very poignant in this regard since the animal patients cannot advocate for themselves. The nursing staff must be conscientious about the therapy being delivered and often need to tailor the process to the individual patient based on their underlying disease process and their tolerance of handling. In addition, it is important to care for pet owners, providing updates on the condition of patients or extending a caring hand whenever possible. Other duties of the critical care nursing team will include oversight of equipment maintenance as well as development and implementation of hospital and patient care guidelines. Appropriate and compassionate nursing care can play a vital role in patient recovery from illness.

Preparedness

A hospital ready area is essential to provide care for patients experiencing critical and potentially life-threatening situations. A ready area should be prepared for incoming patients in a location with easy access for team members (Figure 20.1). A gurney placed near the entrance of the hospital should be available for safe transport of patients.

The ideal location for a ready area will vary between hospitals; in a large ICU, it should be centrally located so that access is maximized for all patients. Additional ready areas may be warranted in sections of the hospital where critically ill patients are kept or where procedures involving sedation or anesthesia are performed. The crash cart should contain all the items required to perform both external and internal cardiopulmonary resuscitation (CPR) (Box 20.1).

It is important that the hospital ready area(s) be well maintained; it must be adequately stocked with necessary supplies and associated equipment and the equipment must be regularly tested for proper function. Ideally, the ready area should be audited twice per day. A check-off list should be created to ensure thorough daily evaluation, and all team members should be aware of the available supplies. If the readiness area is utilized, it should be a priority to return it to its ready state as soon as possible.

The training of new staff members is another important aspect of preparedness. New members of the team can be oriented to the location and purpose of the ready area. Once oriented, they can be assigned to daily inventory duties so that they become familiar with it. An established staff member should be available to provide guidance when necessary. New staff members should be trained in veterinary CPR and established team members should review CPR on a regular basis to maintain cognitive and psychomotor skills. An easy job for inexperienced staff members is the recording of events and drugs during CPR. Figure 20.2 shows an example of a CPR recording sheet.

Cardiopulmonary resuscitation training should include "mock code" situations, which provide invaluable practice for an uncommon and potentially intimidating situation. It is vital to be as realistic as possible when setting up these training situations. The practice session can begin by announcing "code to [hospital area]". As staff arrive, a CPR team leader is established and staff members are assigned to particular jobs such as chest compressions, catheter placement, intubation and respiration, drug administration, recording, and time keeping. Once the code is complete, the team leader and participating staff should have a debriefing session, where the CPR efforts are discussed. The debriefing allows everyone to assess the response to the event both as a team and their individual responses. Chapter 11 discusses how to perform CPR in more detail.

Every patient that is hospitalized should have a preselected CPR code from the owner, such as red (do not resuscitate), yellow (noninvasive resuscitation), and green (all resuscitative efforts including thoracotomy if required). This should be clearly identified on the patient's treatment sheet and cage. If a cardiopulmonary arrest is identified, CPR should be initiated without delay (see Chapter 11). Chest compressions are initiated, while the team is called to the scene. Nursing duties during CPR can be quite varied. Tasks such as contacting the pet owner, performing chest compressions, endotracheal intubation, ventilation, placement of an IV catheter, drug administration, defibrillation, and recording may be assigned to the veterinary nurse. An experienced technician may even lead the CPR efforts when appropriate.

Monitoring and Intervention for the Critically Ill Small Animal: The Rule of 20, First Edition. Edited by Rebecca Kirby and Andrew Linklater.
© 2017 John Wiley & Sons, Inc. Published 2017 by John Wiley & Sons, Inc.

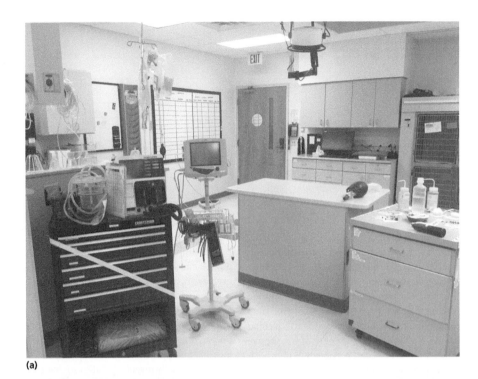

(a)

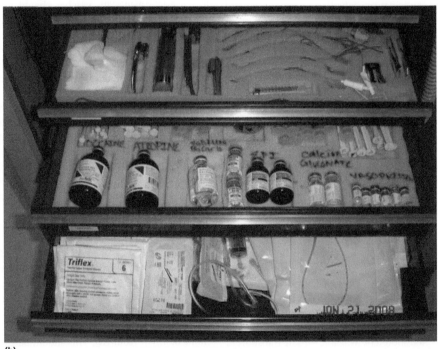

(b)

Figure 20.1 (a) Hospital ready area. Good lighting and central access to equipment and supplies in this area are essential. An examination table can be reserved for emergent patients, with dosing charts, crash cart with supplies (see Table 20.1), materials for IV catheter placement, oxygen source and delivery supplies, monitoring equipment (ECG, ETCO$_2$, pulse oximeter, blood pressure supplies), suction device with Yankauer and whistle-tip apparatus, defibrillator, and AMBU bags all close by. (b) Example of contents that can be located in the first three drawers of a crash cart. The first drawer focuses on airway and breathing, the second on circulation, including medications.

ICU nursing priorities

Triage is the art of prioritizing patients and their treatments based on the severity of their illness. This is an emergency room concept that can also be applied in the ICU environment. When arriving on shift, the ICU nurse technician will review the ICU census sheets, scan the individual treatment sheets, make a general evaluation of each patient, and then triage the patients. Nursing rounds provide vital information used for patient triage and can be done at shift change. At this time, the nurses going off duty can help to prioritize, advise, and direct the oncoming staff regarding patient requirements, treatments, and potential for complications. Organizing the

Box 20.1 Contents of a cardiopulmonary resuscitation (CPR) cart and ready area.

CPR cart contents	Other equipment in the ready area
• Endotracheal tubes of various sizes • Ties • Cuff inflator syringe • Laryngoscope with various blade sizes • Stylets • Drugs: atropine, epinephrine, vasopressin, Na bicarbonate, amiodarone, lidocaine • +/– Drugs for rapid induction of anesthesia or other therapy: etomidate, propofol, benzodiazepines, Ca gluconate, etc. • Syringes of various sizes with 18 G needles attached • Polypropylene catheters and open-ended polypropylene catheter for IT administration of drugs • Saline flushes • Forceps • Sponge forceps – foreign body retrieval	• Suction unit with Yankauer suction tip and whistle tip • Defibrillator • Oxygen source • AMBU bags with PEEP valve or flushed anesthetic machine • IV fluid set-up • IV (+/– IO) catheter materials • Equipment for thoracostomy (open chest CPR) • Sterile gloves • Bandage material • Multiparameter monitor: ECG, ETCO$_2$, blood pressure, SpO$_2$ • Eye lubricant • Thoracocentesis set-up • Recording sheet • Drug dose chart • Scalpel blades • Equipment for open chest CPR

ECG, electrocardiogram; ETCO$_2$, end-tidal carbon dioxide; IO, intraosseous; IT, intratracheal; IV, intravenous; PEEP, positive end-expiratory pressure; SpO$_2$, arterial oxygen saturation.

needs of each patient during rounds allows the technician to make decisions on how to effectively accomplish each of the required tasks. At this time, nursing personnel can be allocated based on the skill level of each member. Prioritizing the needs of each ICU patient will assist in ensuring that the most critical patients are cared for by the most experienced staff.

During cage-side rounds, each treatment sheet and cage card can be reviewed for content, accuracy, and CPR code status. The general physical status of each patient is assessed by reviewing their vital signs and performing a brief physical examination. The veterinary nurse technician will auscultate the thorax, assess pain using the pain scale adopted by the hospital (see Figures 19.2 and 19.3 for an example) and note oral intake, frequency and consistency of urination and defecation, mentation, level of consciousness, and ability to stand. Patients with identified abnormalities of airway, breathing, circulation, level of consciousness or level of pain should be placed strategically in the ICU where they will be observed frequently by all staff members and are treated first. Those with a potential for an impending problem (such as seizures or airway obstruction) should have drug doses precalculated and intervention equipment, such as a laryngoscope and ET tube, set up by the cage. Patients who have transmissible disease should be placed outside of the main flow of traffic and isolated from other susceptible patients.

When using restraint, it is important to determine how much is necessary and whether physical or chemical restraint will be needed to keep everyone safe. A variety of muzzle types and styles made from cloth, plastic or coated wire are commercially available for both dogs and cats. The specific type of muzzle used in a given situation will depend on the patient and disease state. For aggressive animals that cannot be handled without heavy sedation or anesthesia, initial contact may only be possible by administering a sedative that has transmucosal absorption (such as ketamine or buprenorphine) into the mouth or an IM or SC injection of a short-acting anesthetic or tranquilizer. This type of patient should have an Elizabethan collar or cage muzzle placed to protect personnel. A long intravenous fluid line (with extension sets) is attached to the catheter with an injection port located outside the cage for easy access. Direct handling of the animal may be minimal. Treatments and diagnostic procedures for the aggressive patient are prioritized and grouped together with all drugs and equipment ready. This enables everything to be done at the time of sedation, minimizing stress for the patient and protecting the staff from potential injury.

The Rule of 20 for nursing care

The Rule of 20 provides an organized method to evaluate the vital parameters of the small animal ICU patient and anticipate potential complications in preparation for intervention. Many patients enter the ICU with one set of problems but develop additional concerns or complications during their hospitalization.

Nursing notes should be recorded on the medical record or treatment sheet, not only by checking off boxes but also providing a brief but detailed description of the nurse–patient interaction. Recording the times that a treatment is performed and medications administered (Figure 20.3) is important information that will document patient care. Typically, there will be some "default" recommendations for every patient, such as checking an IV catheter every 1–2 hours, daily body weight, and monitoring vital signs (TPR) every 4–6 hours. It is important to group treatments and monitoring procedures together to minimize the handling of the critical patient and utilize nursing staff efficiently. By using the Rule of 20 for nursing care, the staff can prioritize the needs of each patient and provide a balanced approach to patient care.

Perfusion status and fluid balance

The fluid balance in the intravascular (perfusion) and interstitial (hydration) fluid spaces is one of the most important parameters to monitor and maintain in the critical patient. Volume overload can be as detrimental as insufficient fluid volume when the patient has heart or lung dysfunction. Providing fluid therapy is a key component of the care provided in the ICU. Suggestions for IV catheter maintenance and care are provided in Box 20.2.

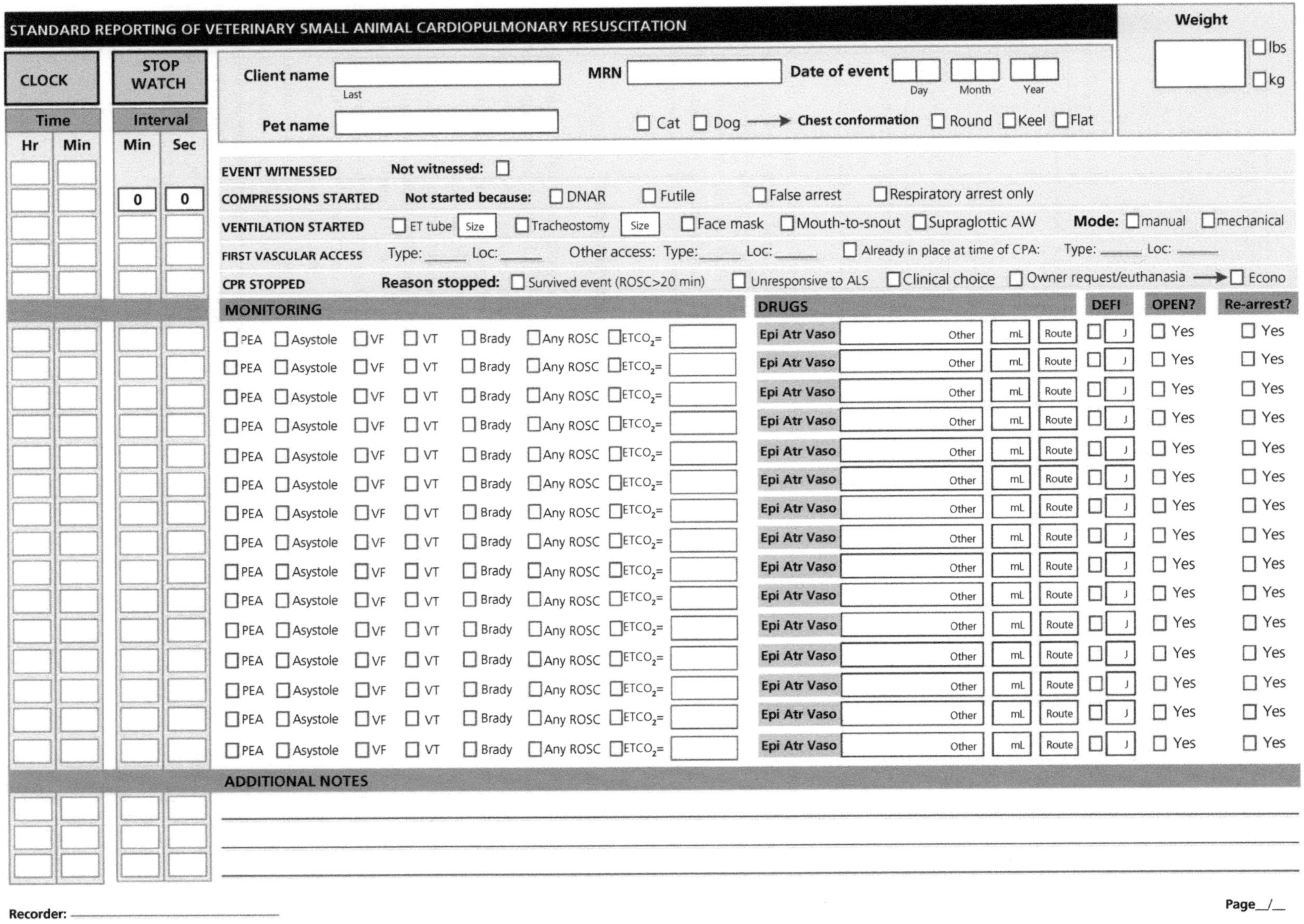

Figure 20.2 Standard case report form for veterinary small animal in-hospital CPR events. ALS, advanced life support; Atr, atropine; AW, airway; Brady, severe bradycardia; CPA, cardiopulmonary arrest; DEFI, defibrillation; Econo, economic; Epi, epinephrine or adrenaline; ET, endotracheal; ETCO₂, end-tidal carbon dioxide; J, joules; Loc, location; MRN, medical record number; OPEN?, was open-chest CPR administered? PEA, pulseless electrical activity; ROSC, return of spontaneous circulation; Vaso, vasopressin; VF, ventricular fibrillation; VT, pulseless ventricular tachycardia. Source: Boeller M, Fletcher DJ, Brainard BM, et al. A Utstein-style guidelines on uniform reporting of in-hospital cardiopulmonary resuscitation in dogs and cats. A RECOVER statement. J Vet Emerg Crit Care 2016;26(1):11–34. Used with permission from Wiley.

STANDARD REPORTING OF VETERINARY SMALL ANIMAL CPR

Date of event ☐☐ ☐☐ ☐☐
       Day Month Year

ADDITIONAL PATIENT INFORMATION

Date of admission ☐☐ ☐☐ ☐☐
       Day Month Year

Disease category at admission (all that apply)

☐ Medical cardiac
☐ Medical non-cardiac
☐ Surgical elective
☐ Surgical emergency
☐ Trauma
☐ DOA
☐ Unknown

Location of CPA (select one)

☐ Out-of hospital
☐ Emergency Room
☐ Intensive Care Unit
☐ Wards
☐ Anesthesia/Surgery
☐ Consult Room
☐ Diagnostic Procedures Area
☐ Waiting Room
☐ Other _____

CPR measures in place at time of CPA (all that apply)

☐ Venous access - peripheral
☐ Venous access - central
☐ Tracheal intubation
☐ ECG monitoring
☐ Arterial catheterization

Client name _____
             Last

Pet name _____

Pet MRN _____

Species ☐ Dog ☐ Cat **Gender** ☐ M ☐ MC ☐ F ☐ FS

Breed _____ **Weight** ☐ kg

Date of birth ☐☐ ☐☐ ☐☐   ☐ lbs
       Day Month Year

Comorbid conditions (all that apply)

☐ Arrhythmia
☐ Congestive heart failure (prior admission)
☐ Congestive heart failure (this admission)
☐ Pericardial effusion/tamponade
☐ Hypotension/Hypoperfusion
☐ Respiratory insufficiency
☐ Pneumonia
☐ Renal insufficiency
☐ Hepatic insufficiency
☐ CNS disease
☐ SIRS

Comorbid conditions (continued)

☐ Sepsis
☐ Infectious disease
☐ Diabetes mellitus
☐ Metabolic or electrolyte disorder
☐ Malignancy
☐ Major trauma
☐ Envenomation
☐ Post-operative
☐ None
☐ Unknown

Pre-arrest severity of illness

APPLE FAST ☐

Pre-arrest functional capacity

Score name: _____

Score: ☐

General anesthesia at time of CPA

☐ Yes
☐ No → **One of the following at time of CPA?** → ☐ Anesthesia induction
                     → ☐ Anesthesia recovery
                     → ☐ Procedural sedation

Previous CPA ☐ Yes: 1 2 3 4 5 x times ☐ No

ADDITIONAL ARREST INFORMATION

Suspected cause of CPA

☐ Life-threatening arrhythmia
☐ Respiratory failure
☐ Heart failure
☐ Trauma
☐ Hemorrhage
☐ Hypovolemia (non-hemorrhagic/non-septic)
☐ Brain disease
☐ Severe sepsis/septic shock
☐ MODS
☐ Metabolic/electrolyte
☐ Toxicity/overdose
☐ Unknown

ADDITIONAL OUTCOME INFORMATION

Duration of sustained ROSC ☐ 20 min – 24 hrs ☐ > 24 hrs

In-hospital event outcome (check one)

☐ Hospital discharge   Date ☐☐ ☐☐ ☐☐   Time __:__
                    Day Month Year   Hour Min

☐ In-hospital death   Date ☐☐ ☐☐ ☐☐   Time __:__
                    Day Month Year   Hour Min

Mode of death after ROSC > 20 min

☐ Euthanasia. Decision based on: →→→→→ ☐ Severity of illness
☐ Re-arrest without CPR →→→ ☐ Terminal illness
☐ Re-arrest w CPR, but w/out sustained ROSC →→ ☐ Economic considerations

Alive at 30 days?

☐ Yes ☐ No → Date of death ☐☐ ☐☐ ☐☐ ☐ Unknown
                            Day Month Year

Post-arrest functional capacity

Extubation: ☐☐ ☐☐ ☐☐
        Day Month Year

    Time __:__

Score name: _____

Score (Time after ROSC): →
→ 1 hour ☐
→ 24 hours ☐
→ Discharge ☐
→ Pre-death ☐

Recorder: _____

Figure 20.2 (*Continued*)

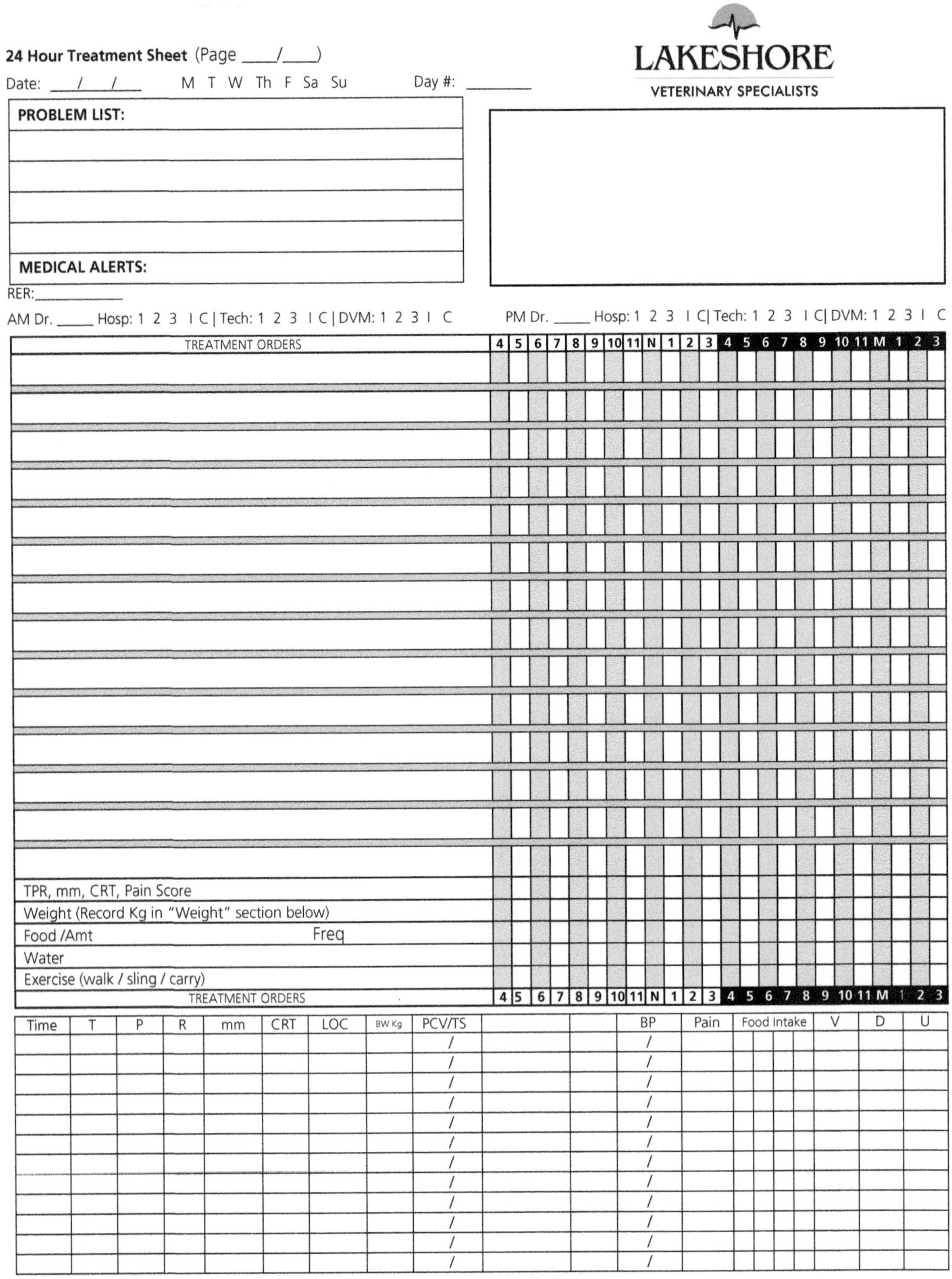

24 Hour Treatment Sheet (Page ____/____)

Date: ___/___/___   M T W Th F Sa Su   Day #: _____

LAKESHORE

VETERINARY SPECIALISTS

PROBLEM LIST:

MEDICAL ALERTS:

RER:_____

AM Dr. _____ Hosp: 1 2 3 I C | Tech: 1 2 3 I C | DVM: 1 2 3 I C   PM Dr. _____ Hosp: 1 2 3 I C | Tech: 1 2 3 I C | DVM: 1 2 3 I C

TREATMENT ORDERS	4	5	6	7	8	9	10	11	N	1	2	3	4	5	6	7	8	9	10	11	M	1	2	3
TPR, mm, CRT, Pain Score																								
Weight (Record Kg in "Weight" section below)																								
Food /Amt Freq																								
Water																								
Exercise (walk / sling / carry)																								
TREATMENT ORDERS	4	5	6	7	8	9	10	11	N	1	2	3	4	5	6	7	8	9	10	11	M	1	2	3

Time	T	P	R	mm	CRT	LOC	BW Kg	PCV/TS			BP	Pain	Food Intake		V	D	U
								/			/						
								/			/						
								/			/						
								/			/						
								/			/						
								/			/						
								/			/						
								/			/						
								/			/						
								/			/						
								/			/						

Figure 20.3 Example treatment (a) and nursing notes sheet (b). Used with permission from Lakeshore Veterinary Specialists.

Fluid infusion involves:
- obtaining the prescribed fluid or combination of fluids
- selection of the best IV drip set (# of drops/mL)
- choosing a method for safe and accurate volume delivery (such as calculation of drops per minute, syringe pump, volumetric pumps, buretrol)
- correctly supplementing the fluids as directed and marking the bags (such as adding glucose or potassium chloride)
- marking the fluid bags with volume versus time to ensure the correct rate and volume of fluid infusion. Stickers are commercially available for marking the fluid bags for volume infused and additives (Figure 20.4).

Catheter / tube	Site	Initial	Date Placed		Patient ID Number:
			/ /		Date:
			/ /		Day # in hospital:
			/ /		Page #: of
			/ /		

Time	Initial	TREATMENTS & OBSERVATIONS

Fluids / Suction														
Time	Initial	Amount	**Total**	Amount	**Total**	Amount	**Total**	Amount	**Total**	Amount	**Total**	Amount	**Total**
	24-Hour totals												

Figure 20.3 (*Continued*)

Often multiple IV lines, tube feeding lines, and a series of pumps are assigned to one patient and must be appropriately labeled. Considerations for fluid therapy in the ICU are discussed in Box 20.3. Formulas and techniques for providing a constant rate of infusion (CRI) for drugs or supplements are provided in Box 20.4.

Once fluid therapy has been initiated, the ICU nurse is assigned the task of monitoring the rate and volume of infusion, as well as the effects of the therapy on the patient. Fluid input should be based on calculated fluid requirements, and reassessed on a regular basis (Table 20.1). Changes in the patient physical peripheral perfusion parameters (heart rate, mucous membrane (MM) color, capillary refill time (CRT), pulse quality) and body temperature often provide the earliest indication of changes in the perfusion and fluid balance.

Box 20.2 Intravenous (IV) catheter protocol [1,2].

IV catheter placement protocol

1. Wash hands with bactericidal soap.
2. Clip hair and perform aseptic skin scrub with chlorhexidine, allowing sufficient skin contact time.
3. Put on gloves; cap, mask, and gown and drape for central venous catheters.
4. Insert catheter into vein.
5. Advance catheter and withdraw stylet.
6. Place injection cap and flush with heparinized saline.
7. Apply topical antibiotic ointment at insertion site.
8. Cover insertion site with sterile gauze or sterile, transparent semipermeable dressing.
9. Use tape to secure catheter to limb or neck.
10. Place support wrap if necessary to protect catheter and maintain flow.

IV catheter maintenance protocol

1. Monitor for patency every 1–2 hours and record fluid volumes.
2. Monitor twice daily for swelling, evidence of hemorrhage, thrombosis or phlebitis. Clinical signs include redness, swelling, heat, discomfort, new fever.
3. Ensure that IV fluids are flowing and/or flush catheter with heparinized saline every 2–4 hours to maintain patency.
4. Monitor for perivascular or limb swelling indicative of fluid extravasation, thrombosis or poor collateral circulation ("fat paw", Figure 21.9).
5. Monitor for occlusions due to venous pressure, patient positioning, viscosity of fluid, tubing occlusion, needle or cannula diameter.
6. Examine IV catheter insertion site once every 24 hours.

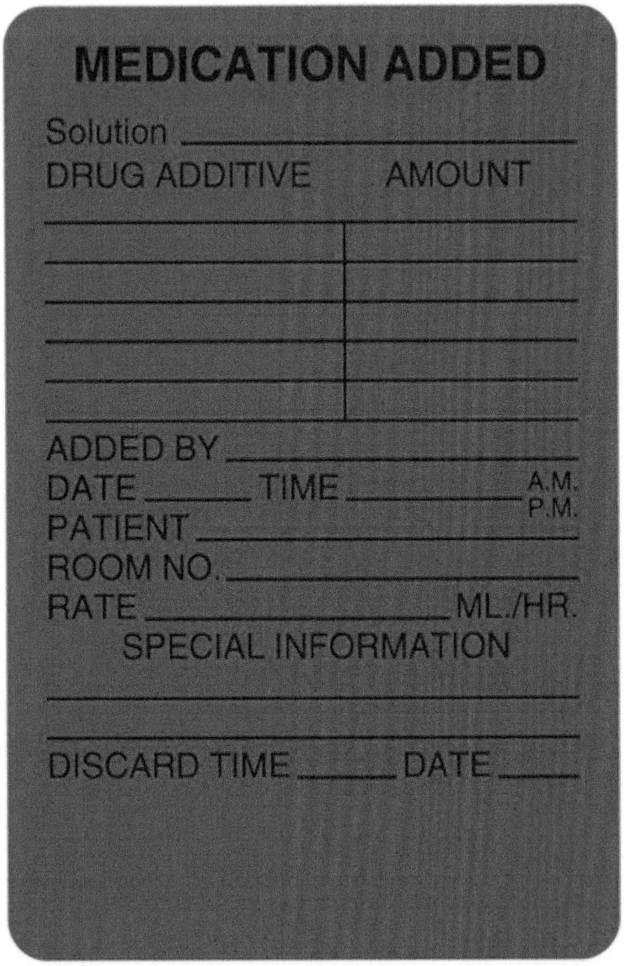
MEDICATION ADDED
Solution ____________
DRUG ADDITIVE AMOUNT
ADDED BY ____________
DATE ______ TIME ______ A.M. P.M.
PATIENT ____________
ROOM NO. ____________
RATE ____________ ML./HR.
SPECIAL INFORMATION
DISCARD TIME ______ DATE ______

Figure 20.4 Fluid additive label. These should be permanently affixed to a fluid bag. Source: United Ad Label, Grand Island, NY. Used with permission.

Box 20.3 Guidelines for properly delivering a fluid therapy plan.

1. Assess patient for fluid deficits or excess:
   Using physical exam findings (see Tables 2.1, 2.2, Box 2.1)
   Using objective data (blood pressure, lactate)
   Using point of care laboratory data (PCV/TP, BUN)
2. Obtain a fluid plan
   Route of administration (IV, IO, enteral, etc.)
   Resuscitate patient (see Box 2.3, Table 2.7)
   Replace deficits
   Monitor for and replace ongoing losses
   Administer maintenance fluids
3. Reassess and adjust fluid plan
   Based on above data
   Account for all "ins": fluids, flushes, drug volumes, enteral intake and blood products
   Account for all "outs": vomiting, diarrhea, urine output, suction from drains
4. Administer IV fluids and medications safely
   Know drug (see Chapter 18) and fluid (see Table 2.9) side-effects
   Determine compatibilities of added drugs and IV fluids
   Monitor the patient for expected or unexpected results
5. Monitor and maintain intravenous catheters (see Box 20.2)
6. Educate and train staff on fluid and drug administration

BUN, blood urea nitrogen; IO, intraosseous; IV, intravenous; PCV, packed cell volume; TP, total protein.

Physical examination findings that reflect the perfusion and hydration status of the patient are listed in Tables 2.1 and 2.2 in Chapter 2. Equipment-based monitoring tools and the results that should trigger concern for decompensation due to fluid imbalance are also discussed. Insufficient fluid balance can result in hypotension and dehydration, which can result in tissue hypoxia. Excessive fluid infusion can cause volume overload with third body fluid spacing and peripheral, lung or brain edema.

Nursing orders are generally carried out every 1–2 hours. Each time a treatment is performed on a patient, the IV fluid infusion rate(s) is rechecked to ensure proper delivery of the prescribed fluids. The fluid line is examined from fluid bag to catheter, as well as examination of the catheterized limb to ensure proper function.

The assessment of the fluid balance over time (24 hours) is dependent upon the quantification of the amount of fluids taken in compared to a careful estimation of the amount of fluids that go out. This should be recorded on the patient flow chart with a progressive total of the volumes noted every 2–4 hours. Fluid input includes oral, IV, tube feedings, and retained irrigants. Fluid output will include urine, wound/tube drainage and loss through vomiting

Box 20.4 A method for calculating a continuous rate infusion for drug delivery. An alternative method is presented in Box 18.3.

1. Simply identify the desired units/minute to determine µg/h or mg/h

$$BW(kg) \times Drug\ dose \times 60\,min/h$$

2. Determine how long your CRI will run based on your determined rate and the total amount of fluids

$$Volume\ of\ fluid\,(mL)/rate\,(mL/h) = \#h$$

3. Now determine the total µg you will use (multiplying step 1 × step 2)

$$µg/h\,(or\,mg/h) \times \#h = \#µg\,(or\,mg)\,to\ add\ to\ bag$$

4. Convert the total mg of the drug into a volume to add to the bag, dividing by the concentration of the drug

$$µg\,(or\,mg)\,total/concentration = \#mL\ to\ add$$

(a volume of fluid should be removed from the fluid bag that is equivalent to the volume of drug being added)

Table 20.1 Common fluid calculations used when caring for the critical patient.

Parameter	Calculation
Daily *maintenance* fluid requirements	(kg$^{0.75}$) x 70 (mL/day) OR 2–4 mL/kg/h (40–60 mL/kg/day)
Daily *replacement* fluid requirements	% dehydration* × 0.6 × kg
Daily *ongoing* fluid requirements	Estimate volumes (mL) lost through tubes, urine, diarrhea, etc.
Daily total fluid requirements	Maintenance + ongoing + replacement
Calculation for drips/sec for manual fluid administration	(mL/h rate) × (#drops/mL)/3600 (sec/h) = # drops/sec

* % dehydration can be estimated as noted in Chapter 2, Table 2.2.

and diarrhea. Voluntary intake should be measured before and after each meal or when fluid is offered. Output can easily be measured if a urinary catheter is in place, with normal urine output in the canine and feline being between 1–2 mL/kg/h. Estimation of the amount of urine in the litter box or excreted on a pad can be made by weighing the material before and after it is placed in the cage. The added weight in grams is approximately the total number of milliliters of urine produced (does not include evaporation).

Assessing the blood volume within the core circulation is an ongoing challenge for the critical care team. The trend of change in the central venous pressure (CVP) can represent the changes in the fluid volume in the central veins in the absence of right heart failure, pneumothorax, mechanical ventilation or pericardial effusion. Normal CVP is 0–5 cmH$_2$O. The target CVP in a patient with normal heart function may be as high as 8–10 cmH$_2$O. A trend of change deviating from the targeted CVP should be reported. CVP measurements can be performed by visual assessment of the pressure with a water manometer or by attaching the manometer to a pressure transducer for an electronic reading.

Blood pressure

Obtaining and recording a baseline blood pressure at the time of admission should be standard of care in the small animal ICU. The consequences of either hypotension or hypertension are detrimental to the critical patient, requiring immediate plans for intervention. There are two techniques for measuring the blood pressure: direct arterial pressure monitoring using an arterial catheter and indirect blood pressure measurement. Monitoring the arterial pressure by the direct method has been the "gold standard" for blood pressure measurement, but it is often not used because of the difficulties in placing and maintaining arterial catheters [3]. A skilled veterinary nurse must place the arterial catheter into one of the peripheral arteries (such as the metatarsal or femoral artery). Most advanced multiparameter monitoring devices (such as SurgiVet®, Waukesha, WI) have a pressure transducer that is connected to the catheter and a monitor to display the systolic, diastolic, and mean arterial pressure numbers as well as the pressure waveform. Materials needed for monitoring direct arterial blood pressure are noted in Figure 3.2, with the supplies and technique for placing and maintaining an arterial catheter in Box 3.2A and Box 3.2B. The steps for measuring the direct arterial blood pressure are listed in Box 3.3.

Noninvasive techniques are more common using an automated oscillometric device or a Doppler ultrasound flow detector. The most common locations to place the Doppler are the palmar arterial arches of the forelimbs and hindlimbs [3], while the tail and pedal arteries can also be used. General guidelines for obtaining indirect blood pressure measurements are provided in Table 3.3 and Figure 3.4. The blood pressure cuff should be 40% of the circumference of the limb being used. When the cuff size is too small, a false elevation in blood pressure will be obtained. Too large a cuff will provide an inaccurate and lower pressure.

The blood pressure should be recorded, noting the position of the patient, the extremity used, and the cuff size to ensure repeatable results. Any variation in these factors can change the blood pressure values obtained. Standard protocol for measurement of noninvasive blood pressure using the American College of Veterinary Internal Medicine consensus statement is noted in Table 3.3, the necessary equipment pictured in Figure 3.4, and the validation criteria listed in Box 3.4.

With every blood pressure measurement, a heart or pulse rate is taken and the results interpreted together. Profound tachycardia can elevate the blood pressure to within a "normal" range in a patient that is unstable and requires IV fluid support. In addition, monitoring the trend of change over time is more important than any single value. Hypotension in a patient that has bradycardia can require different therapeutic intervention than that prescribed for hypotension with tachycardia. Physical examination findings associated with shock are listed in Table 2.1, and further discussion on blood pressure appears in Chapter 3.

Oncotic pull and albumin status

Oncotic pressure (or colloidal osmotic pressure (COP)) is the osmotic pressure exerted by colloids in solution. In the vascular system, the major contributor to the COP is albumin. These large molecules cannot easily pass out of the intravascular space and attract water, maintaining the intravascular fluid volume. Patients at risk for a decrease in the intravascular COP will be prone to fluid shifting from the intravascular to the interstitial space, resulting in peripheral edema (such as conjunctival, hock, facial) and intravascular volume deficits. Clinical signs of low blood protein concentrations are noted in Table 4.3.

The total protein (TP) value from the refractometer can be a rapid and easy means for early identification of changes in blood protein levels. The physical peripheral perfusion parameters are

Hospital name

Patient sticker here

Canine Transfusion Monitoring Record

Pre-transfusion Lab Values:
PCV _____   TP _____   Albumin _____   Platelets _____

Patient Blood Type: _____

Was a Major/Minor Cross Match ordered: Yes   No
Major Cross Match Results: Positive   Negative
Minor Cross Match Results: Positive   Negative
Cross Matched to Donor #: _____

Transfusion Product Type: Whole Blood   FFP   FP   Human Alb
Lyophilized Cryoprecipitate   Lyophilized Albumin   Lyophilized Platelets   PRBC's

Donor ID: _____   **Source:** _____   **Expiration Date:** _____

Was the Patient Pre-medicated?   Yes   No
Pre-medication Name/Amount(mg)/Route of Admin/Time: _____

Date: _____   **Tech:** _____   **DVM:** _____

Vital Signs:

Time		Rate (ml/hr)	Temp	HR	RR	MM	CRT	Transfusion Reactions Signs:
_____	0 min	_____	____	____	____	___	___	_____
_____	15 min	_____	____	____	____	___	___	_____
_____	30 min	_____	____	____	____	___	___	_____
_____	60 min	_____	____	____	____	___	___	_____
_____	90 min	_____	____	____	____	___	___	_____
_____	2 hrs	_____	____	____	____	___	___	_____
_____	3 hrs	_____	____	____	____	___	___	_____
_____	4 hrs	_____	____	____	____	___	___	_____

Remember: Most reactions occur within the first 15-30 minutes of a transfusion. Signs of a possible transfusion reaction include: Fever, Tachycardia, Nausea, Salivation, Vomiting, Facial Edema, Hives, Seizure, Muscle Tremors, Restlessness/Anxiety, Urinary/Fecal Incontinence, Anuria, Coughing, and Increase Respiratory Effort. **If any of these are noted IMMEDIATELY ALERT the DVM overseeing the case.**

***All blood products should be administered w/in 4 hours ***

Post Transfusion Lab Values:
PCV _____   TP _____   Albumin _____   Platelets _____

Figure 20.5 An example template to monitor a patient receiving a transfusion. Used with permission from Lakeshore Veterinary Specialists.

assessed frequently in patients with concern for a low COP for early signs of hypovolemia and poor perfusion.

Decreased albumin production, increased albumin loss, and dilution of plasma proteins with protein-free fluids are all potential causes of a decline in TP and COP. A list of common problems in the small animal ICU patient associated with an altered albumin concentration is presented in Table 4.4. A search for the underlying cause and administration of a synthetic or natural colloid should be pursued. Advantages and disadvantages of synthetic and natural colloid infusion are outlined in Table 4.6 and Table 4.7. A plasma transfusion or administration of canine albumin requires careful monitoring for any signs of a transfusion reaction (Figure 20.5).

Glucose

The small animal ICU patient can experience either hypoglycemic or hyperglycemic episodes, each with their own potential consequences. Monitoring the blood glucose is therefore essential, especially when the underlying problem is known to cause alterations in blood glucose (such as diabetes mellitus, pancreatitis, prolonged seizure activity). Glucose supplementation is an ongoing part of the treatment plan when the patient has liver dysfunction, anorexia has

been prolonged or the patient is young. The amount of blood drawn should be minimized, with the blood used for other tests as well when possible (Table 20.2). The type of glucose analyzer used (such as glucometer, chemistry analyzer, blood gas/electrolyte analyzer) will determine the volume of blood needed, with serial samples best analyzed on the same equipment. Point of care glucometers require small sample volumes, allowing blood to be collected by ear-prick techniques when desired. It must be noted whether the blood glucose sample was taken during fasting or the period of time since feeding.

Patients with hypoglycemia will require IV glucose (typically in the form of dextrose) supplementation. Dextrose is supplied as a 50% solution and is usually diluted prior to administration. However, patients exhibiting seizures, tremors or severe hypotension due to hypoglycemia can require emergent intervention with 0.5 g/kg dose of 50% dextrose. It is better to dilute the solution to 25% for IV bolus administration when possible. The high osmolarity of glucose can cause phlebitis or, if infused outside the vein, perivascular necrosis. Dextrose is not to be administered subcutaneously at any time as the resulting hyperosmolarity may lead to tissue necrosis.

Table 20.2 Considerations for minimizing blood loss from multiple phlebotomies.

Consideration	Rationale
Site of blood collection	Choose vein away from diseased body areas and for optimal patient comfort
Monitoring several parameters	Group requested blood tests together for one blood draw to minimize number of venipunctures
Coagulation status	Use peripheral veins and bandages to minimize hematoma formation in critical body regions
Multiple or repeated blood samples required	Place a catheter to use for blood withdrawal or use an interstitial monitor for glucose
Site and repeated samples	Keep at least one peripheral vein free of venipuncture for IV catheter access should it be required
Patient restraint/sedation	Provide adequate restraint or light sedation to minimize discomfort and complications
Glucose samples	Collect blood from ear veins to save peripheral veins; collection can be done by one person (Figure 5.3). Or consider interstitial monitor instead (Figure 5.4)
Volume of collection	Withdraw the minimal amount of blood needed to run necessary tests
Technique of collection	Use the three-syringe technique with using sampling catheters (Box 10.2)
Apply temporary bandage afterwards	Use to minimize hematoma formation and blood loss

Dextrose that is administered as a CRI should be infused through an IV catheter (peripheral or central). Dextrose is most commonly diluted in crystalloid fluids and administered at a concentration between 1.25% (1.25 g/100 mL) and 5% (5 g/100 mL). A buretrol (Baxter Medical, Deerfield, IL) can be used when short-term dextrose supplementation is anticipated or the concentration of dextrose is likely to change after a few hours. Should a concentration be required that is >5%, it should be administered through a central line. Catheter sites are monitored for signs of perivascular edema or tenderness.

Hyperglycemia associated with diabetes mellitus will necessitate insulin therapy. A CRI of regular insulin is commonly used to initially treat diabetic ketoacidosis or hyperosmolar nonketotic diabetic crises. Frequent assessment of blood glucose is required by collecting blood every 1–4 hours or by placing an interstitial glucose monitor. Adjustments are made to the insulin dose as indicated (see Chapter 5).

Electrolyte and acid–base status

Alterations in blood sodium (Na), potassium (K), ionized calcium (iCa), magnesium (Mg), chloride (Cl), and phosphorus (P) can have important consequences. Causes of specific electrolyte disturbances that commonly occur in the small animal ICU patient are listed in Tables 6.1, 6.2, and 6.3. The clinical signs can be variable and are noted for the specific electrolyte in Table 6.4. The acid–base balance is affected by the electrolyte status and should be assessed by blood gas analysis when an electrolyte disorder has been identified. Blood should be collected in a lithium heparin or serum separator tube. The EDTA anticoagulant in lavender top tubes can alter the K and iCa concentrations. The acid–base analysis must be run immediately after blood collection or the sample stored on ice should a delay in testing be necessary. The procedure for collecting an arterial sample is outlined in Box 8.1. Any residual air in the syringe should be expelled, an air-tight cap placed and the sample stored on ice when transport for analysis is required.

Alterations in blood Na and the treatment for the Na disorder can each cause severe and permanent brain damage when blood Na changes too rapidly. Correction of the Na imbalance begins once perfusion has been restored. The blood Na should be restored to a normal range slowly, at a rate ≤0.5 mEq/h (see Chapter 6).

Hyperkalemia will prolong myocardial cell repolarization, causing ECG changes and affecting perfusion. Medications used to immediately correct the effects of severe hyperkalemia are listed in Table 6.5. Calcium gluconate is infused when clinical signs of hypocalcemia are diagnosed. The ECG is closely monitored when treating hyperkalemia or hypocalcemia, with the electrolyte status rechecked to guide the need for further therapy. Fluid diuresis can result in hypokalemia, causing weakness, ventral flexion of the neck and, if severe, impaired ventilation. Box 6.4 provides a sliding scale for supplementing replacement crystalloid solutions with potassium chloride to prevent hypokalemia associated with IV crystalloid therapy.

Oxygenation and ventilation

Oxygenation describes the ability of the red blood cell to pick up oxygen from the alveoli and transport it to the cell. It is reflected by the PaO_2 and by the saturation of oxygen (SaO_2) from the arterial blood gas and the SpO_2 reading from the pulse oximeter. Ventilation describes the ability of the body to expel carbon dioxide (CO_2). It is reflected by the $PaCO_2$ on the arterial blood gas and the end-tidal CO_2.

Providing a patent airway and ensuring adequate breathing are the first two important interventions in any crisis. The ready area (see Box 20.1, Figure 20.1) will have endotracheal tubes of varying sizes, ties, laryngoscopes, an AMBU bag, and oxygen source available for immediate use. Cage-side oxygen can be delivered through an oxygen cage, oxygen collar or nasal cannula(s) (Box 20.5). Patients with oxygen cages require close monitoring of the environmental temperature, humidity, and concentration of oxygen and CO_2 (see Figure 8.6, Figure 8.7).

Nursing care for patients with oxygenation/ventilation concerns must be completed in a stepwise fashion, providing oxygen and ventilatory support as needed throughout, with minimal stress and ample time for stabilization between handling. The risk–benefit ratio is constantly being examined when performing diagnostic or therapeutic procedures.

It is important to anticipate which patients may be prone to developing a respiratory crisis, initiate appropriate monitoring procedures and prepare ahead of time for rapid intervention. A layrngoscope, endotracheal tubes (see Table 8.8, Table 8.9), tie-in, cuff syringe, rapid induction agents (see Table 8.12), oxygen supply, and AMBU bag should be placed cage side if respiratory failure is possible. Routine monitoring of the respiratory rate and effort, monitoring respiratory pattern, and observing for evidence of orthopnea (see Figure 8.2) are basic monitoring tools. The mucous membrane color is not a reliable indicator of hypoxemia since color change is rare in anemic patients and cyanosis does not appear until severe hypoxemia is present ($PaO_2 < 60$ mmHg). Auscultation of the four quadrants of the thorax (dorso-caudal, dorso-cranial, ventro-caudal, and ventro-cranial) can identify the onset or presence of

Box 20.5 Supplies, placement technique, and oxygen delivery rates for supplemental oxygen therapy [4,5].

Supplies for placing nasal oxygen catheter

- 5, 8, 10, 12 Fr PVC nasal oxygen catheter (Argyle®) or red rubber feeding tube
- Humidifier set-up
- Needle holder
- Suture scissors
- 2-0 or 3-0 monofilament nylon suture
- 22–20 gauge needle
- 2% lidocaine injection, 0.1–0.5 mL (or 0.5% proparacaine)
- 2% lidocaine lubricant
- 1″ waterproof white tape
- O_2 source, flow meter, humidifier, tubing
- Optional: 0.5% phenylephrine drops (to limit bleeding)

Nasal oxygen catheter placement techniques

- Place 0.1–0.5 mL of 2% lidocaine solution into nares.
- Premeasure distance of placement for nasal cannula (from nostril to the vertical ramus of mandible for nasophyarynx, nostril to medial canthus for nasal).
- Place a piece of tape on cannula to mark distance or mark with pen/marker (tape can be used to suture tube in place).
- Apply 2% lidocaine lubricant along tube and on nostril.
- Advance cannula; once in nostril, direct cannula ventrally and slightly medial and advance to mark.
- Secure the tube by inserting a 22–20 gauge needle to pierce the medial septum of the nose. Feed the suture through the sharp end of the needle. Remove needle and place pressure over site if bleeding. Use this suture to secure tube to tape or directly to tube by using a Chinese finger trap or Roman sandal suture technique. This technique decreases the chance of the animal sneezing out the tube.
- Place another suture on the side of face or over the midline of the animal's face and secure the tube to this site (ensure tube cannot rub eye or ear) using Chinese finger trap suturing technique.
- Attach O_2 line with an O_2 tubing adapter or create an adapter from a 1 mL syringe by removing the plunger and cutting off the handle end.
- Use a humidifier to deliver humidified oxygen.
- Keep an Elizabethan collar on at all times.

Oxygen delivery rates

Method	Rate	FiO$_2$
Flow by	2–3 L/min	24–40%
Nasal	1–5 L/min	24–40%
		Or FiO$_2$ = 20% + (4 × O$_2$ rate)
	50–150 mL/kg/min	30–70%
Mask	5–10 L/min	40–60%
Hood	1–2 L/min	30–40%
Incubator	Higher rates	Up to 60%

pulmonary edema or pleural fluid. A pulse oximeter can provide an ongoing assessment of the hemoglobin saturation.

Additional therapeutic intervention for respiratory disorders can vary from providing continuous suction of a thoracic tube, management of trachesotomy tubes, administering nebulization and coupage to, the most challenging, support of the ventilator patient. Suggestions and general guidelines for maintaining and monitoring a critical patient with an oxygenation/ventilation disorder are outlined in Table 20.3.

Neurological status

Repeated neurological examinations are the primary means of detecting neurological decompensation in the ICU patient. The method of performing the examination and the interpretation of the findings should be standardized amongst the critical care team members. A short form should be available to prompt a thorough evaluation and facilitate rapid recording of the findings (Figure 20.6). The modified Glasgow Coma Scale (see Table 12.4) is used when evaluating a small animal with serious intracranial disease (such as head trauma, stupor, coma or other intracranial disease).

The most observable neurological findings are related to the mentation and level of consciousness of the animal. It is noted whether the animal is alert and responsive, depressed, has uncontrolled hyperexcitability (dysphoria or dementia), is obtunded (mild, moderate or severe) or is unconscious (stupor and coma) [6]. The common causes of altered mentation and level of consciousness are listed in Table 12.1. Blood glucose, blood pressure, SpO$_2$, and the list of medications administered are quickly assessed as a possible cause of a sudden decline.

Patients that are agitated, dysphoric or prone to seizures will require extra padding of the cage bottom and sides to minimize trauma. Animals with seizure activity require continuous observation, with anticonvulsant drug and dose predetermined and readily available for immediate intervention, when needed. If seizure activity is frequent or prolonged, a CRI of anticonvulsant medications may be prescribed. The response to the drugs is reported hourly and the guidelines followed for maintaining and monitoring an unconscious patient.

The level of consciousness is reported hourly for the patient that is unconscious or has head injury. The physical peripheral perfusion parameters and blood pressure (BP) are monitored, with signs of hypotension or hypertension warranting immediate reporting and intervention. Many head-injured patients require heavy sedation or anesthesia to prevent thrashing, with the head and neck on a 15–20° incline above the body. Occlusion of the jugular vein is avoided and placement of nasal lines must avoid stimulation of a sneeze response. Decreased tear production is likely and requires regular lubrication of the corneas to prevent drying and corneal ulceration. Monitoring the eyes with the Schirmer tear test, fluoroscein staining, and intraocular pressure may be beneficial, with signs of redness, squinting, ocular pain or abnormal eye discharge reported and treated as indicated. Further nursing guidelines for the unconscious and head-injured small animal patient are often similar to a ventilator patient, and Table 20.3 can be used as a guide.

Patients with limited mobility due to head or spinal disorders require particular care. Small animal patients with a spinal disorder are moved by gurney or carried by supporting the length of the body, under the chest and hips. A sling (Figure 20.7), stanchion apparatus (Figure 20.8) or custom harness (Help 'Em Up Harness®, Denver, CO) can be used for support if the animal is not able to fully bear its own weight. Rehabilitation therapy (such as passive range of motion, massage) may be an important part of the recovery plan.

Patients with musculoskeletal disease (such as tetanus or permethrin toxicity) or neuromuscular disease may be hyperresponsive to touch or sound. A gentle hand is required during patient contact and the environment should be calm and quiet to minimize external stimulation. The respiratory rate and effort are closely monitored in animals with lower motor neuron

Table 20.3 Monitoring and nursing concerns for a sedated and intubated patient (e.g., receiving therapeutic ventilation).

Monitoring/nursing concerns	Frequency	Notes
Electrocardiogram	Continuous	Use adhesive contact pads to avoid skin injury from ECG clips
Pulse oximetry	Continuous	Ensure mucosal surface used is clean and moist; may require frequent repositioning at alternate mucosal sites
End-tidal CO_2	Continuous	Can significantly increase dead space in small animals
Blood pressure	Hourly	Assess perfusion and evaluate need for vasopressors; continuous BP monitoring possible with arterial catheter and pressure transducer
Blood gas (arterial)	q 4–12 h	Maintain $PaCO_2$ 35–60 mmHg and PaO_2 80–120 mmHg
Electrolytes/chemistry	q 4–24 h	Consider central line if frequent blood collections are needed. Be aware of quantity of blood withdrawn (see Table 20.2)
Ventilator settings	q 1 h	Evaluate inspiratory pressure, respiratory rate, tidal volume, FiO_2, need for PEEP; set alarms (see Table 8.13)
Oral care	q 4–6 h	Prevent desiccation, collection of biofilms, pressure sores and ulcerations; can use subglottal suctioning; use only cleaned instruments orally (pulse oximetry probe)
Change ET tube	q 12–48 h	Change when necessary; utilize sterile technique
Deflate cuff and move ET tube	q 4 h	Prevents pressure necrosis of trachea
Move/replace or relieve ET tube tie-in	q 4 h	Replace tie-in every 24 hours; do not use gauze as tie-in since it maintains a moist environment with bacteria
Suction ET tube	q 2–6 h	Preoxygenate, do not occlude ET tube, perform using sterile technique, limit to 15 sec
Chest tube site (if applicable)	q 2–12 h	Monitor bandage for soiling and entry site for evidence of infection
Pleural suction port (if applicable)	Continuously	As above
Humidify airway	q 4–6 h	Instill sterile normal saline into ET tube (0.1–0.2 mL/kg); controversy regarding increased risk of infection (ventilator-associated pneumonia)
Nebulization	Continuous or q 2–6 h	Use of a mechanical device requires changing of filters q 24–48 h; monitor body temperature if heated, could result in hyperthermia; water condensation could increase risk of bacterial colonization/infection
Coupage	q 4–6 h	Avoid if patient prone to pneumothorax or severe chest wall disease; benefit arguable in these patients
Eye lubrication	q 2–4 h	Prevents corneal dryness and resultant ulceration
Musculoskeletal care	q 4–12 h	Provide good surface padding, passive range of motion manipulations, hydrotherapy, rotation of dependent sides and spontaneous breathing trials when indicated
Urinary care	q 4–8 h	Place and maintain sterile urinary catheter or express urinary bladder to monitor urine output
Gastrointestinal care	q 2–12 h	Administration of medications, placement of feeding tube, ulcer prevention can be required
Nutrition	q 1–4 h	Provide a CRI of liquid diet through a feeding tube with regular aspiration of residual gastric contents; oropharyneal suctioning may be required
Tracheostomy tube site	q 6–12 h	Change bandage, clean skin entry site
IV catheter sites	q 1–2 h	Monitor for redness, swelling, discharge, etc. (see Box 20.1)
Fluid totals	q 1–2 h	Total "ins" and "outs"
Temperature	q 2–6 h	Monitor with esophageal or rectal probe for continuous measurements
Oxygenation indices	q 2–12 h	See Table 8.1
Level of sedation	Continuous	Assess needs of patient; a combination of injectable drugs as a CRI is administered. The rate of infusion or drugs can be changed based on the needs of the patient
Ventilator waveforms	Continuous	Identifies drastic short-term changes and trends of change which are important, but interpretation can be difficult
Rule of 20 assessment	q 12 h	Meet the ongoing patient needs

CRI, constant rate infusion; ECG, electrocardiogram; ET, endotracheal; IV, intravenous; PEEP, positive end-expiratory pressure.

disease since hypoventilation is a common complication. Enteral feeding is closely monitored since gastric and esophageal motility may be impaired and contribute to complications such as aspiration pneumonia.

Coagulation

Disorders of coagulation (inadequate clotting or thrombosis) can be part of the presenting complaint or can develop during the course of critical illness. A variety of illnesses can result in altered coagulation (see Box 9.1). There are also several conditions known to be associated with thrombosis (see Table 9.10). A coagulopathy

of some form should be anticipated in animals with the systemic inflammatory response syndrome (SIRS; see Chapter 1).

Monitoring the clotting times can provide the first evidence of hypocoagulation, with the presence of physical signs a much later manifestation. Clinical signs of shock can occur with ongoing hemorrhage, manifested by tachycardia (dogs), bradycardia (cats), tachypnea, weak pulses, dull mentation, prolonged CRT, pale mucous membranes, and altered blood pressure.

Table 9.1 discusses physical examination changes associated with altered coagulation. The presence of ecchymotic hemorrhage (see Figure 9.3) and petechiation (see Figure 9.4) can be a consequence

Mentation:	Posture:
Behavior:	Gait:

Cranial Nerves	Left	Right	Cranial Nerves	Left	Right
Menace (II, VII)			Facial symmetry (VII)		
Visual Placement			Strabismus		
Pupillary Light reflex (II, III)			Nystagmus		
Dark adaptation (II, sympathetic)			Spinal accessory (XII)		
Palpebral reflex (V, VII)			Tongue (XII)		
Corneal reflex (V, VI, VII)			**Other**		
Response to nasal stimulation (V)			Nociception		
Oculovestibular reflex (V, III, IV, VI)			Anal tone/sensation		
Gag reflex (IX, X)			Perineal reflex		
Jaw tone (V)			Tail tone		

Spinal Reflexes	Left	Right	Posautral Reactions	Left front	Right front	Left hind	Right hind
Biceps			Proprioception				
Triceps			Hopping				
Flexor (withdrawal, fore)			Visual placement				
Deep Pain (forelimb)			Tactile placement				
Patellar			Wheelbarrow				
Cranial Tibial			Stairs				
Sciatic			Hemi walk				
Flexor (withdrawl, hind)			Tactile placement				
Gastrocnemius			Extensor postural thrust				
Deep Pain (hind)			Voluntary movement				
X Extensor							
Cutaneous Trunci							

Localization	
Differential diagnosis	

Plans	Diagnostic	Therapeutic	Monitoring

Figure 20.6 Neurological examination form. Used with permission from Lakeshore Veterinary Specialists.

of hypocoagulation. Figures 9.5 and 9.6 demonstrate some changes associated with thrombosis. The 5 Ps can be used to assess a peripheral limb for the presence of thrombosis (such as occurs in feline aortic thromboembolism): Pallor, Pain, Paresis, temPerature (hyPothermia), and Pulselessness.

It is important to minimize blood loss after phlebotomy or surgical procedures in a patient with a coagulation disorder. Bandages should be temporarily placed over any phlebotomy site, and removed when hemostasis is assured. The technique for blood collection in a patient at risk for coagulopathy is outlined in Box 9.2 and Table 20.2. Patients at risk for bleeding should have coagulation testing (see Table 9.2, Box 9.3, Box 9.4) performed prior to invasive procedures (such as surgery, biopsies, aspirates or placement of invasive devices such as central lines). Patients suffering from traumatic hemoabdomen may have abdominal counterpressure placed (see Box 10.5, Figure 10.2) with close monitoring essential (Table 20.3). Clinical signs of hemorrhage will often prompt the administration of a blood transfusion (see Table 10.7).

Red blood cells and hemoglobin

Several physical examination findings can be due to an alteration in the red blood cell (RBC) count (see Table 10.2). A low RBC count (anemia) results in poor oxygen delivery to the tissues. A high RBC count (erythrocytosis) impairs blood flow. The list of causes of increased or decreased RBC count can be found in Tables 10.3 and 10.5. Assessing the physical status of the patient is as important as assessing their laboratory data. Laboratory changes may not occur in patients with acute hemorrhage until after fluid resuscitation.

Minimizing blood loss from the patient by grouping blood draws, using appropriate techniques, and minimizing injury to the vessel (see Table 20.2) is important for avoiding iatrogenic causes of anemia. The three-syringe technique used to collect blood samples from a central catheter is outlined in Box 10.2. Point of care testing will include the PCV, TP, RBC count and blood smear to evaluate RBC morphology and reticulocyte response. The microhematocrit tube will be used to determine the PCV, can demonstrate hemolysis (red) or icterus (yellow) from the color of the serum and provide plasma for determining the TP (see Figure 1.7). Evaluation of blood

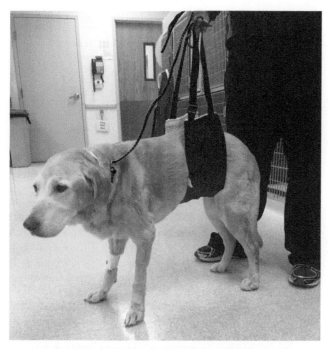

Figure 20.7 Large sling used to support dogs to stand and walk when neurological or orthopedic problems prevent normal mobility; various sizes are available. (Four Flags Over Aspen, St Claire, MN)

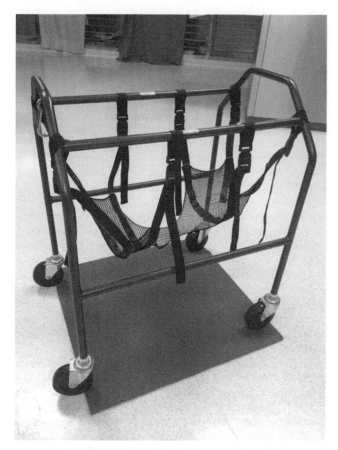

Figure 20.8 A custom-made stanchion used to support larger dogs in a standing position and assist with rehabilitation. Note the stanchion is on wheels resting on a gripping floor surface to prevent accidental rolling.

Table 20.4 Monitoring a patient with external abdominal counterpressure [7].

Monitoring parameters	Frequency
Physical parameters: HR, MM/CRT, RR, RE	Every 15 min when wrap is in place
Oxygen saturation	Every 5 min as wrap is being removed
Indirect systolic BP or MAP (if oscillometric method)	Every 15 min when wrap is in place. Continuously as wrap is removed; if BP drops by more than 5 mmHg, stop unwrapping, evaluate for rebleeding and consider rebinding; determine need for IV fluids or blood transfusion to stabilize perfusion
Urine output	Every 1 h
Temperature – axillary, ear or rectal	Every 1 h
PCV/TP	Every 2–4 h when wrap is in place

BP, blood pressure; CRT, capillary refill time; HR, heart rate; MM, mucous membrane; MAP, mean arterial pressure; RE, respiratory effort; RR, respiratory rate.

smears is critical to identify changes in red cell morphology (see Table 10.7), to accurately identify platelet numbers (see Box 9.3) and morphological changes, performing a reticulocyte count (see Box 10.4) and performing a pretransfusion saline agglutination test (see Box 10.3) or cross-match (Box 20.6). A reticulocyte count is done with new methylene blue stain.

When anemia causes clinical signs, a blood transfusion is warranted. Most commonly, blood is delivered as component therapy, giving only that portion of the blood that is necessary for the patient. Acute blood loss typically requires both RBCs and plasma, given in the form of whole blood or packed RBCs (pRBC) in combination with plasma. Animals with prolonged clotting times but without anemia may only require plasma transfusions. Pretransfusion testing such as a blood type and cross-match is important but does not rule out the possibility of a transfusion reaction. The set-up for component transfusion and guidelines for monitoring for transfusion reaction are noted in Figure 20.5.

Occasionally, blood is collected from the thoracic or abdominal cavity and administered back to the patient, called an autologous blood transfusion (ABT). Collection of ABT is performed in a sterile fashion with a centesis or in surgery, and the blood administered through a filter. The ABT is discussed further in Chapter 10.

Heart Rate, contractility, and rhythm

The goal is to assess whether or not the cardiac output is adequate for delivering sufficient quantities of oxygen to the tissues in light of the ongoing disease process. Cardiac output is dependent upon heart rate and stroke volume. The stroke volume is dependent upon preload (IV volume status), contractility (inherent ability of the heart muscle to contract), and afterload (resistance). The heart rate in beats per minute should be appropriate for the species, age, size, and current clinical condition of the animal and is assessed along with other physical perfusion parameters. It is important to be aware of medications that the patient may be receiving that can affect cardiac function and blood pressure (see Table 3.1).

Using a stethoscope, the heart is auscultated for abnormal sounds while palpating the pulses to see if the two are synchronous. The dorsal pedal and femoral pulses are palpated most often. Pulses that are bounding suggest a hyperdynamic state. Weak or absent pulses

Box 20.6 Procedure for performing a donor-recipient cross-match to assess blood transfusion compatibility [8].

1. Obtain an ETDA (lavender top tube) blood sample from the recipient.
2. Obtain an ETDA (lavender top tube) blood sample from the donor or a blood sample in a red top tube from the stored blood to be transfused (citrate anticoagulant present).
3. Centrifuge donor and recipient samples for 10 minutes at 3500 rpm.
4. Set up the following grid (while the blood is spinning) to set the samples on and record the results.

Cross-match grid

	DONOR	RECIPIENT
PLASMA		
RBCs		

5. Remove the plasma from both the donor and recipient samples and place in its own Sedi-Cal tube or StatSpin tube. Label donor tube #1 and recipient tube #2.
6. Remove 0.05 cc of donor red blood cells and place in a Sedi-Cal or StatSpin tube.
7. Repeat the procedure with the recipient red blood cells and place in a separate Sedi-Cal or StatSpin tube.
8. Place 1.2 cc of 0.9% sodium chloride in each Sedi-Cal or StatSpin tube that contain RBCs to make the RBC solution 4%. Label donor suspension #3 and recipient suspension #4.
9. To perform the cross-match, first label your slides #1–4 (or D, R, minor and major). On the appropriate slide, combine drops as indicated below and rock the slide to mix the samples:
   - 1 drop donor plasma and 1 drop donor RBC (serves as donor control)
   - 1 drop recipient plasma and 1 drop recipient RBC (serves as recipient control; this is also a saline agglutination test)
   - 1 drop donor plasma and 1 drop recipient RBC (or minor cross-match)
   - 1 drop recipient plasma and 1 drop donor RBC (or major cross-match).
   Place a coverslip on each slide. After five minutes have passed, observe the slide for macroagglutination, then examine each slide under the 40× objective microscope for signs of agglutination which indicate incompatibility (see Box 10.3).

D, donor; EDTA, ethylenediaminetetraacetic acid; R, recipient; RBCs, red blood cells.
Sedi-Cal tube, Becton Dickinson, Franklin Lakes, NJ.
StatSpin tube, StatSpin Technologies, Norwood, MA.

can reflect a drop in blood pressure and measurement of BP is indicated. The jugular veins are examined and palpated for a pulse or distension associated with an increase in right heart pressure (such as right heart failure, pericardial effusion). Tachycardia, bradycardia or pulse deficits all warrant an assessment of the heart rhythm by electrocardiogram (ECG).

Leads I, II, and III are most commonly assessed in small animal patients, with additional data available from augmented leads: aVR, AVL, aVF. Lead II is used when continuous monitoring of the ECG is needed. The leads can be placed using clips on the skin or adhesive strips with metal tabs for lead attachment. Hair should be clipped and electrode gel placed at the site of lead attachment for better contact. ECG artifact waves can occur from poor lead contact, respiration, movement, and electrical interference. Rates that are less than 60 or greater than 150 (180 in small dogs and cats) or do not have a normal P-QRS-T waveform (see Chapter 11) should be reported and preparation made for intervention, if needed.

Clinical evidence of poor cardiac contractility will vary and can include pulmonary edema, pleural effusion, pericardial effusion, abdominal effusion, weakness, syncope, coughing, labored breathing, poor perfusion, cyanosis, and exercise intolerance. The clinical assessment of cardiac contractility is more difficult. Patients with moderate or severe deficits in the cardiovascular system should be moved via gurney and not forced to walk. Echocardiography can be performed at the cage side and can give an impression of heart chamber size, pericardial fluid or mass, ejection fraction, and contractility. Pericardial effusion can exert pressure on the right heart and prevent adequate preload. Ultrasound-guided pericardiocentesis will be required with continuous ECG monitoring and fluid support. The administration and monitoring of drug therapy for stabilizing cardiac disorders (such as dobutamine, nitroprousside, antiarrhythmic drugs) require careful drug dose calculation and administration set-ups, as well as close monitoring of ECG, BP, and physical perfusion parameters.

Any extreme change in any of the parameters monitored in the Rule of 20 can be a sign of impending decompensation and warrants preparation for CPR. Some of the more common warning signs of an impending cardiac arrest are listed in Table 20.5.

Renal function

The urinary tract status is important to many components of the Rule of 20, including fluid, electrolyte and acid–base balance, excretion of metabolic wastes, reabsorption of important compounds (glucose, aminio acids), RBC production, drug excretion, and BP. Blood tests that reflect renal function include the serum BUN and creatinine. The urinalysis with specific gravity and sediment will demonstrate the concentrating ability of the kidneys, cast formation or evidence of inflammation within the urinary tract.

Azotemia is often classified as prerenal, intrarenal, or postrenal. Prerenal azotemia is caused by a decrease in blood flow to the kidneys and is often completely reversible with restoration of adequate renal perfusion. Problems associated with prerenal, renal, and postrenal azotemia are listed in Table 13.1. A list of drugs that are potentially nephrotoxic is provided in Table 13.8. Patients receiving one or more of these drugs require careful monitoring for evidence of acute kidney injury. Several methods for staging patients with kidney disease are available (Tables 13.5, 13.6, and 13.7) and can be used as an objective assessment of the renal status for patients.

Estimation of the fluid balance (see Chapter 2) is essential, including perfusion and hydration physical parameters and body weight. Oliguria (decreased urine formation) can manifest with signs of fluid overload such as edema, bounding pulses, increased respiratory effort and rate, chemosis, and serous nasal discharge. Monitoring the amount of fluid going in and coming out can provide insight into the fluid balance of the patient with urinary tract disorders.

Urine output can be monitored through a variety of techniques. Weighing blankets or urinary pads to estimate urine production is a noninvasive means of estimation. The placement of an indwelling urinary catheter allows for quantitation of urine production and assurance of urine outflow and helps to maintain the hygiene of the patient. Materials needed, methods of placement, and care of the urinary catheter and collection system are outlined in Box 20.7 and Box 20.8. Appropriate placement of a urinary catheter can be confirmed with ultrasound or radiographs.

Table 20.5 Clinical signs of impending cardiopulmonary arrest [9].

Parameter	Common changes	Description/notes
Change in breathing pattern	Agonal – gasping motions in an unconscious patient	Ineffective reflex respiratory motions
	Cheyne–Stokes – rhythmic waxing and waning of respiratory rate and effort	Severe generalized cerebral cortical disorder, typically unconscious patient, insufficient for oxygenation and ventilation
	Apneustic – nonrhythmic changes in respiratory rate and effort	Severe brainstem lesion in unconscious animal
Change in HR or ECG	Bradycardia	HR <50 bpm (dogs) and <100 bpm (cats) can reduce cardiac output and predispose to cardiac arrest
	R on T phenomenon	
	Torsades de pointes	Prefibrillatory heart rhythms
	(tachyarrhythmias)	Most rhythms of cardiac arrest; patient is unconscious
	Ventricular fibrillation, pulseless electrical activity, sinus arrest, pulseless ventricular tachycardia	
Blood pressure	Dramatic drop or no obtainable indirect BP reading	
Physical perfusion parameters	Late decompensatory stage of shock (terminal stage)	Cerebral hypoxia, swelling, hemorrhage or herniation
	Declining level of consciousness, unresponsive	Severe shock, insufficient cardiac output, poor peripheral perfusion
	Weak or absent pulse pressure	
	CRT >3 sec or absent	Shunting blood flow to brain and heart
	Hypothermia	Anemia, severe shock
	Pale or white MM color	$PaO_2 < 60$ mmHg
	Blue MM color	
Body posture	Decerebrate or decerebellate rigidity	Brain herniation likely, severe increase in intracranial pressure

CRT, capillary refill time; HR, heart rate; MM, mucous membranes; BP, blood pressure; ECG, electrocardiogram.

Box 20.7 Guidelines for placing urinary catheters in male and female dogs and cats [10].

Urinary catheterization of males

- Choose appropriate catheter size and style.
- Administer sedation/anesthesia as necessary.
- Place in lateral or dorsal recumbency.
- Clip long hairs around prepuce and rinse clean with diluted iodine solution.
- Use 1 person to extract penis and second person to prepare the site and place the urinary catheter.
- Clean tip of penis with dilute iodine or chlorhexidine solution and sterile water.
- Wear sterile gloves to handle urinary catheter.
- Premeasure catheter from tip of penis to the urinary bladder trigone and mark for length to be inserted.
- Apply sterile lubricant to tip of the sterile urinary catheter.
- Insert catheter tip into urethra and slowly advance catheter. (Cats will require caudal +/- dorsal retraction of penis/prepuce to straighten urethral flexure.)
- Connect to sterile, closed urine collection system.
- Confirm placement with radiograph.
- Inflate balloon if Foley catheter inserted and/or suture other catheter type in place using:
  - butterfly tape tabs around catheter
  - stay sutures on both sides of prepuce
  - suture through butterfly tap and stay sutures
  - secure to side of abdomen or rear leg with adequate "slack" to allow animal to sit or move comfortably.

Urinary catheterization of females

- Choose appropriate catheter size and style (Foley style most common for females).
- Sedate or anesthetize as necessary.
- Place in sternal recumbency with support under caudal abdomen: legs can be hanging off edge of table (cats in lateral recumbency).
- Clip, clean, and rinse vulva with dilute iodine or chlorhexidine solution and sterile saline,
- Place 2% lidocaine jelly around vulva region.
- Wear sterile gloves and premeasure catheter for insertion length.
- One of two techniques is commonly selected for placement in dogs (cats are placed with a blind technique without palpation).
  - *Visualization with speculum and light source:* insert lubricated sterile speculum into vagina.
  - Use light to locate urethral opening
  - Insert lubricated sterile urinary catheter and advance to premeasured length or until urine flows.
  - *Blind technique with digital palpation:* insert sterile gloved and lubricated finger into vagina, advancing craniad 2–5 cm while palpating ventral floor to locate urethral opening (papilla).
  - Insert sterile, lubricated catheter into urethral orifice, using inserted finger to guide catheter.
  - Pressing the catheter tip downward with the finger over the urethral papilla, guide the catheter tip into the urethra.
  - Advance the catheter to the premeasured length or until urine flows.
- Connect catheter to a sterile, closed urine collection system.
- Confirm catheter placement with radiograph if desired.
- Inflate balloon of Foley catheter and suture catheter in place:
  - using a butterfly tape
  - stay sutures on either side of the vulva
  - suture through butterfly tap and stay sutures
  - secure tubing to rear leg with adequate "slack" in the line to allow animal to sit or move comfortably.

Immune and white blood cell status, antibiotic stewardship, and maintenance of barrier nursing

The basic nature of critical illness implies that inflammation is occurring in the patient with repeated challenges to their immune systems. The patient may be immunosuppressed either from their disease process or from medications, have been exposed to

infectious agents in the ICU or have had invasive procedures done (such as surgery, IV catheters), each increasing the risk of hospital-acquired infection.

The critical care team must remain conscious of their role in minimizing the spread of pathogens between patients and minimizing the risk of developing a hospital-acquired infection. This will include the separate housing of potentially infectious patients and those that are immunocompromised. Hand washing with antibacterial soap between patients is the number one barrier technique to be utilized, even when gloves are worn during patient handling. Box 20.9 outlines common practices and procedures that each team member should utilize when treating the ICU patient.

Bacterial resistance to antibiotics is common in the ICU environment, requiring practical but stringent guidelines for antibiotic selection and usage in the ICU. Monitoring bacterial resistance to specific antibiotics through use of the antibiogram can become an important responsibility of the critical care team (see Figure 14.5). Obtaining the appropriate samples for culture and susceptibility testing is critical and suggested procedures are outlined in Table 14.1. Participating in hospital surveillance for nosocomial pathogens is an important component of critical care nursing.

Following trends in the white blood count (WBC) can provide an indication of the inflammatory and immune response of the patient. Steps for evaluating a peripheral blood smear are provided in Box 14.2, with steps for reporting the WBC differential in Box 14.3. The general patterns of WBC response to inflammation are listed in Table 14.5 and Table 14.6. Common causes of elevations or decreases in specific WBC lines are listed in Table 14.6.

Gastrointestinal tract status

The gastrointestinal (GI) tract is lined with a mucosal layer that forms a barrier between the body and the luminal environment. The lumen not only contains nutrients but also is full of potentially

---

Box 20.8 Guidelines for the nursing care of urinary catheters in male and female dogs and cats [10].

- Use a sterile closed collection system that limits or avoids disconnection.
- Wash hands and wear sterile gloves immediately prior to handling the system.
- Attach fluid collection bag to urinary outflow line to allow collection and measurement of urinary output.
- Place sign alerting staff to avoid closing urinary system tubing in cage door (causing kink in line or disconnection).
- Place bag in a clean pan, on a clean pad or attach it to lower cage – do not place urine collection bag on floor.
- Measure and empty urine from bag every 4–6 hours; remove urine using aseptic technique.
- Inspect system for occlusion each time staff interacts with patient or q 4h.
- Avoid flushing fluid into the system.
- Remove catheter as soon as possible.
- Keep prepuce or vulvar region clean and dry.
- Clean the external components of the urinary collection system with dilute chlorhexidine solution if soiled.
- Replace the urinary collection system every 72h or if occluded.
- Monitor urine for evidence of new infection and submit urine for culture and susceptibility if concern for catheter-related or other urinary tract infection.

Box 20.9 Barrier nursing techniques for the general patient population with additional procedures for patients with transmissible diseases or immunocompromise.

General ICU patient population

- Wash hands with antibacterial soap before and after handling each patient.
- Wear gloves when placing or maintaining invasive devices (such as IV, urinary catheters).
- Wipe IV injection port with alcohol pad prior to injection or collection of blood.
- Provide appropriate "sterile" preparation of any area having a catheter placed (such as prepuce, vulva, skin).
- Make appropriate antibiotic selection (see Chapter 14).
- Cover areas where nonintact skin is exposed (such as catheters, wounds, surgical site).
- Regularly inspect sites where skin is not intact for signs of inflammation or infection.
- Clean equipment, tables, cages, and other surfaces between every patient using appropriate cleaning products (quaternary ammonium) with sufficient contact time.

Patients with transmissible disease or immunocompromise

- Initiate the procedures listed above.
- Wear gloves, disposable waterproof gowns/suits, mask and goggles or face shield, shoe covers.
- Provide separate isolation area for patients with transmissible disease.
- Provide a separate isolated area for immunosuppressed patients.
- Place visible signs alerting staff and visitors to possible transmissible disease or immunocompromised patient.
- Limit transport of patients through hospital (consider using gurney).
- Reserve equipment used for infectious or immunocompromised patients for the duration of hospitalization, and decontaminate appropriately when no longer needed.
- Limit consumable items brought into isolation or immunocompromised patient area; unused items should be discarded when no longer needed.
- Dispose of waste material and items from patients with possible zoonotic diseases or chemotherapy patients into red disposal bags and other appropriate hazardous waste containers. Dispose of hazardous waste as required by state regulations.
- Alert appropriate authorities regarding transmissibile diseases as required by local government (such as rabies).

hostile microorganisms and toxins. Many factors in the ICU patient can change the GI dynamics. The stress of illness can decrease mucosal blood flow, altering mucosal barrier function and leading to erosion and ulceration.

Medications administered can alter GI transit time and affect absorption. Clinical signs of GI tract problems can be obvious, such as drooling or licking with nausea, vomiting, retching, diarrhea, and abdominal distension. Important signs of GI distress can be more insidious, such as restlessness, shivering, abnormal posture, vocalizing or decreased appetite.

Patient hygiene can become a challenge when the patient has frequent diarrhea or vomiting. Nasogastric tube suctioning can decrease nausea and minimize the fluids being vomited. Frequent walks for elimination are helpful in ambulatory patients. The tail can be wrapped to minimize soiling and long hair in the perineal region clipped to maintain a more sanitary environment. The use of grates in the cage can reduce the amount of fluids and materials in direct contact with the animal. When bathing is required, the patient must be dry before returning to cage.

Nutrition

Most patients in the hospital are not interested in eating, due to stress, pain, primary or secondary GI disease or simply being in an unfamiliar environment. A lack of adequate nutrition can depress the immune system, delay tissue healing, alter drug metabolism, and have a negative effect on GI barrier function.

The body condition score (BCS) and muscle condition score (see Figures 16.3 and 16.4) charts should be posted in the ICU and patients scored when entering the ICU and at discharge. When providing nutrition, it is best to remember, "If the gut works, use it." The nutritional goal is to ease the animal onto their caloric resting energy requirement (RER; see Box 16.3) by enteral feeding. A list of available veterinary critical care enteral diets and their caloric content is provided in Table 16.8.

The voluntary oral intake of food is ideal, with the amount and frequency recorded to ensure adequate caloric intake. When anorexia is present, forced feeding or tube feeding is prescribed. Syringe feeding is challenging to administer and can lead to food aversion. Common feeding tubes include nasoesophageal, nasogastric, esophagostomy, gastrostomy, and jejunostomy. The care and maintenance of feeding tubes are outlined in Table 20.6. Large volumes of diet retrieved by tube aspiration suggest depressed GI motility. Motility modifiers or a reduction in the volume of diet fed may be indicated.

Parenteral nutrition provides nutrition by the intravenous route, bypassing the GI tract. Total parenteral nutrition (TPN) is meant to eventually provide the daily caloric and protein requirement. A dedicated central catheter or multilumen catheter is placed and maintained under strict aseptic procedures. The components of the TPN diet formulation should be combined within a laminar flow hood to minimize the chance of bacterial contamination. The animal is closely monitored for signs of sepsis, hyperglycemia, catheter site inflammation or mental depression. Partial parenteral nutrition provides fewer calories and nutrients, can go through a peripheral catheter and is meant to transition the animal to TPN or enteral feeding.

Table 20.6 Nursing care of feeding tubes.

Consideration	Rationale/method
Instill 1–2 proparacaine drops in nare(s) (NG tubes)	Use as needed to relieve sneezing
Use Elizabethan collar	Prevent patient from removing tube
Wear gloves when handling tube insertion sites	Prevention of infection
Clean tube insertion site q 24 h or PRN	Remove any discharge, decrease risk of infection at insertion site
Apply antibiotic ointment at insertion site	Decrease risk of infection at insertion site or treatment if evidence of infection
Monitor bandage site	Make sure tube is staying in proper position, observe for bandage soiling or discharge
Monitor for complications	Discharge at insertion site, sneezing (NG), fever, lethargy, inflammation of skin around insertion site
Suction (NG, G tubes) q 2–4 h	Decompress stomach, decrease occurrence of vomiting and hopefully aspiration pneumonia
Flush tube with water prior to feeding and after feeding or q 6 h	Confirm and maintain patency of feeding tube, prevent occlusion
Feeding liquid-only diets through small diameter tubes (NG, J tube)	Prevent occlusion of tube
Add food coloring to liquid diets and using colored tubes	Minimize accidental IV and enteral tube mix-up (colored tubing); recognize aspirated material (food coloring in diet)
Feed based on resting energy requirements (RER), starting slow (1/4 RER, increasing by 1/4 every 6–8 h as tolerated)	Maintaining nutrition while determining tolerance of enteral feeding
Administer only finely ground or liquid medications and flush after	Increase ability to administer oral medications successfully, decreases patient stress caused by oral administration; simple for fractious patients
Pass desired food through an identical testing tube of the same size as tube to be inserted or prior to administration of different diet in tube already inserted	Can help ensure food does not clog tube
Tube obstruction: Instill small amounts of carbonated cola beverage (if stomach can tolerate), let sit for a few minutes then begin pulsing and aspirating water through tube until unobstructed.	The effervescent nature and high acidity content of cola may help dislodge occlusions
Remove tube when appropriate; most insertion sites heal by second intention. Most tubes surgically placed should remain in place for at least 5 days prior to removal to decrease risk of peritonitis	Removal is appropriate when there is another method of feeding

G, gastrostomy; IV, intravenous; J, jejunostomy; NG, nasogastric; PRN, pro re nata.

Body temperature

While most patients are not fond of the rectal temperature, it is still considered the most accurate method of temperature assessment for small animals. Methods for monitoring body temperature are listed in Table 17.2 with conversion between degrees Fahrenheit and Celsius noted in Box 17.1.

Common causes of hyperthermia in the ICU patient are listed in Table 17.4. Iatrogenic hyperthermia can occur in patients in a closed environment (such as an oxygen cage), from excessive supplemental heating or from reactions to medications administered. Hypothermia is commonly associated with exposure to cold environments, poor perfusion, medications administered and sedation or anesthesia. Severe changes in body temperature can have a negative effect and contribute to the decompensation of a patient (see Table 17.3). Continuous temperature monitoring is ideal to prevent overwarming or overcooling in the patient with extreme alterations.

Preventing hypothermia in patients that are being sedated or anesthetized is essential and a variety of warming devices such as the Bair Hugger® (3 M, St Paul, MN), warm water bottles, IV warmers, warm water circulating blankets or other temperature-controlled electrical blankets may be used. Water bottles should be used cautiously; since their heat is rapidly lost to the environment. Heated rice bags are not recommended since they heat unevenly and may cause burns. Table 17.9 reviews methods of warming hypothermic patients. Reuseable warm air blower blankets can be made from pillow cases.

Treatment of the underlying disease is essential in patients with hyperthermia. Methods of actively cooling patients are discussed in Table 17.7, and are done cautiously, discontinuing cooling when the body temperature reaches 103 °F (39.5 °C).

Drug dosages and metabolism

It is the responsibility of the critical care team to ensure that prescribed drugs are delivered correctly and safely. The "Five Rights" of drug administration are required: right drug, right patient, right dose, right route, and right time [11]. Systems are developed within the ICU environment to minimize the occurrence of drug errors. The order for drug administration should always be written to avoid errors. When verbal communication is required in urgent situations (such as CPR), it should be closed loop: the receiver of the prescription request should repeat the order back to the prescriber. Some drug names sound similar (such as dopamine and dobutamine) and many vials and pill bottles look identical, necessitating that the actual drug label be read each time a medication is dispensed for administration. Every medication drawn up should be confirmed at three separate time points to ensure it is the exact drug prescribed: when the drug is obtained from stock (off the shelf; expiry date should be checked at this time as well), when the amount is being drawn up, and then prior to placing the medication back into stock. Automated drug dispensing machines may help decrease these errors and also help with inventory control.

Creating a formulary of common ICU drugs with drug generic name, trade names, indications, dose for specific species, negative drug–drug interactions, and possible side-effects can aid nursing staff in successfully supporting the "Five Rights." Knowing the desired drug action and possible side-effects in a specific patient will provide an additional means for ensuring that the right drug is being given to the right patient. The dose is written in units (such as mg, g, µg)/kg body weight with the current body weight for that day

noted on the treatment sheet. The route of administration is designated. Any specific desired concentration or directions for drug administration (such as rate of administration, any specific sequence order for drugs administered) are also written on the orders. The amount of drug to administer can then be calculated (calculators should be available throughout the ICU). It is best to use drug names rather than trade names.

A list of medications with an increased risk of serious side-effects should be highlighted by the veterinary staff and posted in the ICU. This list might include drugs such as insulin, digoxin, aminoglycosides, phenothiazines, metronidazole, phenobarbital, and any potent vasoactive drug administered as a CRI (such as dopamine, dobutamine, nitroprusside, norepinephrine, isoproterenol). Drugs that can cause perivascular necrosis if given outside the vein should also be noted. A second person is requested to confirm the drug dose calculation and quantity of medication dispensed prior to administration of any of these drugs. In the ICU, many drugs are administered as a CRI. Formulas used for calculating a drug CRI are presented in Box 20.4.

Some drugs may not be physically compatible with another drug, but may be prescribed for administration at the same time, for example, injectable furosemide and injectable diltiazem; another example is injectable diazepam, which is not compatible with many medications. These medications should not be mixed in the same syringe or IV line. Much of this information is available either online or in the drug package insert. In addition, some medications may have a more negative effect when given at the same time as another drug. Medscape provides a simple tool to check for common drug interactions (not compatibilities) at: http://reference.medscape.com/drug-interactionchecker.

In addition, some drugs have reversal agents that may be available if an adverse drug reaction occurs. The reversal agent, dose, and route of administration should be noted and the amount of drug precalculated and posted in a highly visible location in case intervention is required.

Pain management

Pain, stress, and anxiety can cause increased heart rate, increased blood flow to skeletal muscles, elevation in glucose metabolism, and activation of the inflammatory response. Pain is easy to identify when a patient is vocalizing, guards or becomes aggressive when an area is palpated. However, most clinical signs of pain are much more subtle. Pain scales have been identified for the dog and cat (see Figures 19.2 and 19.3), and should be standardized and used by the critical care team when evaluating the level of pain.

Analgesics are often administered in the early stages of patient assessment as signs of pain are similar to signs of shock. However, some drugs (such as opioids) may interfere with neurological assessment. Analgesics are continued at appropriate doses and intervals throughout hospitalization. A list of common analgesic agents used in the small animal ICU is available in Table 19.1. Methods of administration include oral, transmucosal, transdermal, and local or intravenous injection. Intermittent injections or a CRI may be prescribed. The effectiveness of analgesia is evaluated using the pain scale, with the trend of change being important. Should the response to the analgesic be inadequate, a change in drug dose, administration interval, route of administration, or class of drug, or the addition of an additional medication can be required. Gentle handling and being attentive to the underlying problem are essential to minimize the development of further pain or injury during hospitalization.

Often, specialized catheters are placed for the local delivery of analgesic drugs. Wound soaker catheters, epidural catheters, or pleural or abdominal catheters can allow infusion of pain medication at the specific site of injury. Lidocaine and fentanyl patches must be applied to clipped and clean skin for optimal transdermal absorption of the drug. Specific recommendations may be available for handling a specific drug or for protecting the site of application.

Wound care and bandages

Several types of wounds can be part of the presenting problem for the ICU patient, such as bite wounds, penetrating injuries, burns, severe abrasions, and lacerations. However, the therapy (such as IV catheter placement, surgical intervention, chest tube insertion) can create wounds that need to be bandaged, monitored, and treated, as well.

Underestimating the severity of a wound can lead to mismanagement, with inflammation and necrosis of the surrounding tissues a potential consequence. Gloves are worn when working with wounds to prevent introduction of bacteria and protect the staff from exposure to unknown sources of blood that may be present. Sedation, analgesia or anesthesia is necessary to care for most traumatic wounds. Appropriate monitoring is necessary during sedation or anesthesia since complications with sedation (including cardiac arrest) are possible. Advanced preparation for intubation, reversal of sedatives, IV catheter placement for resuscitation, and monitoring should be made.

Care of any wound involves protecting the exposed tissues and clipping and cleaning the areas around the wound. Any areas of skin necrosis or bruising should be outlined with a nontoxic permanent marker or documented with a picture to monitor progression or resolution. A complete description of the wound, the dimensions and the presence of drains, sutures or other material are reviewed by the critical care nursing team. Almost all wounds are bandaged, and the purpose (such as support, debridement, protection, compression) of the bandage should be reviewed. Bandages must be protected from being soiled by the patient or the environment. In addition, the bandage should not move or restrict the circulation to the affected area. Tips for providing exceptional nursing care for bandages are provided in Table 20.7.

Burns affecting more than 20% of the total body surface area can cause significant fluid and protein loss. Cardiac, respiratory, and immune system dysfunction should be anticipated with close monitoring initiated for signs of sepsis. With burn wounds, the skin and underlying tissue damage may continue after the initial injury. The management of burn wounds requires additional care as outlined in Table 20.8.

Nursing status

Overseeing the staff and placing the right person for the right job in the right place will help improve efficiency. Managing staff when it is busy (or slow) in the ICU is also a vital part of nursing care. Slow times may allow for development of protocols, maintenance of equipment, checking the crash cart, and restocking so that when it does become busy, everything is ready to go. All equipment should be carefully maintained and set up for immediate use. Inventory management is an essential part of technical care. Logging of controlled medications is vital within guidelines dictated by government agencies.

Veterinary nurse technicians bring different levels of education and experience to nursing care and it is important to provide

Table 20.7 Tips for optimizing bandage care by the veterinary nursing team.

Sites to be covered	• Incisions created by surgery • Catheter or tube insertion sites • Draining wounds
Bandage monitoring	• Ensure bandage remains in appropriate position and is covering the site • Ensure bandage is clean (no strike-through); will lead to wicking and contamination • Ensure there is no swelling around or distal to the bandage that may indicate it is too tight
Frequency of bandage changes	• Change bandage covering an open wound every 6–12 h, decreasing frequency as discharge from wound decreases • Change when strike-through appears • Change when a new fever develops, to inspect wounds
Preparation for bandage change	• Provide analgesics and restraint when removing adhesive bandages since it can be uncomfortable • Wear gloves • Change bandages on a clean, dry surface (such as a clean towel or disposable diaper pad) to prevent contamination of wound(s) • Prepare all materials in advance

guidance on the job. Guidance can come from more experienced nurse technicians, veterinarians or staff members who are experts in a specific area. It is important to discuss the deeper nuances of disease processes and patient care in rounds as time permits. An in-house training program should be instituted so that technicians continue to expand their knowledge and technical skill base. Attending continuing education programs is vital to keep technicians up to date on the current trends in practice.

The critical care team can also help develop protocols for reporting and managing medical errors. Investigation regarding how or why the error occurred and further instruction to avoid such errors in the future are a necessary part of managing a critical care team.

Tender loving care – patients and staff

An important goal of ICU patient care is to minimize stress on the patient while not impeding the ability to provide the required medical care. The nurse–patient relationship is enhanced when providing the patient with much-needed tender loving care (TLC). Each animal is different, with not only the species and breed a distinction, but the personality, home environment, past human interactions, illness, and treatment needs special for that patient. Information from the owners regarding the personality, routines, reactions to other animals and people and other normal at-home behaviors of their pet will guide the critical care nursing team in their approach to the patient. Cage cards should be posted to alert staff regarding any individual traits of the patient (such as cage-jumper, dog-aggressive, fear-biter) to allow adequate caution or restraint at the onset of any interactions.

Learning key aspects of animal behavior is essential to identifying patients that may be aggravated, stressed, scared or painful. Table 20.9 provides a list of frequently observed behaviors of dogs and cats in the ICU environment with possible interpretations and intervention. In general, allowing the animal to see the critical care team member and hear their voice prior to approaching the patient avoids a startled response. A slow, gentle approach with the hands while speaking kindly and softly to the animal can reduce anxiety and allow the

Table 20.8 Nursing management of thermal burns [12].

Problem	Etiology	Nursing care
Ineffective airway clearance	Tracheal edema due to inhalation injury	• Monitor oxygen saturation every hour, arterial blood gas (as needed), thoracic radiographs • Assess respiratory rate, character, noises and depth and level of consciousness every hour; breath sounds every 4 h • Place suction apparatus, ET tubes with tie-in, oxygen source, AMBU bag and rapid induction anesthetic plan by cage side
Impaired gas exchange	Interstitial pulmonary edema, pneumonia	• Administer humidified oxygen as ordered • Suction oropharynx (or ET tube) every 1–2 h or as needed • Monitor sputum characteristics and amount • Turn patient frequently to mobilize secretions
Fluid volume deficit	Fluid shifts, diuresis or evaporative water loss (fluid losses increase with increased body surface area injured)	• Monitor: vital signs and urine output q 1 h until stable; mental status every hour for at least 6 h • Titrate fluid requirements to maintain urinary output and hemodynamic stability • Record daily weight and hourly intake/output measurements; evaluate trends • Monitor PCV, TP, BP, and physical perfusion parameters
Altered tissue perfusion	Fluid losses; impaired vascular perfusion of extremities that have circumferential burns	• Assess peripheral pulses every hour for 72 h. Notify the veterinarian of changes in pulses, CRT, MM color, BP or intensity of pain • Elevate upper and lower extremities • Be prepared to assist with escharotomy or fasciotomy procedure that might be needed to reduce subfascial pressures
Risk for infection	Invasive therapy and loss of integument	• Assess temperature and vital signs and characteristics of urine and sputum every 1–4 h • Monitor white blood cell count and characteristics, burn wound healing status and invasive catheter sites • Ensure appropriate protective isolation and barrier nursing techniques; provide meticulous wound care; educate visiting clients on burn guidelines
Hypothermia	Decreased heat production and increased heat loss secondary to thermal injury	• Monitor and document rectal or core temperature every 1–2 h; assess for shivering • Minimize skin exposure; maintain environmental temperatures • For temperature <99.5 °F (<37.5 °C), institute rewarming measures
Pain	Thermal injury	• Monitor physiological responses to pain (such as increased BP and HR, restlessness) and nonverbal cues. Use validated pain scales to assess pain and anxiety (see Chapter 19) • Assess response to analgesics or other interventions • Administer analgesic and anxiolytic medication as ordered • Medicate patient before bedding changes, dressing changes, and major procedures, as needed
Altered nutrition	Increased metabolic demands	• Place feeding tube for gastric decompression in patients with >20% TBSA burns • Assess abdomen and bowel sounds every 8 h • Assess NG aspirate (color, quantity, pH, occult blood); monitor stool for blood • Administer stress ulcer prophylaxis • Initiate enteral feeding, and evaluate tolerance • Provide high-calorie and protein supplementation • Record all oral intake and track caloric intake compared to estimated RER • Schedule interventions and activities to avoid interrupting feeding times • Monitor weight twice a day
Impaired skin integrity	Thermal injury	• Perform active and passive range of motion exercises to extremities every 2 h when awake and as tolerated. Reinforce importance of maintaining proper joint movement, function, and alignment • Elevate extremities • Provide pain relief measures before manipulating the patient and physical rehabilitation

BP, blood pressure; CRT, capillary refill time; ET, endotracheal tube; HR, heart rate; MM, mucous membranes; NG, nasogastric; PCV, packed cell volume; RER, resting energy requirement; TBSA, total body surface area; TP, total protein.

initial contact with the patient. Using chemical sedation may be necessary to safely care for patients and improve their level of stress or anxiety.

Interacting with the animal when treatments do not need to be performed and walking the animal allows some one-on-one time for patient–nurse bonding when time allows. Providing a place for the patient to hide, such as a box for cats or blanket on the cage door, can minimize stress for some patients when their medical condition allows. Turning the lights down in the ICU to coincide with night time when possible is important for maintaining the circadian rhythm of animals.

Patient mobility and muscle strength can decline rapidly during critical illness and should be addressed in the treatment orders.

Animals that are able to ambulate should be walked several times daily. Harness type leashes are ideal to avoid pulling or compression of the trachea by neck leads. Patients with paresis or paralysis can be encouraged to stand by using towel or commercial slings and spending time in a support stanchion. The nursing team or rehabilitation staff can provide massage and passive range of motion exercises.

If a patient is recumbent, a body rotation schedule is instituted with the patient body position changed every two to four hours, including a sternal position. Close monitoring for cleanliness is necessary since urine and fecal scalding can lead to problems with the skin. Heavy padding of the cage is necessary to avoid pressure necrosis of the skin, with bedding changed and bathing and drying

Table 20.9 Behavior change in animals in the ICU due to stress or anxiety, with possible steps for intervention. All behavioral changes should be reported to the veterinarian immediately. A complete physical examination of the animal is done to identify any underlying changes that could be detrimental to the animal.

Behavior change due to stress, anxiety or depression	Nursing intervention
Decreased or loss of appetite	Assess patient for pain. Encourage patient to eat by giving very palatable foods. Monitor weight twice a day and % RER of voluntary intake. Discuss with veterinarian plan for feeding tube placement. Limit syringe feeding (may cause food aversion). Consider having owners bring favorite foods
Decreased energy or activity level	Monitor for pain and assess vital signs for perfusion deficits. Encourage patient to stand and move to prevent muscle fatigue. Walk outside or around ICU every 6h. Discuss whether drug therapy could be contributing to signs
Hiding	Decrease external stimuli (such as loud noises) in the ICU. Give animals a safe place in their cage or place in a less stressful area of the hospital if possible
Increased shedding or bald patches, excessive scratching or licking of the body	Patient may be overgrooming due to anxiety, boredom, discomfort or pain. Discuss patient exercise programs and owner visitation plans. Place Elizabethan collar to prevent self-mutilation if indicated. Carefully inspect skin areas for signs of inflammation, trauma, swelling or infection
Reluctance or difficulty in getting up or down	Monitor pain parameters. Encourage owners to visit to help get patient up to improve muscle strength and improve any symptoms of depression. Use slings and stanchion to support larger patients
Abnormal vocalization (whining or crying, hissing), sudden aggression	Symptoms may be due to anxiety, nausea or pain. Monitor pain parameters and assess patient for physical changes. If not changed, try to reduce noise and lights in ICU. Discuss sedative or pain medications with veterinarians

provided to keep the patient clean. The urinary bladder may require expressions for urination in these patients and is best accomplished while the animal is in the sling or stanchion.

Owner visits are an important component of patient TLC. This not only provides a continued bonding experience for the owner and the pet, but is an opportunity for the critical care team to develop their relationship with both the pet and the owner. Visits can be arranged in a dedicated room, in the ICU or in an exam room. The owners should be made comfortable and encouraged to hold, touch, and interact with their pet. Favorite toys, blankets, and other personal items can be kept with the patient, but it is not uncommon for such items to be misplaced during hospitalization (if they get soiled and washed, for example).

Information regarding the behavior traits and tips for handling the patient should be shared during rounds at shift change. This can help make the transition to different caretakers easier for everyone and promotes an environment of caring.

Table 20.10 Quality of life questionnaire with point scale used to assess the quality of life of the ICU patient. Each parameter is subjectively assessed on a scale of 0–10, with 0 = could not be worse to 10 = considered ideal or normal for that patient. The owner should consult with the critical care team when completing the questionnaire. Any quality of life scoring system should take into account the current disease(s) and prognosis: many critically ill patients will score low, but many of these patients recover from their disease.

Criterion	Score
Pain – is pain adequately controlled or can analgesia be adjusted?	0–10
Respiratory distress – are there any breathing difficulties?	0–10
Appetite – is the patient physically able to eat? If a feeding tube is present, is it intended to be permanent or temporary? What is the appetite?	0–10
Hydration – is the patient willing or able to drink? Do they or will they require supplemental fluids?	0–10
Hygiene – is the patient urinating or defecating on themselves? Can the pet perform normal grooming procedures?	0–10
Happiness – will the pet be able to enjoy favorite activities?	0–10
Mobility and neurological status – can the patient ambulate in some fashion, even if assisted? Are there frequent seizures that cannot be controlled?	0–10
More good days than bad	0–10
Total – a patient with a score of 35 or higher is generally acceptable	

Source: Adapted from Villalobos A. Canine and Feline Geriatric Oncology: Honoring the Human–Animal Bond. Ames: Blackwell Publishing, 2007 [13]. Used with permission.

Quality of life and euthanasia

Assessing the "quality of life" for a critically ill dog or cat can be difficult since the patient cannot verbalize their level of pain or emotional condition. Quality of life surveys can be introduced to owners during this difficult time in the life of their pet (Table 20.10). This issue can be discussed with the owners in light of the medical problems, prognosis, and ability to make the animal comfortable. Details regarding future at-home care can have an impact on the decision-making process. Unfortunately, the financial commitment for ongoing care of the animal might factor into the prognosis of the patient.

When euthanasia is a viable option, the family should be informed of the euthanasia process. Owners need to decide whether staying with the pet during the procedure is the best way to say good-bye or if they would like to leave before the procedure is performed. The family should be encouraged to grieve in their own way and develop their own methods of closure. Often giving the family a paw print or hair from their animal friend provides comfort. Counseling services, books, and websites for pet owners suffering the loss of their pet are available (see Further reading).

Compassion fatigue

Compassion fatigue is defined as fatigue, emotional distress or apathy resulting from the constant demands of caring for others. It affects caregivers such as veterinary nurse technicians, veterinarians, and other paramedical staff who are continuously exposed to emotional situations centered around patients with poor prognoses or who are dying. While caring for others, the caregiver fails to care for themselves. There are negative consequences such as isolation, depression, and substance abuse. Information on the syndrome and resources for intervention is available through counseling, books (see Further reading) and websites such as:

- www.compassionfatigue.org
- www.aafp.org/fpm/2000/0400/p39.html
- www.stress.org (American Institute of Stress).

References

1. O'Grady P, Alexander M, Burns A, et al. Guidelines for the prevention of intravascular catheter-related infections. Clin Infect Dis. 2011;52(9):e162–93.
2. McCallum L, Higgins D. Care of peripheral venous cannula sites. Nurs Times. 2012;108(34-35):12, 14–15.
3. Battaglia AM. Small Animal Emergency and Critical Care: A Manual for the Veterinary Technician. Ithaca: WB Saunders, 2001: pp 17–18.
4. Richmond M. Oxygen therapy in small animal patients. VNTCPD. 2010;4(3):2–7.
5. American Thoracic Society. Inpatient Oxygen Therapy. Available at: www.thoracic.org/copd-guidelines/for-health-professionals/exacerbation/inpatient-oxygen-therapy/oxygen-delivery-methods.php (accessed 7 June 2016).
6. McCurnin DM, Bassett JM. Clinical Textbook for Veterinary Technicians, 5th edn. Philadelphia: WB Saunders, 2002: p 67.
7. Devey J. Traumatic emergencies. In: Small Animal Emergency and Critical Care for Veterinary Technicians. St Louis: Elsevier, 2016: pp 247–67.
8. Giger U. Blood typing and crossmatching to ensure compatible transfusions. In: Kirk's Current Veterinary Therapy XIII Small Animal Practice. Bonagura JD, ed. Philadelphia: WB Saunders, 2000: pp 396–9.
9. Elliott M, Coventry A. Critical care: the eight vital signs of patient monitoring. Br J Nurs 2012;21(20):621–5.
10. Bassett JM, Thomas, JA, eds. Clinical Textbook for Veterinary Technicians, 8th edn. St Louis: Elsevier Saunders, 2014: pp 607–9.
11. Lehne RA. Pharmacology for Nursing Care. St Louis: Elsevier Saunders, 2010: p 5.
12. Greenfield E. The pivotal role of nursing personnel in burn care. Indian J Plast Surg. 2010;43(Suppl):S94–S100.
13. Villalobos A. Canine and Feline Geriatric Oncology: Honoring the Human-Animal Bond. Ames: Blackwell Publishing, 2007.

Further reading

Sife W. The Loss of a Pet, 3rd edn. Hoboken: Howell Book House, 2005.
Teater M, Ludgate J. Overcoming Compassion Fatigue: A Practical Resilience Workbook. Eau Claire: PESI Publishing and Media, 2014.

CHAPTER 21

Wounds and bandages

Jennifer J. Devey[1], Andrew Linklater[2] and Rebecca Kirby[3]

[1] Fox Valley Animal Referral Center, Appleton, Wisconsin
[2] Lakeshore Veterinary Specialists, Milwaukee, Wisconsin
[3] (Formerly) Animal Emergency Center, Gainesville, Florida

Introduction

A wound is a type of injury in which skin is torn, cut, or punctured (an *open* wound), or where blunt force trauma causes a contusion (a *closed* wound). The skin has many functions that include epidermal turnover, immune function, wound healing, vascular responsiveness, thermoregulation, barrier function, sebum production, and sensory perception. As wounds are caused by various types of external forces, internal injury may be present even when there is no evidence of significant external wounds.

The etiology of wounds can be quite varied, with most naturally occurring wounds caused by some form of trauma and most hospital-acquired wounds resulting from therapeutic intervention, such as placement of catheters or drainage tubes, and surgery. Minor injuries can include cuts, lacerations, abrasions, and contusions. Problems under the skin can become apparent when pathogens, such as parasites (bot fly larvae), bacteria (abscess formation), fungi or migration of a foreign object, cause inflammation of the skin and deeper tissues. All open wounds caused by bites or projectiles (such as sticks, iron rods, bullets, arrows) should be assumed to have substantial trauma to the underlying tissues.

Complex mechanisms and forces come together to cause wounds. In general, the mechanism of injury is categorized as penetrating, blunt or thermal trauma, with a combination of mechanisms possible. Forces exerted on the tissues to cause wounds include compression (squeezing or condensing of tissues), shearing (tissues sliding over adjoining surfaces), torsion (rotation along fixed point), tension (pulling or drawing apart), and bending (impact in middle while ends are stable). Usually two or more mechanical forces are acting on tissues at any one time.

Wounds resulting from traumatic injury can be classified by several methods, including the etiology, location, type of injury, wound depth and tissue loss or clinical appearance of the wound. Specific types of wounds can have a separate classification of their own, such as burns (Rule of 9s), surgical wounds, and general wounds. General wounds are classified as superficial (loss of dermis only), partial thickness (involving the epidermis and dermis), and full thickness (involving the dermis, subcutaneous tissues, and sometimes bone). Surgical wound classifications are generally based on the degree of wound contamination and are described in Table 21.1 [1]. The class of wound has been shown to be a strong predictor for development of infection [2–4]. Open fractures can also be classified based on the degree of injury:

- Type I – wound <1 cm, injury occurs more frequently from bone penetrating through the skin and retracting

- Type II – wound >1 cm, injury occurs more frequently from outside forces with external penetration of skin (Figure 21.1)
- Type III – visible bone with extensive soft tissue injury [5].

The healing process for surgical or traumatic wounds will go through at least four stages. Within the first few minutes of injury, there is vasoconstriction of the local vessels and platelets from the blood begin to stick to the injured site. This results in the activation of coagulation and the formation of a clot that slows or stops further bleeding (hemostasis stage). The inflammatory and debridement stages occur within minutes of the initial injury and can extend over several days. During this phase, damaged and dead cells, bacteria, and other pathogens or debris are removed by phagocytosis. Vasodilation and cytokine release allow fibrinogen and neutrophils in the area to form a scab, remove debris, and initiate angiogenesis. Platelet-derived growth factors are released into the wound and cause the migration and division of cells during the following proliferative phase. This phase promotes the growth of new tissue. In this phase, angiogenesis, collagen deposition, granulation tissue formation, epithelialization, and wound contraction occur. This phase begins a few days after the wound occurs and can last for weeks. Finally, the maturation phase starts many days after the initial injury and can continue for years. Collagen is realigned along tension lines, and cells that are no longer needed are removed by programmed cell death.

There are several patient factors that can affect the ability of the wound to heal. Age, obesity, poor nutritional status, dehydration, inadequate blood supply, depressed immune response, and the presence of chronic disease can all have a negative impact on wound healing. Malignancies can alter the cellular structure of tissues and negatively influence the healing process.

Most wounds, whether natural or hospital acquired, will require a bandage (also called external coaptation) as part of the treatment plan. Almost every hospitalized patient will have some form of bandage, from a simple bandage protecting a peripheral catheter to a more complex dressing for open wounds or a splint or cast. The proper care of the bandages can promote wound healing and prevent the development of a new secondary problem.

The presence of wounds can have a significant impact on morbidity and mortality in the ICU small animal patient. The loss of fluids, electrolytes, and proteins through wound effusions can be substantial, affecting fluid balance and albumin status. Massive tissue damage can lead to systemic inflammation and the systemic inflammatory response syndrome (SIRS), and wound complications, such as necrotizing fasciitis or overwhelming sepsis, can lead to life-threatening hemodynamic alterations. Even the improper

Monitoring and Intervention for the Critically Ill Small Animal: The Rule of 20, First Edition. Edited by Rebecca Kirby and Andrew Linklater.

Table 21.1 Surgical wound classification adapted by the Centers for Disease Control and used by the American College of Surgeons [1].

Classification	Description
Clean	Uninfected surgical wound with no inflammation and internal tracts (respiratory, GI, genital, urinary tract) are not entered; includes surgical wound incisions made after nonpenetrating trauma, if it meets the above criteria
Clean-contaminated	Surgical wound in which internal tracts are entered under controlled conditions and without unusual contamination; no signs of infection and no major break in technique occurs.
Contaminated	Open, fresh, accidental wounds; surgical procedures with major break in sterile technique (such as open cardiac massage) or gross spillage from GI tract; incision with acute nonpurulent inflammation is included
Dirty or infected	Old traumatic wounds with retained or devitalized tissue; wounds with existing infection or perforated viscera; suggests organisms causing postoperative infection were present in the wound before surgical procedure

GI, gastrointestinal.

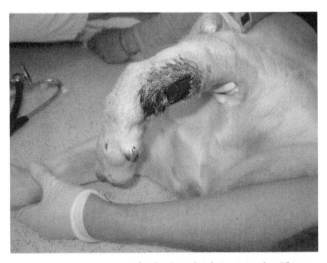

Figure 21.1 A traumatic open distal radius ulna fracture in a dog. This would be classified as a type III open fracture.

application of a bandage or insufficient bandage maintenance can contribute to patient morbidity. Pain associated with the wound or banadage can lead to mutilation of the area by the animal. Because of the negative impact that wounds and bandages can have, appropriate diagnostic investigation to define the cause and nature of the wound and adequate monitoring procedures to optimize recovery should be instituted.

Diagnosis and monitoring procedures

Because the small animal ICU patient is likely to have a long list of medical problems, the presence of a wound or bandage may not be a priority at the time of initial admission. However, it is vital that the nature and classification of any wounds present are known and the plans regarding wound care and bandage support are clearly

defined. Information from the history and physical examination may reveal underlying concerns that may affect wound healing. Clinicopathological laboratory testing and diagnostic imaging may be required to better define the extent and characteristics of the wound. The wound size, shape, and progress toward healing must be monitored.

History and physical examination

The history begins with the signalment (age, sex, breed). Wound healing may be impaired with older age. Both skin and muscle lose their tone and elasticity with age. Metabolism slows and circulation may be altered. Past medical problems become important since health problems such as malignancies, autoimmune diseases, hyperadrenocorticism, diabetes mellitus, and skin diseases can impact wound healing. A list of recent and current medications, to include injectable, oral, and topical drugs, can identify those (such as glucocorticosteroids) that might delay wound healing. The animal's diet becomes important for assessing nutritional status and potential effects on wound healing.

If a wound is present at admission, it should be determined if the skin defect was induced by trauma or developed spontaneously. Progression, regarding the time frame of wound development, changes in the wound character and overall changes in the health of the animal should be obtained. A history of trauma or possibility of bite wounds warrants careful examination for wounds hidden by hair or fur.

The physical examination should include vital signs and an assessment of the perfusion and hydration status of the animal. Immediate identification of external hemorrhage is essential and hemostasis should be rapidly provided with application of a temporary compression bandage. Hyperdynamic perfusion (compensatory stage of shock) or severe hypotension can be a consequence of hemorrhage, significant fluid loss from effusive wounds, infection or systemic inflammation from massive tissue trauma. High body temperatures can be a result of systemic inflammation or infection secondary to dirty or contaminated wounds. Lower body temperatures can be a reflection of cold exposure (frostbite wounds) or poor circulation.

The location of the wound will impact the likelihood of serious secondary complications. The hair or fur must be generously clipped from any body region that might have been affected. The skin is carefully examined for evidence of punctures, lacerations, subcutaneous emphysema, swelling or bruising. Wounds found around the head and neck raise concerns for bleeding, swelling or disruption of tissue within the nasal sinuses, brain, pharynx, larynx or trachea. Wounds over the chest region raise concerns for hemothorax, pneumothorax, pneumomediastinum, and lung parenchymal hemorrhage. Abdominal wounds raise concerns for rupture or perforation of an abdominal organ and abdominal hemorrhage. The limbs are examined for concurrent muscle, tendon, nerve or bone damage.

Close examination of any wound is essential and the size, depth, tissue involvement, evidence of infection or debris, and underlying etiology (which may include parasites, foreign material) should be documented. Skin that is cool to the touch may be indicative of altered perfusion that may be secondary to an embolic event, compartment syndrome or necrosis. Bite wounds require specific attention because a significant injury deep to the skin wound is often present.

For patients that are hospitalized, routine examination of any treatment-induced wound (such as IV catheter, tube placement, incision site) and the evaluation of bandages are an important component of the physical examination performed each shift. Development of a new fever, pain, swelling or redness should stimulate the examination of catheter sites or unwrapping of a bandaged wound to address problems.

Point of care and clinicopathological laboratory testing

Point of care (POC) testing provides immediate information at the cage side and will include packed cell volume (PCV), total protein (TP), creatinine, blood glucose, blood lactate, blood electrolytes, acid–base balance, blood smear for platelet estimate, coagulation profile, and urinalysis. The PCV and TP can imply blood loss, anemia or hypoproteinemia. Evaluation of the clotting profile, with the platelet estimate, can identify a coagulopathy that might be contributing to bruising, bleeding or swelling from a wound. A low blood glucose can be a result of wound-related sepsis and a high blood glucose may be a stress response but if it persists, warrants investigation for diabetes mellitus which can impair healing. A high blood lactate suggests poor tissue oxygenation and anaerobic metabolism, harmful to wound repair. An elevated creatinine can be a result of dehydration or renal impairment, both potentially negatively impacting wound healing.

A complete blood cell (CBC) count and serum biochemical profile should be submitted to assess for underlying diseases or conditions that can affect wound healing in patients with significant wounds. Samples can be collected from an impression smear, skin scraping, wound drains or aspirates of a swollen area. Cytology and gram staining of samples collected can be examined for pathogens, debris or abnormal cell types and may be useful in guiding the initial empirical antibiotic therapy. Wounds that are grossly infected (such as abscesses) or contaminated (such as bite wounds) warrant collection of samples for bacterial culture and susceptibility to help direct antibiotic therapy (see Chapter 14).

Depending on the geographic location, specific diagnostic testing for fungal disease, such as blastomycosis or coccidioidomycosis, may require collection of samples for fungal titers, fungal cultures, and urine antigen testing. When wounds are not healing with appropriate wound management or are associated with swellings or masses or are located at mucocutaneous junctions, then collection of incisional or excisional tissue biopsies for histopathology or macerated tissue culture may be indicated to investigate for underlying etiologies (such as resistant infections, neoplasia or autoimmune skin diseases).

Diagnostic imaging

Imaging techniques (radiographs or ultrasound focused assessment with sonography for trauma (FAST) exams) for examination of inappropriate collections of fluid or air within cavities or wounds may be indicated, particularly in those patients suffering from significant trauma. Chronic wounds may warrant imaging studies to determine if there is involvement of underlying tissues. Occasionally, contrast studies (such as a fistulogram for chronic draining tracts) or advanced imaging (computed tomography (CT) or magnetic resonance imaging (MRI)) may be ordered to investigate the extent of a wound, vascular supply, for neuroorthopedic disease that is identified on examination or to identify the presence of foreign material.

Patient monitoring

Patient monitoring includes frequent assessment of the physical perfusion parameters (heart rate, pulse intensity, capillary refill time (CRT), mucous membrane color, temperature) and hydration parameters (skin turgor, mucous membrane moistness, eye position within socket). Skin wounds usually need to be inspected at least once daily to ensure healing is progressing appropriately. Exceptions to this include wounds that have hydrocolloid dressings (generally changed every 5–7 days) and bandages over skin grafts (usually changed every 3–5 days). Gloves should be worn whenever wounds are exposed to help prevent contamination and nosocomial infection. The skin around the wound should be assessed for evidence of swelling, crepitus, heat, pain, odor, and discharge. By outlining any affected skin areas with a nontoxic permanent marker, it is possible to determine if the damage is progressing or resolving.

Covering catheter and other hospital-acquired wound sites with external coaptation and regular bandage maintenance is necessary. Venipuncture sites and catheter (long- and short-term) sites should be inspected daily. Every catheter (vascular, epidural), tube (tracheostomy, thoracostomy, feeding), and drain (Penrose, suction) site should be assessed by direct visualization and palpation at least once daily. Hourly examination of vascular catheter sites for swelling, pain or heat should be part of the critical care nursing routine (see Chapter 20) when fluids or drugs are being infused at that site.

Each time a limb bandage is changed, sensation should be assessed on the lateral and medial aspects of the limb. Blood flow can be evaluated based on tissue color and temperature, bleeding, and the presence of pulses. If there is any concern for arterial blood supply, a Doppler ultrasonic flow probe should be placed over the regional arteries and flow subjectively assessed. Significant swelling of distal extremities accompanied by rapid bleeding with a needle prick in patients that have experienced crush-type injuries is consistent with venous congestion that may lead to significant complications. The temperature of the surrounding skin can be assessed using infrared thermometry. If there is a significant difference in temperature between the healthy skin and the affected area, the animal should be carefully examined to ensure this is a local rather than a more diffuse problem.

General wound care

The goals of wound care are to preserve viable tissue, restore damaged tissue to a normal condition and function, provide an environment that maximizes the development of wound strength, and avoid problems such as infection that interfere with wound healing. Factors that promote good wound healing include:

- a good blood supply to the affected tissues
- no bacteria, foreign material or necrotic material present
- good apposition of the tissues
- no tension on the suture line
- minimal dead space
- no movement of the wound area
- keeping the wound moist [6–8].

Healing of wounds requires diligent care of the whole patient. Emphasis should be placed on fluid balance, oxygenation, immune status, nutrition, and nursing care from the Rule of 20. The animal may have varying degrees of immune system dysfunction secondary to underlying disease, immunosuppressive drugs and malnutrition, each potentially increasing the risk of infection [4,6,7]. Patient morbidity can also be attributed to inappropriate wound management. Sepsis can occur secondary to wounds and is usually due to a combination of one or more of the following factors: inadequate debridement of necrotic tissue, insufficient irrigation, inappropriate choice of antibiotics, and inadequate patient resuscitation.

Initial wound management

Urgent wound care includes patient stabilization, appropriate analgesia (examples include fentanyl 2–5 μg/kg IV, hydromorphone 0.05–0.1 mg/kg IV, methadone 0.1–0.3 mg/kg IV) (see Chapter 19), and hemostasis. Once these are achieved, a sterile, water-soluble lubricant is applied directly to an open wound, followed by the removal of surrounding hair and cleansing of the surrounding skin. Further injury can be prevented by bandaging, immobilizing the area, and placing an Elizabethan collar on the patient. Administration of antibiotics in the early stages may be warranted in traumatic wound care.

A sterile dressing should be placed on every wound as soon as possible to minimize the risk of nosocomial infection. Wounds should never be handled unless gloves are worn. Hand washing with an antibacterial soap or an alcohol-based rub is required prior to donning gloves. Sterile instruments and sterile suture should be used when treating all wounds.

It may not be possible to perform definitive wound care immediately after urgent wound stabilization. A delay in definitive care can have advantages, such as allowing time to stabilize the patient and time for tissues to "declare" themselves. Disadvantages, such as increased risk of bacterial contamination, can be minimized with timely and appropriate initial wound management. In general, wounds that are kept moist will maintain overall tissue hydration, which helps prevent cell death, encourages angiogenesis, phagocytosis and growth factor production, improves the rate of epithelialization, and may be less painful [9]. Wounds should not be allowed to form a crust as a wound with no crust will epithelialize almost twice as fast [8].

Definitive management

Definitive wound care includes hemostasis, debridement, irrigation, antisepsis, drainage, and closure. The procedures and extent of intervention will vary depending on the nature and extent of the wound.

Hemostasis

Hemostasis during wound care is important during all stages of wound healing. The presence of blood in the wounded tissues can delay healing by inhibiting the migration of fibroblasts, inhibiting angiogenesis, and facilitating colonization with organisms.

Various mechanical, thermal, and chemical methods are available to decrease the flow of blood into the wound site. Without adequate control, bleeding from transected or penetrated vessels or diffuse oozing from large denuded surfaces may interfere with the view of underlying structures. Achieving complete hemostasis before wound closure also will help prevent formation of postoperative hematomas. Collections of blood or fluid in the incision can prevent the direct apposition of tissues necessary for complete union of wound edges. The presence of blood provides an ideal culture medium for microbial growth and can lead to serious infection. When clamping or ligating a vessel, care must be taken to avoid creating excessive tissue damage.

Debridement and congestion

Necrotic tissue increases the risk of infection [9] and should be debrided back to bleeding edges. Surgical debridement of devitalized tissues is usually performed using sharp dissection with a scalpel blade or scissors. Scissors are generally avoided in skin debridement because they have a tendency to crush tissue.

Healthy muscle edges may not bleed but will typically contract when incised. Embedded debris should be removed from exposed tissues and bone by gently scraping the tissues or bone with the edge of a scalpel blade. Minor debridement can be performed using certain dressings including wet-to-dry, honey and sugar bandages [10–12].

Crush injuries with venous or tissue congestion often experience delayed healing. Leeches are an effective method of reducing excessive venous congestion while the tissues are healing [13]. Figure 21.2 shows leeches on a wound and discusses application.

Irrigation

Irrigation is always indicated after debridement and may be warranted whenever a bandage covering an open wound is changed. Sterile isotonic fluids are preferred. There is conflicting evidence regarding the use of antiseptics in irrigation fluids, as they may interfere with wound healing [15]. Irrigation with chlorhexidine at 0.05% has not been shown to negatively impact wound healing in dogs [16] and may actually aid wound healing [17]. The appropriate concentration (0.05%) of chlorhexidine must be used since higher concentrations have been shown to interfere with wound healing [18]. Tap water has been used to irrigate larger wounds without complications [19], and can be used as a first step when large wounds are present. Antibiotics should not be added to irrigation fluids since this is not effective and can lead to bacterial resistance.

The ideal pressure for irrigation systems is unknown. Excessive pressure can lead to tissue trauma and infection [7]. One study demonstrated that use of a 35 ml syringe and needles from 16 to 22 G in size routinely generated pressures well above 15 PSI, which could lead to tissue trauma [20].

Most surgeons agree on a pressure of 8–12 PSI, the pressure necessary to dislodge bacteria [21]. Irrigation can be performed with mechanical lavage systems or by using a 1 L fluid bag pressurized to

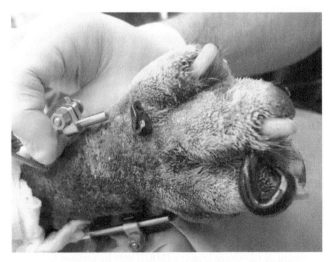

Figure 21.2 Medicinal leeches applied to a wound where significant venous congestion and tissue swelling are noted. Application of leeches: (1) leeches are obtained from a medicinal leech source, (2) the skin is cleaned with chlorhexidine and rinsed with saline, (3) the leech may be held in place with a syringe case until attachment occurs, (4) the leech is left in place until it is full and detaches (10–30 minutes, but it may be longer). Some evidence supports that one leech can decongest and increase perfusion to approximately 2 cm² area of skin, removing approximately 5 mL of fluid each. Leech species include *Hirudo*, *Hirudinaria*, and *Macrobdella* [14].

300 mmHg with any size of needle or catheter [20]. The ideal volume of irrigation is also unknown, although 50–100 mL of irrigation fluid per cm of laceration or cm³ of wound has been recommended [22]. Irrigation should not be done blindly into puncture wounds since this may force foreign material or bacteria further into the wound or into healthy tissues.

Antisepsis

The classification of the wound based on the degree of contamination (see Table 21.1) has been shown to be a strong predictor for development of infection [2–4]. Wounds become infected secondary to the environment or due to the migration of endogenous bacteria, with the majority coming from the latter source [23].

Factors shown to provide an additional risk for wound infection include inadequate skin disinfection, inadequate preparation of the surgical team, hypothermia during the surgical procedure, and prolonged anesthetic and surgical time [6,23,24]. The size of the laceration and the presence of contamination has also been shown to increase the risk of infection [7,25,26]. Potential risk factors and options to minimize their impact are listed in Table 21.2.

Appropriate bandage care and wound debridement is more important than administration of topical or systemic antimicrobials. However, contaminated wounds (Class III) or obviously infected wounds (Class IV) may warrant systemic antibiotic administration (see Chapter 14). Common bacteria in wounds include *Staphylococcus* spp., *Streptococcus* spp., *Escherichia coli*, *Enterococcus*, *Proteus* spp., and *Pseudomonas*; anaerobic infections may include *Bacillus* spp., *Clostridium*, and *Corynebacterium* spp. *Pasteurella* spp. may be more prominent in cat bites. Confirmation of an infection with a resistant bacterium should prompt questioning to confirm the source and discussion with owners

Table 21.2 Risk factors for wound contamination and infection and methods to decrease those risks.

Risk factor	Methods to minimize
Inadequate skin disinfection and preparation	When preparing for surgical manipulation of a wound, cleansing the area with a chlorhexidine or iodine solution is necessary
Inadequate preparation of surgical team	The surgical team should be fully prepared, having necessary monitoring, surgical and bandage equipment, appropriate clipping and preparing as well as surgical materials
Hypothermia during the procedure	Use a variety of warming devices (warm air blowers, warm IV fluids, circulating warm water blankets) to minimize
Prolonged anesthetic time	Having an experienced surgeon and anesthetist with necessary materials "at the ready" will help minimize surgical time
Size of injury	Only necessary incisions should be made
Presence of contamination	Contamination should be minimized with appropriate preparation of the area and appropriate irrigation
Inappropriate sterility of materials	When performing surgery on a wound, all team members in the room should wear caps and masks and the person(s) handling the wound should wear sterile gloves; sterile surgical equipment and suture should be used
Malnutrition or underlying disease	Underlying disease should be identified and treated as possible; delayed healing and additional surgery may be necessary in severe cases

regarding appropriate handling of the pet during the healing process.

Skin antisepsis is extremely important. Commercial and natural antisepsis agents used for wound care with advantages and disadvantages are listed in Table 21.3. Detergents (scrubs) should never be used in wounds since they will damage tissue and facilitate wound infection. Product labels should be carefully read and close attention paid to the concentration of antiseptic that can be applied. Complications can arise from using a solution that is too dilute or too concentrated [27,28].

Drains

Dead space in a wound results from separation of portions of the wound beneath the skin that are not able to be sutured together, or from air or fluid trapped between layers of tissue. Dead space can be effectively eliminated using compression bandages or suction drains. Suturing dead space in infected wounds has been shown to be associated with a worse outcome and is not recommended [15].

Penrose drains are the most common type of passive drain. The drain should only exit from the most gravity-dependent area of the wound through an incision made away from the original injury or wound closure site. Because bacteria and environmental contaminants can ascend along the drain, a sterile bandage should protect it whenever possible. Warm wet compresses can be used to loosen any exudate that has accumulated around the external aspect of the drain and adjacent skin. The skin is then disinfected and dried. A thin film of broad-spectrum antibiotic ointment may be used around the exit site if desired.

Active drainage is provided through drains attached to suction bulbs that continuously evacuate air or fluid. The drain exit site from the skin should be inspected, disinfected, and rebandaged 1–2 times daily. The suction bulb is emptied at that time, or more frequently if needed. The volume and character of the fluid should be recorded. If the suction bulb does not maintain suction over time then an air leak from the drain skin exit site is likely or the drain may have a hole in it. An additional suture can be placed in a purse-string fashion to attempt to close the leak or antibiotic ointment can be placed at the site to make a seal. If pockets of fluid are accumulating despite the presence of active suction, the drain may be occluded.

The decision to remove drains should be based on the amount of fluid being produced rather than the number of days the drain has been present. Seromas are more likely to develop when the drains are removed before fluid accumulation is <0.2 mL/kg/h [29]. Cytology of the drainage fluid can provide information regarding the degree of active inflammation and the presence of bacteria, but it is unclear whether drain removal should be based on these findings. Fluid can be cultured if there are concerns for infection.

Wound closure

One of the more difficult decisions is determining whether or not the wound should be closed since closure at an inappropriate stage of healing can lead to dehiscence. A wound that dehisces is often more difficult to manage than the original wound. Reasons to delay wound closure include:

- debridement fails to remove all potentially necrotic or infected tissue
- the wound is older than 12 hours and could not be converted to a fresh wound
- the wound is infected
- there is too much tension on the suture lines.

Table 21.3 Antisepsis agents used in wound care.

Agent	Manufacturer	Advantages	Disadvantages
Detergents	Many	None	Can damage tissues and facilitate infection
Chlorhexidine 0.05% solution (diluted 1:20 of 2% solution)	Henry Schein, Dublin, OH	Promotes wound healing at 0.05% concentration	Higher concentrations cause tissue damage
Povidone-iodine 1.0% solution	Henry Schein, Dublin, OH	Used around mucous membranes, near ocular regions, and for the prepuce and vulva	Can be toxic (even at 0.5%) to growth of fibroblasts and impair wound healing
Sodium hypochlorite (Dankins) 0.5% solution	Henry Schein, Dublin, OH	Effective at killing bacteria and liquefying necrotic tissues. Broad spectrum of activity against bacteria, spores, mycobacteria, fungi, and biofilms	Damaging to neutrophils, fibroblasts, endothelial cells
Hydrogen peroxide 3% solution	Henry Schein, Dublin, OH	Dislodges bacteria and debris by effervescence. Effective sporicide	Ineffective against most organisms at 3% solution. Higher concentrations damaging to tissues
Chloroxylenol	Technicare® (Care-Tech Laboratories, St Louis, MO)	Broad-spectrum activity against bacteria and fungi. Not cytotoxic and safe to use in eyes, ears, mucous membranes. Might augment wound healing	Use in wounds for 2–3 minutes and irrigate
Unpasteurized honey (applied on wounds, covered with dry occlusive dressing)	Manuka Fill® (Links Medical Products Animal Health, Irvine, CA)	Nontoxic. Used for degloving injuries, contaminated or infected surgical wounds or burns. Spectrum includes gram negative, gram positive bacteria, and yeast. Wounds heal faster treated with honey	Medical-grade honey has more predictable antimicrobial spectrum and is preferred over standard commercial honey
Granulated sugar (layer at least 2 cm thick is applied with bandage changes 1–2 times daily)	Many	Used for degloving injuries, contaminated or infected surgical wounds or burns. Spectrum includes gram negative, gram positive bacteria, and yeast. Osmotic action pulls macrophages into wound to enhance bactericidal action. Increases rate of sloughing of devitalized tissues	Sugar should always be dry. Must change bandage if strike-through occurs. Wound must be irrigated and dried before applying more sugar

Deep puncture wounds may become infected if they are closed [30].

Wounds can be closed by one of three methods: primary intention, second intention or delayed primary closure. Wounds that are sutured initially heal by primary intention. An incision that heals by primary intention does so in a minimum of time, with no separation of the wound edges, and with minimal scar formation.

Wounds that heal without being sutured are considered to have healed by second intention. Healing by second intention is selected when there is infection, excessive trauma, tissue loss, or imprecise approximation of tissue. The wound may be left open and allowed to heal from the inner layer to the outer surface. Granulation tissue forms and myofibroblasts help to close the wound by contraction. This process is much slower than primary intention healing. Excessive granulation tissue may build up and require treatment if it protrudes above the surface of the wound, preventing epithelialization.

Delayed primary closure applies to wounds that are left open for 3–5 days and then closed. This is considered by many surgeons to be a safe method of management of contaminated, as well as dirty and infected traumatic wounds with extensive tissue loss and a high risk of infection. Nonviable tissues are debrided and the wound is left open, inserting gauze packing or other commercial bandage material, which is changed twice a day (Figure 21.3). After 3–5 days, if there is no sign of infection and granulation tissue is present then the wound edges are approximated using adhesive strips, sutures or staples. However, if infection persists or granulation tissue is insufficient, then the wound is allowed to heal by second intention.

Management of hospital-acquired wounds

Most hospital-acquired wounds occur at a site that originally had the hair clipped and the skin aseptically prepared. The skin site should be examined daily. If there is any exudate at the skin entry site, the exudate should be evaluated microscopically. A culture and sensitivity are indicated if bacteria are noted on cytological examination. If there is moderate to severe inflammation, the wound site should be inspected and disinfected three times daily and the catheter, tube or drain removed if signs worsen. If infection is confirmed, the catheter, tube or drain should be promptly removed and replaced if needed. If removal is not possible then careful disinfection three times daily, application of sterile dressings, and culture and sensitivity of the discharge are essential.

Vacuum-assisted closure

Vacuum-assisted closure (VAC) is used primarily to help with second intention healing and skin grafts. Blood flow has been shown to improve by up to fourfold, formation of granulation tissue is enhanced, and bacteria numbers are decreased [31,32]. An open cell foam (KCI, Wimborne, Dorset, UK) is placed in the wound and sealed with an adhesive drape which is attached to a vacuum system set at 125 mm subatmospheric pressure.

Vacuum-assisted closure dressings should be checked hourly to ensure the pressure is being maintained. The foam under the dressing should appear shrunken. Commercial units have alarms that will sound when an air leak is detected. Loss of the vacuum is caused by an air leak, usually due to loosening of the adhesive

drape. If this occurs, the wound edges should be checked to make sure they have been clipped adequately since the adhesive drape will not stick to fur. Adhesive spray, followed by application of adhesive paste (Stomahesive®, Convatec, Skillman, NJ) prior to applying the adhesive drape, will help ensure a good seal. Bandages are usually changed every 48–72 hours although occasionally they are left in place for up to five days, depending on the underlying reason for the VAC placement. Daily bandage changes may be necessary in contaminated wounds to allow debridement. Care should be taken when the bandage is changed to make sure the egress tube is not in contact with any of the tissues since the negative pressure that is applied will lead to necrosis. Figure 21.4 demonstrates placement of a VAC bandage on a necrotic wound on a distal limb of a dog.

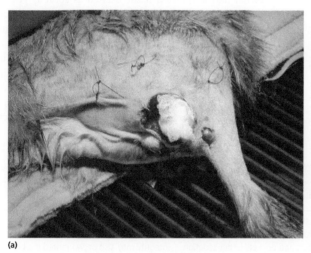
(a)

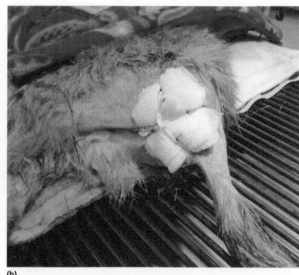
(b)

Figure 21.3 A tie-over bandage on the perineal region of a cat. These are useful for bandaging challenging anatomical regions. (a) A perineal wound on a cat extending down the base of the tail, with gauze, as part of a wet-to-dry bandage, placed inside the wound. Note the loops of suture placed around the wound. (b) The tie-over bandage is completed using gauze and umbilical tape passed through suture loops to keep the gauze in place.

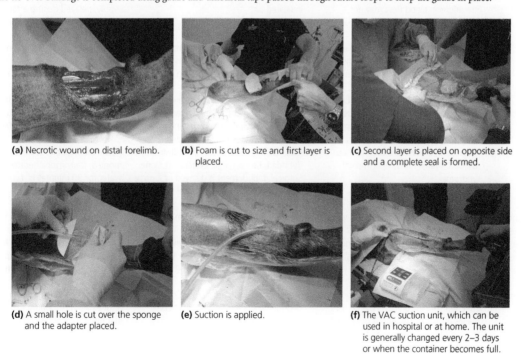

(a) Necrotic wound on distal forelimb.

(b) Foam is cut to size and first layer is placed.

(c) Second layer is placed on opposite side and a complete seal is formed.

(d) A small hole is cut over the sponge and the adapter placed.

(e) Suction is applied.

(f) The VAC suction unit, which can be used in hospital or at home. The unit is generally changed every 2–3 days or when the container becomes full.

Figure 21.4 Placement of a vacuum-assisted wound closure device (KCI, Wimborne, Dorset, UK). Care should be taken when placing this device on a limb to "sandwich" two pads over the limb rather than using a circumferential technique, which may limit blood flow.

Management of different wound types

Characteristics of different wounds and how this difference impacts wound management are outlined in Table 21.4. When wounds are not healing as expected, it is likely that one or more of the wound management goals is not being met and the treatment plan should be thoroughly reassessed (Figure 21.5). Residual foreign material in particular can be a problem in penetrating trauma and advanced imaging using ultrasonography or CT may be indicated in chronic draining wounds.

Special attention is required for burns, frostbite, necrotizing fasciitis, and compartment syndrome

Burns

Burns can occur as a result of exposure to excess heat (flame, sun, water), electricity or toxic chemicals and are classified (first through fourth degree) according to the depth of tissue injured. First-degree burns affect the epidermis, second-degree burns affect the epidermis and varying layers of the dermis, third-degree burns affect all layers of the skin and may involve deeper tissues, and fourth-degree burns involve muscle or bone. Each will be accompanied by different co-morbidities depending on the underlying cause of the burn. Analgesia and fluid therapy in patients with significant burns can be particularly challenging due to a combination of water, electrolyte, and protein losses (see Chapters 2, 19, and 20). Third- and fourth-degree burns carry a more guarded prognosis and must be closely monitored for tissue necrosis.

Patients with burns to more than 20% of their total body surface area (TBSA) are at high risk of metabolic derangements and burns to more than 50% TBSA carry a grave prognosis. Estimating TBSA of a burn can be done using the "Rule of 9 s", where each portion listed is approximately 9% of the TBSA: each forelimb, head and neck, half of each hindlimb, one-quarter of the trunk (Figure 21.6) [33].

Burns should be cleansed with 0.05% chlorhexidine. Spray hydrotherapy is also commonly used in human medicine. In order to reduce the risk of infection, all blisters should be drained of fluid and all eschar and devitalized tissue excised as soon as possible [34]. Systemic antibiotics are required for hemolytic streptococcal and *Pseudomonas aeruginosa* infections that can lead to septicemia and death.

Silver sulfadiazine (1%) is recommended for all skin burns, but superficial and partial-thickness burns heal faster when medical grade honey is used [35]. The burns are dressed with gauze thick enough to prevent seepage to the outer layers. Bandages are changed at least twice daily or more frequently if strike-through is evident. Wounds are gently debrided as needed at each bandage change.

Table 21.4 Differences in the character and management of different types of wounds compared to general wounds.

Wound type	Difference from general wounds	Management differences	Note
Bite and puncture	Tissue damage that is not evident on surface is likely present below skin level; potential for dead space. Residual foreign material a common problem	Clean the skin surface and do not flush into puncture holes; use sterile probe to explore tracts and pockets under sedation or anesthesia. Pockets >1–2 cm should be surgically explored	Most bite wounds warrant surgical exploration. Assessment of internal organ integrity may also be warranted if a bite occurred over the abdomen or chest
Big dog–little dog	Bite wounds on surface and internal crushing injuries below the surface. Smaller dog is often picked up and shaken	Surgical exploration indicated. Multiple traumatic injuries to head, neck, limbs, abdomen, and thorax are possible	Other injuries such as head and neck trauma, tracheal tears, and rupture of abdominal organs possible
Degloving	Tissue damage may be visible but alterations in blood flow may not. Contaminated but not infected. Foreign debris likely	Surgical exploration and debridement indicated	Dehiscence may occur with loss of blood supply; delayed closure after initial wound care is an option (to determine blood flow)
Blunt force	Extensive force applied over large area. Significant underlying tissue damage, ± bone damage not visible from skin level	Careful and repeated monitoring since damage may not be obvious on skin surface. Venous congestion can be treated with leeches	Hemorrhage from parenchymous organs (liver and spleen most common); surgical control of hemorrhage may be difficult
Burns	Damage depends upon depth of burn and TBSA affected (Rule of 9s). Serious fluid, electrolyte, and protein losses. Septicemia anticipated with >50% TBSA affected	Blisters are debrided, spray hydrotherapy helps debridement. Wounds treated with silver sulfadiazine. Superficial and partial thickness heal faster with honey dressing	Fever is not a useful sign of infection since it may persist until wound is closed. See additional reading and Table 20.8
Frostbite	Progression is edema, blistering then necrosis. Watch for compartment syndrome	Clear blisters are drained, torn blisters are debrided, hemorrhagic blisters left alone. Surgical debridement is delayed as long as possible, unless compartmental syndrome develops	Tissue damage can continue for 2–3 months. Daily hydrotherapy with 40 °C water for 30 minutes is recommended. Do not massage tissues
Surgical wounds	Form of deliberate trauma. Clean wound with debridement complete	Usually primary closure if minimal tension	Uncomplicated healing with minimal scarring anticipated
Exposed bone	Poor blood supply to exposed bone if periosteum is damaged or bone is fragmented	Can drill small holes into medullary cavity using 0.045 to 0.062 Kirschner wire, approximately 5 mm apart	Blood clots must be flushed from wound. Nonadherent dressing on exposed bone not changed for first 48–72 h, then every 3–5 days [27]
Necrotizing fasciitis	Sudden onset with rapid progression of infection spreading across the fascial planes in the subcutaneous tissue with sparing of muscle. Very painful	Immediate and aggressive surgical debridement and IV antibiotic therapy required. Amputation of affected limb might be required	Will cause death without rapid and aggressive intervention. Commonly staphylococcal and streptococcal spp. bacteria, though other species possible

TBSA, total body surface area.

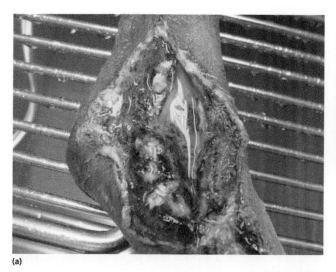

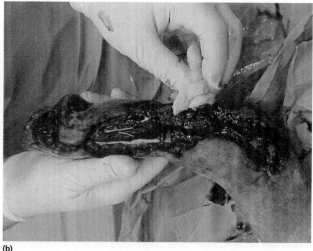

(a)

(b)

Figure 21.5 (a) A wound that has received inadequate debridement (day 3). Note the gray discoloration of devitalized (necrotic) tissues at the edges and within the wound and lack of a normal granulation bed. (b) A wound that has received appropriate wound care and debridement (day 5). Note the lack of gray or discolored tissues; the general red color indicates adequate removal of devitalized tissue and a good blood supply for wound healing.

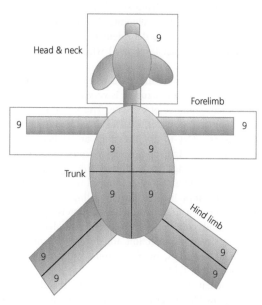

Figure 21.6 The Rule of 9 s is used to determine the total body surface area affected by burns in dogs and cats. The head and neck region = 9%; each forelimb = 9%; each quadrant of the trunk = 9%; half of each hindlimb = 9%.

Oral burns are managed in a similar fashion although surgical debridement should not be performed until the devitalized tissue is clearly demarcated as minor lesions will usually heal by second intention. Chlorhexidine solution for oral use may be helpful as an antiseptic. Topical lidocaine gel applied to affected areas may help decrease the pain that accompanies these lesions [36]. Attention must be paid to oral intake as often patients will not drink or eat due to the pain (see Chapter 16). More detailed information regarding the treatment of burn wounds can be found in the supplemental reading.

Frostbite

Frostbite is caused by freezing and crystallization of fluids in the interstitial and intracellular spaces. There is direct damage to the cells and tissues due to the cold and crystallization, combined with vasoconstriction, endothelial damage, and thrombosis. The thawing process leads to reperfusion injury and can be extremely painful. Intensive pain control is indicated (see Chapter 19). Edema is normal during the first 48–72 hours, and is followed by blistering and then necrosis. Tissue damage can continue for a period of 2–3 months. However, the absence of edema or the development of hemorrhagic blisters has been associated with a worse prognosis. Blisters with clear fluid should be aspirated to reduce the presence of inflammatory mediators and torn blisters should be debrided. Hemorrhagic blisters should be left alone.

Surgical debridement of tissue should be delayed as long as possible, often months, to allow adjacent tissue to heal as much as possible [37]. Debridement should be performed immediately if compartment syndrome develops. Daily hydrotherapy with water at 40 °C (104 °F) for 30 minutes is recommended [37]. Massage of affected areas should be avoided. The use of aloe vera over blisters may be helpful. Light padded bandages should be used to protect the wound and changed as needed. Nursing care is noted in Table 20.8.

Necrotizing fasciitis

Necrotizing fasciitis (NF) is a rare infection of the deeper layers of skin and subcutaneous tissues, easily spreading across the fascial plane within the subcutaneous tissue. Many types of bacteria can cause NF, with streptococcal and staphylococcal spp. identified in dogs [38,39].

Necrotizing fasciitis has a sudden onset and progresses rapidly. The infection begins locally at the site of trauma; even minor trauma (abrasion) may be sufficient. The most consistent feature of NF is necrosis of the subcutaneous tissue and fascia with relative sparing of the underlying muscle. Signs may not be evident initially if the infection lies deep within the tissues. Signs of inflammation, fever, and tachycardia will occur, with the affected tissues becoming progressively more swollen, reddened, and painful. Crepitus may be present and a discharge oozing through the skin may be evident.

Immediate and extensive surgical debridement and intravenous antibiotics are indicated [40]. Often amputation of an affected limb is required to save the life of the patient. Delay in surgical treatment has been associated with higher mortality. Hyperbaric oxygen may be a viable adjunct to therapy. Without surgical and medical intervention, the infection will rapidly progress, ending in death.

Compartment syndrome

Swelling in a confined space can lead to compartment syndrome. In osseofascial compartments, this can occur secondary to trauma such as a crush injury, complex fracture, soft tissue injuries or surgery. Thick layers of fascia separate groups of muscles and inside each layer is a confined space, called a compartment. The compartment includes the muscle tissue, nerves, and blood vessels. The layers of fascia do not expand, so any swelling in a compartment will lead to increased pressure in that area, compressing muscles, blood vessels, and nerves. If the pressure is high enough, blood flow to the compartment will be blocked. This can lead to permanent injury to the muscle and nerves and if the pressure lasts long enough, the muscles may necrose.

Measurement of the compartment pressure should be performed by inserting an 18 G needle attached to a water manometer into the affected area. If the pressure is greater than 40 mmHg ($54.4 cmH_2O$) subtracted from the patient's mean arterial pressure, then the compartment needs emergency exploration and fasciotomy [41]. The resulting incisions need to be treated as an open wound for at least 48–72 hours. Delaying surgery can lead to permanent damage.

Adjunctive therapy

Hyperbaric oxygen therapy has been used as an adjunct to wound therapy in dogs and cats to promote healing [42,43]. It involves placing patients in an airtight chamber and raising the atmospheric pressure and oxygen concentration so that oxygen is dissolved in the blood and delivered to tissues at higher levels than possible under normal atmospheric conditions. The few studies in veterinary medicine have found it to be a safe procedure if performed properly. There are good indications for benefit as an adjunct to wound therapy in humans [44].

Low-level impulse laser therapy (LLLT) has been applied focally to stimulate acupoints and topically over wounds, joints, and other tissues to increase circulation and promote healing in animals [45]. LLLT is reported to reduce inflammation and muscle spasms, increase blood perfusion, and encourage clearance of free radicals and healing in abscessed tissues. More veterinary-based clinical studies are needed to better define the role of LLLT as an adjunctive treatment for wounds.

Acupuncture has been used as an adjunct or stand-alone treatment for wounds, but there are few clinical studies in the veterinary literature [46]. The technique involves the placement of needles either transversely or obliquely along the edge of the lesion and directed toward the center. The technique is known as "circle or surround the dragon." This is combined with acupoints proximal and/or distal on the Channel(s) where the wound is located [47]. Acupuncture may serve to increase blood flow to regions as well as help alleviate patient discomfort.

External coaptation (bandages)

There are several goals of external coaptation, including promoting moist wound healing, protecting the wound and surrounding tissue, immobilizing injured areas, providing compression for hemorrhage, and decreasing pain. All bandages should have three layers: a contact layer, an intermediate layer, and an outer layer. The injury must be assessed and a decision made regarding the role each layer needs to play.

The contact (or *primary*) layer may have one or more functions, including debridement of tissue, delivery of medications, transmission of wound exudate away from the wound, and forming an occlusive seal. The ideal dressing would take the place of epithelium while new epithelium is developing. An adherent contact layer should be used when wound debridement is indicated, in contrast to a nonadherent contact layer used when granulation tissue is present.

Wet-to-dry dressings are indicated when minor debridement is desirable, when the wound exudate is very viscous or if the wound is exuding small volumes of exudate. The initial layers of sterile gauze should be soaked in sterile 0.9% saline; this is then covered by dry sterile gauze. Dry-to-dry dressings are indicated when the volume of exudate is high and not very viscous.

Commercial dressings are preferred although they should be used with caution in heavily contaminated wounds. Advantages of commercial dressings include faster healing because of a more rapid formation of a granulation bed and thus epithelialization, improved wound contraction, more efficient debridement that avoids healthy tissue, less infection, and decreased pain [8,48]. A list of commercial dressings, manufacturers, indications, and comments is provided in Table 21.5.

The intermediate (or *secondary*) layer is the absorbent layer. It is designed to draw blood, serum, exudate, debris, and bacteria away from the contact layer. Because this is the layer that provides padding, it also helps to prevent movement of the contact layer against

Table 21.5 Commercial dressings commonly used in contact layer of bandages.

Dressing	Product name (manufacturer)	Indication	Note
Calcium alginate	Kendall™ (Covidien, Mansfield, MA)	Highly exudative wounds. Promotes hemostasis, absorbs up to 20× its weight	Not recommended with anaerobic infections. Not used in dry wounds
Foams (polyurethane and others)	Kendall AMD™ (Covidien, Mansfield, MA), Tegaderm™ (3M, St Paul, MN)	Wounds with deeper defects. Highly absorbent	Not used in dry wounds. Not recommended in wounds needing frequent inspection
Hydrocolloid	Kendall™ (Covidien, Mansfield, MA)	Used with moderate exudate. Absorbs exudate, forms protective gel	Not ideal for dry wounds or if highly exudative. Not used if exposed bone or tendon. Not used in infected wounds
Hydrogel	Kendall™ (Covidien, Mansfield, MA)	Used in dry wounds	Gel can develop odor and consistency similar to exudate

the wound, thus protecting new epithelial cells, provide mild compression to help prevent seroma formation, and provide comfort to the patient. The thickness of this layer will depend on the degree of exudate the wound is producing as well as the amount of padding that is desired.

The outer (or *tertiary*) layer holds the other two layers in place and protects them from the environment. It is usually made of water-repellant material.

Ideally, all wounds, including all surgical incisions, should be covered for at least the first 24–48 hours while a fibrin seal forms. A patch dressing may be all that is needed for incisions as long as there is no need for protection of the underlying tissues.

All bandages should be protected from the patient and from the environment. Protecting the bandage from the patient usually requires the use of Elizabethan collars. Bitter-tasting sprays can also be used. Protecting the coaptation from the environment can be done in a variety of different ways. Paper surgical drape material or absorbent cage pads loosely wrapped or pinned over the top of the bandage can provide additional protection against soiling. Indwelling urinary catheters should be placed in animals that are recumbent or poorly ambulatory. T-shirts or stockinette can be used over thoracic or abdominal bandages as protection as well as to hold the ends of drains and tubes away from cage doors (Figure 21.7). Plastic bags or commercial bandage protectors should

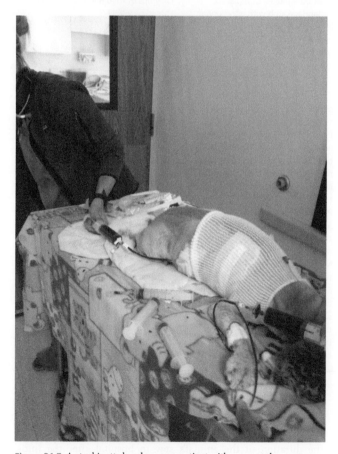

Figure 21.7 A stockinette bandage on a patient with a recent thoracotomy. This tertiary layer helps hold the linear adhesive dressings in place on the right side of the thorax: Telfa pad (Kendall™, Covidien, Mansfield, MA) covered by Hypafix® adhesive dressing.(Hypafix, Smith and Nephew, St Petersburg, FL) in place on the right side of the thorax.

be placed on limbs before the dog is walked outside and removed once the dog is indoors.

Evaluation of the external coaptation

Each goal of bandage placement should be assessed every time the bandage is evaluated, with adjustments made as needed. The frequency of bandage evaluation will vary with the reason the bandage was placed. Common problems found with external coaptation (bandages, splints, casts, slings) and suggestions for remedy and monitoring are provided in Table 21.6. Bandages, splints or casts that are placed too tightly can lead to vascular compromise and subsequent tissue necrosis; some cases may be severe enough to require amputation (Figure 21.8).

Peripheral catheter bandages should be inspected every 1–4 hours to ensure the catheter is patent, the fluid line is tightly connected to the catheter without leakage of liquid into the bandage, and there is no swelling of the proximal or distal limb (Figure 21.9). Circumferential neck bandages protecting central lines, esophagostomy tubes or wounds (Figure 21.10) should be placed loosely and checked at least three times a day for slippage, soiling, and constriction.

The proximal aspect of a circumferential limb bandage should be evaluated to ensure it is not too tight. Whenever possible, there should be approximately 5 mm of the intermediate layer visible beyond the outer layer of the bandage. It should be fairly easy to insert a finger between the third and fourth digits of the foot. A bandage that is too tight can result in impaired circulation and tissue necrosis. Should swelling be evident, the bandage should be removed or altered (Figure 21.11) and the site of the injury closely inspected, in case ongoing hemorrhage into a muscle or infection might be the cause of the limb swelling. If a cast is involved, it will need to be cut into two halves to permit removal. A decision will then need to be made as to whether or not the bivalve cast can be replaced and held together with a gap between the halves or whether a new cast needs to be applied.

Tie-over dressings (see Figure 21.3) are useful for areas that are more challenging to place and should be checked at least twice daily. In addition to standard evaluation for swelling, bleeding, and exudate, attention should be paid to ensuring that there is no excess tension on the suture loop grommets that could lead to necrosis around the suture loops. Bandaging axillary or groin regions can be challenging as well.

Bandage changes

The frequency of bandage change will depend on the type of bandage, the underlying injury, and the patient. Some bandage changes occur easily and without patient discomfort or pain, but removal of some bandages can be painful and adequate analgesia must be provided. Sedation and appropriate monitoring are provided for anxious patients, those that require more restraint, and when immobilization is desirable.

Every bandage should be changed within 24 hours of initial placement. If adhesive tape is holding a bandage in place, the tape layer adhering to the skin should not be removed when the bandage is changed unless it is soiled. Instead, the bandage should be carefully cut, leaving the original tape in place. A new bandage is placed and adhesive tape is placed on top of the original tape to secure it in place. This will help minimize skin irritation.

If strike-through is seen, the bandage should be changed immediately and a thicker intermediate layer may need to be

Table 21.6 Common problems with external coaptation and suggestions for remedy.

Problem	Effect	Remedy	Monitor
Bandages			
Too tight	Alters blood supply, impairs wound healing, causes tissue necrosis	Loosen, adjust or replace bandage	Temperature and pulse of tissues around bandage; check for swelling above or below bandage
Strike-through	Wicking of environmental contaminants into wound	Replace bandage, improve thickness and choice of intermediate bandage layer	Monitor for wetness on bandage and foul odor
Wet bandages	Tissue maceration, increased bacterial growth, breakdown of skin barrier	Apply appropriate covering. Ensure adequate walks for urination, consider urinary catheter if recumbent	Examine bandage hourly for wetness, discoloration, odor
Too loose	Abrasive motion can disrupt epithelialization of open wound	Rebandage with better fitting secondary and tertiary bandage layers. Ensure tape support and stirrups are adequate	Slipping two fingers under bandage rim should find a snug fit. Gently palpate bandage and observe for excessive movement and proper positioning of bandage
Circumferential bandages too tight	Impaired ventilation and oxygenation (neck, chest or abdomen); compression of jugular veins can increase ICP (neck); increased intraabdominal pressure (abdominal). Limb bandages can impair flow to digits and cause digit necrosis. Digit swelling	Incise all layers of bandage on site away from wound (usually dorsum) and retape in place, providing >2–3 mm of new added space between cut bandage edges or replace bandage. If the bandage is a neck splint or spica bandage, these must be removed or replaced. Rebandage limb with appropriate length and padding	Check as soon as patient is awake and mobile; should be able to easily slip two fingers between bandage and skin. Should be able to slip two fingers between third and fourth digits on limb with bandage. Limb bandages are checked every 4–8 h. Only tips of third and fourth digits should be visible
Insufficient padding or bandage not extended enough (limb)	Bandage may be placed too tight, excessive movement, insufficient padding and wicking of exudate	Replace bandage with sufficient padding	Patient mobility, bandage for strike-through
Splints/casts/slings			
Excessive padding	Movement under cast, delayed fracture healing	Cut cast, rebandage with less padding and reapply cast as bivalve cast or recast	Patient comfort. Limit patient mobility
Too tight Placing cast too soon after injury, continued soft tissue swelling in confined environment	Vascular compromise, pressure sores; skin abrasions; secondary infection; worst case can require further debridement or amputation	Place external coaptation that can be adjusted in response to swelling or careful monitoring to change cast in response to changes in swelling. Minor skin problems treated with topical antiseptics	Observe for swelling at site where the cast starts and ends on the body; observe for animal shaking or trying to chew over cast site
Too loose Placing cast at peak of soft tissue swelling or hematomas, swelling resolves and cast becomes loose	Skin abrasions, pressure sores, secondary infection	Place external coaptation that can be adjusted in response to swelling or careful monitoring to change cast in response to changes in swelling. Minor skin problems treated with topical antiseptics	Observe for excessive space between cast and skin at sites where the cast starts and ends on the body; observe for animal shaking or trying to chew over cast site. Observe for skin irritation from movement of cast
Padding present where not indicated (Ehmer, Velpeau)	Slippage of flexion sling	Remove padding and re-sling. Ensure each joint is not in full flexion; extend wrap past the metacarpal-phalangeal or metatarsal-phalangeal joint	Examine digits for cold or swelling (impaired perfusion)
Skin irritation or abrasions in groin or axillary areas (spica splint)	Tape in sensitive areas irritates skin	Limit patient mobility early. Topical creams or ointments, antiseptics	Monitor skin regions for redness, swelling, abrasions

placed or the bandage should be changed more frequently. Bandages should be checked at least three times daily for slippage and soiling and should be changed immediately if either is evident. Some animals will chew any bandage given the opportunity. The bandage, sling or cast should be immediately inspected since chewing and self-mutilation can be an indication of an underlying problem.

Surgical incisional bandages may not need to be changed for the duration of the animal's stay in hospital after the initial change at 24 hours unless there is strike-through. Bandages for open abdominal drainage should be closely inspected every 1–4 hours for signs of slipping, soiling, and strike-through due to the risk associated with ascending contamination. The bandage material should be weighed before it is placed and again at the time of removal to help determine the amount of fluid loss (1 g = approximately 1 mL) into the bandage.

Wet-to-dry dressings should be changed 1–2 times daily depending on the underlying wound or any evidence of strike-through. The bandage must be removed in its dry form, which removes debris and necrotic tissue. Soaking the bandage to permit easier removal is not done since this defeats the purpose of the wet-to-dry bandage. These bandages are painful to remove and analgesics are essential, with sedation recommended.

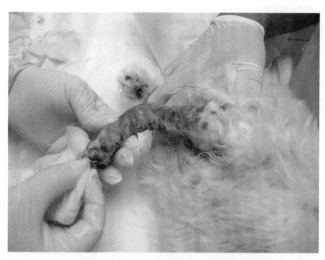

Figure 21.8 A splint and bandage was applied too tightly to this forelimb of a dog and led to compromise of the vascular supply to the distal limb; redness of the more proximal limb is bruising from the initial injury.

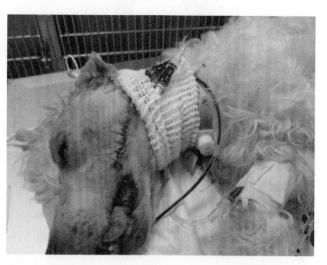

Figure 21.10 A loose cervical circumferential wrap on this patient who had major orofascial surgery, a central venous catheter, and a tracheostomy. Two fingers can easily pass under this bandage and it is not restricting venous flow or breathing.

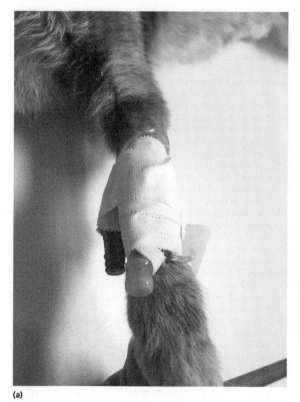

(a)

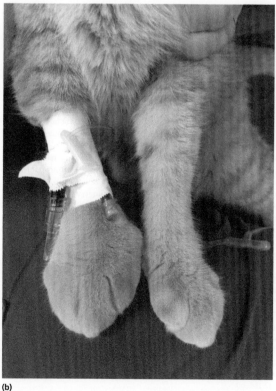

(b)

Figure 21.9 Figure of a newly placed catheter in the left forelimb of a cat (a) and cat with a right forelimb that has developed "fat paw" (b). Fat paw is limb swelling distal to a catheter bandage; this may develop from excessive pressure of the catheter bandage impairing venous and/or lymphatic drainage, extravasation of fluids or thromboembolism. Treatment may involve rewrapping the tape on the limb to make it looser, bandaging the entire limb to prevent further swelling, or removing the catheter if it is no longer functional. Source: Photo courtesy of Dr Annie Chih.

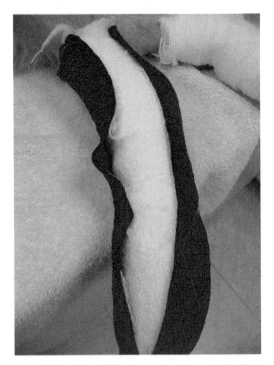

Figure 21.11 A circumferential bandage protecting a peripherally inserted central catheter was incised. Initially placed too tightly, this bandage was cut along one length and retaped as an alternative to bandage replacement.

References

1. National Research Council Division of Medical Sciences Ad hoc Committee of the Committee on Trauma. Postoperative wound infections: the influence of ultraviolet irradiation of the operating room and of various other factors. Chapter III Organization, Methods, and Physical Factors of the Study. Ann Surg. 1964;160(Suppl 2):19–31.

2. Mangram AJ, Horan TC, Pearson ML, et al. Guideline for prevention of surgical site infection. Centers for Disease Control and Prevention (CDC) Hospital Infection and Control Practices Advisory Committee. Am J Infect Control. 1999;27:97–132.

3. Haley RW, Culver DH, Morgan WM, et al. Identifying patients at high risk of surgical wound infection. A simple multivariate index of patient susceptibility and wound contamination. Am J Epidemiol. 1985;121:206–15.

4. Culver DH, Horan TC, Gaynes RP, et al. Surgical wound infection rates by wound class, operative procedure, and patient risk index. National Nosocomial Infections Surveillance System. Am J Med. 1991;91:152S–157S.

5. Millard RP, Towle RA. Open fractures. In: Veterinary Surgery Small Animal, vol. 1. Tobias KM, Johnston SA, eds. St Louis: Elsevier Saunders, 2012: p 572.

6. Nicholson M, Beal M, Shofer F, et al. Epidemiologic evaluation of postoperative wound infection in clean-contaminated wounds: a retrospective study of 239 dogs and cats. Vet Surg. 2002;31:577–81.

7. Hollander JE, Singer AJ, Valentine SM, et al. Risk factors for infection in patients with traumatic lacerations. Acad Emerg Med. 2001;8:716–20.

8. Nickerson D, Freiberg A. Moisture-retentive dressings: a review of the current literature. Can J Plast Surg. 1995;3:35–8.

9. Haury B, Rodeheaver G, Vensko J, et al. Debridement: an essential component of traumatic wound care. Am J Surg. 1978;135:238–42.

10. Mathews KA, Binnington AG. Wound management using honey. Compend Contin Educ Pract Vet. 2002;24:53–60.

11. Bischofberger AS, Dart CM, Perkins NR et al. The effect of short- and long-term treatment with manuka honey on second intention healing of contaminated and noncontaminated wounds on the distal aspect of forelimbs in horses. Vet Surg. 2013;42:154–60.

12. Mathews KA, Binnington AG. Wound management using sugar. Compend Contin Educ Pract Vet. 2002;24:41–50.

13. Hendrix CM, Shealy PM. The changing role of leeches in veterinary medicine. Compend Contin Educ Pract Vet. 1991;13:447–54.

14. Sobczak N, Kantyka. Hirudotherapy in veterinary medicine. Ann Parasitiol. 2014;60(2):89–92.

15. Berk WA, Welch RD, Bock BF. Controversial issues in clinical management of the simple wound. Ann Emerg Med. 1992;21:72–80.

16. Lozier S, Pope E, Berg J. Effects of four preparations of 0.05% chlorhexidine diacetate on wound healing in dogs. Vet Surg. 1992;21:107–12.

17. Swaim SF, Lee AH, Hughes KS. Heating pads and thermal burns in small animals. J Am Anim Hosp Assoc. 1989;5:155–62.

18. Thomas GW, Rael LT, Bar-Or R, et al. Mechanisms of delayed wound healing by commonly used antiseptics. J Trauma 2009;66:82–91.

19. Moscati R, Mayrose J, Fincher L, et al. Comparison of normal saline with tap water for wound irrigation. Am J Emerg Med. 1998;16:379–81.

20. Gall TT, Monnet E. Evaluation of fluid pressures of common wound-flushing techniques. Am J Vet Res. 2010;71:1384–6.

21. Longmire AW, Broom LA, Burch J. Wound infection following high-pressure syringe and needle irrigation. Am J Emerg Med. 1987;5:179–81.

22. Chisholm CD, Cordell WH, Rogers K, et al. Comparison of a new pressurized saline canister versus syringe irrigation for laceration cleansing in the emergency department. Ann Emerg Med. 1992;21:1364–7.

23. Reichman DE, Greenberg JA. Reducing surgical site infections: a review. Rev Obstet Gynecol. 2009;2:212–21.

24. Beal MW, Cimino Brown D, Shofer FS. The effects of perioperative hypothermia and the duration of anesthesia on postoperative wound infection rate in clean wounds: a retrospective study. Vet Surg. 2000;29:123–7.

25. Demetriou J, Stein S. Causes and management of complications in wound healing. In Pract. (J Br Vet Assoc.) 2011;33(8):392–400.

26. Frank M, Schmucker U, Hinz P, et al. Not another 4th of July report: uncommon blast injuries to the hand. Emerg Med. 2008;25:93–9.

27. Devey JJ. Antiseptics, disinfectants, and sterilization. In: Advanced Monitoring and Procedures for Small Animal Emergency and Critical Care. Burkitt-Creedon JM, Davis H, eds. Chichester: Wiley-Blackwell, 2012: pp 719–27.

28. Kramer SA. Effect of povidone-iodine on wound healing: a review. J Vasc Nurs. 1999;17:17–23.

29. Shaver SL, Hunt GB, Kidd SW. Evaluation of fluid production and seroma formation after placement of closed suction drains in clan subcutaneous surgical wounds of dogs: 77 cases (2005–2012). J Am Vet Med Assoc. 2014;245:211–15.

30. Percival NJ. Classification of wounds and their management. Surgery 2002;20:114–17.

31. Morykwas MJ, Argenta LC, Shelton-Brown EI, et al. Vacuum-assisted closure: a new method for wound control and treatment: animal studies and basic foundation. Ann Plast Surg. 1997;38:553–62.

32. Kirkby KA, Wheeler JL, Farese JP, et al. Vacuum-assisted wound closure: application and mechanism of action. Compend Contin Educ Pract Vet. 2009;12:568–76.

33. Garzotto CK. Thermal burn injury. In: Small Animal Critical Care Medicine, 2nd edn. Silverstein DC, Hooper K, eds. St Louis: Elsevier Saunders, 2015: p 744.

34. Vaughn L, Beckel N, Walters P. Severe burn injury, burn shock, and smoke inhalation injury in small animals. Part 2: diagnosis, therapy, complications and prognosis. J Vet Emerg Crit Care 2012;22:187–200.

35. Wijesinghe M, Weatherall M, Perrin K, et al. Honey in the treatment of burns: a systematic review and meta-analysis of its efficacy. N Z Med J. 2009;122:47–60.

36. Mathews KA. Burn injury and smoke inhalation. In: Veterinary Emergency and Critical Care Manual, 2nd edn. Guelph: Lifelearn Inc., 2006: pp 682–9.

37. Reamy BV. Frostbite: review and current concepts. J Am Board Fam Pract. 1998;11:34–40.

38. Weese JS, Poma R, James F. Staphylococcus pseudointermedius necrotizing fasciitis in a dog. Can Vet J. 2009;50:655–6.

39. Jenkins CM, Winkler K, Rudloff E. Necrotizing fasciitis in a dog. J Vet Emerg Crit Care 2001;11(4):299–305.

40. Jain A, Varma A, Mangalanandan K. Surgical outcome of necrotizing fasciitis in diabetic lower limbs. J Diabetic Foot Compl. 2009;4:80–4.

41. Mars M, Hadley GP. Raised intracompartmental pressure and compartment syndromes. Injury 1998;9:403–11.

42. Kerwin S, Lewis C, Elkins DD, et al. Effect of hyperbaric oxygen treatment on incorporation of an autologous cancellous bone graft in a nonunion diaphyseal ulnar defect in cats. Am J Vet Res. 2000;61:691–8.

43. Hosgood G, Jodgin EC, Strain CM, et al. Effect of deferoxamine and hyperbaric oxygen on free autogenous full thickness skin grafts in dogs. Am J Vet Res. 2005;56:41–7.

44. Eskes AM, Ubbink DT, Lubbers MJ, et al. Hyperbaric oxygen therapy: solution for difficult to heal acute wounds? Systematic review. World J Surg. 2011;35(3):535–42.

45. Petermann U. Comparison of pre-and post-treatment pain scores of horses with laminitis treated with acupoint and topical low level impulse laser therapy. Am J Trad Chin Vet Med. 2011;6(1):13–25.

46. Mayo E. Acupuncture and wound healing. Am J Trad Chin Vet Med. 2012;7(2):45–51.

47. Xie H, Preast V. Xie's Veterinary Acupuncutre. Ames: Blackwell Publishing, 2007: pp 244–5.

48. Campbell BG. Managing degloving and shearing injuries. Clin Brief 2011;10:75–9.

Further reading

Haberal M. Abali AES, et al. Fluid management in major burn injuries. Indian J Platic Surg. 2010 Sep;43(Suppl):S29–360.

CHAPTER 22

Anesthesia of the critical patient

Susan E. Leonard

Northeast Veterinary Referral Hospital, Plains, Pennsylvania

Introduction

Anesthesia is an induced, temporary state with one or more of the following features: analgesia, paralysis, amnesia, and unconsciousness. Anesthesia is used to perform medical procedures that would otherwise cause severe or intolerable pain in an awake and conscious patient. General anesthesia works through the central nervous system (CNS) and results in unconsciousness and total lack of sensation. Sedation or dissociative anesthesia inhibits both anxiety and the creation of long-term memories. Local or regional anesthesia causes loss of sensation in the targeted body part.

An anesthetic is an agent that causes anesthesia. The anesthetic drugs are selected and the dose determined to achieve the type and degree of anesthesia appropriate for the procedure and the specific patient. The best anesthetic is the one with the lowest risk to the patient while still achieving the endpoints required to complete the procedure. The types of drugs that can be selected include general anesthetics, hypnotics, sedatives, neuromuscular-blocking drugs, narcotics, and analgesics. Many of the anesthetic drugs can depress cardiac contractility, cause hypotension through vasodilation, and reduce the normal drive to ventilate.

The need for anesthesia in the critical small animal patient is common for diagnostic sampling, invasive therapeutic procedures, surgical correction of underlying problems or maintaining amnesia, analgesia, and immobility while healing occurs (such as traumatic brain injury, severe burn injury). Unfortunately, these patients also have the highest risk of complications. Factors related to the health of the patient, the complexity of the procedure being performed, and the type of anesthetic administered contribute to the likelihood of adverse anesthetic events.

A careful anesthetic plan must be created that includes preanesthetic patient evaluation and stabilization, premedication, anesthetic induction and maintenance, monitoring, and postanesthetic recovery. Risk factors for complications need to be recognized early in the process and steps taken to prepare for intervention should complications occur.

Preanesthetic evaluation

The first step of any anesthetic procedure is the preanesthetic patient evaluation for potential risk factors for anesthetic complications. The health of the animal prior to the anesthesia has a great bearing on the probability of a complication occurring. A comprehensive history and thorough physical examination will reveal most of the immediate risk factors. A review of the point of care (POC) laboratory data and clinicopathological laboratory results can demonstrate additional factors that can be of concern. Occasionally, diagnostic imaging is required prior to anesthetic induction to better characterize a potential or immediate problem that might affect recovery from anesthesia.

Several scoring systems have been proposed to assess the risk of perioperative mortality [1]. A simple stratification system developed by the American Society of Anesthesiologists (ASA) can be utilized for classification of the patient's anesthetic risks. However, it is not designed to provide a prediction of mortality (Table 22.1) [2].

Every parameter of the Rule of 20 can have an impact on anesthesia. Preexisting problems that can affect the anesthetic event will include breed-specific anatomical anomalies, cardiovascular disease, hemorrhage or anemia, hypoglycemia, acid–base imbalances, hypo- or hyperthermia, hypertension, hypotension, increased vagal tone, pain, and severe systemic disease. The Rule of 20 provides an ideal "check-off" list when performing the preanesthetic evaluation. The sample form provided in Figure 22.1 can be adapted to meet the needs of the specific patient and the critical care team.

History

Review of the history begins with the signalment (age, sex, breed). Older animals have a higher risk of metabolic or structural abnormalities that could impact the delivery of anesthesia. Breed-related problems such as brachycephalic syndrome, tracheal hypoplasia or sensitivity to anesthetics (such as sight hounds) must be factored into the anesthetic plan.

A review of past medical problems should look for cardiac disease, hypertension, coagulation disorders, liver disease, renal insufficiency, hypothyroidism, hypoadrenocorticism, and pulmonary disorders that could affect the delivery, maintenance, metabolism of anesthetic drugs as well as recovery from anesthesia. The complete list of prescribed and over-the-counter medications is reviewed for evidence of drugs that might affect cardiac function, blood pressure, clearance of anesthetic agents or clotting ability. Patients that may have an impaired immune response or are immunocompromised (through disease or medications) are identified since perioperative antibiotics can be an important part of their anesthetic and surgical plan [3].

Since it is ideal to have the patient fasted prior to anesthetic induction, the time since the last meal or free access to water becomes important. A careful review of the patient problems list and current therapy is crucial to avoiding anesthetic problems. Knowledge of therapies that should continue throughout the anesthetic procedure,

Monitoring and Intervention for the Critically Ill Small Animal: The Rule of 20, First Edition. Edited by Rebecca Kirby and Andrew Linklater.

© 2017 John Wiley & Sons, Inc. Published 2017 by John Wiley & Sons, Inc.

Table 22.1 American Society of Anesthesiologists Classification of Physical Risk Factors for Anesthesia.

Category	Physical status	Examples
I	Normal healthy patient	Sterilization surgery
II	Mild systemic disease	Fracture in a stable patient without identified systemic injury or disease (cardiac disease, hyperadrenocorticism, etc.)
III	Severe systemic disease	Fever, anemia, shock
IV	Severe systemic disease that is a constant threat to life	Severe shock, uncompensated cardiac disease, uremia, GDV, etc.
V	Moribund patient not expected to survive with or without surgery	Severe uncompensated systemic disease (trauma, infection, malignancy, etc.)
VI	Brain-dead patients to be used as donors	Does not apply to veterinary medicine

Source: Adapted from Thurmon JC, Short CE. History and overview of veterinary anesthesia. In: Lumb and Jones' Veterinary Anesthesia and Analgesia, 4th edn. Tranquilli WJ, Thurmon JC, Grimm KA, eds. Ames: Blackwell Publishing, 2007: p 17 [2]. Used with permission of Wiley.

Parameter	Patient	Target	Intervention	Parameter	Patient	Target	Intervention
Fluid balance				Heart rate, rhythm, contractility			
Blood pressure				Neurological status			
Oncotic pull /albumin				Urinary tract status			
Glucose				WBC, immune status, antibiotics			
Electrolytes				Gastrointestinal status			
Acid–base				Nutritional status			
Oxygenation and ventilation				Drugs, dosage, metabolism			
Coagulation				Pain			
RBCs				Wounds, bandages			
Temperature				Nursing care			

RBC, red blood cell; WBC, white blood cell.

Figure 22.1 Rule of 20 form to use in performing the preanesthetic evaluation of the critical small animal patient. This form should be amended to meet the needs of the specific ICU patient and critical care team.

such as fluid therapy, oxygen supplementation or inotropic support, should be clearly identified and plans made to provide the needed support. Medications that could complicate the anesthetic event, such as insulin infusions or intravenous potassium supplementation, should be recognized and decisions made whether to discontinue these drugs during anesthesia.

Physical examination

Any patient that is being anesthetized should have a recent and accurate body weight; however, some patients may require an estimated lean body weight if obese. The vital signs (temperature, heart rate, pulse intensity, mucous membrane (MM) color, capillary refill time (CRT)) begin the examination. The initial body temperature is important since most animals receiving anesthesia are at risk for hypothermia. An increased risk occurs in patients that are very young or geriatric, have small body size or poor body condition.

Hypoglycemia, prolonged anesthesia times, high inhalant gas flow rates, procedures requiring open body cavities or large shaved areas, and vasodilation provide increased risks of hypothermia in the anesthetized patient.

The physical peripheral perfusion parameters (heart rate, pulse intensity, MM color, CRT) can reflect hyperdynamic (tachycardia, red MM, CRT <1 second, bounding pulses) or hypodynamic (tachycardia (dogs), pale MM, CRT >2 seconds, weak or absent pulses) perfusion associated with hypovolemia, poor cardiac function or lack of vascular tone. Dehydration is observed through loss of skin turgor, dry MM and corneal moisture, and the sunken position of the eye within the orbit. In patients with interstitial deficits, procedures such as central line and feeding tube placement can be more challenging due to increased friction from interstitial tissues. Rehydration prior to anesthesia may improve ease of placement. Overhydration may be evidenced by peripheral edema, conjunctival edema or pulmonary crackles or rales.

The heart rate and pulse rate are compared to identify pulse deficits suggestive of cardiac arrhythmias. Muffled heart sounds or jugular distension might reflect pericardial effusion that could impact cardiac performance under anesthesia.

The respiratory rate and effort, breathing pattern, and lung auscultation can demonstrate most immediate problems causing abnormal oxygenation or ventilation. Significant breathing patterns and abnormal sounds identified on auscultation should be investigated before anesthetic induction (see Chapter 8). Severe respiratory disease may warrant rapid intervention so the airway can be secured and ventilation with oxygen initiated.

A complete neurological examination is performed to assess the level of consciousness and mentation and identify any deficits that might impact the choice of anesthetic. This also provides a baseline for comparing pre- and postanesthetic neurological status.

Auscultation and palpation of the abdomen will aid in assessing gastrointestinal (GI) motility. The GI motility and function can be altered by critical illness as well as by anesthesia. Anesthesia can cause gastric paresis and distension, which can impair ventilation and decrease venous return as well as put the patient at risk for aspiration pneumonia. Ileus is another common complication resulting from anesthesia and can cause a physiological bowel obstruction and mucosal ischemia.

Point of care and laboratory testing

A review of patient blood work and cage-side point of care testing within 12 hours of anesthesia is ideal for preanesthetic screening. The POC testing should consist of packed cell volume (PCV), total protein (TP), blood glucose, blood urea nitrogen (BUN) or creatinine, electrolytes, blood gas analysis, blood lactate, coagulation profile, buccal mucosal bleeding time (BMBT), blood smear for platelet estimate, and urinalysis. The complete blood count and serum biochemical profile can demonstrate high white blood cell (WBC) counts (inflammation), low WBC counts (immune compromise), characterize anemia or erythrocytosis, and provide evidence of disorders of various organs.

The PCV and TP will be used to determine the need for pre- or intraoperative blood products. The PCV should be >20% for adequate oxygen-carrying capacity during anesthesia. A high PCV (erythrocytosis) impairs blood flow and necessitates either fluid dilution or blood letting prior to anesthesia. Patients at risk of requiring blood products during anesthesia should have their blood typed and cross-matched to donor blood. A low TP or hypoalbuminemia warrants plasma or synthetic colloid administration to maintain the intravascular colloidal osmotic pressure. The role of protein binding in the pharmacokinetics of the drugs used for induction and anesthesia maintenance is considered when determining the need for plasma or albumin administration.

A normal blood glucose is ideal for anesthesia. Hypoglycemia will contribute to hypotension, impaired compensatory responses to anesthesia, and depressed mentation. Hyperglycemia can cause fluid imbalance and alter mentation. An elevation in blood lactate suggests anaerobic metabolism and poor tissue oxygenation, requiring improved perfusion prior to anesthetic induction.

Acid–base disorders should be corrected prior to administering the respiratory and cardiovascular depressing agents that are used for sedation and anesthesia. Oxygenation and ventilation, sodium (free water), chloride, phosphorus, uremia, proteins, lactate, and unmeasured anions can all impact acid–base status (see Chapter 7).

Alterations of sodium, potassium, ionized calcium, and magnesium can be associated with changes in fluid balance, cardiac arrhythmias, mental depression, neuromuscular irritability, and prolonged bleeding. Oxygen supplementation, ventilation, fluid therapy, and electrolyte supplementation may be required to establish and maintain an acceptable electrolyte and acid–base status prior to anesthetic induction.

Patients undergoing anesthesia are at risk for hypotension, which can cause or exacerbate preexisting renal conditions. An elevated BUN or creatinine and isosthenuria bring concern for renal disease. Anesthetic drugs that will affect renal blood flow or that require renal excretion should be used judiciously or avoided in patients with preexisting renal disease. Placement of a urinary catheter with a closed collection system before anesthesia will allow monitoring of urine output and fluid balance during anesthesia. A low BUN can be a reflection of poor liver function. If liver dysfunction is suspected, drugs requiring hepatic metabolism should be minimized or avoided.

Coagulation abnormalities are common in the critical animal and anesthetic-related events such as hypothermia or surgery may exacerbate an underlying clotting disorder. Prior to surgical procedures, the platelet number, platelet function (BMBT), and coagulation system are evaluated. Prolonged hypothermia associated with anesthesia must be avoided since it can cause coagulopathies (see Chapter 9), and coagulation factor dilution or inhibition resulting from aggressive fluid therapy (crystalloids and hydroxyethyl starches) can also impair the ability to clot normally.

Diagnostic imaging

Survey chest radiographs should be evaluated for evidence of airway, lung parenchymal or pleural space disorders that could affect oxygenation and ventilation or potentially patient prognosis. Pleural fluid or air should be evacuated prior to anesthetic induction. Focused assessment with sonography in trauma (FAST) techniques for the thoracic and abdominal cavities may help to rapidly identify evidence of hemorrhage or other catastrophic consequences of trauma prior to anesthesia.

An electrocardiogram (ECG) is evaluated prior to anesthetic induction. The presence of arrhythmias can warrant preoxygenation, antiarrhythmic agents or a change in anesthetic drug selection.

Patient preparation

The information from the history, physical examination, and blood testing is used to establish a plan for patient preparation and make a selection of premedication drugs. Interventions to consider include volume resuscitation (crystalloids, colloids, blood components), pain control (narcotics, adjunctive therapies), antiarrhythmic drugs, positive inotropes, vasopressors, and specific steps to normalize metabolic, electrolyte, and acid–base derangements. Patients at risk for adverse cardiovascular events will benefit from having cardiovascular drug doses (such as continuous rate infusion doses of vasopressor agents or positive inotropes) precalculated for rapid intervention if required.

Patients with traumatic injuries, gastric dilation-volvulus, airway disease, respiratory dysfunction or cardiovascular disorders can decompensate rapidly or respond negatively to the anesthetics or other medications administered. The anesthesia monitoring devices, including blood pressure, ECG, and pulse oximetry, should be placed on the animal during the patient preparation phase of anesthesia to allow continuous monitoring throughout all phases.

Catheter placement is essential in critically ill patients both for monitoring and therapy. At least one intravenous or intraosseous catheter is necessary prior to induction of anesthesia. A second catheter should be placed if blood administration or rapid, large-volume fluid administration is anticipated during anesthesia. Placement of catheters such as a central line, direct arterial line, urinary catheter, nasal oxygen and nasogastric tube prior to induction will minimize anesthetic time. However, the procedures may be more challenging and uncomfortable in the awake patient, making placement shortly after induction in these animals another option.

Patients with intravascular volume deficits should have the deficit corrected through resuscitation with the appropriate fluid(s) prior to induction of anesthesia. Additional monitoring procedures such as urinary output and central venous pressure can help assess and maintain an adequate fluid balance during the anesthetic period. Administration of crystalloids is considered standard of care for patients throughout general anesthesia, and is recommended at a dose of 5–10 mL/kg/h. However, fluid choices and infusion rates may need to be altered for short or prolonged anesthetic procedures depending on the fluid balance, cardiac function, and blood pressure of the patient.

Examples of patients that may require preoxygenation include those with pulmonary, pleural or chest wall disease, neurological disease, obese patients, and patients with abdominal distension (including ascites, pregnancy, and pyometra). Those patients with preexisting increase in work of breathing, brachycephalic breeds and patients with anemia would benefit as well. Preoxygenation for 3–5 minutes can increase the alveolar concentration of oxygen. This will provide a slightly longer time for hemoglobin desaturation than without preoxygenation. Preoxygenation can serve as a safeguard during rapid induction and intubation or during patient transfer into the surgery suite [4].

Arrhythmias should be treated prior to anesthetic induction when one or more of the following criteria are met: (1) the arrhythmia is impacting cardiac output and compromising tissue perfusion, (2) if the high heart rate is negatively impacting coronary perfusion, and potentially causing further arrhythmias or (3) prefibrillatory rhythms are noted (such as torsades de pointes, multiform ventricular beats or R-on-T phenomenon). If any of these are present, preoxygenation is instituted and specific pharmacologialc intervention is indicated (see Chapter 11). For bradyarrhythmias, atropine or glycopyrrolate is usually the first drug of choice. For ventricular tachyarrhythmias, lidocaine, procainamide or magnesium sulfate are common drug options.

Anesthesia can reduce GI motility and delay gastric emptying. An appropriate time of fasting prior to anesthesia is desired to decrease the amount of gastric contents. When this is not possible, the administration of antiemetics and prokinetics in the perianesthetic period may decrease the risk of aspiration pneumonia. A nasogastric tube can be placed and used to remove gastric fluid and air to reduce the stimulus for vomiting.

Medical management for an elevation in intracranial pressure should be considered prior to anesthetic induction in any patient with altered mentation, head trauma or a recent history of seizures (see Chapter 12). Interventions can include preoxygenation, maintaining a normal blood pressure, maintaining $PaCO_2$ between 35 and 45 mmHg and ensuring adequate glucose levels. The head and shoulders can be elevated up to 15–20° and jugular vein occlusion is avoided. Hypoventilation leading to hypercapnia will alter cerebral vasomotor tone and predispose to altered intracranial pressures. Drugs such as opioids, dissociative anesthetics, and phenothiazines can induce hypoventilation. Some inhalant anesthetics, particularly halothane and nitrous oxide, can disrupt cerebral autoregulation and increase cerebral metabolic rate and oxygen consumption [4].

Altered drug pharmacokinetics, including drug absorption, distribution, metabolism, and excretion, can occur in critical patients associated with changes in fluid balance, cardiovascular function, albumin concentration, hepatic function, and renal function. Depending on the drug and the pharmacokinetic changes, drug doses or intervals may need to be altered or drug combinations used. Changes in the magnitude and duration of drug effects should be anticipated and adjustments made as indicated.

A flow sheet should be prepared for every patient undergoing anesthesia with precalculated doses of emergency, anesthetic, and vasoactive drugs available for that specific patient in case urgent intervention is required. The clinician should be familiar with side-effects of all medications administered. A list of common sedatives, analgesics, anesthetics, drug reversal agents, and cardiopulmonary resuscitation drugs, their recommended dose and common side-effects is provided in Table 22.2.

One of the overall goals of the anesthetic plan is to minimize the time that the patient is required to be under anesthesia. Methods to consider for saving anesthetic time for patients are listed in Table 22.3. During the premedication phase of anesthetic preparation, the critical care team must prepare the anesthesia and monitoring equipment as well as the procedural or surgical suite. An example of a preanesthetic check-off list is provided in Table 22.4. Equipment, drugs, and materials should be set up for immediate use prior to inducing anesthesia in the patient.

Premedication

Premedication is the administration of drugs prior to anesthesia to prepare the patient for anesthesia and provide optimal conditions for the procedure or surgery. The goal is to reduce pain and anxiety, promote amnesia, decrease postanesthetic nausea and vomiting, allow restraint, and accomplish other patient-specific targets. These drugs are administered any time within 15 minutes to two hours before the induction of anesthesia and can be given by intramuscular or intravenous routes.

Medications can include tranquilizers or sedatives such as benzodiazepines and phenothiazines, opioid analgesic medications, dissociative agents, alpha-2-agonists and local anesthetics. Benzodiazepines are ideal to reduce anxiety and provide some amnesia and light sedation. Drugs such as lorazepam and midazolam may allow a lighter depth of anesthesia by reducing the risk of awareness during the procedure (see Table 22.2). Antiemetics such as maropitant (0.6–1 mg/kg SC or IV), ondansetron (0.5–1 mg/kg, slow IV), or metoclopramide (0.2–0.4 mg/kg IV) can be given to reduce postanesthetic nausea and vomiting. Prokinetics such as or metoclopramide or cisapride should be avoided in patients with gastrointestinal obstruction.

When anesthetics or sedatives are used in combination, lower doses of each medication may be used to decrease the side-effects of any individual drug. An opioid may be combined with the benzodiazepine if analgesia is desired prior to the induction of anesthesia. Common analgesic premedications include pure mu-agonists such as hydromorphone, methadone, fentanyl or morphine. The combination of medications such as a constant rate infusion (CRI) of fentanyl, lidocaine, and ketamine can provide a balanced plan for analgesia. Lidocaine has the added advantage of decreasing some ventricular

Table 22.2 Common sedatives, analgesics, anesthetic medications, reversal drugs, and CPR drug doses and common side-effects. Doses are suggestions and may vary depending on drug combinations used and individual patient health status.

Drug name by class	Dose and route	Common side effects/Notes
Anticholinergics		
Atropine	0.02–0.04 mg/kg IM, half dose IV	Increased heart rate and myocardial oxygen demand
Glycopyrrolate	0.005–0.01 mg/kg IM, IV	As above
Alpha-2-agonists		
Dexmedetomidine	3–40 µg/kg IM or IV then CRI 0.5–2.0 µg/kg/h (125–375 µg/m²; CRI 25 µg/m²/h)	Vasoconstriction, bradycardia, decreased contractility, may cause vomiting
Barbiturates		
Thiopental	4–20 mg/kg IV	Respiratory depression, vasodilation, arrhythmias, local reaction, CV depressions
Pentobarbital	2–4 mg/kg slow IV; CRI 1–4 mg/kg/h	Prolonged recovery, seizures with recovery
Benzodiazepines		All can be given as anticonvulant, muscle relaxer or in combination with an opioid as neuroleptanalgesia
Diazepam	0.2–0.5 mg/kg IM, IV; CRI 0.1–0.5 mg/kg/h	Does not mix well with many medications, may cause phlebitis; dysphoria
Midazolam	0.07–0.4 mg/kg IM, IV; CRI 0.1–0.5 mg/kg/h	Can be administered IM if necessary
Zolazepam/tiletamine	1–4 mg/kg IM, IV	
Dissociatives		
Ketamine	1–5 mg/kg IV, IM (induction); CRI 0.1–0.5 mg/kg/h; 2–10 µg/kg/min	Tachycardia, may increase intracranial pressure
Tiletamine/ zolazepam	1–4 mg/kg IM, IV	
Opioids		Bradycardia, respiratory depression,
Butorphanol	0.1–0.4 mg/kg IM, IV; CRI 0.1–02 mg/kg/h	kappa-agonist, mu-antagonist, only for mild pain
Buprenorphine	0.005–0.02 mg/kg IM, IV	Partial mu, slower onset, difficult to reverse
Fentanyl	2–10 µg/kg IM, IV; CRI 2–10 µg/kg/min	Urine retention
Hydromorphone	0.05–0.2 mg/kg IV, IM; CRI 0.01–0.04 mg/kg/h	Panting, dysphoria
Methadone	0.05–0.2 mg/kg IV, IM; CRI 0.13 mg/kg/h	Panting, dysphoria
Morphine	0.2–1.0 mg/kg IM; CRI 0.1 mg/kg/h	Panting, anaphylaxis IV
Oxymorphone	0.05–0.2 mg/kg IV, IM	Dysphoria, decreased GI function
Remifentanil	3 µg/kg IV; CRI 0.05–0.3 µg/kg/min	
GABA agonist induction agents		
Alfaxalone	2–3 mg/kg (dog), 4–5 mg/kg (cat) slow IV or IM; CRI 0.1–0.15 mg/kg/min	Respiratory depression
Etomidate	0.5–2.0 mg/kg IV; CRI 0.02–0.1 mg/kg/min	Vomiting, apnea, clonic twitching, cortisol deficiency; minimal effects on cardiovascular system, use with benzodiazepine
Propofol	2–8 mg/kg IV; CRI 0.05–0.5 mg/kg/min	Apnea, hypotension, short duration
Local anesthetics		
Lidocaine	1–2 mg/kg IV loading then 25–75 µg/kg/min	Avoid use in cats
Paralytic agents		
Succinylcholine	70–100 µg/kg IV	Hypoventilation; no analgesic effects
Atracurium	0.1 mg/kg IV; CRI 3–8 µg/kg/min (reversal neostigmine 0.02–0.04 mg/kg IV or edrophonium 0.1–0.2 mg/kg IV with atropine)	Paralysis will cause apnea; patient must be ventilated; no analgesic effects
Phenothiazines		
Acepromazine	0.01–0.1 mg/kg IM, IV (maximum dose 3 mg/dog, 1 mg/cat)	Vasodilation; no specific antagonist
Volatile (inhalant) anesthetics		All cause cardiovascular depression, which is dose dependent; no analgesic effects
Halothane	*MAC 0.87	Malignant hyperthermia, arrhythmias
Isoflurane	*MAC 1.3	
Sevoflurane	*MAC 2.3	Rapid recovery (may be too rapid in some cases)
Nitrous oxide	*MAC 188	Should not be used alone nor with closed cavity gas-containing disease
Reversal agents		
Flumazenil	0.01–0.02 mg/kg IV	Reverses benzodiazepines
Atipamezole	Equivalent volume of dexmedetomidine 0.09–0.4 mg/kg	Reverses dexmedetomidine
Naloxone	0.02–0.04 mg/kg IM, IV	Reversal of mu-agonists, multiple doses may be necessary due to short duration

(Continued)

Table 22.2 (*Continued*)

Drug name by class	Dose and route	Common side effects/Notes
CPR medications		
Atropine	0.04 mg/kg IV	Tachycardia
Epinephrine (low dose)	0.01 mg/kg IV	Hypertension and tachycardia
Vasopressin	0.4–0.8 U/kg IV	Hypertension
Lidocaine	2–4 mg/kg IV	Neurological side-effects (cats more susceptible)
Amiodarone	5 mg/kg IV	
External defibrillation	4–6 J/kg monophasic; 2–4 J/kg biphasic	Only appropriate conductive gel should be used; alcohol may ignite. Caregivers must NOT be in direct contact with patient
Internal defibrillation	0.5–1 J/kg monophasic; 0.2–0.4 J/kg biphasic	

* MAC is the minimum alveolar concentration at which 50% of patients will not show a response to a noxious stimuli. This will be lower when used in combination with analgesic agents.
CPR, cardiopulmonary resuscitation; CRI, constant rate infusion; CV, cardiovascular; GABA, gamma-aminobutyric acid; GI, gastrointestinal.

Table 22.3 Procedures that can be performed prior to anesthetic induction to reduce time under anesthesia.

Method	Benefit
Ensure equipment is ready and functioning (catheters, anesthesia machine, monitors, fluid pumps, surgical table, warming device, suction, defibrillator, chest tap set, ventilator settings preset)	Shorter patient preparation time Shorter transit time to the surgical suite
Prepare endotracheal tubes, eye care. Several sizes available, cuff inflation mechanism tested, inflation syringe and tie-ins laid out, corneal lubricant available	Allows rapid intubation, cuff inflation, and tie-in with appropriate tube size
Shave prior to anesthetic induction	Done after premedication
Cross-match or blood typing	Speeds delivery of blood products when needed
Calculate and print emergency/anesthetic drug doses based on weight	Speeds delivery of medications
Shave over both chest and abdomen when surgery of both cavities could be required (trauma, esophageal foreign body)	Saves time in patients with transdiaphragmatic problems
Prewarm lavage fluids	Saves time and improves patient temperature
Prepare a preanesthetic check-off list	Promotes complete patient care
Keep surgical supplies sterile, organized, and readily available	Prevents surgical delays due to equipment nonavailability
Use additional staff when available	Can scrub in for surgical procedures, help the person(s) monitoring, get necessary equipment, care for newborns in C-section
Lay out surgical attire (gloves, gowns) and equipment in advance	Shortens anesthetic time
Have the surgeon help initial set-up of patient in surgical suite. Staff does final patient scrub while surgeon scrubs and gowns	Shortens anesthetic time

Table 22.4 Example anesthesia check-off list.

Material to set up	Notes
Gas anesthesia machine	Ensure oxygen hooked up, tubes hooked up, appropriate size reservoir bag, leak test, ensure sufficient volatile agent
Surgical prep area	ET tubes of appropriate sizes, check cuffs, check separate anesthetic machine if used, eye lube, laryngoscope, ET tube cuff syringe and tie-in
Surgical and prep table	Warming units turned on, clippers and scrub ready, eye lube, ET tube tie, cuff inflator, laryngoscope
Anesthetic and emergency drug list	Printed and ready, drugs nearby with syringes and needles. Anesthesia related drawn up prior to induction
Monitoring sheet	Monitoring and recording vital parameters every 3–5 minutes, along with start and stop time of anesthesia and surgical procedures and all drugs recorded
Surgical equipment laid out	Gloves, gowns, caps, masks, surgical instruments, sutures, warm lavage, scalpel blades, cautery, additional equipment
Materials for anticipated procedure	Examples: thoracocentesis set for trauma patient, meds and towels for puppies/kittens, feeding tubes, bandages, suction, defibrillator, etc.
Anesthetic or therapeutic ventilator	Check that settings are appropriate and test prior to connecting patient
Monitors ready	ECG, SpO$_2$, oscillometric or Doppler blood pressure, ETCO$_2$, arterial line and necessary set-up
Patient preparation	Necessary IV or other catheters, presurgical diagnostics (bloodwork, clotting times, radiographs), stable for anesthesia (pain medications, fluid resuscitation, preoxygenation, etc.)

ECG, electrocardiogram; ET, endotracheal.

arrhythmias, acute kidney injury, and hospitalization time in dogs with gastric dilation-volvulus [5]. Some critically ill patients can be induced and intubated with higher doses of premedications.

Anesthetic induction

Rapid-sequence anesthetic induction and endotracheal intubation techniques are employed in patients with critical illness. The purpose is to minimize the time between loss of consciousness and endotracheal intubation, allowing airway and ventilation. The patient is preoxygenated and injectable anesthetics such as propofol, etomidate-midazolam, ketamine-midazolam or alfaxolone are titrated until the patient loses the gag reflex. The injectable agents are often used in combination for several reasons: (1) when combining different mechanisms of action, analgesic effects can be increased, (2) adding drugs that work by different mechanisms can allow a lower dose of some anesthetics, including volatile agents, and (3) lower doses will decrease unwanted side-effects of any single agent (see Table 8.12).

Endotracheal intubation is immediately performed, followed by cuff inflation, oxygenation, ventilation, and securing of the endotracheal tube with ties. A complete description of how to perform endotracheal intubation and techniques to assure proper tube placement within the trachea is provided in Chapter 8, with tube sizes in Table 8.8 and Table 8.9. The endotracheal tube should have a thin coat of sterile water-based lubricant applied to the tip prior to placement, confirmed with auscultation, visualization and $ETCO_2$ measurement and secured with a tie. A back-up plan for intubation should be in place in case standard tracheal intubation is not possible (such as brachycephalic abnormalities, intraoral or pharyngeal disease, or unable to open mouth). Using a stylet or guidewire, endoscopic visualization, transtracheal catheter or tracheostomy may be required. In addition, suction should be available to clear regurgitated GI contents, large volumes of tracheal fluid or salivary secretions. An oropharyngeal and laryngeal exam is performed in every patient at the time of intubation to evaluate for any masses, polyps or laryngeal dysfunction.

When the airway is confirmed and secured, the patient is ready for maintenance of anesthesia with volatile anesthetics or constant rate infusion of injectable anesthetic and sedative drugs. Monitoring devices should be immediately connected to the patient and assessed to ensure an adequate level of anesthesia is achieved and the initial vital parameters are within acceptable limits. Careful patient monitoring is required throughout the entire anesthetic preparation and maintenance period.

Anesthetic maintenance

Balanced anesthesia involves the administration of different drugs to target anesthesia, analgesia, and neuromuscular relaxation. Often opioids are given during induction for analgesia with benzodiazepines for neuromuscular relaxation and volatile anesthetic agents used to maintain the desired plane of anesthesia.

Anesthesia drugs are a contributing factor to negative physiological changes in the animal since certain drugs, e.g. inhalant anesthetics, phenothiazines, and propofol, can cause vasodilation. This will decrease preload and can cause hypotension. Anesthetic agents will also depress the respiratory drive. Manual or mechanical ventilation should be employed for any critical patients undergoing general anesthesia.

Analgesic drugs in combination with sedatives can obtain neuroleptanalgesia. When used in combination with anesthetic drugs, neuroleptanalgesics can decrease the required dose for all medications since many of the drugs are synergistic. Local anesthetic techniques can also minimize the need for systemic analgesia and reduce the depth of anesthesia required.

The five stages of anesthesia are listed in Box 22.1 along with questions that the anesthetist should consider when assessing the anesthetized patient in Box 22.2 [7]. The physical monitoring parameters that aid in determining the plane of anesthesia are listed in Table 22.5. Physical parameters such as jaw tone, palpebral and corneal reflexes, presence or absence of voluntary movement to

---

Box 22.1 Classic stages of anesthesia.

Stage I	Not anesthetized
Stage II	Excitatory phase, not anesthetized
Stage III	Plane 1 – light anesthesia
	Plane 2 – moderate anesthesia (surgical plane)
	Plane 3 – deep anesthesia
Stage IV	Overdose
Stage V	Death

Box 22.2 Questions used to assess the anesthetized patient [7].

1. Is the animal adequately anesthetized?
2. Is there adequate analgesia?
3. Is the animal adequately immobilized?
4. What are the physiological consequences of the anesthetic state?
5. Are any of the identified abnormalities serious enough to warrant specific intervention?

Table 22.5 Physical monitoring parameters to determine a patient's level of anesthesia. The classic stages of anesthesia are noted in Box 22.1.

Parameter	Too light a plane of anesthesia	Appropriate plane of Anesthesia	Too deep a plane of anesthesia
Jaw tone	Normal or mild resistance with opening	Decreased resistance to opening	Absent
Eye position	Central	Ventro-medial	Central
Swallowing	Present	Absent	Absent
Palpebral/corneal reflex	Present, normal	Diminished	Absent
Voluntary motion without stimulation	Present	Absent	Absent
Voluntary motion with surgical stimulation	Present	Absent	Absent

Table 22.6 Patient parameters to monitor under sedation or general anesthesia with methods to monitor and normal values. Patients are at high risk of adverse events during initial induction and recovery periods; diligent monitoring is essential.

Parameter	Normal values	Physical monitoring	Electronic monitoring	Comments
Blood pressure	BP 120/80 (100) mmHg; minimum acceptable value 80/40 (60) mmHg	Pulse palpation (rate, rhythm, quality), MM, CRT. However, these do not adequately reflect blood pressure	SpO_2, blood pressure (direct or indirect Doppler or oscillometric)	Some continuous monitoring of circulation is considered mandatory
Heart rate	Rate 80–120 bpm dogs, 120–180 bpm cats	Pulse palpation, (rate, rhythm, quality), auscultation (transthoracic, esophageal)	Electrocardiogram	Continuous monitoring is considered mandatory
Oxygenation	$SpO_2 > 96\%$, $PaO_2 > 400$ mmHg (on 100% O_2)	MM color (inadequate on its own)	Pulse oximetry, arterial blood gas monitoring	MM color does not change to cyanotic until hemoglobin-oxygen saturation is critically low
Ventilation	$ETCO_2$ 35–45 mmHg, $PaCO_2$ 35–45 mmHg; RR 10–20 bpm, inspiratory time 1–1.5 sec; expiratory time 2–3 sec	Thoracic wall movement (or breathing bag/ventilator when thorax cannot be visualized) stethoscope	Capnography ($ETCO_2$), arterial blood gas, respirometry	Hypoventilation is common in anesthetized patients
Temperature	99–102 °F (37.2–38.9 °C)	Palpation (considered inadequate)	Rectal or esophageal temperature probe	Hypothermia is common in anesthetized patients; prevention is key with warming methods, continue to monitor in the postop period
Neuromuscular blockade		Reaction to noxious stimuli	Spirometer or peripheral nerve stimulator	Essential to control ventilation in these patients
Record keeping		Monitor every 3–5 min and record	Monitor every 3–5 min and record	Record all drugs and doses administered
Recovery period		Respiratory rate and pattern, MM, CRT, pulse palpation, behavior changes, level of consciousness	Temperature, BP, SpO_2 and $ETCO_2$ are possible in many patients	Consider perioperative bloodwork (electrolytes, PCV/TP, blood gas)

Source: Adapted from ACVAA Small Animal Monitoring Guidelines Update [8] and Ko [9].
BP, blood pressure; CRT, capillary refill time; MM, mucous membrane; PCV, packed cell volume; RR, respiratory rate; TP, total protein.

surgical stimulation and eye position are used to assess the plane or depth of anesthesia.

Anesthetized patients are often moved between locations within the hospital over the course of their anesthetic event (such as between the imaging suite, surgery prep area, surgery suite, and back to the imaging suite). In addition, it is common for perioperative procedures to take longer than expected, requiring a longer anesthetic time than initially anticipated after the patient is transferred. It is *crucial* that one person is dedicated to monitoring the patient during this time to make sure that there are no significant changes in physiological parameters or depth of anesthesia.

The "destination site" must be set up in advance (see checklist in Table 22.4). When transferring patients, the critical care team should be utilized to carry the needed equipment and get the patient positioned in the new location. One person should be charged with keeping the endotracheal tube stable during transfer. The use of a gurney will minimize the possibility of injury to the patient during transfer. It is best to try and prevent hypothermia with a variety of methods such as warm water blankets, warmed intravenous fluids, and forced warm air blowers. Minimizing contact time with cold surfaces and time that large cavities are open will also help minimize hypothermia.

Monitoring

Monitoring begins the moment that the animal is taken from the cage in preparation for premedication. The ability of the patient to respond appropriately to anesthesia-induced physiological changes is influenced not only by the anesthetic agents administered but also by the underlying disorder that makes the animal critical and the events that occur during anesthesia (such as surgery or biopsy). The American College of Veterinary Anesthesia and Analgesia (ACVAA) has published guidelines for anesthetic monitoring (www.acvaa.org), emphasizing the importance of close anesthetic monitoring for every patient [8,9]. These guidelines encompass the monitoring of circulation and oxygenation/ventilation parameters at regular 3–5 minute intervals. Documentation of the anesthetics and anesthetic events is emphasized. Guidelines regarding recording temperature and neuromuscular blockade, as well as personnel and sedation guidelines are presented. Table 22.6 lists the parameters to monitor under anesthesia with methods of monitoring and normal values, as recommended by the ACVAA [8,9]. Trends of change over time are more important than a single value, and any one parameter is interpreted in light of other parameters (such as heart rate and blood pressure being monitored together).

Arterial blood gases provide the gold standard for monitoring oxygenation and ventilation, but samples can be difficult to collect in the anesthetized patient without a preplaced arterial catheter. The procedure for placing an arterial catheter is outlined in Box 3.2 and Box 3.3 in Chapter 3. Oxygenation is routinely monitored during anesthesia with pulse oximetry and ventilation with end-tidal CO_2. Causes of hypoxemia during anesthesia and recommendations for intervention are outlined in Table 22.7. Possible differential diagnosis for altered end-tidal CO_2 during anesthesia are listed in Table 22.8 with suggestions for intervention. These monitoring procedures are always combined with observation of respiratory rate and thoracic excursion, along with auscultation of the lungs.

Table 22.7 Differential diagnoses and intervention for hypoxemia (SpO_2 <96%).

Differential possible causes	Intervention
Hypoventilation	• Employ manual or mechanical ventilation if not already done • Check ventilator settings and oxygen flow/connection • Check tubes, valves on ventilator • Check connections to patient including endotracheal tube • Check patient (auscultate lungs, ensure intubation, adjust or change ET tube, etc.)
Low inspired concentration of oxygen (FiO_2)	Increase oxygen flow rate or concentration rate (if on mechanical ventilator, change ventilator settings)
Ventilation/perfusion mismatch	Treat the underlying etiology
Diffusion abnormality	Treat underlyling etiology
Low cardiac output/blood pressure	Improve cardiac output (fluids, positive inotropes)
Increased oxygen consumption	Treat the underlying disorder, check temperature
Severe anemia	Administer blood products
Inappropriate probe placement	Correct probe placement, moisten mucous membrane (if appropriate), try alternate site or probe
Poor signal quality	Check for hypotension
Cardiac arrest	Institute CPR immediately

CPR, cardiopulmonary resuscitation; ET, endotracheal.

Table 22.8 Differential diagnosis and intervention for altered end-tidal CO_2.

Change in $ETCO_2$ and differentials	Intervention
Increased ETCO2 (>45 mmHg)	
Increased metabolism (hyperthermia)	Check body temperature; cooling is not usually essential, but discontinue active warming and monitor for malignant hyperthermia
Rebreathing CO_2	Check there is adequate fresh gas flow and that soda lime scavenger is not exhausted; check there is not a machine malfunction (such as expiratory valve)
Impaired alveolar ventilation	Make sure the patient is intubated correctly (that there is not one-lung inbutation or airway obstruction), ensure no development of pneumothorax or pneumomediastinum; thoracocentesis may be necessary
Low respiratory rate or tidal volume	Employ manual or mechanical ventilation if not already done and check settings on ventilator
Sodium bicarbonate administration	Discontinue administration or increase respiratory rate or tidal volume
Decreased ETCO2 (<35 mmHg)	
Hyperventilation	Decrease respiratory rate or tidal volume
Low cardiac output	Check other vital parameters (HR, ECG, blood pressure) and correct as necessary
Apnea	Employ manual or mechanical ventilation
Inappropriate (esophageal) intubation	Replace ET tube into esophagus
Hypothermia	Employ warming measures
Airway obstruction	Relieve obstruction
Cardiac arrest	Institute CPR immediately

CPR, cardiopulmonary resuscitation; ECG, electrocardiogram; ET, endotracheal; HR, heart rate.

Patients undergoing sedation only without intubation should be provided flow-by oxygen during sedation.

When an increase in respiratory rate is noted, important causes to consider include too light a plane of anesthesia, pain, hypoxemia, hypercarbia, hyperthermia, hypotension, and drug administration. A decreased respiratory rate may be due to a deep plane of anesthesia, hypothermia, neuromuscular paresis or paralysis (primary or due to metabolic disease), anesthetic drug-induced hypoventilation, endotracheal tube obstruction or ventilator malfunction.

Since inhaled anesthetic agents are very potent vasodilators, monitoring ECG and blood pressure is vital for assessing the cardiovascular status of the anesthetized patient. Physical parameters to monitor include peripheral pulse strength, regularity and quality, palpation of an apical heart beat, auscultation of the heart, mucous membrane color and CRT. Cardiac abnormalities observed during anesthesia are listed in Table 22.9 with suggestions for therapeutic intervention. Both hypotension and hypertension are detrimental to the anesthetized animal. Blood pressure abnormalities common to the anesthetized patient and potential methods of intervention are provided in Table 22.10.

Using a balanced approach to anesthesia will help minimize volatile anesthetic dose and can have a positive impact on cardiac function and blood pressure. Specific therapy using vasopressor drugs (such as dopamine) can be indicated in patients with persistent vasodilation not responsive to appropriate volume resuscitation or decreasing the anesthetic concentration (see Chapters 2 and 3).

Trends of change in heart rate and rhythm, pulse quality, and blood pressure will also indicate changes in depth of anesthesia. Patients that are critically ill and under anesthesia may not be able to mount the typical cardiovascular response to hypotension or pain, requiring that abnormalities be identified and addressed rapidly.

The body temperature of patients undergoing anesthesia can be monitored with esophageal or rectal thermometry. Patients that are under anesthesia will often have increased heat loss from (1) conductive loss on cold tables, (2) evaporative losses from open cavities and endotracheal intubation, (3) the inability to maintain a normal body temperature through normal physiological changes, and (4) the use of drugs that cause active vasodilation. Hypothermia can be managed with forced air warming, warm

Table 22.9 Heart rate abnormalities for patients under anesthesia with possible causes and methods of intervention.

Parameter abnormality/ possible causes	Suggested intervention
Tachycardia	
Anesthetic plane too light	Additional injectable or inhalant anesthesia
Hypotension	Administration of IV fluids, inotrope or vasopressor
Pain	Increased dose of analgesics or addition of other medications; advise surgeon to temporarily discontinue painful procedures
Hypoxemia	Evaluate anesthetic delivery system from oxygen connection, fresh gas flow, valves, tubes, and patient
Anemia	Consider transfusion
Drug administration (anticholinergics or vasoactive drugs)	Discontinue or taper use, reversal agent if available
Anaphylaxis	May require use of epinephrine, diphenhydramine, and/or steroid use
Hypercarbia	Evaluate equipment for rebreathing, inappropriate gas flow, malfunction, exhausted scavenging system, respiratory rate, tidal volume
Arrhythmias	Depending on the type and severity of arrhythmias, antiarrhythmic medications may be necessary (see Chapter 11)
Bradycardia	
Anesthetic plane too deep	Decrease volatile and/or injectable medications, ensuring patient remains immobile and has sufficient analgesia
Vagal stimulation	Depending on surgical procedure (i.e. ocular or cervical pressure, thoracic or abdominal organ manipulation), discontinue manipulation and/or consider anticholinergic if affecting cardiac output or blood pressure
Hypertension	Consider antihypertensive medications such as nitroprusside (see Chapter 3), evaluate for intracranial disease; if present, consider mannitol and furosemide, consider hyperventilation; avoid occlusion of jugular vein, mechanical ventilation if not already employed
Hypothermia	Warming methods if not already employed
Hypoglycemia	Dextrose infusions
Hypoxemia (prolonged)	This will be a prearrest sign, so correct hypoxemia immediately – employ positive pressure ventilation immediately and determine underlying cause and correct
Drug related	Alter or discontinue contributing drugs
Arrhythmia	Evaluate ECG, discontinue arrhythmogenic drugs, consider antiarrhythmic medications.

ECG, electrocardiogram.

Table 22.10 Blood pressure abnormalities for patients undergoing anesthesia with possible causes and methods of intervention.

Parameter abnormality/ possible causes	Suggested intervention
Hypotension	
Anesthetic plane too deep	Lighten anesthetic plane, ensuring adequate analgesia and depth
Bradycardia	Correct arrhythmia, often with anticholinergics, or lighten plane of anesthesia
Decreased contractility or stroke volume	Consider use of positive inotrope (dobutamine)
Decreased venous return	Administration of fluids, blood products, pressors or surgical/ centesis relief of obstruction
Arrhythmias	Treat arrhythmia for bradycardia, anticholinergics may be utilized; lidocaine for ventricular tachyarrhythmias
Hypoglycemia	Administer dextrose
Hypokalemia	Supplement potassium
Drug induced	Decrease dose, discontinue or administer reversal agent
Hypovolemia	Administer volume with crystalloids, colloids or blood products
Systemic vasodilation	Administration of vasopressor agents
Hypertension	
Anesthetic plane too light	Titrate increases in anesthetic drug(s)
Pain (with tachycardia)	Increase dose of analgesics or administer additional analgesics
Recent use of anticholingerics or other sympathomimetics (associated with tachycardia)	Discontinue administration
Fever	External cooling, dantrolene and/or discontinue volatile anesthesia if associated with malignant hyperthermia
Hypercarbia	Initiate mechanical ventilation if not employed and check ventilator settings (RR, tidal volume, etc.)
Hypervolemia	Taper or discontinue IV fluid administration; furosemide or dialysis

RR, respiratory rate.

water bottles, water circulating heating pads, warmed IV fluids, cavitary lavage with warmed fluids, and covering exposed areas of the patient [8,9]. Drug reversal or lightening the plane of anesthesia may also be necessary if hypotension and hypothermia are a persistent problem.

Hyperthermia is much less common in anesthetized patients; causes of hyperthermia associated with anesthesia include inappropriate use of external heating devices, heavy-coated breeds, histamine release, and breeds predisposed to malignant hyperthermia or genetic hyperthermia syndromes (Greyhound, Rottweiler). Hyperthermia can impact coagulation and vascular tone and is best treated with cooling methods or discontinuing procedures that may be contributing factors. Malignant hyperthermia is treated with dantrolene (1 mg/kg IV) and discussed in Chapter 17.

Intraoperative monitoring of coagulation, PCV, TP, blood lactate, and blood glucose can be critical, especially if there are negative anesthetic events. Estimating blood loss by weighing or counting sponges (dry versus blood soaked) and keeping track of suction canister contents compared to lavage fluid volume can provide valuable information. Patients with cavitary hemorrhage may have their blood collected during surgery for possible autologous blood transfusion (see Chapter 10). Diligent intraoperative hemostasis will help prevent blood loss and development of consumptive coagulopathies. Lactate is assessed as a measure of anerobic metabolism. Serial measurement during anesthesia provides another method for evaluating tissue oxygenation.

Recovery period

One of the most critical periods of the anesthetic event is during recovery from anesthesia:

- the patient is often being moved from one location to another
- monitors are often disconnected or inadvertently removed
- staff can be distracted by other tasks
- sedated patients are at high risk of adverse events such as hypoventilation, aspiration, etc.

During the recovery period it is important not only that the inhalant gas must be discontinued but also the system should be flushed with oxygen to ensure removal of the volatile gases from the tubing. Hypoventilation during this time is common and can be immediately life threatening if not recognized and managed. Patients should be allowed to develop a normal to slightly elevated $PaCO_2$ at the end of the procedure to stimulate normal respiration. Electronic monitoring (SpO_2, $ETCO_2$, ECG, blood pressure) should continue though the recovery period.

Patients can be extubated when they have some mental responsiveness, have a strong gag or swallow reflex and are able to lift their head or maintain sternal recumbency. Patients with dysphoria associated with their analgesic or anesthesia drugs should be kept in a dim, quiet environment with minimal stimuli. Reversal agents may be administered or additional sedatives if deemed necessary and safe.

The Rule of 20 is an essential part of patient evaluation during anesthetic recovery. A pain scale can be used to monitor perioperative pain (see Chapter 19). Varied therapeutic interventions may be indicated and treatment sheet orders completed as a result of the procedure(s) performed. These may reflect a need for analgesics or monitoring of fluid or air production from a tube, etc.

Patients with prolonged recoveries from anesthesia should have the following biochemical assessment: glucose, arterial blood gas or oxygenation, electrolytes and/or ammonia levels, PCV/TP, blood pressure, ECG, and temperature. Correction of any identified abnormalities may hasten recovery. The need for drug reversal agent(s) should be assessed. It is common for patients recovering from anesthesia to be hypothermic, and warm IV fluids, fluid line warmers, forced air blowers, warm water circulating blankets, and warmed water bottles can be used to maintain body temperature during recovery.

Monitoring can be discontinued only when vital parameters have been normal for at least two cycles, five minutes apart. However, when multimodal pain management or sedation continues in the postanesthetic period, some monitoring should continue (such as SpO_2, ECG, blood pressure). Careful monitoring of organ function with blood work, urine output, and other methods are required if hypotension occurred under anesthesia.

Anesthesia can slow intestinal transit time and impair GI function. A feeding tube (such as nasogastric, nasoesophageal, esophagostomy or gastrostomy tubes) can be placed prior to full anesthetic recovery to reduce nausea and vomiting and provide nutritional support. It is important that drains, wounds or incisions are covered to prevent contamination and nosocomial infection.

Nursing care for the anesthetic patient is critical, particularly for long-term anesthetic candidates (such as those requiring long-term ventilation or prolonged surgical procedures). The goal is to minimize patient discomfort, ensure the patient is clean, and assist the patient in a smooth anesthetic recovery.

Anesthesia for cesarean section

During the patient preparation phase, placement of an intravenous catheter and preoxygenation are essential for the pregnant animal since ventilation may be impaired due to the distended abdomen. Anesthetic drugs and doses are carefully selected with the goal of minimizing effects on the fetus and the mother. The estimated lean body weight of the pregnant patient is used for drug dose calculations since there are large volumes of fluid and fetuses, which add weight and can alter volume of distribution. Shaving the fur and performing the initial surgical scrub of the abdomen can occur during the premedication phase, prior to induction of anesthesia. An epidural may be used to reduce the use of anesthetic drugs that could affect the fetus.

Rapid induction with short-acting drugs such as propofol will minimize the anesthetic effects on the fetus. Local anesthetics such as lidocaine or bupivacaine can be used to block over the midline abdominal incision site to minimize drug effects on the fetus. Maintenance of anesthesia with isoflurane is commonly recommended [10].

Drugs that have been associated with decreased puppy vigor include ketamine and barbiturates such as thiopental and thiamylal. Drugs associated with increased fetal mortality include methoxyflurane and alpha-2-agonists (such as xylazine) [10]. Drugs that can be reversed (such as mu-agonist opioids reversed by naloxone) are a reasonable option for pregnant animals since they can be reversed in the fetus immediately after birth. Some clinicians prefer not to administer opioids to the mother until the fetuses have been removed.

The critical care team should be prepared for neonatal resuscitation. The fetuses are often removed one at a time from the dam and should be immediately handed to a member of the neonatal resuscitation team. Neonatal resuscitation includes drying, stimulation (with gentle rubbing), removing the fetal membranes from the body, suctioning the airway, and stimulation of respirations. Further information pertaining to fetal resuscitation can be found in the Further reading list.

References

1. Moonesinghe SR, Mythen MG, Das P, et al. Risk stratification tools for predicting morbidity and mortality in adult patients undergoing major surgery: qualitative systematic review. *Anesthesiology* 2013;119(4):959–81.
2. Thurmon JC, Short CE. History and overview of veterinary anesthesia. In: *Lumb and Jones' Veterinary Anesthesia and Analgesia*, 4th edn. Tranquilli WJ, Thurmon JC, Grimm, KA, eds. Ames: Blackwell Publishing, 2007: p 17.
3. Brown DC. Wound infections and antimicrobial use. In: *Small Animal Veterinary Surgery*, vol. 2. Tobias KM, Johnston SA, eds. St Louis: Elsevier Saunders, 2012: pp 135–9.
4. Brainard BM, Hofmeister EH. Anesthesia principles and monitoring. In: *Small Animal Veterinary Surgery*, vol. 1. Tobias KM, Johnston SA, eds. St Louis: Elsevier Saunders, 2012: pp 248–90.
5. Bruchim Y, Itay S, Shira BH, et al. Evaluation of lidocaine treatment on frequency of cardiac arrhythmias, acute kidney injury and hospitalization time in dogs with gastric dilation and volvulus. *J Vet Emerg Crit Care* 2012;22(4):419–27.
6. Hartsfield SM. Anesthetic machines and breathing systems. In: *Lumb and Jones' Veterinary Anesthesia and Analgesia*, 4th edn. Tranquilli WJ, Thurmon JC, Grimm, KA, eds. Ames: Blackwell Publishing, 2007: p 480.
7. Haskins SC, Monitoring the anesthetized patient. In: *Veterinary Anesthesia*, 3rd edn. Thurmon JC, Tranquilli WJ, Benson GJ, eds. Baltimore: Williams and Wilkins, 1996: 409–24.
8. ACVAA Small Animal Monitoring Guidelines Update. 2009. Available at www.acvaa.org. Original guidelines published: *J Am Vet Med Assoc.* 1995;206(7): 936–7.

9. Ko J. Anesthesia monitoring and management. In: *Small Animal Anesthesia and Pain Management*. London: Manson Publishing, 2013: pp 123–62.

10. Fransson BA. Ovaries and uterus. In: *Small Animal Veterinary Surgery*, vol. 2. Tobias KM, Johnston SA, eds. St Louis: Elsevier Saunders, 2012: pp 1886–7.

Further reading

Campoy L, Read MR. *Small Animal Regional Anesthesia and Analgesia*. Ames: Wiley-Blackwell, 2013.

Drobatz KJ, Costello MF. *Feline Emergency and Critical Care Medicine*. Ames: Wiley-Blackwell, 2010.

Grimm KA, Tranquilli WJ, Lamont LA. *Essentials of Small Animal Anesthesia and Analgesia*, 2nd edn. Ames: Wiley-Blackwell, 2011.

Mathews KA. *Veterinary Emergency and Critical Care Manual*. Ontario: Lifelearn, 2006.

Muir WW, Hubbell JA. *Handbook of Veterinary Anesthesia*, 5th edn. St Louis: Elsevier Mosby, 2013.

Seymour C, Duke-Novakovski T. BSAVA Manual of Canine and Feline Anaesthesia and Analgesia, 2nd edn. Gloucester: BSAVA, 2011.

Index

Page numbers in **bold** indicate tables and/or boxes; page numbers in *italics* indicate figures